Non-Steroidal Antioestrogens

LUDWIG SYMPOSIA

---

1. Non-Steroidal Antioestrogens: Molecular Pharmacology and Antitumour Activity
   R.L. SUTHERLAND and V.C. JORDAN (Eds)

2. Nucleosides and Cancer Treatment: Rational Approaches to Antimetabolite Selectivity and Modulation
   M.H.N. TATTERSALL and R.M. FOX (Eds)

Non-Steroidal Antioestrogens

Molecular Pharmacology and Antitumour Activity

Edited by

Robert L. Sutherland

Ludwig Institute for Cancer Research
University of Sydney

and

V. Craig Jordan

Ludwig Institute for Cancer Research
Inselspital, Universitat Bern

1981

ACADEMIC PRESS

A Subsidiary of Harcourt Brace Jovanovich, Publishers

Sydney New York London Toronto San Francisco

Printed in Australia

National Library of Australia Cataloguing-in-Publication Data

Non-steriodal antioestrogens.

Bibliography
Includes index
ISBN 0 12 677880 9

1. Breast—Cancer. 2. Cancer—Chemotherapy.
I. Sutherland, Robert L. (Robert Lindsay).
II. Jordan, V. Craig (Virgil Craig).
(Series: Ludwig symposia; no. 1).

616.99'449061

Library of Congress Catalog Card Number: 81-67869

This book is dedicated to the memory of Dr A. L. Walpole

Preface

It is now more than twenty years since the first report of an effective non-steroidal antioestrogen, MER 25, was published. This original work inspired many research groups to synthesize and test related compounds as potential antifertility agents. However, the only compounds to reach the clinic (clomiphene and tamoxifen) proved to be inducers of ovulation and are now used routinely in sub-fertile patients.

The work by Dr Elwood V. Jensen and others, which suggested some human breast cancers were directly dependent on oestrogen, led to the initiation of clinical trials with synthetic antioestrogens. Encouraging preliminary results with nafoxidine were offset by a high incidence of troublesome side-effects. However, the successful introduction of tamoxifen for the treatment of advanced breast cancer has resulted in a renewed interest in the pharmacology and mechanisms of action of these drugs.

The exponential increase in the number of research articles on anti-oestrogenic mechanisms throughout the 1970s prompted us to attempt to summarize the wealth of available data in a single volume. As a basis, much of the information published in this book was presented at an Antioestrogen Workshop held at the Ludwig Institute for Cancer Research, University of Sydney, Australia between the 4th and 6th February, 1980. Due primarily to limitations of space we have only been able to include those areas of antioestrogen research that relate to the development and action of antioestrogens as anticancer agents. For this reason a substantial literature on the effects of antioestrogens in reproductive and behavioural biology has not been included.

The untimely death of Dr Arthur L. Walpole in 1977 unfortunately did not allow him to witness the world-wide acceptance of tamoxifen as an effective therapy for advanced breast cancer. Tamoxifen was developed by Drs M. J. K. Harper, D. Richardson and A. L. Walpole as part of the fertility control programme at Imperial Chemical Industries Ltd, Pharmaceutical Division, but it was Dr Walpole's deep interest in cancer research that led to its ultimate introduction as an antitumour agent. On a personal note, Dr Walpole was known as a scientist who helped and encouraged young investigators, including one of the editors of this volume (V.C.J.). It is for these reasons that we have dedicated this volume to his memory.

The keen interest shown by the UICC, Imperial Chemical Industries Ltd, Eli Lilly and Co. and Upjohn Pty Ltd in both the Antioestrogen Workshop and the preparation of this volume is gratefully acknowledged.

Finally we would like to thank Christine Cook, Elaine Heffernan, Leigh Murphy, Anne Whybourne, Terry Foo, Mike Green, Roger Reddell and Colin Watts without whose help this venture would not have been possible.

Rob Sutherland
Craig Jordan

Contents

3 Structure–Activity Relationships amongst Non-Steroidal Antioestrogens

V. Craig Jordan, E. R. Clark and Karen E. Allen

4 A Review of the Pharmacokinetics and Metabolism of "Nolvadex" (Tamoxifen)

H. K. Adam

5 Binding of Tamoxifen and its Metabolites 4-Hydroxytamoxifen and N-Desmethyltamoxifen to Oestrogen Receptors from Normal and Neoplastic Tissues

R. L. Sutherland and A. M. Whybourne

6 Metabolism and Binding of Non-Steroidal Antioestrogens in Mammals and Chickens

H. Rochefort, F. Capony and J. L. Borgna

16 Effects of Antioestrogens in Carcinogen-Induced Rat Mammary Cancer

V. Craig Jordan, C. J. Dix and Karen E. Allen

17 Biochemical Basis of Tamoxifen Action in Hormone-Dependent Breast Cancer

R. I. Nicholson, N. M. Borthwick, C. P. Daniel, J. S. Syne and P. Davies

18 Antioestrogen Action in Ovarian-Dependent and Ovarian-Autonomous Experimental Mammary Tumours

Benita S. Katzenellenbogen, Ten-Lin S. Tsai and Ellen A. Rorke

19 Binding of Non-Steriodal Antioestrogens to Saturable Binding Sites Distinct from the Oestrogen Receptor in Normal and Neoplastic Tissues

L. C. Murphy, M. S. Foo, M. D. Green, B. K. Milthorpe, A. M. Whybourne, Z. S. Krozowski and R. L. Sutherland

23 Effects of Antioestrogens on the Growth and Cell Cycle Kinetics of Cultured Human Mammary Carcinoma Cells

M. D. Green, A. M. Whybourne, I. W. Taylor and R. L. Sutherland

24 Steriod Receptors and Response to an Antioestrogen in Postmenopausal Endometrial Carcinoma and Metastatic Breast Cancer

P. Robel, R. Mortel, C. Levy, M. Namer, and E. E. Baulieu

25 Changes in Endocrine Status Following Antioestrogen Administration to Premenopausal and Postmenopausal Women

A. Manni, B. Arafah, and O. H. Pearson

List of Contributors

Numbers in parentheses indicate the pages on which the authors' contributions begin.

H. K. Adam (59), Safety of Medicines Department, ICI Pharmaceuticals Division, Alderley Park, Macclesfield, Cheshire, SK10 4TG, U.K.

D. J. Adams (339), Department of Medicine/Oncology, University of Texas Health Science Center, San Antonio, Texas 78284, U.S.A.

S. C. Aitken (365), Medicine Branch, National Cancer Institute, Bethesda, Maryland 20205, U.S.A.

J. C. Allegra (365), Medicine Branch, National Cancer Institute, Bethesda, Maryland 20205, U.S.A.

K. E. Allen (31, 261), Department of Pharmacology, The Worsley Medical and Dental Building, The University of Leeds, LS2 9JK, U.K.

B. Arafah (435), Department of Medicine, Case Western Reserve University, School of Medicine, Cleveland, Ohio 44106, U.S.A.

E. E. Baulieu (177, 249, 413), Unité de Recherches sur le Métabolisme Moléculaire et la Physio-Pathologie des Stéroides, INSERM U 33, Medical School, University of Paris-Sud. Lab Hormones, 94270 Bicêtre, France.

N. Binart (177), Unité de Recherches sur le Métabolisme Moléculaire et la Physio-Pathologie des Stéroides, INSERM U 33, Medical School, University of Paris-Sud. Lab Hormones, 94270 Bicêtre, France.

J. L. Borgna (85,355), Unité d'Endocrinologie Cellulaire et Moléculaire (INSERM U 148), 60 rue de Navacelles, 34100 Montpellier, France.

N. M. Borthwick (281), Tenovus Institute for Cancer Research, Welsh National School of Medicine, Heath Park, Cardiff CF4 4XX, U.K.

F. Capony (85, 215), Department of Pharmacological Sciences, Health Sciences Center, State University of New York at Stony Brook, Stony Brook, New York 11794, U.S.A.

M. G. Catelli (177), Unité de Recherches sur le Métabolisme Moléculaire et la Physio-Pathologie des Stéroides, INSERM U 33, Medical School, University of Paris-Sud. Lab Hormones, 94270 Bicêtre, France.

E. R. Clark (31), Department of Pharmacology, The Worsley Medical and Dental Building, The University of Leeds, LS2 9JK, U.K.

J. H. Clark (113), Department of Cell Biology, Baylor College of Medicine, Houston, Texas 77030, U.S.A.

E. Coezy (355), Unité d'Endocrinologie Cellulaire et Moléculaire (INSERM U 148), 60 rue de Navacelles, 34100 Montpellier, France.

C. P. Daniel (281), Tenovus Institute for Cancer Research, Welsh National School of Medicine, Heath Park, Cardiff CF4 4XX, U.K.

P. Davies (281), Tenovus Institute for Cancer Research, Welsh National School of Medicine, Heath Park, Cardiff CF4 4XX, U.K.

C. J. Dix (261), Department of Pharmacology, The Worsley Medical and Dental Building, The University of Leeds, LS2 9JK, U.K.

D. P. Edwards (339), Department of Medicine/Oncology, University of Texas Health Science Center, San Antonio, Texas 78284, U.S.A.

C. W. Emmens (17), Department of Obstetrics and Gynaecology, University of Sydney, N.S.W. 2006, Australia.

R. W. Evans (165), Worcester Foundation for Experimental Biology, Shrewsbury, Massachusetts 01545, U.S.A.

E. R. Ferguson (95), Department of Physiology and Biophysics, University of Illinois, and School of Basic Medical Sciences, University of Illinois College of Medicine, Urbana, Illinois 61801, U.S.A.

M. S. Foo (195, 317), Ludwig Institute for Cancer Research, University of Sydney, N.S.W. 2006, Australia.

C. Geynet (177), Unité de Recherches sur le Métabolisme Moléculaire et la Physio-Pathologie des Stéroides, INSERM U 33, Medical School, University of Paris-Sud. Lab Hormones, 94270 Bicêtre, France.

S. R. Glasser (113), Department of Cell Biology, Baylor College of Medicine, Houston, Texas 77030, U.S.A.

M. D. Green (317, 397), Ludwig Institute for Cancer Research, University of Sydney, N.S.W. 2006, Australia.

R. Hähnel (177), University of Western Australia, King Edward Memorial Hospital, Subiaco, W.A. 6008, Australia.

J. R. Hayes (95), Department of Physiology and Biophysics, University of Illinois, and School of Basic Medical Sciences, University of Illinois College of Medicine, Urbana, Illinois 61801, U.S.A.

W. H. Hendry III (165), Worcester Foundation for Experimental Biology, Shrewsbury, Massachusetts 01545, U.S.A.

V. C. Jordan (31, 261, 473), Department of Human Oncology, Wisconsin Clinical Cancer Center, 600 Highland Avenue, University of Wisconsin, Madison, Wisconsin 53792, U.S.A.

B. S. Katzenellenbogen (95, 303), Department of Physiology and Biophysics, University of Illinois, and School of Basic Medical Sciences, University of Illinois College of Medicine, Urbana, Illinois 61801, U.S.A.

J. A. Katzenellenbogen (95), Department of Chemistry, University of Illinois, and School of Basic Medical Sciences, University of Illinois College of Medicine, Urbana, Illinois 61801, U.S.A.

J. L. Keene (231), Department of Physiology, St. Louis University Medical Center, St. Louis, Missouri 63104, U.S.A.

Z. S. Krozowski (317), Department of Biochemistry, Royal Prince Alfred Hospital, Camperdown, N.S.W. 2050, Australia.

N. C. Lan (95), Department of Physiology and Biophysics, University of Illinois, and School of Basic Medical Sciences, University of Illinois College of Medicine, Urbana, Illinois 61801, U.S.A.

C. B. Lazier (215), Department of Biochemistry, Dalhousie University, Halifax, Nova Scotia, B3H 4H7, Canada.

W. W. Leavitt (165), Worcester Foundation for Experimental Biology, Shrewsbury, Massachusetts 01545, U.S.A.

M. C. Lebeau (249), Unité de Recherches sur le Métabolisme Moléculaire et la Physio-Pathologie des Stéroides, INSERM U 33, Medical School, University of Paris-Sud. Lab Hormones, 94270 Bicêtre, France.

L. J. Lerner (1), Departments of Obstetrics and Gynaecology and Pharmacology, Jefferson Medical College, Thomas Jefferson University, Philadelphia, Pennsylvania 19107, U.S.A.

C. Levy (413), Universidad de Buenos Aires, Instituto de Oncologia "Angel H. Roffo", Avenida San Martin 5481, Buenos Aires, Argentina.

M. E. Lippman (365), Medicine Branch, National Cancer Institute, Bethesda, Maryland 20205, U.S.A.

S. A. McCormack (113), Department of Cell Biology, Baylor College of Medicine, Houston, Texas 77030, U.S.A.

W. L. McGuire (339), Department of Medicine/Oncology, University of Texas Health Science Center, San Antonio, Texas 78284, U.S.A.

A. Manni (435), Department of Medicine, Case Western Reserve University, School of Medicine, Cleveland, Ohio 44106, U.S.A.

B. M. Markaverich (113), Department of Cell Biology, Baylor College of Medicine, Houston, Texas 77030, U.S.A.

L. Martin (143), Department of Hormone Physiology, Imperial Cancer Research Fund, P.O. Box 123, Lincoln's Inn Fields, London WC2A 3PZ, U.K.

N. Massol (249), Unité de Recherches sur le Métabolisme Moléculaire et la Physio-Pathologie des Stéroides, INSERM U 33, Medical School, University of Paris-Sud. Lab Hormones, 94270 Bicêtre, France.

J. Mešter (177), Unité de Recherches sur le Métabolism Moléculaire et la Physio-Pathologie des Stéroides, INSERM U 33, Medical School, University of Paris-Sud. Lab Hormones, 94270 Bicêtre, France.

B. K. Milthorpe (317), Ludwig Institute for Cancer Research, University of Sydney, N.S.W. 2006, Australia.

R. Mortel (413), Milton S. Hershey Medical Center, Hershey, Pennsylvania, U.S.A.

L. C. Murphy (317), Ludwig Institute for Cancer Research, University of Sydney, N.S.W. 2006, Australia.

M. Namer (413), Centre A. Lacassagne, 36, Voie Romaine, 06054 Nice, France.

R. I. Nicholson (281), Tenovus Institute for Cancer Research, Welsh National School of Medicine, Heath Park, Cardiff CF4 4XX, U.K.

J. S. Patterson (453), Clinical Research Department, ICI Pharmaceuticals Division, Alderley Park, Macclesfield, Cheshire SK10 4TG, U.K.

O. H. Pearson (435), Department of Medicine, Case Western Reserve University, School of Medicine, Cleveland, Ohio 44106, U.S.A.

V. Puri (177), All India Institute of Medical Sciences, New Delhi 110016, India.

P. Robel (413), Unité de Recherches sur le Métabolisme Moléculaire et la Physio-Pathologie des Stéroides, INSERM U 33 and CNRS ER 125, Medical School, University of Paris-Sud. Lab Hormones, 94270 Bicêtre, France.

D. W. Robertson (95), Department of Chemistry, University of Illinois, and School of Basic Medical Sciences, University of Illinois College of Medicine, Urbana, Illinois 61801, U.S.A.

H. Rochefort (85, 355), Unité d'Endocrinologie Cellulaire et Moléculaire (INSERM U 148), 60 rue de Navacelles, 34100 Montpellier, France.

E. A. Rorke (303), Department of Physiology and Biophysics, University of Illinois, and School of Basic Medical Sciences, University of Illinois College of Medicine, Urbana, Illinois 61801, U.S.A.

P. Ross Jr. (231), Department of Physiology, St. Louis University Medical Center, St. Louis, Missouri 63104, U.S.A.

T. S. Ruh (231), Department of Physiology, St. Louis University Medical Center, St. Louis, Missouri 63104, U.S.A.

N. Savage (339), Department of Medicine/Oncology, University of Texas Health Science Center, San Antonio, Texas 78284, U.S.A.

D. Seeley (177), Department of Population Sciences, Harvard School of Public Health, Boston, Massachusetts 02115, U.S.A.

R. L. Sutherland (75, 177, 195, 317, 397, 473), Ludwig Institute for Cancer Research, University of Sydney, N.S.W. 2006, Australia.

J. S. Syne (281), Tenovus Institute for Cancer Research, Welsh National School of Medicine, Heath Park, Cardiff CF4 4XX, U.K.

T. Tatee (95), Department of Chemistry, University of Illinois, and School of Basic Medical Sciences, University of Illinois College of Medicine, Urbana, Illinois 61801, U.S.A.

I. W. Taylor (397), Ludwig Institute for Cancer Research, University of Sydney, N.S.W. 2006, Australia.

T.-L. S. Tsai (303), Department of Physiology and Biophysics, University of Illinois, and School of Basic Medical Sciences, University of Illinois College of Medicine, Urbana, Illinois 61801, U.S.A.

S. Upchurch (113), Department of Cell Biology, Baylor College of Medicine, Houston, Texas 77030, U.S.A.

F. Vignon (355), Unité d'Endocrinologie Cellulaire et Moléculaire (INSERM U 148), 60 rue de Navacelles, 34100 Montpellier, France.

B. Westley (355), Unité d'Endocrinologie Cellulaire et Moléculaire (INSERM U 148), 60 rue de Navacelles, 34100 Montpellier, France.

A. M. Whybourne (75, 317, 397), Ludwig Institute for Cancer Research, University of Sydney, N.S.W. 2006, Australia.

D. L. Williams (215), Department of Pharmacological Sciences, Health Sciences Center, State University of New York at Stony Brook, Stony Brook, New York 11794, U.S.A.

K. I. H. Williams (165), Worcester Foundation for Experimental Biology, Shrewsbury, Massachusetts 01545, U.S.A.

D. M. Wood (231), Department of Physiology, St. Louis University Medical Center, St. Louis, Missouri 63104, U.S.A.

1

The First Non-Steroidal Antioestrogen — MER 25

LEONARD J. LERNER

I. INTRODUCTION

The ability of one chemical compound to antagonize the activities of another compound has importance not only for clinical utility but also for the study of basic physiological mechanisms. One of the first demonstrations of competitive antagonism was that the bacteriostatic effect of the compound sulphanilamide could be inhibited competitively by the compound para-aminobenzoic acid to which it is structurally related (Woods, 1940; Harris and Kohn, 1941).

Hisaw *et al.* (1954) demonstrated that the weak oestrogen oestriol administered concomittantly with oestradiol inhibited the full expression of the uterotrophic activity of the more potent oestrogen in rats. This report showed that it was possible for a less potent compound of the same biological and chemical class to inhibit, at least at one end point, the biological activity of

NON-STEROIDAL ANTIOESTROGENS
ISBN 0 12 677880 9

a more potent compound of the same class. Previously, investigators reported that uterotrophic and vaginal cornification induced by the natural steroids oestradiol and oestrone could be modified by various non-oestrogenic steroids.

If a weak oestrogenic steroid could block the effect of a potent oestrogenic steroid at a particular target site of oestrogenic action, would a weak non-steroidal oestrogen do the same thing? All of the materials to test this hypothesis were present at the Merrell Laboratories. These included an ongoing uterotrophic activity screen in mice, and a number of di- and triphenylethylene compounds that had been synthesized in the program that led to the development of the sucessfully marketed oestrogen chlorotrianisene (TACE) (Fig. 1). The screening of a number of these compounds, in my laboratory, demonstrated that some of these weak oestrogens could partially antagonize the uterotrophic response to oestradiol and oestrone as well as to hexoestrol and diethylstilboestrol.

This partial success increased the enthusiasm for continuing the search for more potent antagonists, possibly having reduced inherent oestrogenic potency. Certainly, it was thought, such a product could have utility in breast and uterine cancers and menstrual disorders, and could possibly be useful, through alterations of hormonal balance, for inhibiting or increasing fertility. Moreover, if a very weak oestrogen could express its oestrogenity at some oestrogen target tissues but not at others, and even antagonize oestrogen at some sites, several useful therapeutic agents could be envisaged. Among those that we thought to be feasible, in addition to the anti-tumour, menstrual disorder and fertility regulation areas, were the regulation of blood lipids and inhibition of atherosclerosis and the effects on behaviour. In addition, the

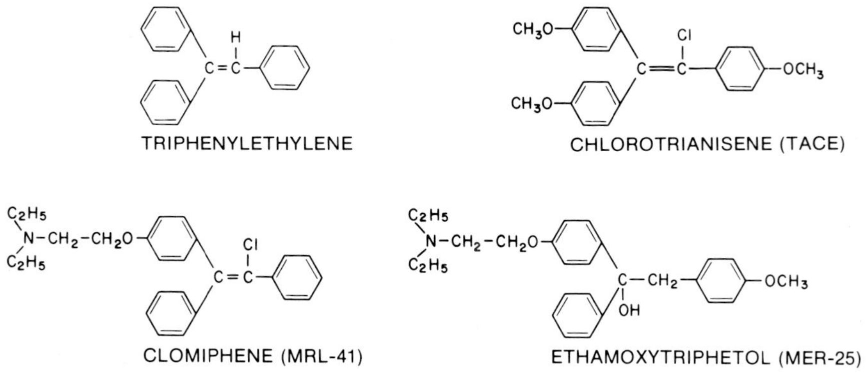

TRIPHENYLETHYLENE

CHLOROTRIANISENE (TACE)

CLOMIPHENE (MRL-41)

ETHAMOXYTRIPHETOL (MER-25)

Fig. 1. Chemical structures and commonly used designations of several triphenylethylene oestrogens and antioestrogens.

availability of such a compound would allow for studies of the requirements for oestrogen in many biological processes and for the mechanism of oestrogenic action. Eventually a number of these utilities were realized through the use of this new class of compounds.

As 1954 was drawing to its end a triphenylethanol compound was synthesized, not for the purpose of investigation for oestrogen antagonism but for testing by the cardiovascular research section at Merrell since it had been reported that a related compound had some effect on blood flow. A request for a sample of that compound for study as a possible oestrogen antagonist was answered by the cardiovascular system pharmacologist with his entire supply since it was essentially inactive in his studies. This compound, 1-p-2 (diethylamino)-ethoxyphenyl-2-(p-methoxyphenyl)-1-phenylethanol was tested in immature mice at the arbitrary 3-day screening dose of 5 mg. It was administered subcutaneously twice daily for three days alone or in combination with 0.3 μg of oestradiol benzoate, and the uterine weight and intraluminal fluid served as the end points to be measured on the day after the last treatment. The results of this study were highly questioned since neither the uteri of the mice administered the compound alone or the uteri of the animals receiving the compound plus oestrogen were significantly heavier than those of controls treated with olive oil vehicle alone. It was thought that this was a "bad study". The compound, however, was retested and the results were identical to those of the first study. The increase in uterine weight and intraluminal fluid by oestradiol treatment was completely prevented by simultaneous administration of the compound that was eventually to be called MER 25 or ethamoxytriphetol (Fig. 1).

II. ANTIOESTROGENIC PROPERTIES

The compound MER 25 was appealing not only because it completely inhibited the uterine response to oestradiol but also because it was devoid of uterine stimulatory properties (Lerner, 1958, 1959; Lerner *et al.*, 1958). This was an added bonus. Here was a possible tool for the study of oestrogen requirements and involvement in bodily functions.

Was the inhibition of oestrogenic activity competitive or non-competitive? Various doses of MER 25 were studied against a single dose of oestradiol benzoate, and various doses of the oestrogen were studied against a single dose of the antagonist. The results of these studies demonstrated dose response relationships compatible with competitive antagonism (Fig. 2).

Would this compound inhibit the uterine weight increase induced by other oestrogens, steroidal and non-steroidal? MER 25 was effective against several potent and weak steroidal and non-steroidal oestrogens (Lerner *et al.*, 1958).

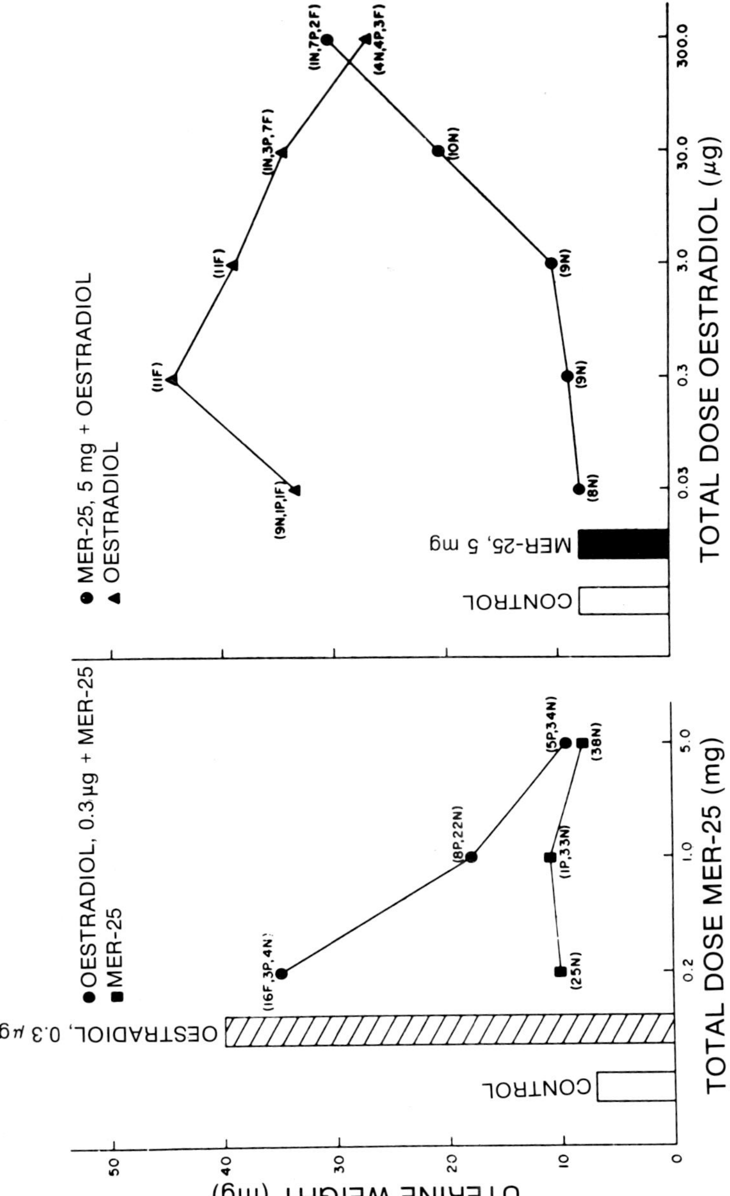

Fig. 2. Antagonism by MER 25 of the uterine effects of oestradiol in immature mice. Numbers preceding letters at each point indicate number of animals per luminal fluid grade, and the letters indicate the grade (F = Full; P = Partial; N = No Fluid).

Was the inhibition of the uterotrophic response limited to effects on oestrogens or could MER 25 also antagonize testosterone and progesterone-induced uterine weight increase? Studies in immature mice showed that MER 25 did not antagonize the uterotrophic effect of testosterone propionate but did cause a small decrease in the progesterone-induced uterotrophic response (Lerner *et al.*, 1958). In contrast, in immature rats MER 25 treatment reduced the uterine weight response to testosterone propionate and slightly augmented the uterine response to progesterone (Lerner *et al.*, 1966b). In any case the effect of this oestrogen antagonist was minimal against androgen and progestogen uterotrophic effects in rodents. In the rabbit, MER 25 did not inhibit the effect of progesterone on the endometrium but it did antagonize the effect of oestradiol on the uterine weight and on uterine histology. Indeed in immature rabbits MER 25 effectively inhibited the "oestrogen priming" effect of oestradiol benzoate required for glandular development which we now know is due to induction of progesterone receptors by the oestrogen (Horwitz and McGuire, 1978; Jordan and Dix, 1979). Moreover, since all of the non-steroidal oestrogen antagonists are weak oestrogens, it is not surprising that tamoxifen stimulated progesterone receptor synthesis (Jordan and Dix, 1979) or that MER 25 could "prime" the immature rabbit uterus and allow for a weak expression of uterine growth and glandular development by subsequent progesterone treatment (Lerner *et al.*, 1958).

To study the effect of this compound on endogenous oestrogen activity, a study was performed in immature mice administered pregnant mares serum (PMS) since the resultant uterotrophic response is effected by stimulation of ovarian steroidogenesis. MER 25 induced a dose-dependent inhibition of the uterine weight augmentation and increase in its intraluminal fluid resulting from the PMS treatment (Lerner *et al.*, 1958). Another study employed daily oral administration of MER 25 to adult rats for one month. The resultant weights of the uteri of the treated rats were only 40% that of the animals receiving the oil vehicle only (Lerner *et al.*, 1958). These studies showed that the compound MER 25 was effective in blocking the uterotrophic activity of both endogenous and exogenous oestrogens regardless of the chemical structure of the hormones.

The effect of MER 25 on uterine biochemistry and histology in the presence or absence of oestradiol was studied in immature rats (Adam *et al.*, 1960; Lerner, 1964; Lerner *et al.*, 1966a, 1966b). The antagonist by itself induced little or no changes with the exception of a small increase in RNA and phospholipids after 4 days of treatment. When MER 25 was administered together with a total 4 day dosage of 2 μg oestradiol benzoate, it suppressed the oestrogen-induced elevations of total RNA and DNA and the RNA/DNA ratio as well as glucose-6-phosphate dehydrogenase and NADP-malic enzyme activities (Table I). It is interesting to note that, in studies where MER 25 was administered in a single dose and a time course for uterine biochemical events was followed, some changes were found. This compound produced a short-lived increase in glucose-6-phosphate dehydrogenase, glucose isomerase and total lipids in the uterus which was no longer evident by 24 hours post treatment. In combination with oestradiol-17β, MER 25 inhibited the oestrogen-induced biochemical changes in the uterus. Similar effects were found in the rat oviduct (Harris *et al.*, 1968).

In 1959, at a conference on the "Biochemical Activities of Steroids in Relation to Cancer", Jensen and Jacobson (1960) presented their findings on specific binding of oestrogen to target tissues such as the uterus and vagina and non-specific binding to liver and kidney. This research led to the concept of specific proteins in the cell cytoplasm that bind and translocate the steroid to the nucleus. Here the protein and nucleic acid synthesis required for growth is initiated. These investigators also reported that 9α-fluoro-11β-hydroxyprogesterone not only reduced the uterotrophic response of the rat uterus to oestradiol but also reduced the incorporation of tritiated oestradiol

TABLE I
Effect of MER 25 and Oestradiol Benzoate on Uterine Weight, Nucleic Acids and Enzyme Activities in the Immature Rat[a]

Treatment	Total dose (μg)	MER 25 Total dose (mg)	Final body weight (g)	Uterine weight (mg)	Uterine RNA	
					μg/mg	μg/uterus
Control	—	0	66.7 ± 1.1[a]	40.4 ± 2.3	5.25 ± 0.34	212 ± 14
	—	0.8	60.4 ± 1.4[e]	39.5 ± 1.0	6.56 ± 0.37[e]	259 ± 15[e]
	—	4	60.2 ± 1.1[e]	38.0 ± 0.9	6.80 ± 0.20[e]	258 ± 8[e]
	—	20	52.9 ± 1.2[f]	37.2 ± 1.1	6.52 ± 0.16[e]	243 ± 6[e]
	—	100	54.5 ± 0.8[f]	37.5 ± 1.0	7.07 ± 0.23[f]	265 ± 9[f]
Oestradiol benzoate	2.0	0	63.8 ± 1.5	147.3 ± 4.6	7.15 ± 0.46[f]	1053 ± 68[f]
	2.0	0.8	58.7 ± 1.2[f]	126.2 ± 3.9[f]	7.02 ± 0.36	886 ± 45
	2.0	4	58.0 ± 1.4[f]	91.9 ± 3.0[f]	7.51 ± 0.45	690 ± 41[h]
	2.0	20	54.6 ± 1.0[f]	47.0 ± 0.8[f]	6.82 ± 0.20	321 ± 9[h]
	2.0	100	48.9 ± 0.7[f]	41.0 ± 1.4[f]	6.60 ± 0.12	271 ± 5[h]

[a] Methodology has been described previously (Lerner *et al.*, 1966b) and data are presented as mean ± S.E.M.
[b] Glucose-6-phosphate dehydrogenase.
[c] Isocitric dehydrogenase.
[d] Malic enzyme.

to 50% of that in controls. I suggested that MER 25 might be a better agent for such studies and Jensen subsequently compared the effect of 9α-bromo-11-ketoprogesterone with MER 25. The results of this study demonstrated that both compounds reduced uterine incorporation of tritiated oestradiol but that MER 25 was more potent and consistent in this activity (Jensen, 1960). Jensen suggested that the progestational compound might be inhibitory through a mechanism different from that of MER 25. This study was the first to demonstrate that the antiuterotrophic effect of MER 25 was probably a consequence of blocking oestrogen incorporation.

Oestrogens, however, affect many tissues. The end point of vaginal cornification is equal to uterine weight increase in its use as a measure of oestrogenic activity. This end point was studied in a variety of experiments. MER 25 did not induce cornification in ovariectomized mice or rats even at very high doses, however it did antagonize this vaginal response to oestradiol (Lerner, 1958; Lerner *et al.*, 1958). Moreover, when administered to cycling rats it blocked the cyclic changes in vaginal cytology, but cyclicity returned in 2–6 days after cessation of the month long treatment (Lerner *et al.*, 1958). In

Uterine DNA		RNA/DNA	Enzyme activities (μmoles NADP/min/mg DNA)		
μg/mg	μg/uterus		G6PD[b]	ICD[c]	ME[d]
8.68 ± 0.49	351 ± 20	0.62 ± .05	0.176 ± 0.016[a]	0.270 ± 0.024	0.039 ± 0.001
8.75 ± 0.77	346 ± 30	0.77 ± .08	0.138 ± 0.012	0.271 ± 0.024	0.038 ± 0.004
8.69 ± 0.39	330 ± 15	0.79 ± .03[e]	0.159 ± 0.016	0.269 ± 0.027	0.044 ± 0.011
8.11 ± 0.75	302 ± 28	0.82 ± .05[e]	0.165 ± 0.018	0.295 ± 0.044	0.041 ± 0.005
8.41 ± 0.62	315 ± 23	0.81 ± .04[e]	0.184 ± 0.025	0.302 ± 0.043	0.043 ± 0.004
4.49 ± 0.44[f]	661 ± 65[f]	1.63 ± .17[f]	0.869 ± 0.180[f]	0.512 ± 0.085[e]	0.214 ± 0.031[f]
4.39 ± 0.51	554 ± 64	1.60 ± .05	0.711 ± 0.118	0.549 ± 0.072	0.187 ± 0.031
5.10 ± 0.38	469 + 35[g]	1.45 ± .03	0.496 ± 0.087	0.508 ± 0.078	0.137 ± 0.011
5.00 ± 0.29	235 + 14[h]	0.97 ± .05[g]	0.324 ± 0.029[g]	0.482 ± 0.066	0.072 ± 0.006[g]
5.24 ± 0.18	215 + 7[h]	0.92 – .07[g]	0.330 – 0.036[g]	0.468 – 0.049	0.053 – 0.004[g]

[e] $p < 0.05$ versus control.
[f] $p < 0.01$ versus control.
[g] $p < 0.05$ versus oestradiol benzoate.
[h] $p < 0.01$ versus oestradiol benzoate.

these animals the weights of the uteri, ovaries and pituitaries were also decreased, but after cessation of treatment the weights of these organs returned to control levels.

The decrease in ovarian weight was confirmed in longer term treatment studies and, indeed, was not unexpected since MER 25 is structurally related to the triphenylethylene class of oestrogens. In a number of studies using various dosages, it was observed repeatedly that at the lower part of the dose-response curve, MER 25 had a real uterotrophic effect showing that a small amount of oestrogenic activity was still retained. Indeed, similar to very weak oestrogens, MER 25 was shown to be a weak inhibitor of gonadotrophins (Lerner *et al.*, 1958). Moreover, it did not antagonize the gonadotrophin inhibitory activity of oestradiol. It did, however, prevent the degranulation of the pituitary gonadotrophs by the oestrogen (Lerner *et al.*, 1958).

MER 25 did not decrease ovarian weight in puberal rats administered the compound for four days with or without oestradiol benzoate (Table II). Paradoxically, the oestrogen antagonist treatment resulted in a 50% increase in ovarian weight and concomittant oestrogen administration antagonized this effect (Lerner, L. J., Michel, I., Bianchi, A., Hilf, R., unpublished observations). This hypertrophy of the gonad was similar to, but more moderate than, that resulting from human chorionic gonadotrophin (hCG) treatment. Human chorionic gonadotrophin and MER 25 also were similar in the stimulation of ovarian glucose-6-phosphate dehydrogenase, NADP-isocitric dehydrogenase and NADP-malic enzyme activities. Administration of oestradiol together with the oestrogen antagonist prevented the MER 25 induced augmentation of these enzyme activities. In contrast, hCG, MER 25 and oestradiol increased ovarian RNA in relation to the weight of this organ whereas DNA was largely unaffected by treatment.

III. OESTROGENIC PROPERTIES

The oestrogenic property of MER 25 was evident and even expected because of its chemical structure, but its manifestation was often puzzling. It was weakly uterotrophic but only at low dosages. A single injection induced a small increase in uterine weight within 48 hours after injection, but this effect was not seen thereafter even though inhibition of the uterotrophic effect of oestradiol benzoate by MER 25 was seen for 120 hours (Lerner *et al.*, 1958). A similar observation was reported by Jensen (1960).

MER 25 was also compared with oestradiol for effects on uterine and oviduct phospholipid metabolism. Like oestradiol the antagonist induced an increase in phospholipids and total lipids in these organs, although when administered together with oestradiol MER 25 partially inhibited the increase

TABLE II

Effect of MER 25, Oestradiol Benzoate and Human Chorionic Gonadotrophin on Ovarian Weight, Nucleic Acids and Enzyme Activity in the Puberal Rat.[a]

Treatment daily dose/animal			Final body weight (g)	Ovarian weight (mg)	DNA (μg/ovary)	RNA (μg/ovary)	RNA/DNA	Enzyme activity (μ moles NADP/min/mg)		
Oestradiol benzoate (μg)	MER 25 (mg)	hCG I.U.						G-6-PD[b]	ICD[c]	ME[d]
—	—	—	101 ± 1.8	27.1 ± 2.0	190.1	128.0	0.673	0.063	0.134	0.058
0.5	—	—	98 ± 2.8	35.5 ± 2.8	213.7	182.0	0.852	0.101	0.159	0.067
—	1.25	—	106 ± 1.1	40.3 ± 1.8	208.9	186.8	0.894	0.132	0.320	0.127
0.5	1.25	—	97 ± 1.9	28.1 ± 2.4	197.9	142.1	0.718	0.076	0.167	0.063
—	—	10	111 ± 2.3	54.5 ± 3.9	247.8	297.2	1.199	0.153	0.299	0.149

[a] MER 25 and oestradiol benzoate were dissolved in sesame oil and administered subcutaneously once daily for 4 days to groups of 10 Charles River C-D rats weighing 90-95g at the start of the study. Human chorionic gonadotrophin in a saline vehicle was administered subcutaneously in a single dose on day 4. Animals were sacrificed on day 5. Ovaries were pooled in two pools of 5 animals (10 ovaries each) for nucleic acid and enzyme studies. The biochemical methodology has been described previously (Lerner *et al.*, 1966b).

[b] Glucose-6-phosphate dehydrogenase.

[c] Isocitric dehydrogenase.

[d] Malic enzyme.

induced by the oestrogen (Lerner *et al.*, 1966a, Harris *et al.*, 1968). This antioestrogen also behaved as an oestrogen on several enzyme activities involved in carbohydrate metabolism. A single intraperitoneal injection of MER 25 elevated uterine glucose-6-phosphate dehydrogenase and glucose phosphate isomerase activities 8–24 hours post-treatment and then these activities returned to lower levels (Harris *et al.*, 1968).

Oestrogens in low doses stimulated the superficial cells of the rodent vagina to mucify. Larger doses induced cornification of the vaginal epithelium thereby overriding the mucification stage. Weak oestrogens, including low dosages of oestriol, induce mucification but frequently cannot advance the epithelium to the stage of stratification and cornification. MER 25 did not induce vaginal cornification in rats and mice even at very large doses. However, it did induce vaginal mucification in ovariectomized rats (Lerner *et al.*, 1958).

A further expression of the weak and limited oestrogenicity of MER 25 was its ability to advance the time of vaginal opening in immature rats (Lerner *et al.*, 1958; Lerner, 1964). Although other mechanisms cannot be ruled out, MER 25 might be producing this effect by acting on the hypothalamic-pituitary-ovarian axis to increase gonadotrophin release and/or increase ovarian sensitivity to the low levels of gonadotrophins.

Many other studies in male and female animals of several species and stages of maturity were performed to survey the effects of MER 25 and define areas of utility for its weak oestrogenic, antioestrogenic and gonadotrophin inhibitory qualities (Lerner, 1958, 1964; Lerner *et al.*, 1958).

IV. ANTIFERTILITY PROPERTIES

Since this compound demonstrated both antioestrogenic and gonadotrophin inhibitory activities, it was obvious that studies on effects on reproduction were in order. MER 25 was administered at various times prior to and after mating. These studies (Lerner *et al.*, 1958; Lerner, 1964), showed that MER 25, probably through its antioestrogenic or gonadotrophin inhibitory activities prevented mating. It may have inhibited nidation and ova transport since no foetuses were recovered when treatment was initiated on day one of pregnancy. Treatment on days 4–7 after mating prevented blastocyst implantation. When treatment was delayed until day 13 of pregnancy, the rats gave birth to live young but parturition was prolonged, delayed and difficult.

These antifertility effects of MER 25 were confirmed by other investigators (Segal and Nelson, 1958; Chang, 1959; Emmens and Finn, 1962; Clark and Jordan, 1976). None of the antioestrogenic compounds, however, have been shown to be sufficiently efficacious in primates, although they can inhibit ovum implantation in the uteri of monkeys (Morris *et al.*, 1967). The effect on fertility may result from either the antioestrogenic or oestrogenic property of this compound.

V. EFFECTS ON LIPIDS

A study of the chick demonstrated that oestradiol but not MER 25 could elevate plasma phospholipids as well as oviduct weight, and when both these compounds were administered together, the antioestrogen completely prevented these oestrogen-induced effects (Lerner *et al.*, 1958). In most species, as plasma phospholipids increase with oestrogen administration cholesterol levels decrease or remain unchanged. In spite of the lack of effect of MER 25 on plasma phospholipids in the chick, it was of interest to investigate the effects of MER 25 and related compounds for their effect on plasma cholesterol in young male rats (Lerner, L. J. and Yiacas, E., unpublished observations). After ten days of treatment with daily subcutaneous doses of 0.04 to 5.0 mg the plasmas were analysed for cholesterol concentration. MER 25, MRL 41 (clomiphene citrate) and MER 29 (triparanol) decreased cholesterol concentration. MER 25 and MRL 41 were equipotent, and MER 29 was approximately five times as potent as the former agents (Table III). In this same study only MRL 41 inhibited testicular growth; only MER 25 and MRL 41 reduced ventral prostate weights; but all three reduced seminal vesicle weights, the most potent for this effect being MRL 41 and the least effective being MER 29. Adrenal weights were unaffected by these treatments and only the highest dose of each compound moderately retarded body weight gain. Studies *in vitro* using liver homogenate preparations demonstrated that the two antioestrogens, MER 25 and clomiphene, effectively inhibited the conversion of [^{14}C]mevalonate to cholesterol whereas MER 29 and TACE did not (Lerner, L. J. and Januska, J. P., unpublished observations). MER 29 produces its major block between desmosterol and cholesterol, so that while cholesterol concentration decreases desmosterol accumulates (Steinberg *et al.*, 1961). MER 29 also prevents some conversion at earlier steps in the biosynthesis of cholesterol but after mevalonic acid (Holmes and DiTullio, 1962). The problems which were associated with the accumulation of desmosterol might have been avoided if one of the compounds of the ethamoxytriphetol or clomiphene series had been chosen for development rather than the close relative, triparanol. The oestrogenic, antioestrogenic or other qualities of the compounds related to MER 25 or clomiphene, however, may have introduced a new problem.

TABLE III
Effect of MER 25, MRL 41 and MER 29 on Plasma Cholestrol Concentration and Weights of the Testes, Seminal Vesicles, Ventral Prostate and Adrenals of Young Rats[a]

Compound	Daily dose (mg/animal)	Plasma cholesterol (mg/100 ml)	Testes (g)	Seminal vesicles (mg)	Ventral prostate (mg)	Adrenals (mg)
MER 25	5.0	41.4	1.29	45.9	55.4	29.0
	1.0	63.0	1.33	53.3	86.5	25.3
	0.2	65.1	1.32	60.9	94.1	28.1
	0.04	76.6	1.27	52.3	79.9	25.4
	0.0	75.9	1.34	53.6	86.9	26.0
MRL 41	5.0	40.0	0.94	20.9	30.7	28.4
	1.0	68.5	1.05	26.8	48.1	24.4
	0.2	65.1	1.15	33.3	63.7	26.2
	0.04	67.7	1.25	61.3	96.5	28.5
	0.0	77.9	1.29	63.7	91.7	26.9
MER 29	5.0	31.4	1.41	51.8	81.1	28.7
	1.0	43.3	1.41	57.0	80.4	28.3
	0.2	65.6	1.36	66.5	86.0	27.5
	0.04	80.0	1.33	67.3	99.0	26.4
	0.0	78.1	1.38	59.8	96.2	28.2

[a] Sprague Dawley rats (65–70g) were administered the compounds in sesame oil subcutaneously once daily for 10 days. Control animals were assigned to each compound treatment series and received the vehicle only (3 groups). Plasma and organs were removed for analyses on day 11.

VI. CLINICAL APPLICATIONS

A. The Ovary

In the mid-1950s we thought that a possible clinical use of a compound like MER 25 could be the treatment of polycystic or cystic ovaries. As a graduate student with James H. Leathem it would have been difficult not to have been exposed to his experiments in which hypothyroid rats were made cystic with hCG treatment. A study was therefore performed using this model but the results were far from satisfactory. MER 25 antagonized the uterine hypertrophy induced by the hyperactive ovary and moderately decreased ovarian weight, but cystic follicles were still evident. These results were communicated to Dr Leathem and he and his graduate students repeated and extended the study. In these experiments, MER 25 prevented the induction of cystic ovaries and alteration in ovarian ascorbic acid concentrations (Adams *et al.*, 1960). Dr James T. Bradbury suggested that the nymphomaniac cow with its high oestrogen producing cystic ovaries could be studied by R. M. Melampy and W. Hansel in Iowa. A full study was never set up but a few nymphomaniacal cows were treated with a low dose of MER 25 and these animals ceased to display the abnormality, but no observations on ovarian function were reported.

R. Kistner, R. Hertz, and E. Tyler studied MER 25 in several pathological conditions including anovulatory patients. Kistner and Smith (1960) reported that, in patients that had endometrial hyperplasia or carcinomas, MER 25 treatment resulted in increased excretion of oestrogen and gonadotrophin in the urine. At the same time Tyler *et al.* (1960), studying patients with secondary amenorrhea, found that treatment with the antioestrogen resulted in ovulation in 6 of 18 women. These experiences stimulated R. Greenblatt to investigate the MER 25 and TACE related compound clomiphene citrate (Fig. 1) for similar activity. Clomiphene (MRL 41), a weak oestrogen and gonadotrophin inhibitor (Holtkamp *et al.*, 1960) and antioestrogen (Lerner, 1964) proved to be a more potent ovulation inducer than MER 25 (Greenblatt *et al.*, 1961).

B. The Breast

Other clinical applications that were suggested by the biological properties of MER 25 were those associated with the ovary-mammary gland or pituitary-ovary-mammary gland axes. Animal studies, however, were not particularly encouraging. Little or no changes were seen in rat mammary glands after treatment, although some animals on high doses exhibited reduced proliferation of the glandular epithelium. One study in rats bearing the Walker 256 carcinosarcoma demonstrated that MER 25 was weakly inhibitory, but this tumour was not a good model for the study of an oestrogen antagonist. A better model was the R3230AC mammary adenocarcinoma in rats that is responsive to oestrogens (Hilf *et al.*, 1966). This tumour responds to oestrogen by increasing enzyme synthesis and decreasing growth. MER 25 administered together with oestradiol antagonized the changes induced by the oestrogen (Hilf, 1973). Another tumour which is oestrogen-dependent is the dimethylbenzanthracene (DMBA)-induced mammary adenocarcinoma in the rat. The MER 25 related antioestrogen tamoxifen partially inhibits the growth of the DMBA-induced tumour and the binding of tritiated oestradiol to the receptors in the tumour (Jordan and Dowse, 1976).

The first studies of an antioestrogen in mammary gland disorders were performed by Dr Roy Hertz in several patients with metastatic breast cancers and by Dr Robert Kistner in patients with chronic cystic mastitis and breast carcinomas. Hertz reported (personal communication) that the patients had relief from pain and other positive responses with MER 25 treatment, but treatment had to be terminated due to some signs of toxicity including hallucinations. Kistner and Smith (1960) reported that 16 of 18 women with chronic cystic mastitis had relief from pain while on MER 25 treatment. They also reported that these patients' breasts decreased in size and there was a reduction in glandular proliferation. However, treatment caused anorexia and probably was the cause of nightmares in one of the patients. In this same publication, Kistner and Smith reported that 2 of 4 patients with carcinomas of the breast experienced relief from pain and a reduction in calcium excretion during MER 25 therapy. While the unwanted biological activities, especially those of the central nervous system, prevented the development of MER 25 for use in breast cancer, it stimulated the pharmaceutical industry to synthesize and study many related compounds for potential use in mammary and uterine cancers and for ovulation induction. A notable success in the use of antioestrogenic activity for treatment of breast cancer was achieved with the use of tamoxifen.

VII. CLUES TO FUTURE DEVELOPMENTS

The undesired central nervous system activity of MER 25 seen in patients in the late 1950s and early 1960s was the first indication that antioestrogens could be used for gaining information on the role of oestrogens on behaviour. The antioestrogen interrupted the oestrous cycle in rats and lengthened the menstrual cycle in monkeys (Lerner *et al.*, 1958). The vaginal smears of rats were devoid of cornified cells and the percentage of cornified cells was severely decreased in the monkey. It was to be expected, therefore, that MER 25 would inhibit mating behaviour and this was demonstrated by a number of investigators (Arai and Gorski, 1968; Meyerson and Lindstrom, 1968; Feder and Morin, 1974; Södersten, 1974; Roy and Wade, 1977). Effects of hormones and antihormonal compounds on other behaviours have also been noted.

Adrenal and gonadal function and the hormones of these glands can influence several experimental aggressive states in mice and rats (Conner and Levine, 1969; Leaf *et al.*, 1969; Sigg, 1969). Administration of antihormonal compounds may also influence aggressive states. In the muricidal rat model administration of MER 25, clomiphene and several other oestrogen antagonists have suppressed the mouse killing (Lerner, L. J., unpublished observations).

Antioestrogens could also be useful in the treatment of menstrual disorders, especially if those disorders are caused by hormonal imbalances. The oedemas in such disfunctions might be altered by inhibiting oestrogens and the resultant sodium retention. Similarly, the effect of oestrogen on uterine contraction could be alleviated by an antioestrogen. MER 25 inhibits oestrogen-induced uterine contractions in an *in vitro* rat preparation (Cutler *et al.*, 1961).

Similarity between the uterine response to oestrogen and the hyperaemia, oedema and hypertrophy of inflammation led to a comparative study of anti-inflammatory drugs such as indomethacin with oestrogens and anti-oestrogens (Lerner *et al.*, 1975). Clomiphene and diethylstilboestrol were anti-inflammatory in carrageenan-induced hind leg oedema in rats although they were weaker than indomethacin. MER 25 and MER 29 were only marginally effective as anti-inflammatory agents. These compounds were also studied for inhibition of prostaglandin synthesis (Lerner *et al.*, 1975). Clomiphene proved to be as potent a suppressor of prostaglandin synthesis as indomethacin but, surprisingly, diethylstilboestrol was also potent for this activity. MER 25 and MER 29 were very weak inhibitors.

The possible uses of MER 25 and other antioestrogenic compounds as therapeutic agents and for the study of basic mechanisms is still unexhausted even twenty-five years after the initial finding of a competitive oestrogen antagonist. It is gratifying to have observed the many developments with antioestrogens which have increased our understanding of the role of oestrogens in many physiological functions. It has also been satisfying to witness the use of this class of compounds in therapy.

REFERENCES

Adams, W. C., France, E. S., and Leathem, J. H. (1960). *Proc. Penn. Acad. Sci.* **34**, 155.

Arai, Y., and Gorski, R. A. (1968). *Physiol. Behav.* **3**, 351–353.

Chang, M. C. (1959). *Endocrinology* **65**, 339–342.

Clark, E. R., and Jordan, V. C. (1976). *Br. J. Pharmacol.* **57**, 487–493.

Conner, R. L., and Levine, S (1969). *In* "Aggressive Behaviour" (S. Garattini and E. B. Sigg, eds), pp. 143–149. Exerpta Medica, Amsterdam.

Cutler, A., Ober, W. B., Epstein, J. A., and Kupperman, H. S. (1961). *Endocrinology* **69**, 473–482.

Emmens, C. W., and Finn, C. A. (1962). *J. Reprod. Fert.* **3**, 239–245.

Feder, H. H., and Morin, L. P. (1974). *Horm. Behav.* **5**, 63–71.

Greenblatt, R. B., Barfield, W. E., Jungok, E. C., and Ray, A. W. (1961). *J. Am. Med. Assoc.* **178**, 101-104

Harris, D. N., Lerner, L. J., and Hilf, R. (1968). *Trans. N. Y. Acad. Sci.* **30**, 774–782.

Harris, J. S., and Kohn, H. I. (1941). *J. Pharmacol. Exptl. Therap.* **73**, 383–385.

Hilf, R. (1973). *Enzyme.* **14**, 318–324.

Hilf, R., Michel, I., Bell, C., and Carrington, M. J. (1966). *Cancer Res.* **26**, 1365–1370.

Hisaw, F. L., Velardo, J. T., and Goolsby, D. M. (1954). *J. Clin. Endocr. Metab.* **14**, 1134–1143.

Holmes, W. L., and DiTullio, N. W. (1962). *Am. J. Clin. Nutr.* **10**, 310–322.

Holtkamp, D. E., Greslin, J. G., Root, C. A., and Lerner, L. J. (1960). *Proc. Soc. Exp. Biol. Med.* **105**, 197–201.

Horwitz, K. B., and McGuire, W. L. (1978). *J. Biol. Chem.* **253**, 2223–2228.

Jensen, E. V. (1960). Discussion of the C. W. Emmens, R. I. Cox and L. Martin paper. *In* "Biological Activities of Steroids in Relation to Cancer" (G. Pincus and E. P. Vollmer, eds), pp. 415–466. Academic Press, New York.

Jensen, E. V. and Jacobson, H. I. (1960). *In* "Biological Activities of Steroids in Relation to Cancer" (G. Pincus and E. P. Vollmer, eds), pp. 161–178. Academic Press, New York.
Jordan, V. C., and Dix, C. J. (1979). *J. Steroid Biochem.* **11**, 285–291.
Jordan, V. C., and Dowse, L. J. (1976). *J. Endocr.* **68**, 297–303.
Kistner, R. W., and Smith, O. W. (1960). *Surgical Forum.* **10**, 725–729.
Leaf, R. C., Lerner, L., and Horovitz, Z. P. (1969). *In* "Aggressive Behaviour" (S. Garattini and E. B. Sigg, eds), pp. 120–131. Excerpta Medica, Amsterdam.
Lerner, L. J. (1958). *Fedn Proc.Am. Socs Exp. Biol.***17**, 388
Lerner, L. J. (1959). *Ann. N. Y. Acad. Sci.* **75**, 460–462.
Lerner, L. J. (1964). *Recent Progr. Horm.Res.* **20**, 435–490.
Lerner, L. J., Holthaus, F. J., Jr., and Thompson, C. R. (1958). *Endocrinology* **63**, 295–318.
Lerner, L. J., Harris, D. N., Hilf, R., Bianchi, A., and Raskin, B. K. (1966a). *In* "Proceedings of the Second International Congress of Hormonal Steroids" (L. Martini, F. Fraschini and M. Motta, eds), pp. 628–636. Excerpta Medica, International Congress Series No. 132.
Lerner, L. J., Hilf, R., Turkheimer, A. R., Michel, I., and Engle, S. L. (1966b). *Endocrinology* **78**, 111–124.
Lerner, L. J., Carminati, P., and Schiatti, P. (1975). *Proc. Soc. Exp. Biol. Med.* **148**, 329–332.
Meyerson, B. J., and Lindstrom, L. (1968). *Acta Endocr.* **59**, 41–48.
Morris, J. M., Van Wagenen, G., McCann, J., and Jacobs, D. (1967). *Fertil.Steril.* **18**, 18–34.
Roy, E. J., and Wade, G. N. (1977). *Brain Res.* **126**, 73–87.
Segal, S. J., and Nelson, W. O. (1958). *Proc. Soc. Exp. Biol. Med.* **98**, 431–436.
Sigg, E. B. (1969). *In* "Aggressive Behaviour" (S. Garattini and E. B. Sigg, eds), pp. 143–149. Excerpta Medica, Amsterdam.
Södersten, P. (1974). *Horm. Behav.* **5**, 111–121.
Steinberg, D., Avigan, J., and Feigelson, E. B. (1961). *J. Clin. Invest.* **40**, 884–893.
Tyler, E. T., Olson, H. J., and Gotlib, M. H. (1960). *Int. J. Fertil.* **5**, 429–436.
Woods, D. D. (1940). *Brit. J. Exptl Pathol.* **21**, 74–90.

2

Early Work on Antioestrogens

C. W. EMMENS

I. INTRODUCTION

This chapter is confined to remarks on the non-steroidal synthetic compounds mostly developed during the late 1950s and extensively studied during the 1960s. Some of these compounds already existed (e.g. dimethylstilboestrol) but their antioestrogenic properties had not been discovered. The earlier work was primarily biological, leading to speculations which, later, more biochemical work has in some instances amply confirmed. Much of this biological interest was stimulated not only by scientific curiosity, but also by the then prevalent belief that antioestrogens were likely to be useful as contraceptive agents. This followed from studies of rodent implantation (cf. Shelesnyak, 1957), which showed that a rise in circulating oestrogen precedes and is necessary for implantation to occur. Oddly, although some of the compounds studied are indeed potent antifertility agents, those most successful and active in this regard would not seem to be so because of their antioestrogenic properties, or because of their oestrogenicity.

NON-STEROIDAL ANTIOESTROGENS
ISBN 0 12 677880 9

Although the classical antagonists of oestrogens are androgens and progesterone (Smith, 1926; Parkes and Bellerby, 1926), synthetic compounds having the same actions as these have been until very recently confined to the steroids. The antioestrogens of interest in this book are related to the synthetic oestrogens themselves, not to the steroids. Some of the isomers of diethylstilboestrol and other di-p-hydroxyphenyl alkanes and alkenes inhibited proliferation or cornification of the rodent epithelium in tests by Bárány *et al.* (1955), Miquel *et al.* (1958), Emmens and Cox (1958) and also α-ketoglutarate production in suspensions of human placenta in the presence of oestradiol-17β (Villee, 1957). However, only intravaginal application worked in the rodent, and only very high doses in the studies *in vitro*. The related compound, MER 25 (ethamoxytriphetol) was extensively investigated at this time by Lerner *et al.* (1958), and it blocked reponses to oestrogens even when given systemically, although milligram amounts were needed. Stone (1964) and others showed that this compound blocks the early uptake of oestradiol in the rodent reproductive tract.

II. TESTS OF OESTROGENIC AND ANTIOESTROGENIC ACTIVITY

The classical tests of oestrogenic activity, vaginal smear tests and uterine weight tests, were supplemented early by intravaginal smear methods (Freud, 1939; Muhlbock, 1940) and later by vaginal mitosis and epithelial thickness (Martin and Claringbold, 1960), vaginal tetrazolium reduction (Martin, 1960) and tritiated uridine uptake by the uterus (Miller and Emmens, 1967). These tests enabled the segregation of antioestrogens into two biologically different types, those which inhibited all responses to varying degrees, and those which only inhibited responses occurring many hours after administration of the oestrogen. Emmens *et al.* (1962) thought that the former class of antioestrogens would compete with oestrogens at a common site and thus interfere with the earliest responses, whereas the latter would modify only secondary responses. It was of great interest that only non-steroids were at that time found to occupy the first class. This class could also be subdivided into those compounds first discussed by Bárány *et al.* (1955), which were only active locally, and those introduced by Lerner *et al.* (1958), which were active parenterally.

With carefully timed local application of dimethylstilboestrol, Martin *et al.* (1961) showed that it was an inhibitor only when applied intravaginally within a few minutes of the oestrogen. It was concluded that the oestrogen (steroidal or otherwise) reached the site of action rapidly and that dimethylstilboestrol acted by blocking it, but could not displace it once it was at the site of action, or could do so only after the hormone had set in train the series of events leading to a response. This would also explain the ineffectiveness of dimethylstilboestrol and similar compounds as systemic inhibitors of naturally produced oestrogens, which, circulating all the time, would not be susceptible to such blocking.

Martin (1969) also showed that if dimethylstilboestrol, known to be a weak oestrogen by conventional tests, was given at hourly intervals, it elicited responses in the mouse vagina comparable to those to oestradiol-17β, just as oestriol does. Thus, after displacing an oestrogen from the site of action, it would seem that a single dose of dimethylstilboestrol does not stay there long enough to complete its action.

We thus had the concept of one class of antioestrogens, usually "weak" oestrogens, competing for receptor sites when given simultaneously with more potent oestrogens, synthetic or otherwise, but which left the sites shortly afterwards and thus at best gave rise to an abortive oestrogenic stimulus. Such antioestrogens would be effective when administered locally, but might be poorly effective or ineffective by the parenteral route. A second class of antioestrogens, which included the steroids, was effective by both routes but did not interfere with initial uptake, acting instead at some later stage or stages. Effects on receptor induction and the like were not at that time considered.

When the assay of oestrogens by tritiated uridine uptake and its incorporation into the uterine RNA was developed, Miller and Emmens (1967) studied the duration of response to single injections. It was found that initial responses to various natural and synthetic oestrogens were very similar, and that stilbene or bibenzyl derivatives, which inhibited the action of oestradiol-17β by local administration, elicited responses typical of oestrogens, some at the same dosage level as diethylstilboestrol. However, they differed from typical oestrogens (except oestriol) in failing to maintain the response for more than a few hours. This was regarded as a further confirmation of the ideas outlined above.

In the tetrazolium assay of Martin (1960) both true oestrogens and pro-oestrogens were more effective by subcutaneous than by intravenous administration. However, the difference between the routes of administration was greater with a pro-oestrogen, and for some, such as mesobutoestrol, ethylstilboestrol and η-propylstilboestrol, the intravenous dose-response slopes were very low (Stone, 1964). These observations might be explained by both a low receptor affinity of the pro-oestrogens or their metabolites and a more rapid clearance by the intravenous route.

It may be noted in passing that the apparent pro-oestrogenic properties of these compounds might be due to the same phenomenon, i.e. an affinity for receptors so weak that the body has to be saturated with the compounds before a sustained stimulus is achieved. With other compounds, a transformation to an oestrogen in the body, probably in the liver, is still the most likely explanation for a lack of high local potency.

Various early studies of the uptake and retention of oestrogens in target organs supported these concepts. Oestradiol-17β and *meso*-hexoestrol showed similar patterns, and labelled oestradiol was displaced by other oestrogenic compounds in approximate proportion to their oestrogenic potencies in a variety of tests (see summary by Emmens and Miller, 1969). However, the isomer, *dl*-hexoestrol, an inhibitor, was not selectively retained in the uterus or vagina of the mouse after 2 hours.

III. TYPES OF ANTIOESTROGEN

Despite the interesting properties of compounds of the stilbene series, they lack parenteral activity as antioestrogens and exhibit only their oestrogenic potencies when administered by routes other than the local one. However, the very weak parenteral activity of MER 25 gave a clue to the possibilities of similar compounds, the triarylalkanes and alkenes. The presence of a dialkylaminoethoxy side chain seemed desirable, and many series of compounds were investigated in different laboratories. These compounds usually exhibited a spectrum of activities, demonstrating weak oestrogenic, antioestrogenic and anti-fertility activities in varying degrees.

Callantine (1967), using CN 55,945-27 (CI 628) as an example, discussed the various substances then under investigation (see Fig. 1 for these and some other compounds) and commented on their common property of antagonizing certain oestrogen actions while themselves being mildly oestrogenic (mainly in uterine weight tests). CI 628 acts as a mild oestrogen when given orally to the ovariectomised rat but antagonizes the action of oestradiol if given at the same time, as assessed by uterine weight and nucleic acid synthesis assays. It is an "impeded" oestrogen since the small increase in uterine weight it induces does not increase with dosage. However, its antagonistic effect on oestradiol-induced uterine weight increases is dose-dependent. Similar observations were made with clomiphene. Clinically, clomiphene, and MER 25, are said to cause reversal of endometrial hyperplasia and of carcinoma of the breast and endometrium. These and other actions in the human were taken to indicate predominantly antioestrogenic activity in the intact subject, yet clomiphene releases gonadotrophins in the human, and stimulates ovulation (Roy *et al.* 1963), which are oestrogenic responses.

Terenius and Ljingkvist (1972), aided by the beginning of effective research on receptor substances, later grouped the antioestrogens as follows.

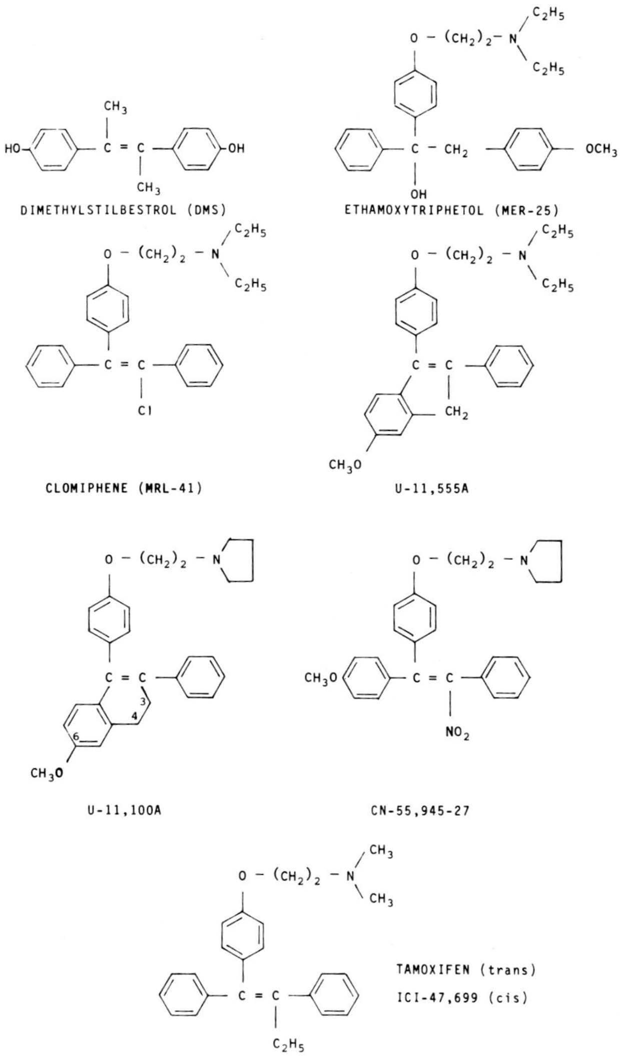

DIMETHYLSTILBESTROL (DMS)

ETHAMOXYTRIPHETOL (MER-25)

CLOMIPHENE (MRL-41)

U-11,555A

U-11,100A

CN-55,945-27

TAMOXIFEN (trans)

ICI-47,699 (cis)

Fig. 1. Some of the compounds discussed in the text.

A. Uterotrophic Effects

Normal responses to *cis*- and *trans*- clomiphene, tamoxifen and U 11,555A impeded responses to oestriol, DMS and *ent*-oestradiol, partial responses to nafoxidine and CI 628, and practically none to MER 25. Stone and Emmens (1964) have since shown that, in the rat, positive vaginal smears are seen after 40 mg of MER 25.

B. As Antioestrogens

Impeded oestrogens are fairly inactive, but those with partial or no response oestrogenically are more active. This conclusion seems rather odd, particularly since Terenius and others have found MER 25 to be oestrogenically inactive. They were able to trace this difference to differences in the interaction between the compounds and oestradiol-17β in the uterus. Impeded oestrogens were said to have high affinity for receptors but were easily lost to the circulation, whereas the others had lower affinity but remained on the receptors for longer.

Note that Terenius and Ljingkvist (1972) classified CI 628 as giving a partial response (whatever that means) rather than an impeded response.

Thus, biological work prior to about 1970 had demonstrated the essence of the antioestrogen problem: there are different types of antioestrogens, detectable in both uterine weight and vaginal smear tests and also in other tests; different test methods and different species may give different results; and a single definition of an antioestrogen is not possible. It was clear, however, that competition for receptor sites occurs or may occur in one series (mainly the non-steroids), and that weak oestrogenic activity of one sort or another is usually involved.

IV. SPECIFIC COMPOUNDS

For various reasons, research both in the laboratory and in the clinic has centred on a few compounds, obviously not always the best available. They will be discussed at length in this book, and are clomiphene (MRL 41), nafoxidine (U 11,100A), CI 628 (CN 55,945-27), and tamoxifen (ICI 46,474). All but nafoxidine are closely related to triphenylethylene and all have an alkylaminoethoxy side chain. I propose to discuss the earlier work with these compounds and with the series of compounds in which they fall.

A. Clomiphene

Clomiphene, first described by Holtkamp *et al.* (1960) as an anti-fertility agent with some oestrogenic and antioestrogenic effects, came into prominence with MER 25 because of its capacity to induce ovulation in the human. It was also reported by several investigators to cause a rise in urinary gonadotrophin excretion in both sexes (cf. Callantine, 1967, for a useful summary). In animals, small doses were found to stimulate gonadotrophin release and large doses to inhibit it. Those of us who followed these results at the time were inclined to feel that perhaps all of these effects reflected clomiphene's weak oestrogenic activity. However, further work suggested that clomiphene acts in some way other than simply as a weak oestrogen, although there does not appear to be any reason to believe that its antioestrogenic properties are concerned in its actions on the normal reproductive tract apart from in the mammary gland. Present-day opinion would, I think, opt for a primary action of the hypothalamus, followed by gonadotrophin release and ovulation, a typical oestrogenic effect. It is thus most useful in patients showing evidence of hyposecretion of gonadotrophins.

When clomiphene is given to patients with breast or uterine hyperplasia or carcinoma, presenting a different picture hormonally from that of the hyposecreting women of low fertility, its antioestrogenic action comes into prominence. This was appreciated during the 1960s and was attributed to the capacity of clomiphene to displace the more potent natural oestrogen and to exert, therefore, a lower degree of oestrogenicity. Laboratory studies supported such conclusions. For example, Wood *et al.* (1968) concluded that MER 25, clomiphene and CI 628 all act as competitive inhibitors of oestradiol-17β. This was on the basis of biological observations — uterine water, glycogen and glucose responses.

B. Nafoxidine

Other antifertility compounds followed MER 25 and MRL 41 and the series to which they belong, notably U 11,555A (Duncan *et al.* 1962) and U 11,100A (Duncan *et al.* 1963), the latter being nafoxidine. U 11,555A is an interesting compound, but it is unstable and also causes photosensitization of the recipient, so interest centred on U 11,100A instead. The antioestrogenic properties of these compounds were thought to be responsible for their antifertility effects in rodents, and were more impressive than their uterotrophic or gonadotrophin suppressing activities. Ericsson (1966) also demonstrated the capacity of nafoxidine to suppress spermatogenesis and libido in rabbits, but did not seem to suspect that this might be due to oestrogenic activity, while Emmens and Martin (1965) found it to be oestrogenic in rats and mice at approximately ED_{50}s of 0.5 and 0.05 mg respectively, in vaginal smear tests, acting as an impeded oestrogen with weak antioestrogenicity. These authors also found that its antifertility action in the female mouse was in line with its oestrogenic potency and that antioestrogenic activity was not an explanation of its action.

C. CI 628

CI 628 was introduced by Callantine *et al.* (1966) as an oestrogen antagonist interfering with reproduction in the rat. Some of its properties have already been discussed. It is a weak oestrogen in the mouse with no detectable antioestrogenic activity in systemic vaginal smear tests (Collins *et al.* 1971) and it also has weak antifertility activity. The range of activities of compounds like CI 628, related to triphenylethylene, can only be appreciated when results like those of Collins *et al.* (1971) are studied. We were surprised to find that relatively few compounds of the CI 628 – ICI 46,474 series had been made, although they were patented, and proceeded to make some 25–30 of them during the late 1960s. Since our primary objective, apart from basic study, was to find useful antifertility compounds, we had not concentrated on tricyclics because of worry about possible carcinogenicity. The application of some members of the series as anticancer drugs at the present time is therefore somewhat ironic.

Comparisons within the series will be made when discussing tamoxifen, but as far as CI 628 is concerned, there does not seem to be much to say about it beyond noting its characteristic impeded oestrogenic activity, and the difference in overt antioestrogenic properties between the rat and the mouse.

D. Tamoxifen

Harper and Walpole (1966, 1967), again primarily interested in fertility control, reported on the properties of the *trans*- and *cis*-isomers of tamoxifen. They found that, in the female rat, the *trans*-isomer (ICI 46,474) prevented implantation, was "weakly and atypically oestrogenic", and antioestrogenic in vaginal cornification and uterine weight tests. By contrast, the *cis*-isomer (ICI 47,699) behaved in all respects like a typical oestrogen and was very much more potent than the *trans*-isomer. In mice, the *trans*-isomer was, however, the more potent in vaginal cornification tests.

In contrast to the above, Collins *et al.* (1971) did not find the two isomers to be very different in oestrogenic potency in either species as far as threshold doses were concerned, but since they had different slopes further comparison was meaningless. However, they agreed with Harper and Walpole (1967) in finding the *trans*-isomer to be an impeded oestrogen, and more potent as an antifertility agent in both species. Neither compound was antioestrogenic in the mouse.

Quite extensive biological tests of 16 compounds of this series (12 triarylalkenes and 4 triarylalkanes) were reported by Collins *et al.* (1971), and other compounds in the series have since been examined. These showed that dose-response lines in vaginal smear tests might reveal an ordinary oestrogenic response (steep line) or an impeded response (shallow line usually not reaching 100% response). Dose-response lines as post-coital antifertility agents were quite normal, as steep as for typical oestrogens, but the relationship between the anti-implantation ED_{50} and the oestrogenic ED_{50} did not follow the rule for oestrogens, i.e. the daily ED_{50} for post-coital antifertility is approximately equal to that for vaginal smear tests. Only three of the compounds showed any antioestrogenic activity in the mouse (rat not tested), and then in doses of 0.5 to 1.0 mg, whereas most of them were potent antifertility agents.

Dissociation between oestrogenic or antioestrogenic activity and post-coital antifertility activity is therefore most apparent in this series. The most potent group, which includes tamoxifen, has compounds with much the same antifertility activity post-coitally, while others are much less potent. Some are shown in Table I for comparison, with figures for subcutaneous activity.

Emmens (1971) discovered that some of the triarylalkenes discussed, including tamoxifen, when given in relatively high dosage prior to vaginal smear tests or prior to fertility tests, act both as antioestrogens and as antifertility agents for several weeks. These long-term effects are much more prominent by injection than gavage, raising the possibility of depot formation or of gut metabolism. However, even a single dose is followed by increasing refractoriness to oestradiol in vaginal smear tests, and although mating occurs in fertility trials, pregnancies are few. These effects are shown in Tables II and III, for the rat and mouse respectively. Histological studies were made by Emmens and Carr (1973) with H 1076 (Table I), a compound which prevents implantation in the mouse in a daily dose of 1.5 μg on days 1–3 post-coitally without detectable effects on tubal transport or endocrine functions. Given prior to mating in the relatively massive dose of 2–5 mg, it has little effect on coitus, but produces prolonged infertility. Initial oestrogenic responses are seen in both uterus and vagina, followed over the next few weeks by antioestrogenic effects. The uterine glands gradually enlarge over a 9 week period (5 mg dose) and later revert to normal. Ovarian weights are not affected, but in mated animals corpora lutea are few and poorly developed. The animals eventually regain fertility. The phenomena suggest interference with ovulation and corpus luteum function, possibly via pituitary or hypothalamic inhibition.

TABLE I
Biological Activities of various Triarylalkenes by Injection in the Mouse

$O-(CH_2)_2-N-R_1$

R_2 — C = C — R_4

R_3

Compound	R_1	R_2	R_3	R_4	ED_{50}(µg) for activity		
					Oestrogenic (vag. smears)	Antifertility daily dose Days 1–3	Days 4–6
ICI 46,474	$(CH_3)_2$	H	C_2H_5	H(trans)	> 250	2.0	5.0
ICI 47,699	$(CH_3)_2$	H	C_2H_5	H(cis)	200	60.0	20.0
H 774	$(C_2H_5)_2$	OCH_3	C_2H_5	OCH_3[a]	2000	6.0	50.0
H 1067	$(C_2H_5)_2$	OCH_3	C_2H_5	OCH_3(trans)	2700	3.0	6.0
H 1076	$(C_2H_5)_2$	OCH_3	$CH(CH_3)_2$	OCH_3[b]	100	2.0	6.0
H 1285	$(C_2H_5)_2$	OH	C_2H_5	OCH_3	100	0.4	1.6
CI 628		OCH_3	NO_2	H	1000	50.0	100.0

[a] cis:trans, 62:38 %
[b] cis:trans, 39:61 %
[c] See CN-55, 945-27 in Fig. 1, p. 21
No compound was antioestrogenic in vaginal smear tests.

TABLE II
The Effects of two Consecutive Daily Injections of Various Compounds on the Response of Spayed Rats to Oestradiol[a]

Compound	Total dose (mg)	Dose of oestradiol (μg)	Percent positive response to 0.3 μg oestradiol after				
			0 weeks	2 weeks	4 weeks	6 weeks	8 weeks
H 774	1	—	65	25	0	15	80
	3	—	85	35	0	15	80
	9	—	75	50	0	5	55
H 774	1	0.3	70	15	10	20	75
	3	0.3	75	60	5	50	60
	9	0.3	75	25	0	5	65
ICI 46,474	1	0.3	90	100	70	80	93
	3	0.3	85	55	15	50	83
	9	0.3	95	90	0	20	50
ICI 47,699	0.1	0.3	95	50	100	75	80
	0.5	0.3	100	85	95	100	90
	2.5	0.3	100	85	100	90	80
	—	0.3	85	—*	100	65	95

[a] The oestradiol was given 2, 4, 6 or 8 weeks after the first administration of the compounds. Initially, each group consisted of ten animals. Data from Emmens (1971).
* Omitted in error.

TABLE III
The Effects of a Single Dose of Various Compounds on the Occurrence of Vaginal Plugs and Resulting Pregnancies in Mice[a]

Compound		Plugs found and litters resulting during the following 10 day periods after injection					
		1–10	11–20	21–30	31–40	Total	%
H 774 (1 mg)	Plugs	13	6	1	0	20	100
	Litters	0	2	1	0	3	15
H 1075 (1 mg)	Plugs	7	6	4	1	18/19	95
	Litters	0	1	3	0	4	21
H 1076 (1 mg)	Plugs	11	8	0	1	20	100
	Litters	0	0	0	1	1	5
Controls (vehicle only)	Plugs	19	1	0	0	20	100
	Litters	17	1	0	0	18	90

[a] Males were introduced on day 3 after injection. Initially, each group consisted of 20 mice. Data from Emmens (1971).

Jordan (1975) followed up these observations with experiments on tamoxifen, of which 3 mg over 2 days produced refractoriness for up to 6 weeks in mouse vaginal smear tests with oestradiol. However, simultaneous administration of the two substances showed no inhibition, in agreement with Emmens (1971). Uptake of tritiated oestradiol-17β was severely inhibited in the uterus and vagina of treated animals, and did not return to normal for about 10 weeks in the uterus and 6 weeks in the vagina. In such circumstances, tamoxifen clearly acts, after a short period of oestrogenicity, as an antioestrogen preventing receptor binding. However, Martin and Middleton (1978) questioned this conclusion, since, in the mouse, such a dose of tamoxifen produced vaginal weight increases, and from 48 hours on, multilayered stratified or cornified epithelia, in contrast to controls, which had thin and atrophic epithelia. Jordan (1975) also recorded vaginal weight increases. Martin and Middleton (1978) feel that this indicates only a prolonged, weak oestrogenic response. However, this is exactly what an antioestrogen which is at the same time weakly oestrogenic does: it hinders the uptake of a normal, potent oestrogen.

Emmens and Carr (1973) did not find vaginal weight increases in intact mice after single doses of H 1076, a compound structurally related to and resembling tamoxifen in action. Instead, vaginal weights decreased significantly up to 6 weeks after 2 mg and up to 9 weeks after 5 mg (Table IV). Within 24 hours, all mice showed pro-oestrous or oestrous smears; by 72 hours, all but one mouse out of 99 had had an oestrous smear. Thereafter, prolonged oestrous cycles occurred, with many predominantly cornified smears. Sections

TABLE IV
Mean Body Weights and Mean Wet Vaginal Weights of Mice after receiving a Single Dose of H 1076[a]

Days after injection	Dose of H 1076					
	0 mg		2 mg		5 mg	
	Body wt. (g)	Vaginal wt. (mg)	Body wt. (g)	Vaginal wt. (mg)	Body wt. (g)	Vaginal wt. (mg)
3	26.8	79.3	27.0	79.0	23.8	76.5
7	25.8	72.0	24.5	58.8	22.0	55.3
21	27.7	84.2	28.3	64.8	25.3	54.0
42	25.5	76.7	29.0	58.8	24.3	56.0
63	24.8	92.7	28.7	64.2	28.7	56.3
84	30.7	112.2	29.7	91.7	30.2	66.2
119	—	86.8	—	72.8	—	82.3

[a] 3 mice per group. After Emmens and Carr (1973).

showed no obvious structural changes other than those characteristic of the oestrous cycle. Argument from ovariectomized to intact mice and from tamoxifen to another (even if related) compound is regrettably invalid, but there would seem to be more to the question than purely oestrogenic stimulation in the mouse.

V. CONCLUDING REMARKS

This brief summary has ignored many early investigations of series of antifertility and antioestrogenic compounds, for reasons of space and time and also because most of them led nowhere. It has concentrated as much on antifertility activity as any other because that was the motivating force more often than not, and this frequently led to scanty and sometimes poor work on antioestrogenicity *per se*. For instance, many compounds were only investigated by the oral route, because that is how it was envisaged they would be used in humans.

Although events such as the thalidomide disaster, and the prohibitive costs of development led to investigators abandoning many such antifertility investigations, the use of promising members of the series as anti-cancer agents was explored. Presumably this was due in part to the use of possibly suspect drugs in cancer research, whereas their use as contraceptives might be hard to justify, and certainly very expensive to develop.

It looks as if the pendulum might swing across in the near future, and if so, there are some existing members among those discussed which might yet turn out to be the key to a new line of contraception. Tamoxifen, for example, is a potent antifertility agent in the mouse at doses which show no oestrogenic or antioestrogenic activity. So are other members of the series to which it belongs.

REFERENCES

Bárány, E. H., Morsing, P., Muller, W., Stalberg, G., and Stenhagen, E. (1955). *Acta Soc. Med. Upsaliensis* **60**, 68–72.

Callantine, M. R. (1967). *Clin. Obstet. Gynaecol.* **10**, 74–87.

Callantine, M. R., Humphrey, R. R., Lee, S. L., Windsor, B. L., Schottin, N. H., and O'Brien, O. P. (1966). *Endocrinology* **79**, 153–167.

Collins, D. J., Hobbs, J. J., and Emmens, C. W. (1971). *J. Med. Chem.* **14**, 952–957.

Duncan, G. W., Stucki, J. C., Lyster, S. C., and Lednicer, D. (1962). *Proc. Soc. Exp. Biol. Med.* **109**, 163–166.

Duncan, G. W., Lyster, S. C., Clark, J. J., and Lednicer, D. (1963). *Proc. Soc. Exp. Biol. Med.* **112**, 439–442.

Emmens, C. W. (1971). *J. Reprod. Fert.* **26**, 175–182.
Emmens, C. W., and Carr, W. L. (1973). *J. Reprod. Fert.* **34**, 29–40.
Emmens, C. W., and Cox, R. I. (1958). *J. Endocr.* **17**, 265–271.
Emmens, C. W., and Martin, L. (1965). *J. Reprod. Fert.* **9**, 269–275.
Emmens, C. W., and Miller, B. G. (1969). *Steroids* **13**, 725–730.
Emmens, C. W., Cox, R. I., and Martin, L. (1962). *Recent Progr. Horm. Res.* **18**, 415–466.
Ericsson, R. J. (1966). *J. Reprod. Fert.* **11**, 107–115.
Freud, J. (1939). *Acta Brevia Neerl. Physiol. Pharmacol. Microbiol.* **10**, 42–44.
Harper, M. J. K., and Walpole, A. L. (1966). *Nature* **212**, 87.
Harper, M. J. K., and Walpole, A. L. (1967). *J. Reprod. Fert.* **13**, 101–119.
Holtkamp, D. E., Greslin, J., Root, C. A., and Lerner, L. J. (1960). *Proc. Soc. Exp. Biol. Med.* **105**, 197–201.
Jordan, V. C. (1975). *J. Reprod. Fert.* **42**, 251–258.
Lerner, L. J., Holthaus, F. J., and Thompson, C. R. (1958). *Endocrinology* **63**, 295–318.
Martin, L. (1960). *J. Endocr.* **20**, 187–197.
Martin, L. (1969). *Steroids* **13**, 1–10.
Martin, L., and Claringbold, P. J. (1958). *Nature* **181**, 620–621.
Martin, L., and Claringbold, P. J. (1960). *J. Endocr.* **20**, 173–186.
Martin, L., and Middleton, E. (1978). *J. Endocr.* **78**, 125–129.
Martin, L., Cox, R. I., and Emmens, C. W. (1961). *J. Endocr.* **22**, 129–132.
Miller, B. G., and Emmens, C. W. (1967). *J. Endocr.* **39**, 473–484.
Miquel, I. F., Bárány, E. H., and Müller, W. (1958). *Arch. intern. pharmacodynamie* **67**, 262.
Muhlbock, O. (1940). *Acta brevia Neerl. Physiol. Pharmacol. Microbiol.* **10**, 42–44.
Parkes, A. S., and Bellerby, C. W. (1926). *J. Physiol.* **62**, 145–155.
Roy, S., Greenblatt, R. B., Mahesh, V. B., and Jungck, E. C. (1963). *Fertil. Steril.* **14**, 575.
Shelesnyak, M. C. (1957). *Recent Progr. Horm. Res.* **13**, 269–322.
Smith, M. G. (1926). *Bull. John Hopkins Hosp.* **39**, 203–214.
Stone, G. M. (1964). *J. Endocr.* **29**, 159–165.
Stone, G. M., and Emmens, C. W. (1964). *J. Endocr.* **29**, 147–157.
Terenius, L., and Ljingkvist, I. (1972). *Gynecol. Invest.* **3**, 96–107.
Villee, C. A. (1957). *Cancer Res.* **17**, 507–511.
Wood, J. R., Wren, R. T., and Bitman, J. (1968). *Endocrinology* **82**, 69–74.

3

Structure–Activity Relationships amongst Non-Steroidal Antioestrogens

V. CRAIG JORDAN, E. R. CLARK AND KAREN E. ALLEN

I. INTRODUCTION

A. Drug–Receptor Interaction

The introduction by Paul Ehrlich of the concept of drug receptors, drawn in part from his earlier experiences with histological staining and immunology, laid the early foundations for an understanding of drug action at the molecular level. A wealth of practical pharmacological knowledge that provides substance to Ehrlich's suggestions has now been accumulated. In the main, evidence for drug receptors has come from (a) studies of the selectivity of drug action in various tissues of the body, (b) an examination of structure–activity relationships, which has allowed, in some instances, the description of a crude receptor map, and (c) the quantitative relationship

NON-STEROIDAL ANTIOESTROGENS
ISBN 0 12 677880 9

between drug dosage, or concentration, and tissue response, which has permitted a mathematical comparison of drugs.

In their simplest form, the current theories of drug interaction with receptors are based upon the fundamental studies by Clark (1926) and Gaddum (1926) who suggested that the response to a drug is proportional to the number of receptors occupied. However, the occupation theory has been modified by Ariens and Simonis (1964) and Stephenson (1956) into two steps: firstly, receptor binding (dependent upon affinity), and secondly, the production of a response (dependent upon the intrinsic activity or efficacy of the drug–receptor complex). Thus within a group of drugs which are all full agonists (i.e. the intrinsic activity $\alpha = 1$) but which have progressively smaller affinity constants, their sigmoidal log dose–response curves would be progressively shifted to the right. However, for a group of drugs with intrinsic activities progressively less than 1.0, the maximal responses in their log dose–response curves would become progressively lower. These compounds are known as partial agonists. When administered with a full agonist, partial agonists do not produce an additive effect but rather an antagonist effect. Within these definitions an ideal antagonist would have high affinity for the receptor, but the complex would have zero intrinsic activity.

The aim of this chapter is to survey the structure–activity relationships of various non-steroidal antioestrogens and compare the findings with the established theories of drug–receptor interaction. However, first it is important to describe something of the basic biology of oestrogens and antioestrogens.

B. Evolution of a Model for Oestrogen Action

The tissue specificity of ovarian extracts was confirmed in castrated laboratory animals by observation of changes in the cells of vaginal smears (Allen and Doisy, 1923). However, the crystallization of active steroids from the urine of pregnant women (Butenandt, 1929; Doisy *et al.*, 1929, 1930) rapidly led to the conclusion that oestradiol-17β (originally referred to as α-oestradiol) was the real hormone and oestrone and oestriol were metabolic products.

The finding by Dodds *et al.* (1939) that *trans*-diethylstilboestrol and the reduced form *meso*-hexoestrol were potent oestrogens proved that non-steroidal compounds could elicit oestrogenic responses. These observations possibly provided the future direction for the identification of an oestrogen receptor system.

The early attempts to demonstrate selective accumulation of synthetic radiolabelled oestrogens in target tissues (uterus and vagina) were frustrated by their low specific activity. In 1959 Glascock and Hoekstra prepared a tritium labelled sample of hexoestrol with high specific activity and demonstrated a selective uptake by the uterus and vagina of immature sheep and goats. However, the report by Jensen and Jacobson (1962) of the selective uptake and retention of [^{3}H]oestradiol in the immature rat uterus and vagina established the concept of a receptor mechanism for the initiation of oestrogen action.

These first reports were followed throughout the 1960s by an enormous number of papers on oestrogen action. Fortunately the subject has been adequately reviewed (Gorski *et al.*, 1968; Jensen and DeSombre, 1973) and only a basic description is necessary for the forthcoming discussion. Unlike the membrane-bound receptor studied at the neuromuscular junction or at adrenergic nerve terminals by the classical pharmacologist, the oestrogen receptor appears to function as a binding and transport protein. Circulating oestrogen binds to the cytoplasmic oestrogen receptor which then becomes activated by an as yet poorly understood transformation reaction, and the resulting complex is translocated to the nucleus where it modulates gene transcription. The initiation of these nuclear events by oestrogen then apparently results in an increase in whole uterine lipid, RNA (via activation of RNA polymerase; Gorski, 1964) and proteins (Aizawa and Mueller, 1961), and finally triggers DNA synthesis and cell division (Kaye *et al.*, 1972). During the protein synthetic phase it has been suggested that cytoplasmic oestrogen receptors are resynthesized (Sarff and Gorski, 1971), although Mester and Baulieu (1975) have suggested that the early phase of oestrogen receptor replenishment may be from the "activation" of pre-formed receptor molecules. Oestrogen action is also known to sensitize the uterus to progesterone, presumably because of the stimulation of progesterone receptor synthesis (Feil *et al.*, 1972; Milgrom *et al.*, 1973).

C. Assay for Antioestrogens

The testing methods for antioestrogens have been developed from the already established methods for assaying oestrogens. These methods are many and varied, so the present discussion will focus upon the uterine responses to oestrogens in laboratory animals.

The increase in uterine wet weight of young castrated rats was used to determine systemic oestrogen activity by Bülbring and Burn (1935). The preparation of castrated animals was found to be an unnecessary step and immature rats or mice are usually used (Lauson *et al.*, 1939; Evans *et al.*, 1941). These methods have been adapted to screen for systemic anti-oestrogenic activity by the simultaneous administration of the test compound and oestrogen.

The first non-steroidal antioestrogen, MER 25, was found to have virtually no intrinsic activity as an oestrogen agonist in rats and mice with the added advantage of apparently no other endocrine activity (Lerner *et al.*,

1958). This conclusion was confirmed by Terenius (1971) although Clitheroe and Leatham (1965) and Wood *et al.* (1968) have reported mild oestrogenic effects in the mouse and rat uterus respectively. These data are in complete contrast to the uterine effects of antioestrogens that are structural derivatives of the oestrogen triphenylethylene. In general these compounds appear to be full oestrogen agonists in the mouse (Terenius, 1970, 1971), pure antagonists in the chick (Sutherland *et al.*, 1977) and partial agonists in the rat (Callantine *et al.*, 1966; Harper and Walpole, 1967) and hamster (Leavitt *et al.*, 1977).

In the present structure–activity relationship study we have used the immature rat as our test system in order to define the partial agonist response of the test compounds. Unless otherwise stated, the method we have used is an adaptation of that described by Rubin *et al.* (1951).

D. Cellular and Subcellular Effects of Antioestrogens

[^{3}H]Oestradiol exchange assay techniques which can determine the concentration of ligand filled oestrogen receptor in uterine nuclei (Anderson *et al.*, 1972) have been used to demonstrate that non-steroidal antioestrogens can provoke the translocation of oestrogen receptors to the nuclear compartment (Clark *et al.*, 1973; Capony and Rochefort, 1975; Katzenellenbogen and Ferguson, 1975). However the suggestion by Clark *et al.* (1974) that non-steroidal antioestrogens inhibit the resynthesis of cytoplasmic oestrogen receptors provoked us to study oestrogen receptor distribution during the 3 day immature rat uterine weight test. Using the antioestrogen tamoxifen, small but effectively antioestrogenic doses were found to produce antioestrogenic effects without depleting the cytoplasmic oestrogen receptor pool (Jordan *et al.*, 1977b). Koseki *et al.* (1977a) came to a similar conclusion using ovariectomized rats. Nevertheless, non-steroidal antioestrogens do produce a dose-related decrease in the cytoplasmic oestrogen receptor pool (Jordan *et al.*, 1978) probably by a continual translocation of receptor complexes to the nuclear compartment. These findings have been confirmed by an examination of the uterine binding of [^{3}H]oestradiol *in vivo* during antioestrogen administration in the uterine weight test (Jordan and Naylor, 1979). Antioestrogenic doses of the compounds do not inhibit the total binding of oestradiol in the uterus or affect the translocation of steroid to the nucleus. The mechanism of action of antioestrogens over the range of the partial agonist dose–response curve must therefore involve an interaction or competition of oestradiol–oestrogen receptor and antioestrogen–oestrogen receptor complexes for sites within the nucleus.

Clearly though, the administration of large doses of an antioestrogen that completely excludes oestrogen from the target tissue by occupying all the receptors will produce the best antagonism of oestrogen action. Under these circumstances any partial oestrogenic activity will reside in the intrinsic activity of the antioestrogen–oestrogen receptor complex.

Kang *et al.* (1975) studied the histological changes and uptake of [^{3}H]thymidine in the rat uterus after the administration of either oestradiol or CI 628 (mixed isomers). In general oestradiol stimulates an increased uptake of [^{3}H]thymidine (as determined by autoradiography) in stromal and luminal epithelial cells, whereas CI 628 does not increase the incorporation of [^{3}H]thymidine in luminal epithelial cells. However, CI 628 stimulates an enormous increase in luminal epithelial cell size. In similar experiments tamoxifen has been shown to produce an increase in luminal epithelial cell size without a large increase in cell division. In contrast, oestradiol benzoate causes a large increase in cell division with hyperplasia of the luminal epithelial layer (Clark *et al.*, 1978; Jordan and Dix, 1979). These events are shown in Figures 1 and 2 where the mitotic activity of tamoxifen and oestradiol benzoate are compared in the luminal epithelial cells of the uterus. The increased size of the luminal epithelial cells (Fig. 1B) is illustrated by representative histological sections (Fig.2). Thus an inhibition of cell division or at least DNA synthesis might be considered as a reliable antioestrogenic endpoint for an assay system.

In the past few years attempts have been made to identify the initial biochemical effects of antioestrogen action. One of the early events in oestrogen action is the synthesis of a specific protein referred to as "the induced protein" (IP) (Notides and Gorski, 1966) and the first reports suggested that antioestrogens were poor inducers of IP (Katzenellenbogen and Ferguson, 1975). Recent evidence suggests, however, that antioestrogens are full inducers of IP (Mairesse and Galand, 1979). Similarly, progesterone receptor synthesis, a well-defined event in oestrogen action, is also stimulated by antioestrogens (Leavitt *et al.*, 1977; Koseki *et al.*, 1977b; Jordan and Prestwich, 1978).

In the light of this brief survey it seems as though the definition of an antioestrogen must be modified to take account of species differences and to refer specifically to the activity of the compound in whole tissue or upon some subcellular response that is equated with oestrogen action.

II. STRUCTURE–ACTIVITY RELATIONSHIPS

A. Geometric Isomers of Substituted Triphenylethylenes

1. Tamoxifen and Clomiphene

The fundamental importance of the geometric shape of a molecule for antioestrogenic activity was first realized after the report by Harper and

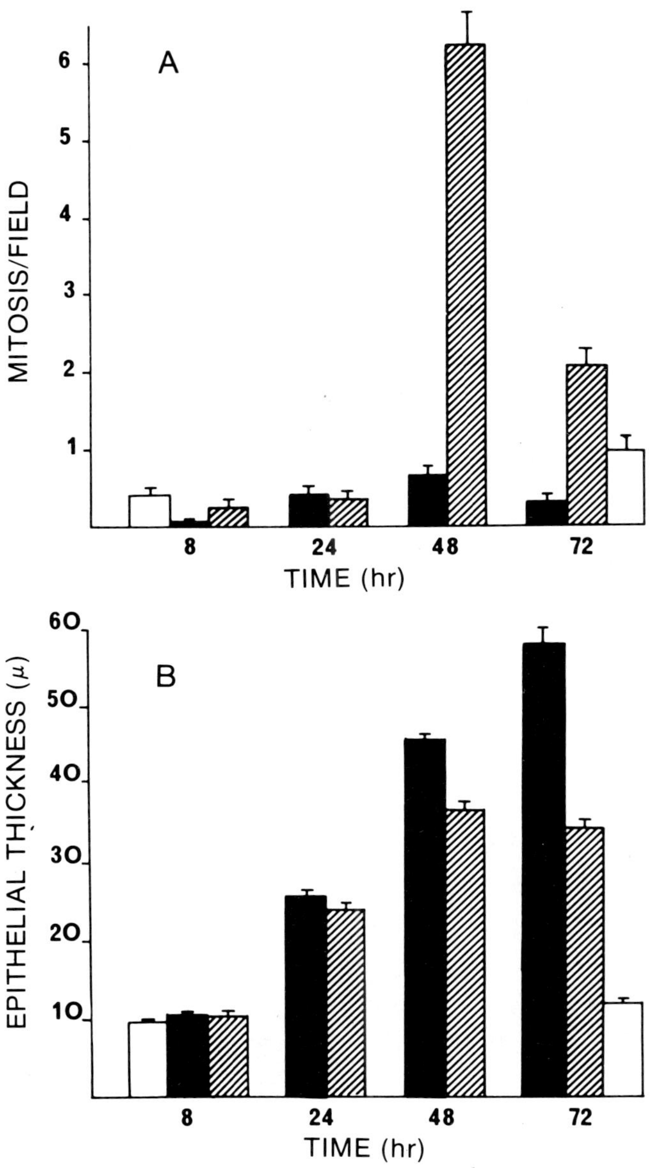

Fig. 1. Effect of tamoxifen (25 μg) (black bars) or oestradiol benzoate (25 μg) (hatched bars) on (A) luminal epithelial mitosis per field of (B) luminal epithelial thickness. Control animals (open bars) received injections of saline (0.9 %). Each animal was injected with colchicine (100 μg in 0.05 ml saline) 7 hours prior to sacrifice. For mitotic determinations N = 50, and for thickness determinations N is not less than 25. From Jordan *et al.* (1980a).

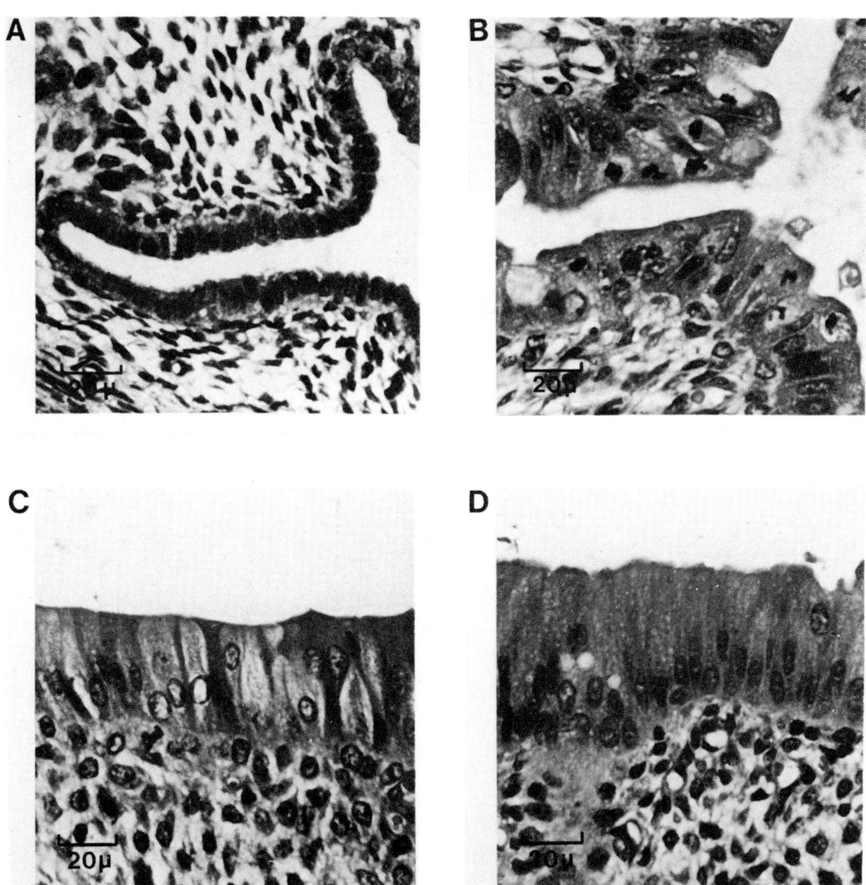

Fig. 2. Effect of tamoxifen (25 µg) or oestradiol benzoate (25 µg) on the histological appearance of immature rat luminal epithelial cells. Control animals received saline (0.9 %). Animals were injected with colchicine (100 µg in 0.05 ml saline) 7 hours before sacrifice. Sections were stained with haemotoxylin and eosin. (A) control; (B) 48 hours after oestradiol benzoate; (C) 48 hours after tamoxifen; (D) 72 hours after tamoxifen. From Jordan *et al.* (1980a).

Walpole (1966) on the contrasting biological properties of the *cis*- and *trans*-isomers of triphenylethylenes. The simultaneous administration of the *trans*-isomer tamoxifen (ICI 46,474) (Fig. 3) with oestradiol prevents the increase in uterine wet weight or vaginal cornification observed with oestradiol alone. In contrast, the *cis*- isomer of tamoxifen, ICI 47,699, is fully oestrogenic (Harper and Walpole, 1967).

Although clomiphene's pharmacology was reported before that of tamoxifen, all the early investigators used a mixture of isomers under the name of either chloramiphene (Holtkamp *et al.*, 1960; Van Maanen *et al.*, 1961) or MRL 41 (Greenblatt *et al.*, 1961). When clomiphene was separated into two geometric isomers (Palopoli *et al.*, 1967) they were unfortunately given the reverse biological designation. This situation led to some confusion

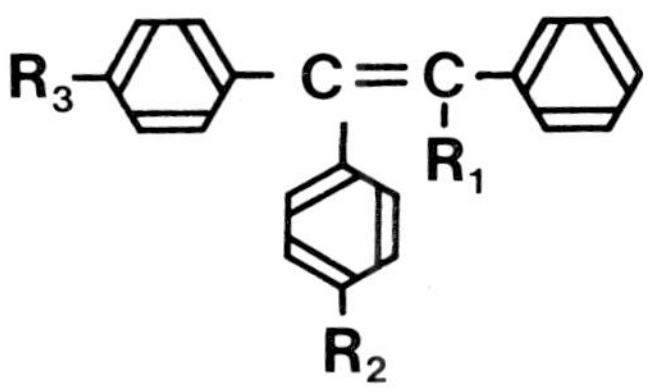

COMPOUND	R_1	R_2	R_3	GEOMETRIC ISOMER
ICI 46474 (TAMOXIFEN)	C_2H_5	H	$(CH_3)_2NCH_2CH_2O$	TRANS.
ICI 47699	C_2H_5	H	$(CH_3)_2NCH_2CH_2O$	CIS.
ICI 79280 (MONOHYDROXYTAMOXIFEN)	C_2H_5	OH	$(CH_3)_2NCH_2CH_2O$	TRANS.
ICI 79280	C_2H_5	OH	$(CH_3)_2NCH_2CH_2O$	CIS.
CI 628	NO_2	OCH_3	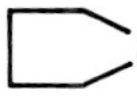 NCH_2CH_2O	TRANS.
CI 628	NO_2	OCH_3	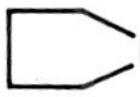 NCH_2CH_2O	CIS.
ENCLOMIPHENE	Cl	H	$(C_2H_5)_2NCH_2CH_2O$	TRANS.
ZUCLOMIPHENE	Cl	H	$(C_2H_5)_2NCH_2CH_2O$	CIS.

Fig. 3. The geometric isomers of substituted triphenylethylenes.

for comparisons of structure–activity relationships. It is now clear that the *trans*-isomer, enclomiphene (originally named isomer B or *cis*-clomiphene), has antioestrogenic properties in the rat, whereas the *cis*-isomer, zuclomiphene (originally named isomer A or *trans*-clomiphene), is oestrogenic. With this revised nomenclature in mind, the reported differences in the biological activities of the isomers in the immature rat uterine weight test (Self *et al.*, 1967), relative activities of the isomers to suppress oestrogen-induced uterine hexokinase activity (DiPietro *et al.*, 1969) and the relative abilities of the isomers to inhibit dimethylbenzanthracene-induced rat mammary tumour growth (Schultz *et al.*, 1971) are consistent with the antioestrogenicity of *trans*-isomers in this group of compounds.

The oestrogenic (Fig. 4). and antioestrogenic (Fig. 5) actions of tamoxifen, enclomiphene, ICI 47,699 and zuclomiphene demonstrate that the minor differences in structure (Fig. 3) do not markedly alter the biological effects or potency. However, one point of interest is the premature plateauing of the zuclomiphene log dose–response curve. This prompted us to extend the dose–response curve for ICI 47,699. Increasing the dose up to 10 mg daily (Table I) decreases the uterine response and antagonizes the full uterotrophic effect of a standard dose of oestradiol benzoate that can produce a maximal uterine response. It therefore appears that the oestrogenic *cis*-isomers can produce "antioestrogenic" actions probably by an ill-defined autoinhibitory effect.

Considering the biological activity of *cis*- and *trans*-isomers at the subcellular level, again the effects are consistent with full and partial agonist actions. ICI 47,699 causes a much higher rise in uterine DNA content than tamoxifen (Fig. 6A) and these whole-tissue determinations are similar to the changes in luminal epithelial cell division (unpublished observation). However, for equal doses, tamoxifen translocates much more of the cytoplasmic oestrogen receptor pool into the nucleus than ICI 47,699 (Fig. 6B). This observation may be related to the higher affinity of tamoxifen for the oestrogen receptor (Skidmore *et al.*, 1972). Nevertheless, the lower nuclear concentrations of the ICI 47,699-oestrogen receptor complex, as previously pointed out, are much more effective at initiating cell division. Therefore, the intrinsic activity of the complex, rather than number of receptors present in the nuclear compartment, is of prime importance for the future development of the cellular response.

2. *Monohydroxytamoxifen and CI 628*

One of tamoxifen's metabolites, monohydroxytamoxifen (Metabolite B; Fromson *et al.*, 1973) (Fig. 3) is a partial oestrogen agonist with potent antioestrogenic activity consistent with its high affinity for the oestrogen receptor (Jordan *et al.*, 1977a). Only the *trans*-isomer (by comparison with tamoxifen's structure) has been used in investigations, and it might be thought from the previous discussion that the *cis*-isomer would be a full oestrogen agonist. However the *cis*-isomer of monohydroxytamoxifen is less potent than the *trans*-isomer but with partial agonist and antagonist properties (Fig. 7). This finding prompted a re-examination of the biological properties of the antioestrogen CI 628 (originally referred to as CN 55,945-27A).

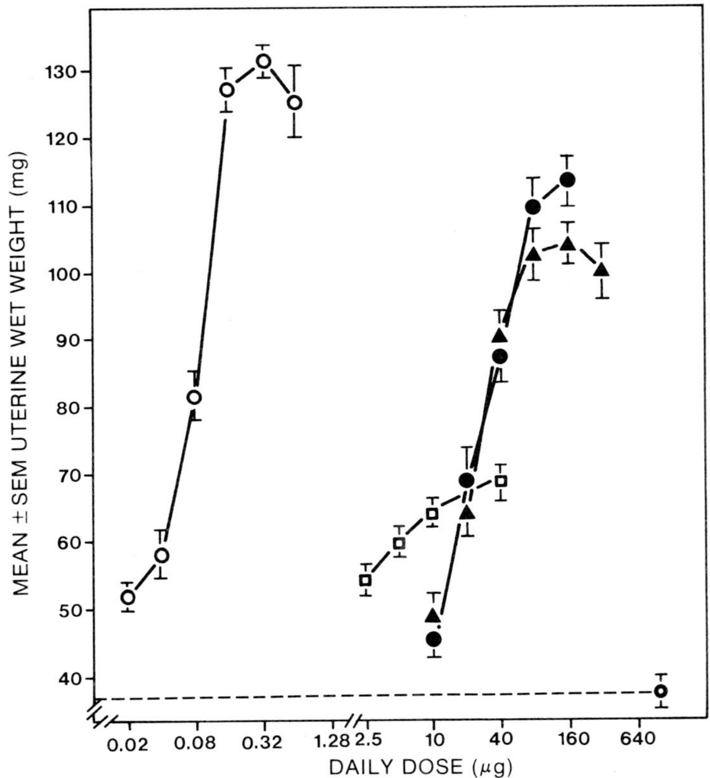

Fig. 4. The uterotrophic effect of oestradiol benzoate (○), zuclomiphene (▲), ICI 47,699 (●) and tamoxifen (□) in the 3 day immature rat uterine weight test. Compounds were dissolved in peanut oil and administered (0.1 ml) on consecutive days. Controls received vehicle alone (---●). Animals were killed on day 4. Eight rats per group. From Jordan *et al.* (1981).

Fig. 5. The oestrogenic (open symbols) and antioestrogenic (closed symbols) effect of tamoxifen (□,■) and enclomiphene (△,▲) in the 3 day immature rat uterine weight test. In antioestrogenic tests, compounds were administered with 0.64 μg oestradiol benzoate daily and compared with oestradiol benzoate alone (○). The procedure was the same as Fig. 4. Controls received vehicle alone (●). Ten rats per group. From Jordan *et al.* (1981).

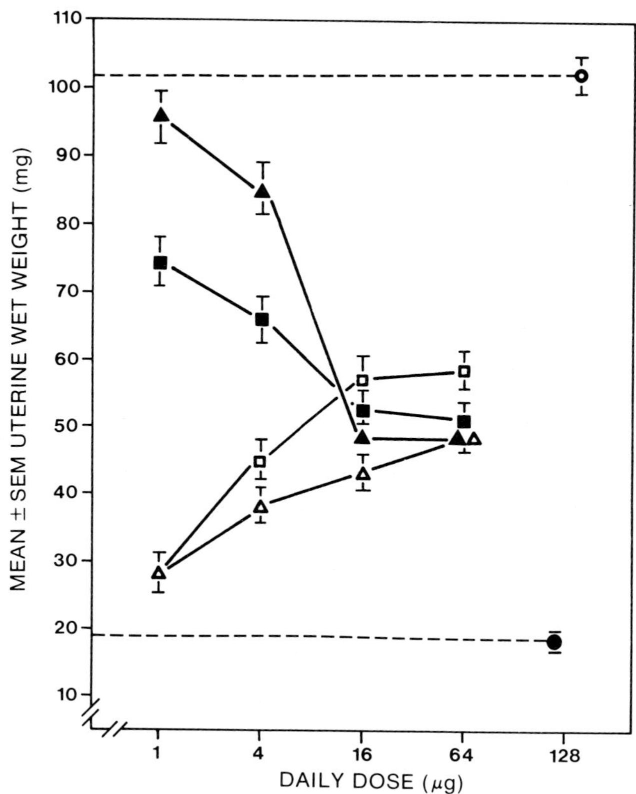

TABLE I
Effect of Increasing Doses of ICI 47,699 Administered with and without Oestradiol Benzoate on Immature Rat Uterine Wet Weight

Daily dose ICI 47,699[a] (mg)	Daily dose of oestradiol benzoate (μg)[b] 0	0.16
0	33.6 ± 2.1	112.0 ± 5.3
0.1	118.7 ± 5.1	128.4 ± 6.0
1.0	100.0 ± 3.6	92.9 ± 3.0[c]
10.0	87.9 ± 5.9[c]	82.0 ± 5.2[c]

[a] Injections were made on 3 consecutive days and animals were sacrificed on day 4.
[b] Results are means ± S.E.M. Eight rats per group.
Comparison of treatment group means with oestradiol benzoate alone.
[c] $p < 0.01$; all other values $p > 0.05$.

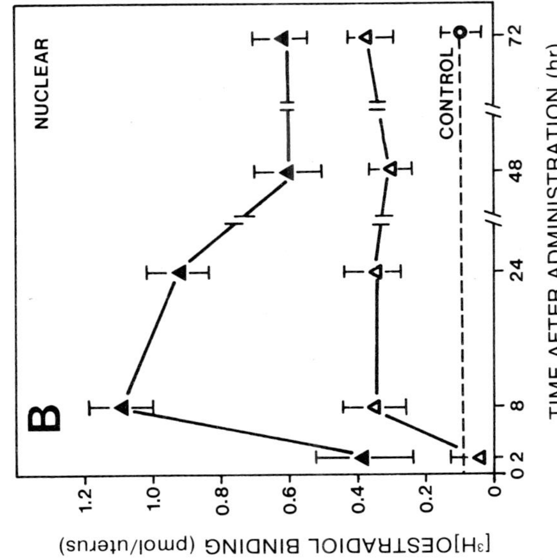

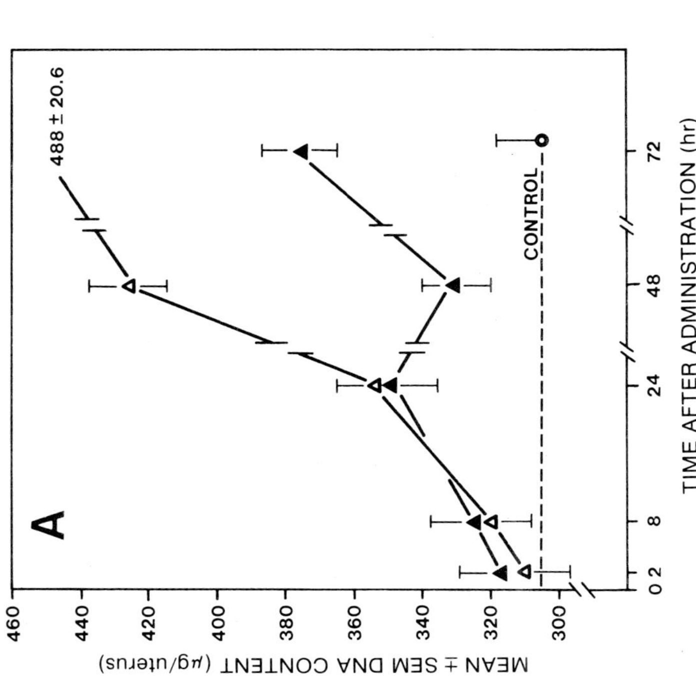

Fig. 6. The effect of a single administration (25 μg) of tamoxifen (▲) or ICI 47,699 (△) on (A) whole uterine DNA and (B) the levels of exchangeable nuclear oestrogen receptors determined by the method of Katzenellenbogen (1975). Eight rats per group. From Jordan *et al.* (1981).

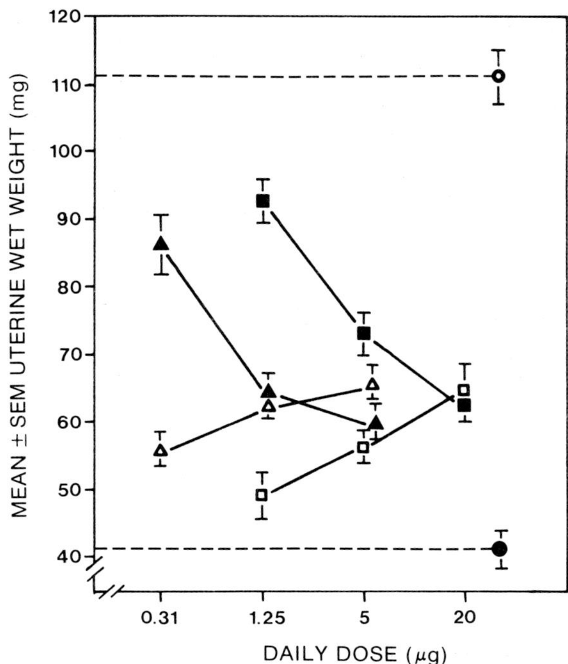

Fig. 7. The oestrogenic (open symbols) and antioestrogenic (closed symbols) effect of *trans*-monohydroxytamoxifen (△▲) and *cis*-monohydroxytamoxifen (□■) in the 3 day immature rat uterine weight test. In antioestrogen tests compounds were administered with 0.16 μg oestradiol benzoate daily and compared with oestradiol benzoate alone (○). The procedure was the same as Fig. 4. Controls received vehicle alone (●). Eight rats per group. From Jordan *et al.* (1981).

CI 628 (mixed isomers) was reported to be a potent antioestrogen in the rat by Callantine *et al.* (1966) and to have antitumour properties in rats with DMBA-induced mammary carcinomata (DeSombre and Arbogast, 1974). From studies with the radiolabelled compound it has been concluded that CI 628 may exert its biological effects via activation to a polar metabolite (Katzenellenbogen *et al.*, 1978). We now report that the *cis*- and *trans*-isomers are both partial oestrogen agonists with antioestrogenic properties (Fig. 8). Certainly this finding is consistent with the results with monohydroxytamoxifen, if CI 628 is demethylated to phenolic compounds prior to binding in the target tissue (Katzenellenbogen *et al.*, 1978). The apparent inconsistency of the biological properties of the *cis*-isomers (ICI 47,699, zuclomiphene, *cis*-monohydroxytamoxifen and *cis*-CI 628) might be explained in several ways. It is possible that the receptor binding of the phenolic

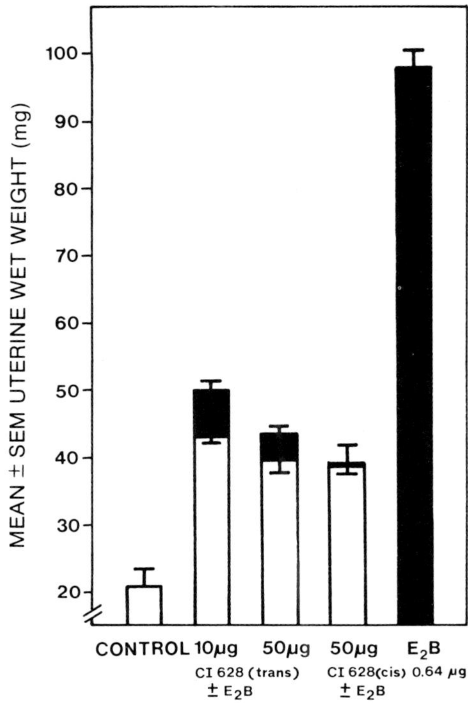

Fig. 8. The oestrogenic (open bars) and antioestrogenic effect (open and black bars) of the *cis*- and *trans*-isomers of CI 628 in the 3 day immature rat uterine weight test. Results are compared with vehicle treated control and oestradiol benzoate alone. Ten rats per group. From Jordan *et al.* (1981).

group may override any structural restrictions to binding in the *cis* structure. In this case, as we have found, the compounds would have lower affinity than their *trans*-isomers but similar efficacy. Alternatively the *cis*-isomers might be all oestrogens but the hydroxylated derivatives may be so unstable that they rapidly convert *in vivo* to a *cis/trans* mixture. The overall pharmacology of the *cis*-isomer would then appear to be as an antagonist. Clearly further study is needed to resolve these problems.

B. Nafoxidine Derivatives

From the previous arguments it appears that the nuclear oestradiol–oestrogen receptor and antioestrogen–oestrogen receptor complexes are fundamentally different. Some support for this view has come from

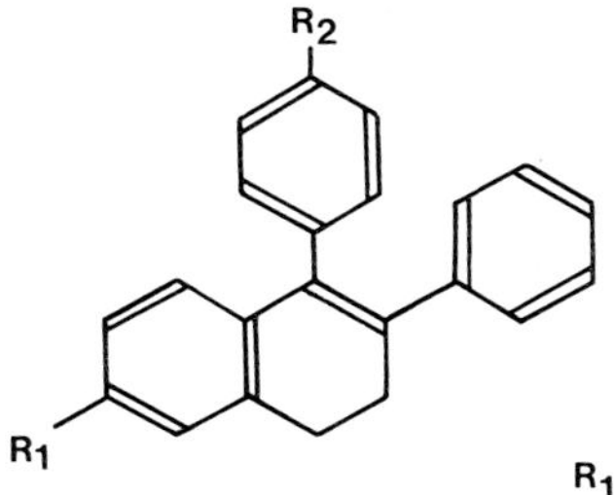

	R_1	R_2
U-11,100A (NAFOXIDINE)	OCH_3	$OCH_2\ CH_2N$[pyrrolidine ring] · HCl
U-22,410A	H	$OCH_2\ CH_2N$[pyrrolidine ring] · HCl
U-10,520	OCH_3	$OCH_2CH_2N(C_2H_5)_2$
U-11,854	OCH_3	H

Fig. 9. Structural derivatives of nafoxidine.

studies of antioestrogen action in cultured human breast cancer cells (MCF 7).

Nafoxidine (Fig. 9) causes a long nuclear retention time for the ligand receptor complex compared with oestradiol (Horwitz and McGuire, 1978). However, the nafoxidine–oestrogen receptor complex does not stimulate incorporation of [^{3}H]thymidine as a prerequisite for DNA synthesis (Lippman *et al.*, 1976) or stimulate progesterone receptor synthesis (Horwitz *et al.*, 1978). Similarly, tamoxifen does not cause incorporation of [^{3}H]thymidine (Lippman *et al.*, 1976), but nuclear retention time of the ligand receptor complex is shorter than nafoxidine's and progesterone receptor synthesis does occur (Horwitz *et al.*, 1978). The inability of an antioestrogen to stimulate progesterone receptor synthesis must be fundamental to pure antioestrogen action. The differences between nafoxidine and tamoxifen with regard to progesterone receptor synthesis may result from a partial conversion of tamoxifen to its oestrogenic *cis*-isomer. The rigid structure of nafoxidine would not permit a similar change.

Apart from the study by Leavitt *et al.* (1977) in the hamster, there is no data *in vivo* about oestrogen receptor effects and progesterone receptor synthesis by nafoxidine with which to compare the data from experiments *in vitro*. We have addressed this question by studying the biological effects of a small series of nafoxidine derivatives (Fig. 9).

As previously reported (Lednicer *et al.*, 1967) U 11,854, without an aminoethoxy side chain, demonstrated potent oestrogenic activity (Fig. 10) although increasing doses were autoinhibitory. The compounds U 10,520 and U 22,410A were both partial agonists with antioestrogenic properties (Fig. 11). U 10,520 with a methoxy group was slightly more active.

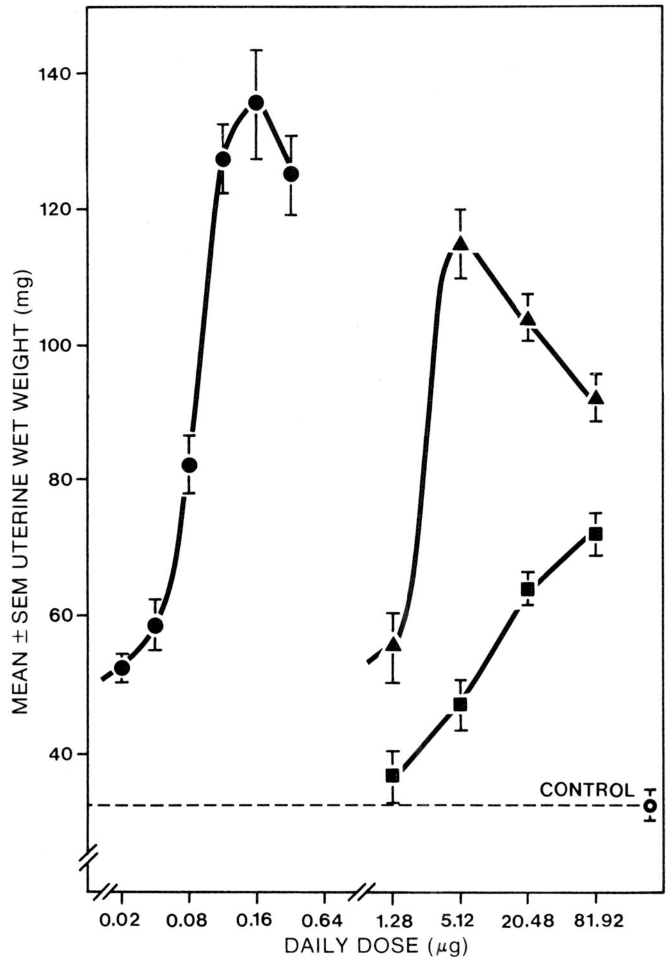

Fig. 10. Mean uterine wet weights for groups of immature rats treated with 3 daily doses of oestradiol benzoate (●), U 11,854 (▲) or U 10,520 (■). Compounds were administered subcutaneously in 0.1 ml peanut oil. The control group (○) received peanut oil alone. Animals were sacrificed on day 4 and the uteri weighed wet. Eight rats per group.

Biochemical studies demonstrated that after U 10,520 administration the nuclear concentration of oestrogen receptors was increased during the first 14 hours but then slowly decreased during the next 56 hours. As nuclear levels decreased, cytoplasmic [^{3}H]R 5020 binding increased. This increase was retarded by early cycloheximide administration (Fig. 12).

In a similar experiment with U 22,410A, the ligand specificity of the rises in uterine [^{3}H]R 5020 binding was determined *in vivo*. Only the progestational agents, progesterone and norethindrone, effectively reduced [^{3}H]R 5020 binding (Fig. 13).

The study demonstrates that progesterone receptor synthesis is a biochemical consequence of the partial oestrogenic activity of these compounds in the immature rat. Thus the suggestion that tamoxifen-stimulated progesterone receptor synthesis *in vitro* is the result of conversion to its oestrogenic *cis*-isomer would seem to be unlikely.

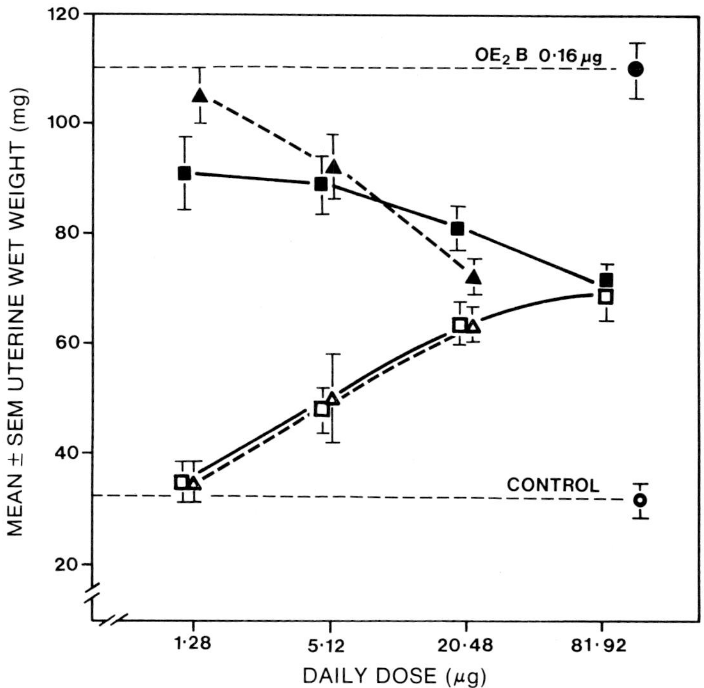

Fig. 11. Mean uterine wet weights for groups of immature female rats treated with 3 daily doses of oestradiol benozoate (0.16 μg), increasing doses of U 10,520 (△) or U 22,410A (□) alone, or increasing doses of U 10,520 (▲) or U 22,410A (■) and 0.16 μg oestradiol benzoate. The procedure was the same as described in Figure 10.

As an alternative explanation for progesterone receptor synthesis, it is possible that the compounds are being metabolized to biochemically more oestrogenic components. One of tamoxifen's metabolites, monohydroxytamoxifen, stimulates progesterone receptor synthesis *in vivo* (Jordan and Dix, 1979), however Horwitz *et al.* (1978) could not detect metabolism of [^{3}H]tamoxifen by MCF 7 cells *in vitro*. In contrast, a single administration of [^{3}H]tamoxifen to immature rats leads to the accumulation of [^{3}H]monohydroxytamoxifen in uterine nuclei (Borgna and Rochefort, 1979). Also, Katzenellenbogen *et al.* (1979) have reported the appearance of metabolites in uterine nuclei after the administration of [^{3}H]U 23,469 (a

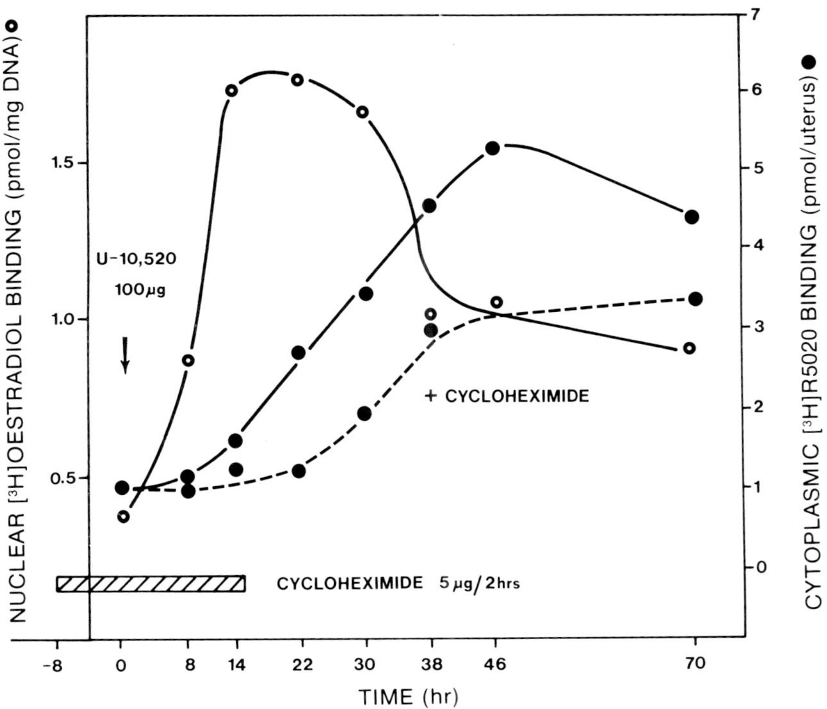

Fig. 12. The effect of a single administration of U 10,520 (100 μg) on the uterine levels of exchangeable nuclear oestrogen receptors measured by the method of Katzenellenbogen (1975) and cytoplasmic [^{3}H]R 5020 binding (progesterone receptors) measured by the method of Vu Hai and Milgrom (1978). In a parallel experiment (5 μg cycloheximide in 0.1 ml 0.9% saline) was administered every 2 hours for 8 hours before and 16 hours after the U 10,520. Points represent the mean of four separate determinations each in duplicate on paired uteri. Data from Jordan *et al.* (1980b).

nafoxidine derivative) to rats. These conflicting results may either reflect the different metabolic capacities of immature rats and MCF 7 cells or truly be an expression of the differences in the hormone receptor regulatory systems.

C. Inhibition of Metabolic Activation

There is much circumstantial evidence to suggest that antioestrogens are metabolically activated prior to binding in target tissues. However, all the experiments to date have only studied the tissue localization of radiolabelled ligands after a single injection. This is clearly not the situation during the treatment of mammary cancer (either in animals or humans) or even in the 3 day immature rat uterine weight test.

The importance of metabolic activation of a drug like tamoxifen really depends upon two major factors, the capacity of the liver to metabolize significant quantities of the drug to active metabolites and the relative importance of metabolic pathways in the species under study. A consideration of the blood levels of tamoxifen will be important because at very high concentrations the parent compound will be the dominant oestrogen receptor

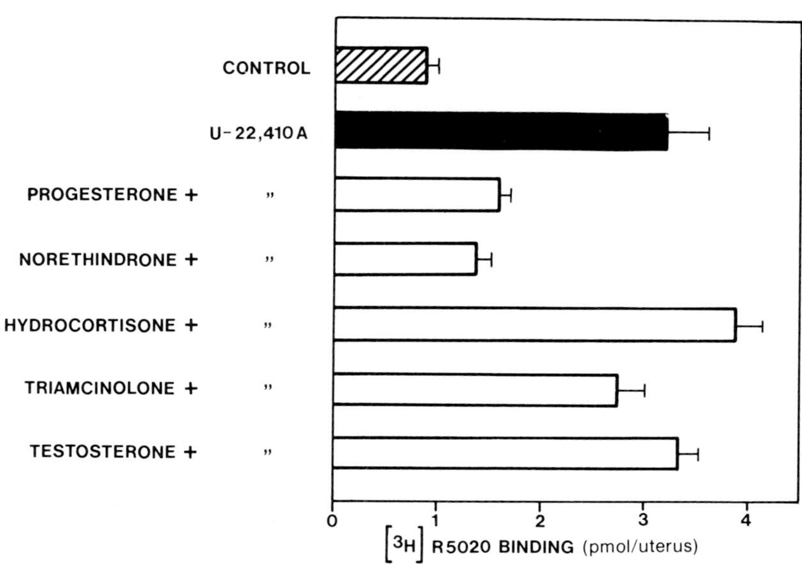

Fig. 13. Effect of various steroids on U 22,410A (100 μg) stimulated rises in immature rat uterine [^{3}H]R 5020 binding 48 hours later determined by the method of Vu Hai and Milgrom (1978). Steroids (1 mg) were administered 3 hours before animals were killed. Results represent mean ± S.E.M. of four determinations, in duplicate on paired uteri.

binding ligand, whereas at low concentrations metabolism may provide a significantly greater proportion of active metabolites for receptor binding. However, the prime factor for consideration will be the relative importance of the major metabolic pathways. In humans it has been suggested that the primary metabolic route for tamoxifen is via N-demethylation to produce desmethyltamoxifen (Adam *et al.*, 1979), although recently some monohydroxytamoxifen has been detected in breast cancer patients on tamoxifen therapy (R. I. Nicholson, personal communication). In the rat the primary route for tamoxifen metabolism is via mono- and dihydroxylation (Fromson *et al.*, 1973); therefore significant amounts of monohydroxytamoxifen would be expected to be produced.

To investigate the contribution of metabolic activation for tamoxifen's actions *in vivo*, we have evaluated the oestrogenic and antioestrogenic properties of a series of structural derivatives of tamoxifen (Fig. 14).

Tamoxifen is approximately equi-active with its p-methyl, fluoro and chloro derivatives in inhibiting [^{3}H]oestradiol binding to rat uterine oestrogen receptor *in vitro*. Similarly, tamoxifen is equi-active with its p-methyl and fluoro derivatives in inhibiting vaginal cornification of ovariectomized rats when administered intravaginally with oestradiol (Allen *et al.*, 1980). All the derivatives of tamoxifen are partial oestrogen agonists when compared with oestradiol benzoate in the immature rat uterine weight test (Fig. 15A), and all the compounds inhibit the uterotrophic activity of oestradiol (Fig. 15B). However, unlike the situation *in vitro*, where the tamoxifen derivatives are equipotent with tamoxifen, *in vivo* the derivatives are at least 1/10 the potency of tamoxifen. This result indicates that the antioestrogenic effect of tamoxifen

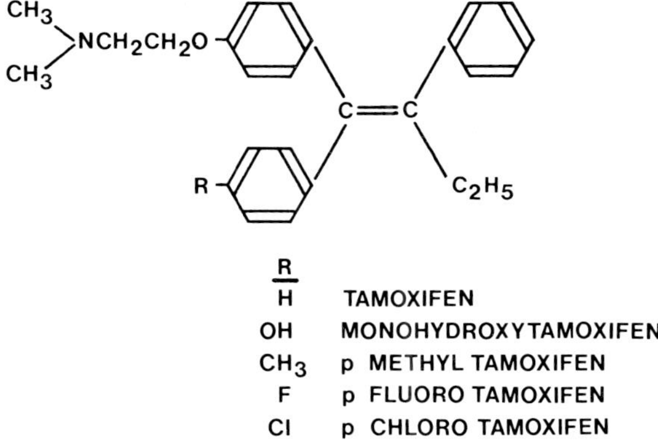

Fig. 14. Structural derivatives of tamoxifen.

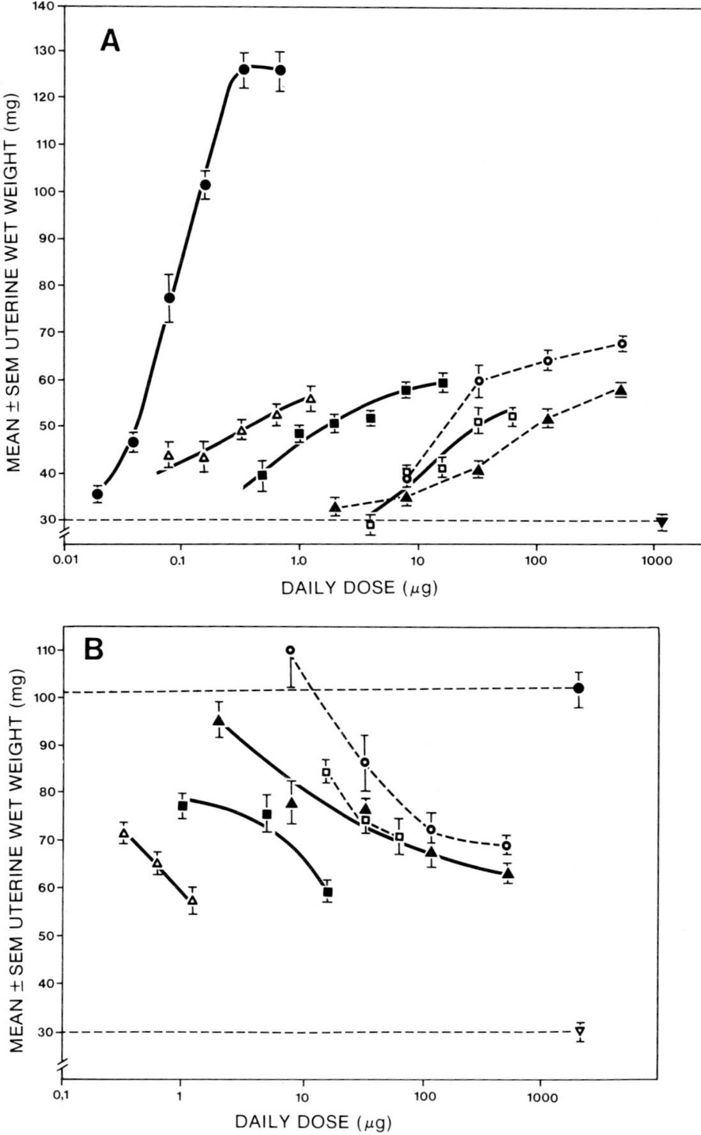

Fig. 15. (A) Oestrogenic and (B) antioestrogenic effect of various derivatives of tamoxifen (monohydroxytamoxifen, △; tamoxifen, ■; fluoro-, ▲, chloro-, □, and methyltamoxifen, ○) in the immature rat uterine weight test. Oestradiol benzoate (●) was used for comparative purposes and in the tests for antioestrogenic activity compounds were administered simultaneously with oestradiol benzoate (0.16 μg daily) and the results compared with oestradiol benzoate alone (---●). Controls (▼) were injected with peanut oil alone. Results represent means ± S.E.M. with at least 7 rats per group. Data from Allen *et al.* (1980).

over the range of the partial agonist dose–response curve is the net result of the parent compound and its metabolites.

Nevertheless, the finding that compounds unable to undergo conversion to monohydroxytamoxifen were still antioestrogenic supports the view of Horwitz *et al.* (1978) that tamoxifen does not have to undergo metabolic transformation before exerting its antitumour effects *in vitro*. In conclusion it appears from this structure–activity relationship study that the metabolic activation of antioestrogens is an advantage, but not a requirement, for activity.

D. Summary: The Antioestrogenic Ligand

It is clear that the structural requirements for antioestrogenic activity are quite precise, and overall the system is consistent with the pharmacological concept of drug–receptor interactions. In the design of antioestrogens several features are dominant:

1. The triphenylethylene structure has proved to be a good molecular "backbone" for the first generation of antioestrogens. However, the increased potency of these compounds compared with the less rigid triphenylethane (MRL 37) and triphenylethanol (MER 25) derivatives is at the expense of low oestrogenic activity, since all the triphenylethylene derivatives are partial agonists.
2. In the triphenylethylene group the *trans* geometric isomers are consistently antioestrogenic.
3. Hydroxylation of a compound like tamoxifen to produce monohydroxytamoxifen increases receptor affinity and antioestrogenic activity, but partial agonist activity remains.
4. The alkylaminoethoxy side chain is essential for activity. Restriction in the number of positions it can adopt in space reduces activity (Clark and Jordan, 1976) and removal increases oestrogenic activity (Fig. 10).

For the future it would clearly be an advantage to develop compounds with high receptor affinity and zero intrinsic activity. Dihydroxytamoxifen (Jordan *et al.*, 1977a) has a high affinity for the oestrogen receptor but poor activity *in vivo*, probably because the catechol structure is chemically unstable and is rapidly conjugated and excreted. Interestingly, however, this compound has very low intrinsic activity. Polyhydroxylated antioestrogens may therefore provide a useful second generation of oestrogen antagonists. At present, examples of these compounds are notably lacking from the literature. If this route of synthesis is to be considered, then the triphenylethylene structure should probably be abandoned because of the instability of hydroxylated derivatives (monohydroxytamoxifen). A rigid structure, based for example upon nafoxidine, could be re-investigated.

As a final consideration, high affinity for the oestrogen receptor and high potency in short-term assay systems should not be developed at the expense of biological half-life. Continuing receptor saturation with antagonists is important. Perhaps the best solution for this pharmacokinetic problem is to design the compounds so that the biologically active ligand is efficiently and exclusively produced by metabolic activation.

III. APPLICATION OF DRUG RECEPTOR THEORIES

The aim of the present survey has been to compare the progress made during the past 20 years in the understanding of antioestrogen action with the established basic concepts in pharmacology. As stated in the introduction, evidence in favour of drug receptors has come from (a) the study of tissue-site specificity, (b) comparisons of structure–activity relationships, and (c) the mathematical comparison of drugs in assay situations that has led to theories of drug action. As we have discussed in the foregoing sections, the non-steroidal antioestrogens satisfy the first two of these pharmacological concepts. It is now perhaps relevant to consider whether the pharmacology of the antioestrogens is consistent with some of the established theories of drug–receptor interaction.

The antioestrogens appear to comply with the concepts implicit in the occupation theory. The intrinsic activity or efficacy of the antioestrogen–oestrogen receptor complex is lower than the oestradiol–oestrogen receptor complex, "spare receptors" are available during maximal agonist activity (Clark and Peck, 1976) and partial agonists produce good dose related inhibition of agonist activity eventually occupying all of the receptor pool (Jordan *et al.* 1977a, 1978; Jordan and Naylor, 1979). In contrast, another theory, the rate theory proposed by Paton (1961) to explain agonist and antagonist action, might not be applicable. It is suggested that agonists have a rapid rate of association and dissociation whilst antagonists have a rapid association rate but a slow dissociation rate. This does not seem to be true for oestrogens and antioestrogens since the latter dissociate from the receptor more rapidly than the former (Capony and Rochefort, 1978). However Thron and Waud have suggested that the information used to derive the rate theory could be artificial and may result from kinetic factors that are inherent in the pharmacological test systems (Waud, 1967; Thron and Waud, 1968). In this case the inability of an antagonist to dissociate from a tissue preparation *in vitro* may not mean slow dissociation from the receptor. This proposal may be fundamental to our understanding of these models since it is interesting to note that many of the antioestrogens have very long biological half-lives, probably because of complete saturation of the system with high protein binding (Fromson *et al.*, 1973; Katzenellenbogen *et al.*, 1978; Jordan and

Allen, 1980). High local tissue concentrations could then set up an effective equilibrium between receptor and non-receptor proteins, which may imply receptor binding is extended.

Unfortunately the rate theory does not really consider descriptive events at the molecular level. It is perhaps relevant, therefore, to consider the application of Koshland's (1958) induced fit theory for enzyme-substrate interaction to drug receptor theory. Briefly, if the structural change in the receptor protein leads to a configuration in which an agonist drug binds less firmly then the rate theory would be satisfied. No structural changes and the formation of a stable complex would produce blocking action. However, the evidence of the interaction of oestrogen antagonists with oestrogen receptor is perhaps not in agreement with this concept.

The affinity of antioestrogens (with the exception of monohydroxytamoxifen) for the oestrogen receptor is much lower than that of oestradiol (Korenman, 1970; Skidmore *et al.*, 1972), and the antioestrogen binding is readily reversed by oestradiol (J. A. Katzenellenbogen *et al.*, 1973). These properties would not be at variance with the rate theory, but, as previously mentioned, the rate of dissociation of oestrogen antagonists is more rapid than oestradiol. Furthermore, Rochefort and Capony (1977) have suggested that oestradiol stabilizes the receptor into a form that is insensitive to antioestrogen binding *in vitro*. However, the situation *in vitro* may not correspond to events *in vivo,* simply because there are new antioestrogenic molecules produced by metabolism. Tamoxifen is a case in point with conversion to monohydroxytamoxifen.

Thus it is possible that different subcellular effects are produced by different forms of the complex. This would seem reasonable since the oestrogen antagonists are really partial agonists. At the molecular level, these events are somewhat similar to Belleau's (1964) macromolecular perturbation theory, which was developed from a consideration of acetylcholine and a series of antagonists at the muscarinic receptor (Belleau and Moran, 1963). With the receptor in a resting state it can bind with an agonist that produces a specific conformational perturbation and a stimulant action. Binding with an antagonist would produce a non-specific conformational perturbation and a partial agonist would produce an equilibrium mixture of the two states. From our survey of structure–activity relationships amongst antioestrogens it is apparent that the aminoethoxy side chain is essential for activity and could be producing the non-specific conformational perturbation in the oestrogen receptor. These suggestions must remain speculative until further progress is made in understanding the biophysics of the receptor protein. With the future development of a high affinity pure antagonist it might be possible to compare the biophysical properties of the antagonist–receptor and the agonist–receptor complexes, and the results could then be used with confidence to develop a mechanistic theory for antioestrogen action.

REFERENCES

Adam, H. K., Douglas, E. J., and Kemp, J. V. (1979). *Biochem. Pharmacol.* **27**, 145–147.
Aizawa, Y., and Mueller, G. C. (1961). *J. Biol. Chem.* **236**, 381–386.
Allen, E., and Doisy, E. A. (1923). *J. Am. Med. Assoc.* **81**,819-821.
Allen, K. E., Clark, E. R., and Jordan, V. C. (1980). *Br. J. Pharmacol.* **71**, 83–91.
Anderson, J., Clark, J. H., and Peck, E. J. (1972). *Biochem. J.* **126**, 561–567.
Ariens, E. J., and Simonis, A. M. (1964). *J. Pharm. Pharmacol.* **16**, 136–157.
Belleau, B. (1964). *J. Med. Chem.* **7**, 776–784.
Belleau, B., and Moran, J. (1963). *Ann. N. Y. Acad. Sci.* **107**, 822–839.
Borgna, J. L., and Rochefort, H. (1979). *C. R. Acad. Sci.* **287**, 1141–1144.
Bülbring, E., and Burn, J. H. (1935). *J. Physiol.* **85**, 320–333.
Butenandt, A. (1929). *Naturwissenschaften* **17**, 879.
Callantine, M. R., Humphrey, R. R., Lee, S. L., Windsor, B. L., Schottin, N. H., and O'Brien, O. P. (1966). *Endocrinology* **79**, 153–169.
Capony, F., and Rochefort, H. (1975). *Mol. Cell. Endocr.* **3**, 233–251.
Capony, F., and Rochefort, H. (1978). *Mol. Cell. Endocr.* **11**, 181–198.
Clark, A. J. (1926). *J. Physiol.* **61**, 530–546.
Clark, E. R., and Jordan, V. C. (1976). *Br. J. Pharmacol.* **57**, 487–493.
Clark, E. R., Dix, C. J., Jordan, V. C., Prestwich, G., and Sexton, S. (1978). *Br. J. Pharmacol.* **62**, 442P–443P.
Clark, J. H., and Peck, E. J. (1976). *Nature* **206**, 635–637.
Clark, J. H., Anderson, J. N., and Peck, E. J. (1973). *Steroids* **22**, 707–718.
Clark, J. H., Peck, E. J., and Anderson, J. N. (1974). *Nature* **251**, 446–448.
Clitheroe, J. H., and Leatham, J. H. (1965). *Endocrinology* **76**, 127–130.
DeSombre, E. R., and Arbogast, L. Y. (1974). *Cancer Res.* **34**, 1971–1976.
DiPietro, S. L., Sander, F. J., and Goss, D. A. (1969). *Endocrinology* **84**, 1404–1408.
Dodds, E. C., Goldberg, L., Lawson, W., and Robinson, R. (1939). *Proc. R. Soc. B* **129**, 140–166.
Doisy, E. A., Veler, C. D., and Thayer, S. A. (1929). *Am. J. Physiol.* **90**, 329–330.
Doisy, E. A., Veler, C. D., and Thayer, S. A. (1930). *J. Biol. Chem.* **86**, 499–509.
Evans, J. S., Varney, R. F., and Roch, F. C. (1941). *Endocrinology* **28**, 747–752.
Feil, P. D., Glasser, S. R., Toft, D. O., and O'Malley, B. W. (1972). *Endocrinology* **91**, 738–746.
Fromson, J. M., Pearson, S., and Bramah, S. (1973). *Xenobiotica* **3**, 693–709.
Gaddum, J. H. (1926). *J. Physiol.* **61**, 141–150.
Glascock, R. F., and Hoekstra, W. G. (1959). *Biochem. J.* **72**, 673–682.
Gorski, J. (1964). *J. Biol. Chem.* **239**, 889–892.
Gorski, J., Toft, D. O., Shyamala, G., Smith, D., and Notides, A. (1968). *Recent Progr. Horm. Res.* **24**, 45–80.
Greenblatt, R. B., Barfield, W. E., Jungck, E. C., and Ray, A. W. (1961). *J. Am. Med. Assoc.* **178**, 101–104.
Harper, M. J. K., and Walpole, A. L. (1966). *Nature* **212**, 87.
Harper, M. J. K., and Walpole, A. L. (1967). *J. Reprod. Fert.* **13**, 101–119.
Holtkamp, D. E., Greslin, J. G., Root, C. A., and Lerner, L. J. (1960). *Proc. Soc. Exp. Biol. Med.* **105**, 197–201.
Horwitz, K. B., and McGuire, W. L. (1978). *J. Biol. Chem.* **253**, 8185–8191.
Horwitz, K. B., Koseki, Y., and McGuire, W. L. (1978). *Endocrinology* **103**, 1742–1751.
Jensen, E. V., and DeSombre, E. R. (1973). *Science* **182**, 126–134.
Jensen, E. V., and Jacobson, H. I. (1962). *Recent Progr. Horm. Res.* **18**, 318–414.
Jordan, V. C., and Allen, K. E. (1980). *Eur. J. Cancer* **16**, 239–252.
Jordan, V. C., and Dix, C. J. (1979). *J. Steroid Biochem.* **11**, 285–291.
Jordan, V. C., and Naylor, K. E. (1979). *Br. J. Pharmacol.* **65**, 167–173.

Jordan, V. C., and Prestwich, G. (1978). *J. Endocr.* **76**, 363–364.
Jordan, V. C., Collins, M. M., Rowsby, L., and Prestwich, G. (1977a). *J. Endocr.* **75**, 305–316.
Jordan, V. C., Dix, C. J., Rowsby, L., and Prestwich, B. (1977). *Mol. Cell. Endocr.* **7**, 177–192.
Jordan, V. C., Rowsby, L., Dix, C. J., and Prestwich, G. (1978). *J. Endocr.* **78**, 71–81.
Jordan, V. C., Prestwich, G., Dix, C. J., and Clark, E. R. (1980a). *In* "Pharmacological Modulation of Steroid Action" (G. Genazzani, F. DiCarlo, and W. I. P. Mainwaring, eds), pp. 81–97. Raven Press, New York.
Jordan, V. C., Haldermann, B., and Allen, K. E. (1981). *Endocrinology* **108**, 1353–1361.
Kang, Y. H., Anderson, W. A., and DeSombre, E. R. (1975). *J. Cell. Biol.* **64**, 682–691.
Katzenellenbogen, B. S. (1975). *Endocrinology* **96**, 289–297.
Katzenellenbogen, B. S., and Ferguson, E. R. (1975). *Endocrinology* **97**, 1–12.
Katzenellenbogen, B. S., Katzenellenbogen, J. A., Ferguson, E. R., and Krauthammer, N. (1978). *J. Biol. Chem.* **253**, 697–707.
Katzenellenbogen, B. S., Bhakoo, H. S., Ferguson, E. R., Lan, N. C., Tatee, T., Tsai, T. L. S., and Katzenellenbogen, J. A. (1979). *Recent Progr. Horm. Res.* **35**, 259–300.
Katzenellenbogen, J. A., Johnson, H. J., and Carlson, K. E. (1973). *Biochemistry* **12**, 4092–4099.
Kaye, A. M., Sheratzky, D., and Lindner, H. R. (1972). *Biochem. Biophys. Acta* **261**, 475–486.
Korenman, S. G. (1970). *Endocrinology* **87**, 1119–1123.
Koseki, Y., Zava, D. T., Chamness, G. C., and McGuire, W. L. (1977a). *Endocrinology* **101**, 1104–1110.
Koseki, Y., Zava, D. T., Chamness, G. C., and McGuire, W. L. (1977b). *Steroids* **30**, 169–178.
Koshland, D. E. (1958). *Proc. Natl Acad. Sci. U.S.A.* **44**, 98–103.
Lauson, H. D., Heller, O. G., Golden, J. B., and Sevringhaus, E. L. (1939). *Endocrinology* **24**, 35–44.
Leavitt, W. W., Chan, T. J., and Allen, T. C. (1977). *Ann. N. Y. Acad. Sci.* **286**, 210–225.
Lednicer, D., Lyster, S. C., and Duncan, G. W. (1967). *J. Med. Chem.* **10**, 78–84.
Lerner, L. J., Holthaus, J., and Thompson, C. R. (1958). *Endocrinology* **63**, 295–318.
Lippman, M., Bolan, G., and Huff, K. (1976). *Cancer Treat. Rep.* **60**, 1421–1429.
Mairesse, N., and Galand, P. (1979). *Endocrinology* **105**, 1248–1253.
Mester, J., and Baulieu, E. E. (1975). *Biochem. J.* **146**, 617–623.
Milgrom, E., Thi, L., Atger, M., and Baulieu, E. E. (1973). *J. Biol. Chem.* **248**, 6366–6374.
Notides, A., and Gorski, J. (1966). *Proc. Natl. Acad. Sci. U.S.A.* **56**, 230–235.
Palopoli, F. P., Feil, V. J., Allen, R. F., Holtkamp, D. E., and Richardson, A. (1967). *J. Med. Chem.* **10**, 84–86.
Paton, W. D. M. (1961). *Proc. R. Soc. B.* **154**, 21–69.
Rochefort, H., and Capony, F. (1977). *Biochem. Biophys. Res. Commun.* **75**, 277–285.
Rubin, B. L., Dorfman, A. S., Black, L., and Dorfman, R. J. (1951). *Endocrinology* **49**, 429–439.
Sarff, M., and Gorski, J. (1971). *Biochemistry* **10**, 2557–2563.
Schultz, K. D., Hazelmayer, B., and Holzel, F. (1971). *In* "Basic Actions of Sex Steroids in Target Organs" (P. O. Hubinont, F. Leroy and P. Galand, eds) pp. 274–299. Karger, Basle.
Self, L. W., Holtkamp, D. E., and Kuhn, W. L. (1967). *Fedn. Proc. Fedn. Am. Socs. Expt. Biol.* **26**, 534.
Skidmore, J. R., Walpole, A. L., and Woodburn, J. (1972). *J. Endocr.* **52**, 289–298.
Stephenson, R. P. (1956). *Br. J. Pharmacol.* **11**, 379–392.
Sutherland, R. L., Mester, J., and Baulieu, E. E., (1977). *Nature* **267**, 434–435.
Terenius, L. (1970). *Acta Endocr.* **64**, 47–58.
Terenius, L. (1971). *Acta Endocr.* **66**, 431–447.
Thron, D. C., and Waud, D. R. (1968). *J. Pharmacol. Exptl Therap.* **160**, 91–105.

Van Maanen, E. F., Greslin, J. G., Holtkamp, D. E., and King, W. M. (1961). *Fedn. Proc. Fedn. Am. Soc. Exp. Biol.* **20**, 419.
Vu Hai, M. T., and Milgrom, E. (1978). *J. Endocr.* **76**, 21–31.
Waud, D. R. (1967). *J. Pharmacol. Exptl Therap.* **148**, 99-114.
Wood, J. R., Wrenn, T. R., and Bitman, J. (1968). *Endocrinology* **82**, 69–74.

4

A Review of the Pharmacokinetics and Metabolism of "Nolvadex" (Tamoxifen)

H. K. ADAM

I. INTRODUCTION

This review is an account of the present state of the art on the pharmacokinetics and metabolism of the antioestrogenic agent "Nolvadex".* Nolvadex tablets contain tamoxifen citrate, equivalent to 10 mg free base, as the active ingredient. Discussions in this review will refer to tamoxifen base. It will cover methods of analysis for the drug and some of its metabolites, and the information generated by these procedures in laboratory animals and in humans. For convenience the metabolism is covered separately, although, as will become apparent, this split is artificial. Finally the discussion section

*"Nolvadex" is a trade-mark, the property of Imperial Chemical Industries Ltd.

NON-STEROIDAL ANTIOESTROGENS
ISBN 0 12 677880 9

considers how the results generated from pharmacokinetic and metabolic studies can assist the clinician in his use of Nolvadex to treat patients and the direction in which future studies could be pointed.

II. METHODS OF ANALYSIS

Before a pharmacokinetic evaluation of any drug can be carried out a prerequisite is a method of analysis which is specific for the chemical entity under consideration and sensitive enough to allow accurate quantification at anticipated levels. Early studies with [^{14}C]tamoxifen (see Section IV, B) had shown that concentrations of unchanged drug of the order of 1–30 ng/ml were obtained after a single therapeutic dose in humans. It was the requirement for sensitivity that proved the stumbling block to further progress. Procedures to extract and chromatograph, either by gas liquid chromatography or on thin layer plates, had been available from the earlier studies but it is only recently that sufficiently sensitive detection procedures have been devised. Three procedures are now available and these will be discussed in turn.

A. Gas Chromatography–Mass Spectrometry

The chromatographic properties of tamoxifen and its metabolites had been used by Fromson *et al.* (1973a, 1973b). The major advance of Gaskell *et al.* (1978) was to combine it with quantitative mass spectrometry.

Plasma samples were extracted with ether and purified by chromatography on a column of Lipidex 5000 and subsequently by further separation on a column of Sephadex LH20. The total recovery throughout the assay was 78%. Quantification was by high resolution mass spectrometry using the molecular ion, with reference to an internal standard added to the plasma before extraction.

In a modification of the procedure (Daniel *et al.*, 1979), the Lipidex column was omitted, the internal standard for tamoxifen was changed and a further internal standard was added to allow quantification of 4-hydroxytamoxifen (see Section IV, A). Although levels of 200 pg could be detected, in practice the limit of accurate quantification for both compounds was 1.0 ng/ml of plasma.

B. Photochemical Conversion and High-Pressure Liquid Chromatography

The photochemical conversion of stilbene and triphenylethylenes to phenanthrene derivatives has been examined by several authors, (Mallory *et al.*, 1962, 1963; Moore *et al.*, 1963; Kan, 1967; and Doyle *et al.*, 1970). The fact that such a conversion for tamoxifen was quantitative and that the fluorescent phenanthrene derivative could be subjected to high-pressure liquid chromatography allowed Mendenhall *et al.* (1978) to develop a sensitive procedure for the drug.

Plasma samples (5 ml) were extracted by either ion-pairing with trifluoroacetate or directly with ether. After removal of the solvent, photochemical conversion to a phenanthrene derivative was achieved by irradiation with ultra-violet light. High-pressure liquid chromatography of the photochemical products allowed quantification of tamoxifen down to 1.0 ng/ml plasma. Slight modifications permitted measurement of both tamoxifen and the 4-hydroxymetabolite to a similar level.

The finding that desmethyltamoxifen (see Section IV, B) was present in human serum in high concentrations after chronic administration of tamoxifen necessitated the modification of this procedure, since the chromatographic conditions used were unable to resolve the phenanthrene derivatives of 4-hydroxytamoxifen and desmethyltamoxifen. The use of an ion-pairing high-pressure liquid chromatography system, with the same extraction procedure and a modified photolysis step, allowed measurement of both metabolites and parent drug down to 0.1 ng/ml (Golander and Sternson, 1980).

C. Thin-Layer Chromatography and Photochemical Conversion

In the early metabolic studies with tamoxifen (Fromson *et al.*, 1973a, 1973b), thin-layer chromatography was used extensively. Combining this technique with the photochemical conversion *in situ* and the use of a densitometer was the basis of the procedure described by Adam *et al.* (1980a).

Serum samples were extracted with a mixed solvent system (hexane-amyl alcohol). The organic extracts, after a suitable volume reduction, were applied to a thin-layer plate. After development of the chromatogram and removal of the elution solvent, the plate was irradiated with ultra-violet light and the fluorescent products quantified, with reference to an internal standard added to the serum before extraction, by a densitometer in the fluorescence mode.

This method allowed measurement of not only tamoxifen but also its non-conjugated metabolites. Indeed it was in the early use of this method that it was discovered that desmethyltamoxifen (see Section IV, B) was the major free metabolite in human serum (Adam *et al.*, 1979a). Using this method, levels of all three compounds could be measured simultaneously with the addition of a single internal standard.

D. Comparison of the Analytical Procedures

From the results discussed in Section III it is apparent that all three procedures give similar results for tamoxifen. A choice between them rests in availability of equipment and the use to which the procedure is to be put.

The gas chromatography–mass spectrometry procedure requires sophisticated, expensive equipment. It also requires the addition of a separate internal standard for each compound to be quantified and two separate chromatographic runs to quantify tamoxifen and its hydroxy metabolite. A brief report suggests that it may also be capable of monitoring the desmethyl metabolite (Nicholson *et al.*, 1979). Its major advantage is its extremely high specificity, since the process of measurement confirms the molecular weight of the compound being analysed. The high specificity of this method arises from the use of the molecular ion at high resolution. However, this in turn leads to a lower sensitivity than would normally be expected from a gas chromatography–mass spectrometry procedure.

The original procedure of Mendenhall *et al.* (1978) suffers from a major drawback as it fails to resolve the desmethyl and hydroxy metabolites, and for any high-pressure liquid chromatography work the revised method must be used if this is desired. Simultaneous measurement of all three compounds down to 0.1 ng/ml (from 5 ml plasma) is possible with the revised procedure. No internal standard is included. The equipment required is one of the most widely used analytical instruments.

The thin-layer densitometric procedure also allows simultaneous estimation of all three compounds and includes an internal standard. A major advantage is that all known unconjugated tamoxifen metabolites, with the exception of metabolite A (Fromson *et al.*, 1973a), which does not form a fluorescent derivative, can be monitored by it. A problem associated with it is that, although desmethyltamoxifen and 4-hydroxytamoxifen are resolved, the presence of high concentrations of the former can cause problems in the quantification of the hydroxy metabolite. Once the ratio of desmethyl to hydroxy metabolite exceeds 20:1 the hydroxy compound cannot be detected. In the light of the results generated by other methods (see Section IV, B, 2) this could be a major drawback if measurement of the hydroxy metabolite is desired. In addition quantitative thin-layer densitometers are relatively unusual tools in most analytical laboratories.

III. PHARMACOKINETICS

A. In Laboratory Animals

Since the analytical procedures for tamoxifen and its metabolites have only become available in recent years, the groups working in this area have concentrated their efforts on human studies. Hence most of the available data from animals are from radiotracer studies and suffer from a lack of specificity.

Fromson *et al.* (1973a) in their metabolic studies examined serum components in several species after administration of [^{14}C]tamoxifen. Unfortunately "it was not possible to distinguish between drug and metabolites on account of the low levels of radioactivity in the blood". Table I summarizes the data these workers obtained.

In all species examined, maximum serum levels (as equivalents of tamoxifen) were low. The apparent terminal half-life from the faecal excretion was long, ranging from 10 to 18 days, but the components which contributed to the apparent terminal half-life could not be determined.

Using [^{3}H]tamoxifen, Major *et al.* (1976) looked at levels of radioactivity in pregnant rats after single oral (0.2 or 0.4 mg/kg) or intravenous (0.2 mg/kg) doses on day 2 of pregnancy. They also examined levels in various tissues and attempted to distinguish between unchanged drug and metabolites in some tissues. Six hours after a single oral dose (0.2 mg/kg), levels in blood, liver, ovary, pituitary, uterus and cerebral cortex were approximately 650, 550, 150, 100, 50 and 40 ng/g respectively (all expressed as tamoxifen equivalents). These workers concluded that radioactivity was retained by all reproductive tissues, with the ovary showing greatest retention. At a higher dose (0.4 mg/kg) they also showed that a decreasing proportion of the uterine radioactivity (50% at 6 hours falling to less than 15% at 72 hours) was unchanged tamoxifen.

Using the gas chromatography–mass spectrometry procedure (Section II, A) Gaskell *et al.* (1978) examined the plasma levels of unchanged tamoxifen in ovariectomized rats after intramuscular dosing. Mean values of 10.6, 97.3 and 244 ng/ml were obtained from 0.9, 8 and 29 mg/kg respectively.

TABLE I
Pharmacokinetic Data in Laboratory Animals[a]

	Species						
	Rat			Mouse	Monkey	Dog	
Route of administration	p.o.	i.p.	i.p.	p.o.	p.o.	p.o.	p.o.
Dose (mg/kg)	40	40	1.3	40	8	1	5
Maximum serum level (μg tamoxifen equivalents/ml)	2.0	1.7	0.5	3.3	0.6	0.5	1.9
"Terminal half-life" (days)[b]	—	—	10	18	12	—	14

[a] From Fromson *et al.* (1973a).
[b] Estimated from excretion rate.

B. In Humans

1. Single Doses

Fromson *et al.* (1973b) examined the profile of total radioactivity in a female patient after a single oral dose of 20 mg [^{14}C]tamoxifen. A peak level of 100 ng tamoxifen equivalents/ml occurred 4 hours after dosing. Concentrations decreased rapidly falling to 40 ng/ml after 24 hours, but thereafter the decay was slower, with detectable levels still present 14 days after dosing. In a further 3 subjects, a similar pattern was observed. By pooling sera from one subject and fractionating the radioactivity on thin layer plates these workers attempted to differentiate between the components present. The fraction which corresponded to unchanged tamoxifen fell from about 30% within the first 4 hours to less than 5% by day 8.

Fromson and Sharp (1974) examined serum and uterine tissue from patients who had received 20 mg of [^{14}C]tamoxifen prior to hysterectomy. The serum results were similar to those in the previous study. In the uterus, concentrations of [^{14}C] material were 2 to 3 times those in the serum and about one half of this material was unchanged drug. The data suggested selective uptake of the drug by the uterus with the mean ratio of concentration in the endometrium to that in serum being 6.2:1. However, control tissue was not available.

With the availability of specific analytical methods, the requirement to utilize radiotracers has disappeared and several studies have examined serum/plasma levels of tamoxifen after a single oral dose.

Mendenhall *et al.* (1978) showed the serum profiles which were achieved in two female patients with breast cancer after a single 10 mg/m^2 dose. In both subjects, a peak value of about 30 ng/ml was obtained after 3 hours. Greater detail on patients was reported by Fabian and Sternson (1979), who found that a median blood concentration of 16 ng/ml was obtained between 3 and 6 hours after dosing. A half-life of 9–12 hours was quoted by these workers. A further amplification of these results (Fabian *et al.*, 1980) showed a wide interpatient spread in plasma levels, the difference between the highest and lowest value being up to 20-fold at 3 hours and about 7-fold at 6 hours after dosing.

In a study of 6 female breast cancer patients, Wilkinson *et al.* (1979) found peak serum levels of between 15 and 25 ng/ml of tamoxifen after a single oral dose and stated that the apparent half-life ranged between 16 and 114 hours.

In a more detailed study of serum profiles, in healthy male volunteers, Adam *et al.* (1980b) monitored serum concentrations for up to 10 days after a single 10 mg dose, (Fig. 1). Peak levels were similar to those seen in other studies and an initial rapid decay was apparent. However, at times greater than 48 hours, it was apparent that a slower terminal elimination phase existed. The half-life of this phase ranged from 91 to 156 hours. These results showed that previous estimates of the tamoxifen half-life had underestimated the true elimination phase because the profile had not been followed for a sufficiently long period.

This study also provided the only evidence on absorption of tamoxifen, when it showed that the drug (formulated in the commercial dosage form "Nolvadex") was as well absorbed as when it was administered in aqueous solution. Absolute bio-availability cannot be calculated as there is no parenteral formulation and the drug is not excreted, to any large extent, in the urine.

2. *Chronic Administration*

In the treatment of advanced breast cancer Nolvadex is administered chronically, usually at 10 or 20 mg b.i.d. Thus, although a single dose situation is of interest, the chronic situation is of more relevance to the clinical usage of the drug.

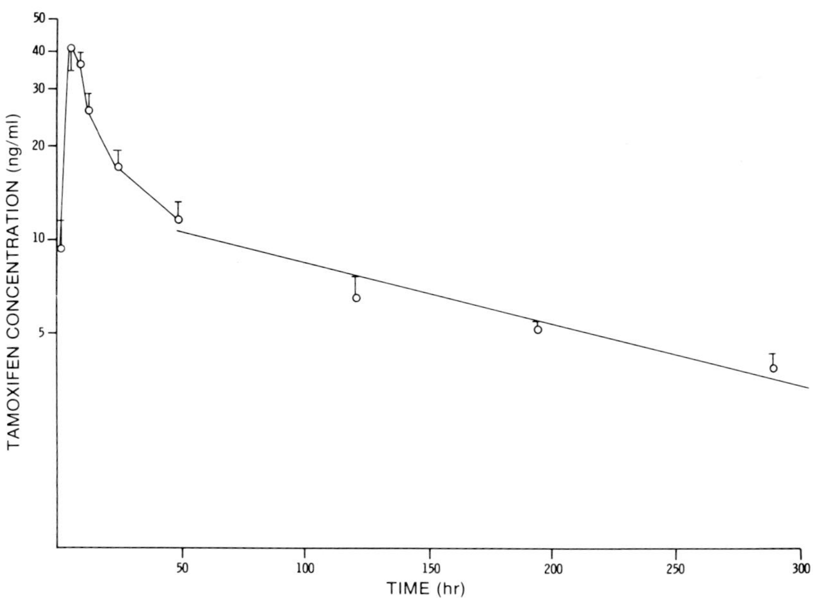

Fig. 1. Tamoxifen serum profile over 10 days after an oral dose of 20 mg (Mean ± S.E.M., n = 6). After Adam *et al.* (1980b).

Several studies have examined the pharmacokinetic profile of tamoxifen in breast cancer patients. After 21 days administration of 10 mg b.i.d. Wilkinson *et al.* (1979) found that serum levels had risen to 150 ± 17 ng/ml compared to a mean peak concentration of 17 ± 2 ng/ml in the same patients after a single dose. In addition, as has been described by Adam *et al.* (1980a) (Fig. 2), once high levels were achieved in these patients (i.e. steady state was approached) the time of sampling in relation to dose was relatively unimportant since little change occurs over a 12 hour dosing interval.

Fabian and Sternson (1979) showed that steady state concentrations were not achieved until 4 weeks after starting on therapy at 10 mg/m^2 b.i.d. and found a median steady state value of 194 ng/ml. In patients in whom the treatment had been discontinued the mean terminal half-life was 5.5 days.

The time scale of approach to steady state and the fact that this value, once achieved, remained constant was also demonstrated by Patterson *et al.* (1980). Figure 3 shows the mean (± S.E.M.) values obtained from 22 breast cancer patients who were examined at regular intervals over 26 weeks therapy with Nolvadex, 20 mg b.i.d. Daniel *et al.* (1979) have also confirmed that tamoxifen concentrations in the range of 100–400 ng/ml were obtained after periods of up to 689 days administration at 20 mg tamoxifen b.i.d.

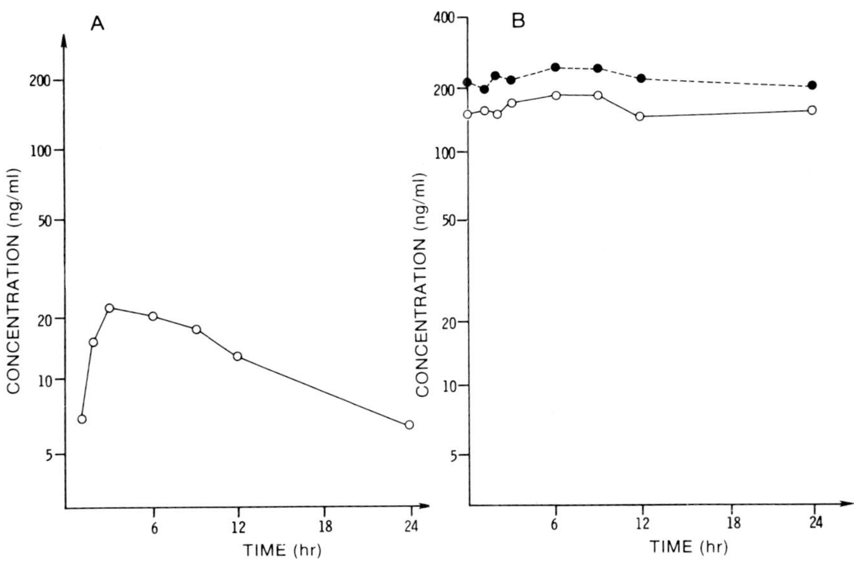

Fig. 2. Concentration of tamoxifen (○) and N-desmethyltamoxifen (●) in a female patient with advanced breast cancer after (A) a single 10 mg dose and (B) after 21 days administration of 10 mg twice daily. After Wilkinson *et al.* (1979).

Thus it appears that all the investigators have shown very similar results from both disparate patient populations and when utilizing different methods of assessing tamoxifen concentrations.

C. Protein Binding

The antioestrogenic activity of tamoxifen is thought to rely on its ability to compete for the intracellular oestrogen receptor protein. Therefore a factor which should be considered in any pharmacokinetic correlation with activity is the fraction of the total tamoxifen (and/or metabolites) which is available to bind to the receptor.

A major contributing factor to this will be the extent to which the compound is bound to protein. Tamoxifen is highly plasma protein bound at therapeutic concentrations, ($\geqslant$ 99%, W. Bastain, personal communication) and studies have been carried out on the possible sites of binding on human albumin (Sjoholm *et al.*, 1979).

Hence any comparison of relative levels of oestrogen and antioestrogen (Daniel *et al.*, 1979) should take the free concentrations in both plasma and the cell into account.

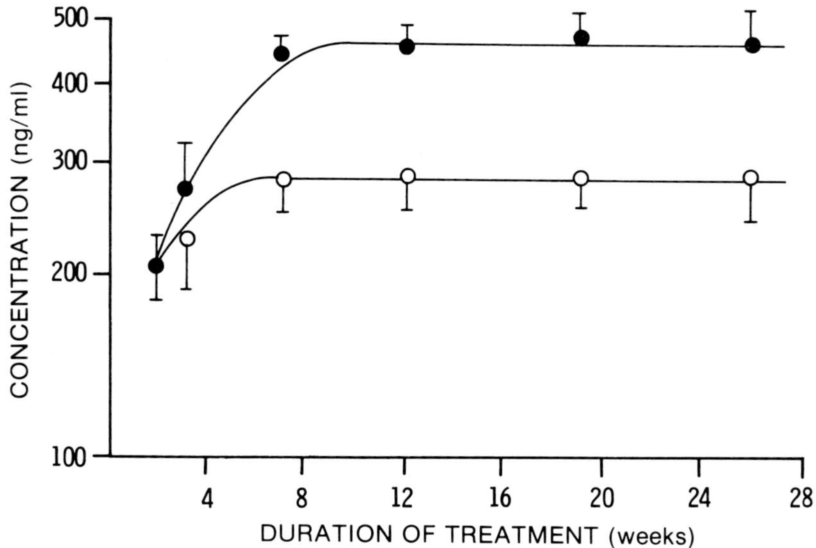

Fig. 3. Concentrations of tamoxifen (○) and N–desmethyltamoxifen (●) in female patients during 26 week treatment with tamoxifen, 20 mg twice daily (Mean ± S.E.M., n = 22). After Patterson *et al.* (1980).

IV. METABOLISM

Metabolic studies with tamoxifen have tried to answer two questions. By what route(s) is the compound (and its metabolites) excreted? What are the biotransformation products?

A. In Laboratory Animals

Using [^{14}C]tamoxifen, Fromson *et al.* (1973a) examined the route of excretion of radioactivity in female rat, mouse, rhesus monkey and dog. Table II summarizes their results. In all species examined, the major route of excretion was via the faeces. It was also demonstrated that, in rats and dogs, this was mainly due to biliary excretion and that reabsorption of the excreted material occurred, leading to extensive enterohepatic recirculation.

In the search for the chemical nature of the excreted material, an examination of urine was not productive. Examination of faecal extracts revealed only traces of unchanged drug, with most of the material being present as polar metabolites. Much of the metabolite isolation work used bile, after hydrolysis with the enzyme glucuronidase. Six different metabolites were identified (Fig. 4). In three cases the structural assignment was by comparison with authentic standard (metabolites A, B and E). In the remaining three cases (metabolites C, D and F) structural assignment was tentative.

In recent studies on rat uterus and chicken oviduct, Borgna and Rochefort (1979) identified 4-hydroxytamoxifen (metabolite B) and, in the rat uterus, hydroxylation products of tamoxifen whose structure(s) have yet to be elucidated.

B. In Humans

In female subjects Fromson *et al.* (1973b) found a similar excretion pattern to that seen in animals (i.e. the major route was via faeces). Overall

TABLE II
Routes of Excretion of Tamoxifen and Metabolites in Laboratory Animals[a]

	Species			
	Rat	Mouse	Monkey	Dog
Route of administration	i.p.	p.o.	p.o.	p.o.
% Dose in faeces	95	79	65	90
% Dose in urine	7	10	19	4

[a] From Fromson *et al.* (1973a).

recovery of radioactivity (see Table III) was low, probably because of an insufficiently long collection period. In the two subjects examined, however, about three-quarters of the total recovery was in the faeces. The [^{14}C] material found therein was mainly polar metabolites, with small amounts of unchanged drug and materials, identified by Rf as metabolites B and F. The quantities of these latter compounds present are difficult to assess as the results were expressed as percentages of extractable [^{14}C] without any indication of the proportion extracted.

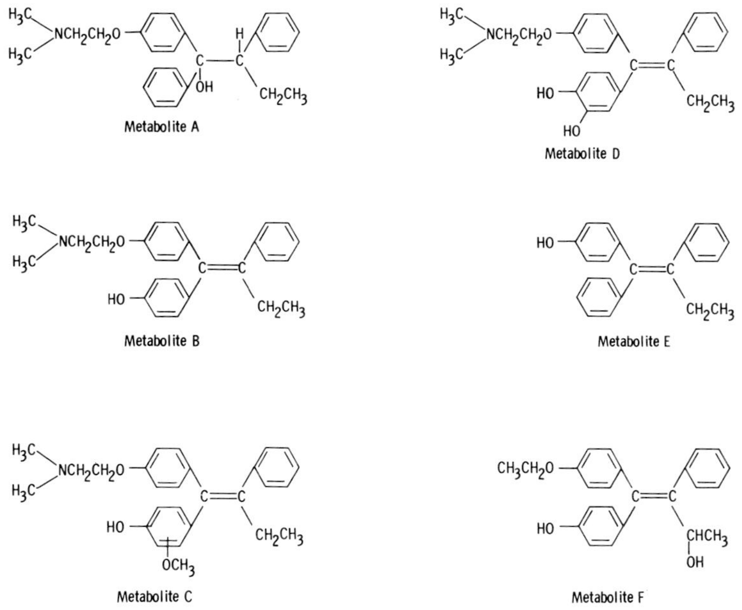

Fig. 4. Metabolites of tamoxifen identified by Fromson. After Fromson *et al.* (1973a).

TABLE III
Routes of Excretion of Tamoxifen and Metabolites in Humans[a]

	Subject	
	1	2
% Dose in urine	9	14
% Dose in faeces	26	51
Collection period (days)	8	13
% of Total recovery in faeces	74	78

[a] From Fromson *et al.* (1973b).

Examination of pooled sera on thin-layer chromatograms led to the identification of a component, whose concentrations ranged from 10 to 20% of the total isotopic content, as 4-hydroxytamoxifen (metabolite B). Most of the [^{14}C] material present in serum did not chromatograph.

Subsequent studies on human metabolism have examined the components in human serum/plasma by one of the procedures outlined in Section II. In the original report of Mendenhall *et al.* (1978) concentrations of "metabolite" were presented. However in the light of present knowledge, the nature of this material must now be in doubt.

In early studies with the densitometric procedure, Adam *et al.* (1979a) showed that the major free metabolite in human serum was desmethyltamoxifen (metabolite X; Fig. 5). It now appears that the metabolite identified by Fromson *et al.* (1973b) as being a major component in human plasma was not, as thought at the time, the 4-hydroxy metabolite, but was in fact this desmethylated product. The chromatographic system used by these workers would not have been able to distinguish between the two compounds.

The desmethyl metabolite, although present in low concentrations after a single dose, accumulates, like the parent drug, on repeated administration. After 21 days administration of 10 mg tamoxifen b.i.d. the ratio of the concentration of this metabolite to that of the parent drug ranged from 0.7 to 2.3. With more prolonged administration the concentration of the metabolite rose even further (Adam *et al.*, 1979b). Figure 3 shows the accumulation pattern in 22 patients over a period of 26 weeks (Patterson *et al.*, 1980). From the single dose data and the pattern of accumulation it appeared that the elimination half-life of the metabolite was about 14 days, i.e. approximately twice that of the parent drug.

Concentrations of 4-hydroxytamoxifen have been measured in 14 subjects during chronic administration (Daniel *et al.*, 1979). In all subjects the steady state concentrations were below 10 ng/ml, indicating that this material is a minor metabolite in the systemic circulation in humans, a finding confirmed by Golander and Sternson (1980).

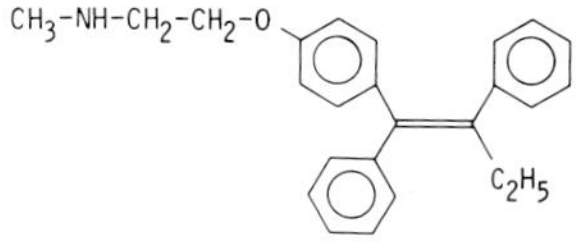

$CH_3-NH-CH_2-CH_2-O$

C_2H_5

Fig. 5. N-Desmethyltamoxifen.

A further possible minor metabolite, whose structure is unknown, other than it appears to be isomeric with metabolite B, has been reported by Daniel *et al.* (1979).

C. Pharmacological Activity of Tamoxifen Metabolites

The finding that the biotransformation in man is a complex process and that some of the non-conjugated metabolites may be present in human serum/plasma in measurable quantities has spurred work on the pharmacological activity of these metabolites.

It has been shown that 4-hydroxytamoxifen is an antioestrogen and that its ability to inhibit [^{3}H]oestradiol binding to oestrogen receptors *in vitro* is greater than that of the parent drug (Jordan *et al.*, 1977).

Recent studies have shown that desmethyltamoxifen has an affinity similar to tamoxifen for oestrogen receptors *in vitro* and have confirmed the higher affinity of the 4-hydroxy metabolite. However, the three compounds were equipotent as antioestrogens in the rat *in vivo* (Wakeling and Slater, 1980).

In the clinical situation, if it can be assumed that tissue concentrations of the three compounds reflect their systemic concentrations, it is likely that both metabolites will play a supportive role to tamoxifen in the production of an antioestrogenic effect. However, it should be noted that studies in rat (Borgna and Rochefort, 1979) suggested that differences exist between the relative concentrations of tamoxifen and its metabolite in the plasma and those in the cell nucleus. It is difficult, therefore, to assess the relative clinical importance of tamoxifen and these metabolites.

V. DISCUSSION

Recent studies with new, sensitive methodology have provided an insight into the pharmacokinetic behaviour of tamoxifen. Healthy male volunteers and females with advanced breast cancer absorb and eliminate the drug in a similar manner. It is well absorbed and peak levels are attained in 3 hours after a single dose. An initial rapid decline is followed by a slower elimination phase. The elimination half-life of between 5 and 7 days, becomes apparent after 48 hours. This long terminal half-life leads to a 10-fold increase in serum levels of tamoxifen during therapy with an accumulation pattern that is in accord with linear pharmacokinetic principles (Van Rossum, 1968; Ballard and Menczel, 1971). The steady state serum value is then maintained over long periods with little variance.

Studies on the metabolism of tamoxifen in man have shown that after repeated administration desmethyltamoxifen is present in concentrations which are 1 to 2 times those of tamoxifen and that 4-hydroxytamoxifen is also present but at much lower concentrations in the plasma ($\leqslant 5\%$ of the parent drug).

Although some questions about the metabolic transformation of tamoxifen inevitably remain, the basic information on the pharmacokinetics of both parent drug and metabolites is now available. How can this knowledge be applied to the therapeutic use of this drug? Measurements of systemic drug levels are a convenient and the most widely used way of determining the absorption, distribution and elimination of the active agent. This basic information is now available on tamoxifen. However, before this information can be utilized a new and critical step must be taken; that is, to attempt a correlation between systemic levels and the therapeutic effect. The first attempts in this direction (Patterson *et al.*, 1980; Fabian *et al.*, 1980) failed to establish any correlation between serum/plasma level and the response to therapy.

For an antioestrogenic agent used in the treatment of advanced breast cancer it is generally accepted that its effect is related to its ability to compete with oestradiol for cytoplasmic oestrogen receptors. Thus, for any individual patient, this effect may be assumed to be related to the amount of the agent which reaches the sensitive target cells and passes through the membrane into the cytoplasm. This may be directly related to the vascular concentration. The factors which govern even this simplistic approach are many. Before any drug can be made available to a particular cell it must first be delivered via the circulation. Thus the vascularity of the target site is important. Once it has attained the site the drug must be free to diffuse from the blood into the target cell. This diffusion will be governed initially by the degree of plasma protein binding, since only unbound material can diffuse, then by the ability of the molecule to diffuse through the potential barriers to its progress.

Once it has attained the cytoplasm it must then compete with other substances for oestrogen receptors, including its own metabolites, whose concentrations are governed by similar considerations. At the same time it must avoid being bound non-specifically to other cell constituents. Once bound to the receptors, of which there may be more than one class, it must be translocated to the nucleus to produce its effect.

All these complex phenomena have been identified as contributing to the final therapeutic effect, manifested by a decrease, or at least no increase, in tumour size. It is probable that most of the processes described above will vary between individuals and may vary at different sites in the same individual. Hence it is perhaps not surprising that the first attempts to correlate levels of antioestrogen in plasma with therapeutic effect across a patient population have failed to produce a clear-cut answer.

However indications of the way ahead can be given. It has been suggested that dosing 10 mg tamoxifen twice daily offers little pharmacokinetic advantage over a single 20 mg daily dose. Clinical studies would be needed to establish that this is the case. If this could be demonstrated it would establish the validity of the pharmacokinetic approach. A similar argument applies to the concept of "loading doses". Preliminary small scale studies (Fabian *et al.*, 1980) have shown that the high tamoxifen concentrations achieved during chronic administration can be attained much earlier by using higher doses initially. However no information is available on the metabolite concentration. Again this concept must be proved clinically with a clear end point of an earlier response. The complex regimen required could also affect patient compliance.

The most fruitful area would appear to be the measurement of tissue levels of drug and/or metabolites. Given the new sensitive procedures available, this is not out of the question. In the therapeutic area under study a unique opportunity exists since the tissues are frequently well defined and, on occasion, available for analysis. Hence it should be possible to obtain samples from "the biophase" or site of action of tamoxifen. Determination of tissue concentrations relative to systemic levels would be enlightening. Furthermore, subcellular fractionation and determination of the concentrations of each active species at the subcellular level may allow a resolution of how these relate to the serum concentration. If this information could be obtained, then the pharmacokinetic input to the therapeutic use of Nolvadex could be considerable.

REFERENCES

Adam, H. K., Douglas, E. J., and Kemp, J. V. (1979a). *Biochem. Pharmacol.* **27**, 145–147.

Adam, H. K., Patterson, J. S., Kemp, J. V., Ribeiro, G., and Wilkinson, P. (1979b). *AACR Abstracts* **20**, 47.

Adam, H. K., Gay, M. A., and Moore, R. H. (1980a). *J. Endocr.* **84**, 35–42.

Adam, H. K., Patterson, J. S., and Kemp, J. V. (1980b). *Cancer Treat. Rep.* **64**, 761–764.

Ballard, B. E., and Menczel, E. (1971). *J. Pharm. Sci.* **60**, 406.

Borgna, J. L., and Rochefort, H. (1979). *C. R. Acad. Sci.* **289**, 1141–1144.

Daniel, C. P., Gaskell, S. J., Bishop, H., and Nicholson, R. I. (1979). *J. Endocr.* **83**, 401–408.

Doyle, T. D., Filipescu, N., Benson, W. R., and Banes, D. (1970). *J. Am. Chem. Soc.* **92**, 6371–6372.

Fabian, C., and Sternson, L. (1979). *ASCO Abstracts* **20**, 326.

Fabian, C., Sternson, L., and Barnett, M. (1980). *Cancer Treat. Rep.* **64**, 765–773.

Fromson, J. M., Pearson, S., and Bramah, S. (1973a). *Xenobiotica.* **3**, 693–709.

Fromson, J. M., Pearson, S., and Bramah, S. (1973b). *Xenobiotica.* **3**, 711–714.

Fromson, J. M., and Sharp, D. S. (1974). *J. Obstet. Gynaecol.* **81**, 321–323.

Gaskell, S. J., Daniel, C. P., and Nicholson, R. I. (1978). *J. Endocr.* **78**, 293–294.

Golander, Y., and Sternson, L. A. (1980). *J. Chromatog.* **181**, 41–49.

Jordan, V. C., Collins, M. M., Rowsby, L., and Prestwich, G. (1977). *J. Endocr.* **75**, 305–316.

Kan, R. O. (1967). *In* "Organic Photochemistry" pp. 219–222. McGraw Hill, New York.
Major, J. S., Green, B., and Heald, P. J. (1976). *J. Endocr.* **71**, 315–324.
Mallory, F. B., Wood, C. S., Gordan, J. T., Lindquist, L. C., and Savitz, M. L. (1962). *J. Am. Chem. Soc.* **84**, 4361–4362.
Mallory, F. B., Gordon, J. T., and Wood, C. S. (1963). *J. Am. Chem. Soc.* **85**, 828–829.
Mendenhall, D. W., Kobayashi, H., Shih, F. M. L., Sternson, L. A., Higuchi, T., and Fabian, C. (1978). *Clin. Chem.* **24**, 1518–1524.
Moore, W. M., Morgan, D. D., and Stermitz, F. R. (1963). *J. Am. Chem. Soc.* **85**, 829–830.
Nicholson, R. I., Daniel, C. P., Gaskell, H., and Bishop, H. (1979). *Cancer Treat. Rep.* **63**, 1151.
Patterson, J. S., Settatree, R. S., Adam, H. K., and Kemp, J. V. (1980). *In* "Breast Cancer — Experimental and Clinical Aspects" (H. Mouridsen and T. Palshof, eds), pp. 89–92. Pergamon, Oxford.
Sjoholm, I., Ekman, B., Kober, A., Ljungstedt-Pahlman, I., Seiving, B., and Sjodin, T. (1979). *Molecular Pharmacology* **16**, 767–777.
Van Rossum, J. M. (1968). *J. Pharm. Sci.* **57**, 2162.
Wakeling, A. E., and Slater, S. R. (1980). *Cancer Treat. Rep.* **64**, 741–744.
Wilkinson, P., Ribeiro, G., Adam, J. K., Kemp, J. V., and Patterson, J. S. (1979). *ASCO Abstracts* **20**, 309.

5

Binding of Tamoxifen and its Metabolites 4-Hydroxytamoxifen and N-Desmethyltamoxifen to Oestrogen Receptors from Normal and Neoplastic Tissues

R. L. SUTHERLAND AND A. M. WHYBOURNE

I. INTRODUCTION

The non-steroidal antioestrogen tamoxifen is extensively metabolized following administration to experimental animals and humans (Fromson *et al.*, 1973a, 1973b). Little is known of the biological properties of these metabolites but it is likely that some of them contribute to the overall antioestrogenic activity of the drug (Wakeling and Slater, 1980). With the recent development of sensitive techniques for measuring the plasma concentrations of tamoxifen and its metabolites, values for the concentrations of these compounds in human plasma have been reported (Daniel *et al.*, 1979; Adam *et al.*, 1980; Patterson *et al.*, 1980). These studies have illustrated that

NON-STEROIDAL ANTIOESTROGENS
ISBN 0 12 677880 9

the major tamoxifen metabolites that accumulate in human plasma are N-desmethyltamoxifen and 4-hydroxytamoxifen. Following chronic administration of tamoxifen, at a dose of 20 mg/day, steady state plasma levels of tamoxifen and its metabolites are reached after 4–8 weeks at which time N-desmethyltamoxifen is the major plasma constituent and is present at about 1.75 times the concentration of the parent drug (Patterson *et al.*, 1980). Contrary to an earlier report (Fromson *et al.*, 1973b), it was found that 4-hydroxytamoxifen was not the major metabolite in human plasma and was present at only about 2.5% of the concentration of tamoxifen itself (Daniel *et al.*, 1979).

In vitro binding studies using 4-hydroxytamoxifen have indicated that this metabolite has a greater affinity for the uterine and chick oviduct oestrogen receptors than tamoxifen itself (Jordan *et al.*, 1977; Rochefort *et al.*, 1979; Binart *et al.*, 1979). Indeed, it appears that 4-hydroxytamoxifen has an affinity for the oestrogen receptor that is similar to or greater than that of oestradiol and about 10 times higher than that of the parent compound tamoxifen (Rochefort *et al.*, 1979; Binart *et al.*, 1979). This enhanced affinity of the monohydroxylated metabolite for the oestrogen receptor has led Borgna and Rochefort (1979) to postulate that it is this compound rather than tamoxifen that is the biologically active antioestrogenic agent *in vivo*.

The affinity of the demethylated metabolite, N-desmethyltamoxifen, for the oestrogen receptor has not been extensively investigated (Wakeling and Slater, 1980). In this study, the binding of N-desmethyltamoxifen, 4-hydroxytamoxifen and tamoxifen to oestrogen receptors extracted from a number of normal tissues and neoplastic cell lines has been investigated.

II. BINDING TO RAT UTERINE AND CHICK OVIDUCT CYTOSOLIC OESTROGEN RECEPTOR

Since neither N-desmethyltoxifen nor 4-hydroxytamoxifen were available in radioactive form, direct binding studies could not be performed. Hence, all binding data reported here are derived from indirect binding studies in which the binding affinity of each ligand relative to that of oestradiol was determined.

Cytosols from immature rat uteri and oestrogen-withdrawn chicken oviducts were prepared as previously described (Sutherland and Baulieu, 1976; Sutherland and Foo, 1979). Aliquots (100 μl) of cytosol were incubated for 16 hours at 4°C with 50 μl [^{3}H]oestradiol (final concentration 0.25 nM) and 50 μl of increasing concentrations of oestradiol, tamoxifen, 4-hydroxytamoxifen or N-desmethyltamoxifen. Following incubation, protein-bound and unbound radioactivity were separated by charcoal adsorption (0.5 ml of 0.5% charcoal, 0.05% dextran for 30 minutes at 4°C) and data plotted as protein-bound radioactivity versus log of the added ligand concentration. The relative binding affinity of each ligand was calculated from the amount of ligand required to displace 50% of the specifically bound tracer oestradiol (Korenman, 1970).

Since tamoxifen and its metabolites are readily adsorbed to surfaces, all solutions, including the tracer and cold oestradiol, were prepared in buffers containing 0.2% bovine serum albumin (BSA) yielding a final concentration of 0.1% BSA in the reaction medium. In addition, all aqueous solutions of tamoxifen and metabolites were prepared and stored in polypropylene tubes and all assays were performed in 4 ml disposable tubes of the same material (Sutherland and Murphy, 1980).

The competition curves for the binding of oestradiol, tamoxifen, 4-hydroxytamoxifen and N-desmethyltamoxifen to oestrogen receptors from rat uterine cytosol and chick oviduct cytosol are illustrated in Figure 1. The mean relative binding affinities from replicate experiments are shown in Table I. Together these data demonstrate that in cytosol from both these target tissues 4-hydroxytamoxifen has a higher affinity for the oestrogen receptor than its natural ligand, oestradiol. Tamoxifen and N-desmethyltamoxifen have similar but significantly lower affinities for the oestrogen receptor sites, i.e. 18–22% that of oestradiol in rat uterine cytosol and 6% that of oestradiol in chick oviduct cytosol. The differences between the relative binding affinities of tamoxifen for receptor sites in these two target tissue cytosols are in agreement with earlier observations from this laboratory (Sutherland and Foo, 1981).

TABLE I
Relative Binding Affinities of Tamoxifen and Metabolites for Oestrogen Receptors from Normal and Neoplastic Tissues[a]

Tissue and fraction	Relative binding affinity (oestradiol = 100)		
	4-Hydroxy-tamoxifen	Tamoxifen	N-Desmethyl-tamoxifen
Rat uterine cytosol	133	22	18
Chick oviduct cytosol	144	6	6
Chick oviduct nuclear extract	95	16	17
MCF 7 cytosol	33	2	2
T 47D cytosol	32	4	4
MCF 7 nuclear extract	73	13	14
T 47D nuclear extract	119	13	14
Mean ± S.E.M.	90 ± 17	11 ± 3	11 ± 2

[a] The relative binding affinities (oestradiol-17β = 100) were calculated according to Korenman (1970).

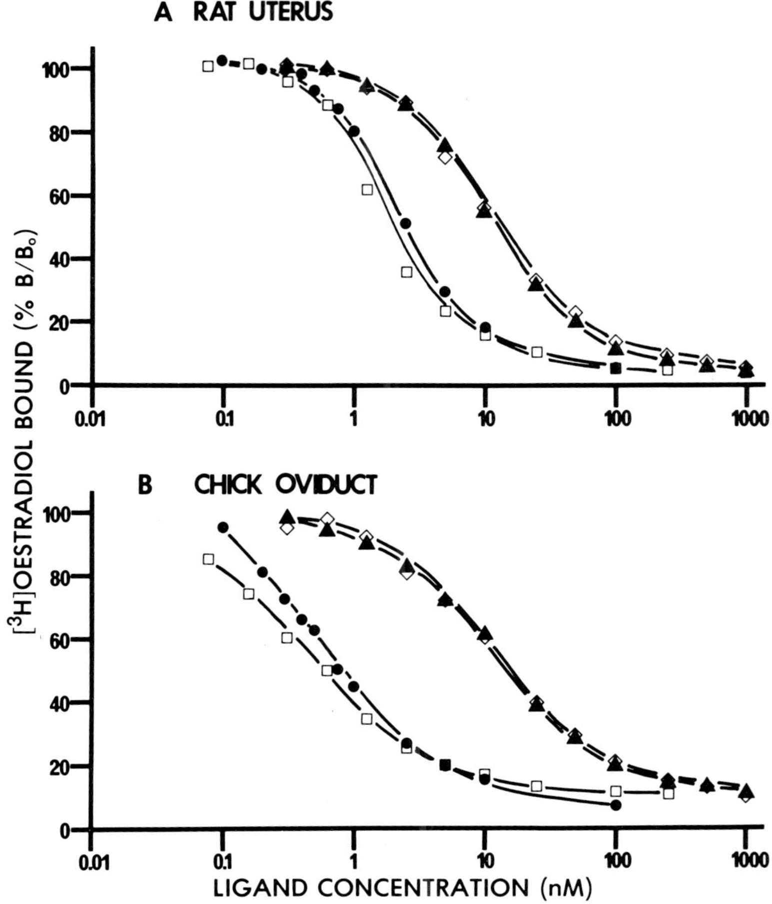

Fig. 1. Competition of oestradiol (●), tamoxifen (▲), 4-hydroxytamoxifen (□) and N-desmethyltamoxifen (◇) for oestrogen receptor sites in (A) immature rat uterine cytosol and (B) oestrogen-withdrawn chick oviduct cytosol. The experimental conditions are described in the text.

III. BINDING TO CHICK OVIDUCT NUCLEAR OESTROGEN RECEPTOR

The nuclear extracts used in this study were prepared from crude oviduct nuclei of oestrogen-stimulated immature chicks, as previously described (Sutherland and Baulieu, 1976). Endogenous oestrogens were removed from the extracts by the method of Best-Belpomme *et al.* (1975). Assays were performed as described above for rat uterine and chick oviduct cytosols and the data are summarized in Table I. Again, the hydroxylated metabolite had at least a 5-fold greater affinity for the receptor than the demethylated metabolite and the parent compound did. However, the affinity of the 4-hydroxytamoxifen for the oestrogen receptor was no greater than that of oestradiol in this material. This is in contrast to the observations made in Figure 1 with rat uterine and chick oviduct cytosol where the potency of 4-hydroxytamoxifen was significantly greater than that of oestradiol.

IV. BINDING TO CYTOSOLIC AND NUCLEAR OESTROGEN RECEPTORS FROM MCF 7 AND T 47D HUMAN MAMMARY CARCINOMA CELLS

The MCF 7 and T 47D cell lines are well characterized human mammary carcinoma lines which express the oestrogen receptor (Soule *et al.*, 1973; Brooks *et al.*, 1973; Keydar *et al.*, 1979). For the experiments described here the cells were grown in two different ways. Nuclear extracts were prepared from the crude nuclear pellets of cells grown in 10 % foetal calf serum while cytosols came from cells that had been grown for at least 4 days in 10 % foetal calf serum which had been treated with dextran-coated charcoal to remove endogenous oestrogen. The removal of oestrogen from the culture medium resulted in a redistribution of oestrogen receptor between the cytoplasm and nucleus so that the oestrogen receptors were located predominantly in the cytoplasm.

In a typical experiment $5–8 \times 10^8$ cells were homogenized in approximately 10 ml of buffer and a cytosol or high salt extract (0.5 M NaCl) of the crude nuclear pellet was prepared using techniques similar to those described by Sutherland and Baulieu (1976). Endogenous oestrogens were not removed. Aliquots of cytosol or nuclear extract were incubated with [^{3}H]oestradiol and increasing concentrations of unlabelled ligand as described above. The data are summarized in Figures 2 and 3 and Table I.

In agreement with data from all tissues in this study, tamoxifen and N-desmethyltamoxifen had similar potencies to each other in the cytosol from both cell lines (Fig. 2). However, these affinities, relative to oestradiol, were markedly reduced in these preparations; cf. all other tissue preparations except chick oviduct cytosol (Table I). Interestingly, the relative affinity of 4-hydroxytamoxifen was also markedly reduced in both these cytosolic preparations where the relative binding affinities were reduced to 33 % of that for oestradiol. A similar reduced affinity of 4-hydroxytamoxifen for the oestrogen receptor was reported by Nicholson *et al.*, (1979) in studies on DMBA tumour cytosol.

The situation was appreciably different when the nuclear extracts from these cell lines were used as the source of oestrogen receptor sites (Fig. 3). Tamoxifen and desmethyltamoxifen had similar relative binding affinities to each other in both cell lines, and these values of 13–14% were in agreement with data from the chick oviduct nuclear extract and rat uterine cytosol (Table I). The relative affinity of 4-hydroxytamoxifen for these sites was again considerably greater than that of the other two ligands, i.e. 5–8 fold higher, but was significantly lower in the MCF 7 line than in the T 47D line (Fig. 3, Table I).

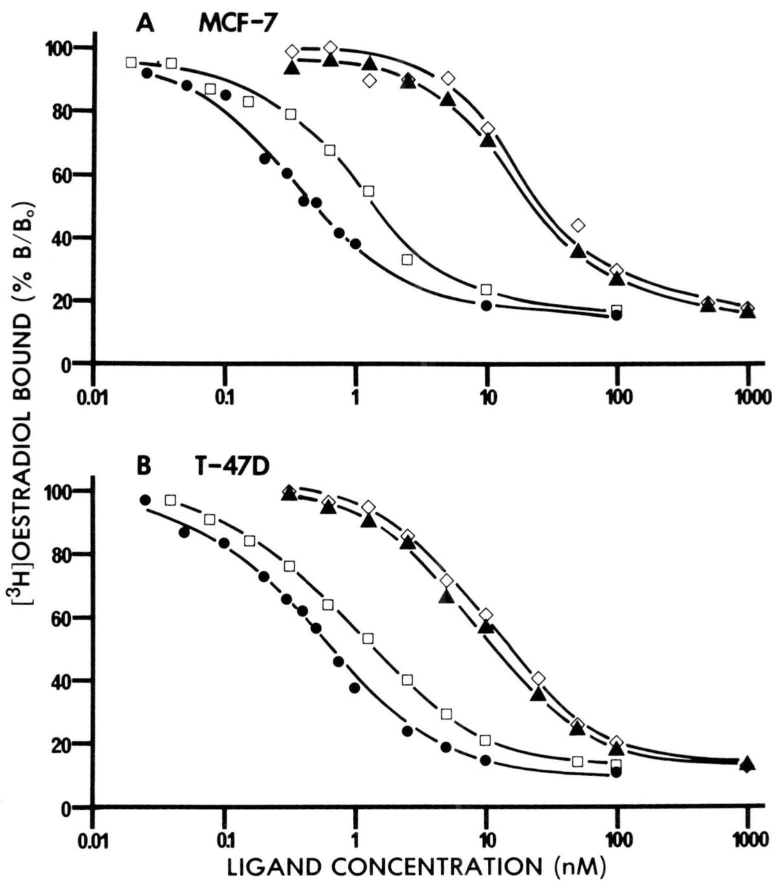

Fig. 2. Competition of oestradiol (●), tamoxifen (▲), 4-hydroxytamoxifen (□) and N-desmethyltamoxifen (◇) for cytoplasmic oestrogen receptor sites from (A) MCF 7 and (B) T 47D cultured human mammary carcinoma cells. The experimental conditions are described in the text.

V. DISCUSSION

The aim of this study was to derive estimates of the affinities of tamoxifen and its metabolites for cytoplasmic and nuclear oestrogen receptors from a number of different oestrogen target tissues. Since these metabolites were not available in radioactive form it was not possible to conduct direct saturation analysis studies similar to those previously described for tamoxifen and CI 628 (Sutherland and Foo, 1979; Sutherland and Murphy, 1980). As a result, indirect competitive binding studies had to be employed (Korenman, 1970).

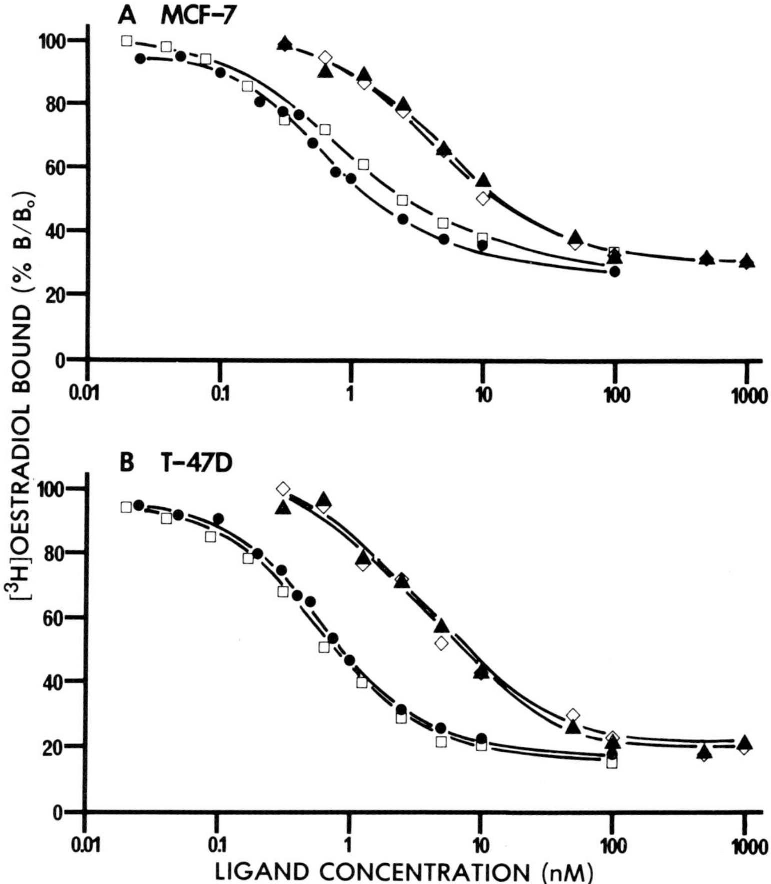

Fig. 3. Competition of oestradiol (●), tamoxifen (▲), 4-hydroxytamoxifen (□) and N-desmethyltamoxifen (◇) for nuclear oestrogen receptor sites from (A) MCF 7 and (B) T 47D cultured human mammary carcinoma cells. The experimental conditions are described in the text.

Such techniques are subject to a number of systematic errors and as a result estimates of affinity, obtained in this way, can only be regarded as first approximations. Rochefort *et al.* (1979) have demonstrated a time and temperature dependence of the competitive ability of antioestrogens in such binding systems, and data from this laboratory indicate that the relative binding affinities of these compounds are influenced by a number of other parameters. These include the oestrogen receptor concentration of the material under study and the concentration of [^{3}H]oestradiol employed (Sutherland and Foo, unpublished observations). However, despite these limitations, very valuable information can be obtained from such assays, particularly when one is comparing the binding of a series of ligands to the same receptor preparation or when different target tissue extracts are assayed under similar *in vitro* conditions, i.e. time, temperature, receptor concentration and [^{3}H]oestradiol concentration.

The most striking result in the present study was the observation that N-desmethyltamoxifen had an affinity for the oestrogen receptor which was identical to that of the parent drug, tamoxifen. This was true for all seven tissue extracts studied despite quite large differences in relative binding affinities between individual tissue extracts (Table I). Such a result is in agreement with the only other published study on the binding of N-desmethyltamoxifen to oestrogen receptors (Wakeling and Slater, 1980).

As had been previously demonstrated (Jordan *et al.*, 1977; Rochefort *et al.*, 1979; Binart *et al.*, 1979; Nicholson *et al.*, 1979), 4-hydroxytamoxifen was bound to the oestrogen receptor with a considerably higher affinity than tamoxifen and N-desmethyltamoxifen. However, the potency of 4-hydroxytamoxifen relative to the other two compounds varied from 5-fold greater in MCF 7 and chick oviduct nuclear extracts to 24-fold higher in chick oviduct cytosol (Table I).

The large differences in relative binding affinities between different tissue extracts were unexpected. Whilst there was reasonably good agreement between the data obtained with rat uterine cytosol and the nuclear extracts from chick oviduct, MCF 7 and T 47D cell lines, the relative binding affinities for tamoxifen and its metabolites, derived from studies with chick oviduct cytosol and to a greater extent MCF 7 and T 47D cell cytosols, were markedly reduced. Although these differences in relative binding affinity between target tissues could be partially explained by factors alluded to above, i.e. oestrogen receptor and [^{3}H]oestradiol concentrations, one should also consider the possibility of metabolic conversion *in vitro* and the influence of an additional high affinity, saturable, antioestrogen binding site (see Chapter 19). More detailed kinetic studies are required to fully understand these binding systems, and this seems unlikely to occur until all ligands are available in radioactive form.

The observation that N-desmethyltamoxifen has an affinity for oestrogen receptors equal to that of tamoxifen has broad implications for future studies on the mechanism of action of tamoxifen *in vivo*. Since N-desmethyltamoxifen accumulates in plasma at almost twice the concentration of tamoxifen following chronic administration to humans (Patterson *et al.*, 1980) and is equipotent with tamoxifen in competing for oestrogen receptor sites *in vitro* and inhibiting implantation *in vivo* (Wakeling and Slater, 1980), it is possible that this metabolite is more important than the parent drug in inhibiting oestrogen receptor mediated events in humans.

The role of 4-hydroxytamoxifen in effecting the action of tamoxifen *in vivo* is controversial. Borgna and Rochefort (1979) have suggested that tamoxifen exerts its effects mainly through hydroxylated metabolites, yet Jordan and Allen (1980) and Wakeling and Slater (1980) have demonstrated that 4-hydroxytamoxifen is a less potent antitumour and antifertility agent *in vivo* than tamoxifen itself. It is clearly evident from the studies reported here (Table I, Figs 1–3) and the work of others (Jordan *et al.*, 1977; Rochefort *et al.*, 1979; Binart *et al.*, 1979; Nicholson *et al.*, 1979; Wakeling and Slater, 1980) that 4-hydroxytamoxifen has a significantly higher affinity for the oestrogen receptor than tamoxifen and this probably accounts for the greater antioestrogenic potency of 4-hydroxytamoxifen *in vitro* (Binart *et al.*, 1979). The lack of correlation between the affinities of 4-hydroxytamoxifen and tamoxifen for the oestrogen receptor *in vitro* and their antioestrogenic potency *in vivo* has been attributed to a shorter biological half-life of the hydroxylated metabolite (Jordan and Allen, 1980). In view of the fact that 4-hydroxytamoxifen is present at about 2.5 % of the concentration of tamoxifen in the plasma of women treated for breast cancer (Daniel *et al.*, 1979) and has lower antitumour and antifertility activity *in vivo* (Jordan and Allen, 1980; Wakeling and Slater, 1980), it seems unlikely that this compound plays the major role in inducing tumour regression in tamoxifen treated patients, unless it is preferentially accumulated at the site of action of the drug.

It is too early, however, to draw definite conclusions about the relative contributions of tamoxifen and its two major metabolites, 4-hydroxytamoxifen and N-desmethyltamoxifen, to tumour regression in humans. Such conclusions must await a detailed study of the antitumour effects of each compound *in vivo*, their antiproliferative properties *in vitro* and accurate estimates of the relative concentrations of tamoxifen and metabolites in the tumours themselves.

REFERENCES

Adam, J. K., Gay, M. A., and Moore, R. H. (1980). *J. Endocr.* **84**, 35–42.

Best-Belpomme, M., Mester, J., Weintraub, H., and Baulieu, E. E. (1975). *Eur. J. Biochem.* **57**, 537–547.

Binart, N., Catelli, M. G., Geynet, C., Puri, V., Hähnel, R., Mester, J., and Baulieu, E. E. (1979). *Biochem. Biophys. Res. Commun.* **91**, 812–818.

Borgna, J. L., and Rochefort, H. (1979). *C. R. Acad. Sci.* **289**, 1141–1144.

Brooks, S. C., Locke, E. R., and Soule, H. D. (1973). *J. Biol. Chem.* **248**, 6251–6253.

Daniel, C. P., Gaskell, S. J., Bishop, H., and Nicholson, R. I. (1979). *J. Endocr.* **83**, 401–408.

Fromson, J. M., Pearson, S., and Bramah, S. (1973a). *Xenobiotica* **3**, 693–709.

Fromson, J. M., Pearson, S., and Bramah, S. (1973b). *Xenobiotica* **3**, 711–714.

Jordan, V. C., and Allen, K. E. (1980). *Eur. J. Cancer* **16**, 239–252.

Jordan, V. C., Collins, M. M., Rowsby, L., and Prestwich, G. (1977). *J. Endocr.* **74**, 305–316.

Keydar, I., Chen, L., Karby, S., Weiss, E. R., DeLarea, J., Radu, M., Chateik, S., and Grenner, H. J. (1979). *Eur. J. Cancer* **15**, 659–670.

Korenman, S. G. (1970). *Endocrinology* **87**, 1119–1123.

Nicholson, R. I., Syne, J. S., Daniel, C. P., and Griffiths, K. (1979). *Eur. J. Cancer* **15**, 317–329.

Patterson, J. S., Settatree, R. S., Adam, H. K., and Kemp, J. V. 1980). *In* "Breast Cancer — Experimental and Clinical Aspects" (H. Mouridsen and T. Palshof, eds), pp. 89–92. Pergamon, Oxford.

Rochefort, H., Garcia, M., and Borgna, J. L. (1979). *Biochem. Biophys. Res. Commun.* **88**, 351–357.

Soule, H. D., Vazquez, J., Long, A., Albert, S., and Brennan, M. (1973). *J. Natl Cancer Inst.* **51**, 1409–1413.

Sutherland, R. L., and Baulieu, E. E. (1976). *Eur. J. Biochem.* **70**, 531–541.

Sutherland, R. L., and Foo, M. S. (1979). *Biochem. Biophys. Res. Commun.* **91**, 183–191.

Sutherland, R. L., and Foo, M. S. (1981). This volume, pp. 195-214.

Sutherland, R. L., and Murphy, L. C. (1980). *Eur. J. Cancer* **16**, 1141–1148.

Wakeling, A. E., and Slater, S. R. (1980). *Cancer Treat. Rep.* **64**, 741–744.

6

Metabolism and Binding of Non-Steroidal Antioestrogens in Mammals and Chickens

H. ROCHEFORT, F. CAPONY AND J. L. BORGNA

I. INTRODUCTION

Non-steroidal antioestrogens display partial agonist-antagonist activities in mammals. According to the period of retention of oestrogen receptors in the nucleus of the target cell, one distinguishes the short acting antioestrogens, such as the dimethylstilboestrol and oestriol, and the long acting anti-oestrogens (Clark *et al.*, 1976), such as the triphenylethylene derivatives currently used in therapy. Conversely, in chick oviduct (Sutherland *et al.*, 1977) or liver (Gschwendt, 1975), the long acting antioestrogens are full oestrogen antagonists. Since it is known that these drugs competitively inhibit the binding of oestrogen to the oestrogen receptor, attempts have been made to predict the antioestrogenic activity of a ligand by characterizing its binding to the cytosol, i.e. oestrogen receptor (Bouton and Raynaud, 1978). However, one first needs to know which of the ligands is actually acting *in vivo* in target cells because administered antioestrogens can be metabolized into compounds having quite different affinities for the oestrogen receptor.

NON-STEROIDAL ANTIOESTROGENS
ISBN 0 12 677880 9

We report here results from our laboratory dealing with (i) the *in vitro* binding characteristics of classical antioestrogens; (ii) the hydroxylated metabolites of tamoxifen formed *in vivo* and *in vitro*; and (iii) the *in vitro* binding characteristics of an hydroxylated metabolite of tamoxifen.

II. *IN VITRO* BINDING OF CLASSICAL ANTIOESTROGENS TO UTERINE CYTOSOLIC OESTROGEN RECEPTOR

It is well known that non-radioactive antioestrogens (nafoxidine, MER 25, CI 628, dimethylstilboestrol, tamoxifen) inhibit the binding of oestradiol to its receptor, competitively, reversibly and totally (Korenman, 1970; Rochefort and Capony, 1972; Clark *et al.*, 1976). However, it is still debated whether this binding inhibition is due to a direct interaction of the drugs with the oestrogen binding site and whether it is responsible for the antioestrogenic effect observed. The availability of [^{3}H]antioestrogens of high specific activity allowed us to study directly the interaction of these antagonists with specific proteins in oestrogen target cells. We have used successively [^{3}H]dimethylstilboestrol (Capony and Rochefort, 1977), a short acting antioestrogen, and [^{3}H]tamoxifen (Capony and Rochefort, 1978), a long acting antioestrogen. Since we found similar results with the two drugs, we will only consider [^{3}H]tamoxifen. By using a dextran-coated charcoal and an hydroxyapatite batchwise assay, [^{3}H]tamoxifen was found to bind with a high affinity ($K_d \simeq$ 2–10 nM) to saturable cytosol proteins in the uterus of the immature rat and lamb.

A. Tamoxifen Binds to the 8S Oestrogen Receptor in Uterine Cytosol

This conclusion was based on several experimental observations originally reported by Capony and Rochefort (1978). The stereo-specificity for binding to the antioestrogen site was similar to that for the oestrogen binding site (Fig. 1). [^{3}H]tamoxifen binding was mainly inhibited by oestrogens and antioestrogens, while tetraiodothyronine, progesterone and cortisol had little ($\simeq 10\%$) or no effect. Androgens competed with [^{3}H]tamoxifen as they were shown to compete with [^{3}H]oestradiol (Rochefort and Garcia, 1976) and in the same order of efficiency. There was mutually exclusive binding of tamoxifen and oestrogen ligands, either on the same binding site (true competition) or on two different but functionally related sites, one for the hormone, the other for its antagonist. The number of tamoxifen binding sites was slightly lower than that of the oestradiol binding sites but this difference could be due to the marked variation in the stability of the two complexes. Sucrose gradient analysis of the binding of [^{3}H]tamoxifen with uterine cytosol proteins revealed a saturable 8S binding peak. A 4S binder was also found intermittently which, unlike the 8S peak, was not displaced by an excess of non-radioactive tamoxifen or oestradiol. Actually, when the oestrogen binding sites were measured by the dextran-coated charcoal assay in each fraction of the gradient after resaturation with [^{3}H]oestradiol (post labelling experiments) more 8S oestrogen receptor sites were assayed. This suggested that some of the 4S binding peak was due to the transfer of [^{3}H]tamoxifen

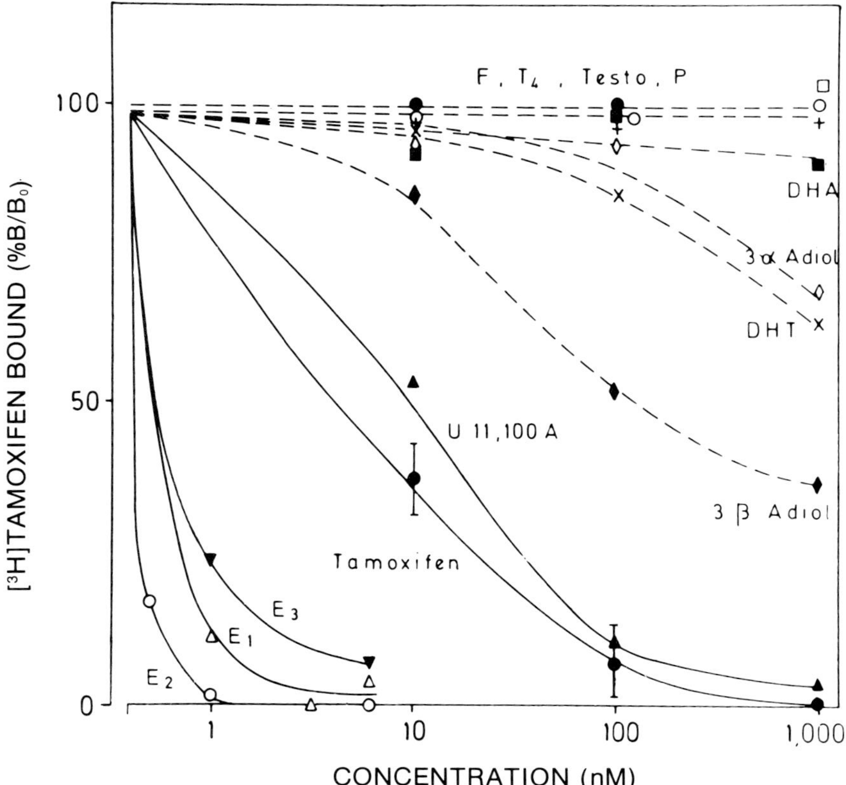

Fig. 1. Binding specificity. The cytosol was incubated at 2°C with [^{3}H]tamoxifen, 7 nM, and various concentrations of the following hormones and antioestrogens: oestradiol (E_2), oestrone (E_1), oestriol (E_3), tamoxifen, nafoxidine (U11,100A), testosterone (Testo), dihydrotestosterone (DHT), dehydroepiandrosterone (DHA), 5α-androstan-3α-17β diol (3α Adiol), 5α-androstan-3β-17β diol (3β Adiol), progesterone (Prog), cortisol (F), thyroxine (T_4). Four hours later, the specific binding of [^{3}H]tamoxifen was assayed by the dextran coated charcoal assay. The 100% value corresponds to the non-inhibited specifically bound [^{3}H]tamoxifen. From Capony and Rochefort, (1978).

during the run from the 8S oestrogen receptor to non-receptor specific 4S binders. Finally, the tamoxifen-oestrogen receptor complex also bound to DNA *in vitro* and was digested by trypsin into a 4S-partially proteolysed oestrogen receptor still able to bind tamoxifen.

B. Differences between Tamoxifen and Oestradiol Binding

A series of differences were found between the *in vitro* binding of tamoxifen and that of oestradiol. First, tamoxifen was found to dissociate from the oestrogen receptor much more rapidly than oestradiol. In the presence of an excess of unlabelled tamoxifen or oestradiol, the [^{3}H]tamoxifen dissociated according to a first order reaction with a half-time of dissociation equal to 0.3 to 2 hours, while the half-time of dissociation of [^{3}H]oestradiol was 10 days at 2°C (Capony and Rochefort, 1978). Occasionally, a second slope of dissociation was observed but the proportion of the slow dissociating complex was always less for tamoxifen (10–15%) than for dimethylstilboestrol (50%) and oestradiol (80%). Second, tamoxifen protects the hormone receptor sites against thermo-inactivation to a lesser extent than oestradiol does. Thus, in studies performed *in vitro* at a temperature above 4°C, it is difficult to reach any conclusion concerning the comparison between the effects of tamoxifen and oestradiol on oestrogen receptor localization. Third, we noticed a time and temperature dependent decrease of competitive efficiency of antioestrogens (Rochefort and Capony, 1977). When [^{3}H]oestradiol and non-radioactive antioestrogens were incubated together with uterine cytosol, one observed a progressive decrease of the inhibition of [^{3}H]oestradiol binding to its receptor. The apparent equilibrium dissociation constant evaluated indirectly by Dixon plot (K_i) was therefore found to increase progressively according to time, while that evaluated by the Scatchard representation (K_d) was much lower and constant with time (Table I).

It is difficult to explain these time-dependent changes of apparent affinities without considering a transformation of the oestrogen receptor by oestradiol. One hypothesis is that, in the absence of ligand, the oestrogen receptor would be in an inactive conformation having a relatively high affinity for tamoxifen. Oestradiol would progressively transform this conformation (induced fit) or displace the equilibrium (allostery) towards a form having either a high affinity for oestradiol or a lower affinity for antioestrogens. However, another hypothesis is that this phenomenon is restricted to low affinity and rapidly dissociating ligands and has nothing to do with the antioestrogenic activities of these ligands. Results described with monohydroxytamoxifen support this last hypothesis (see Section III).

Fourth and finally the [^{3}H]tamoxifen and the [^{3}H]oestradiol binding to the oestrogen receptor were differentially altered by oestrogen receptor

TABLE I
Binding characteristics of Antioestrogens to the Cytoplasmic Oestrogen Receptor[a]

		Oestradiol	Classical antioestrogens (tamoxifen, nafoxidine)	OH tamoxifen
1. Hormone site	K_d(nM)	0.3	2–10	0.3
	k-	slow	rapid	slow
	k-/k+	0.002	2–10	0.002
	Ligand protection	yes	weak	yes
2. Antibody site	K_d decreased	no	yes	no
	Sedimentation shift	yes	—	yes
3. Acceptor site	Nuclear translocation	yes	yes	yes
	DNA binding	yes	yes	yes
	Productive sites	yes	?	?

[a] The binding characteristics of classical antioestrogens have been compared to those of hydroxytamoxifen and oestradiol for three types of sites located on the oestrogen receptor. (1) Hormone site results are from Capony and Rochefort (1978) and Borgna (unpublished). (3) Acceptor site results are from Rochefort *et al.* (1972), Capony and Rochefort (1978) and André (1977). The results concerning OH tamoxifen are from Borgna and Rochefort (1981).

antibodies. These antibodies had been obtained by Greene and Jensen (Chicago) from immunized rabbit and goat and were kindly given to us through the U.S.–French (NIH–INSERM) cooperation on hormones and cancer. While the affinity of oestradiol for the oestrogen receptor was not altered after interaction with the specific oestrogen receptor antibodies (Greene *et al.*, 1977), that of tamoxifen was markedly decreased by the same antibodies without any significant modification of the number of binding sites (Garcia *et al.*, 1979). The antibodies of non-immunized animals had no effect. These results indicated that tamoxifen was directly interacting with the oestrogen receptor and suggested that oestrogen receptor antibodies might be an interesting probe to differentiate oestrogenic and antioestrogenic ligands.

III. *IN VIVO* AND *IN VITRO* METABOLISM OF TAMOXIFEN TO HYDROXYLATED DERIVATIVES

Even though several metabolites of tamoxifen have been identified in plasma (Adam *et al.*, 1979; Daniel *et al.*, 1979), bile and faeces (Fromson *et al.*, 1973), no data are available on the metabolites accumulated in target tissues and more precisely at the oestrogen receptor sites. We therefore attempted to determine which compounds (tamoxifen or its metabolites) were concentrated at the oestrogen receptor sites. After *in vivo* administration of [^{3}H]tamoxifen to immature female rats, the ethyl acetate extracts of plasma, cytosol and KCl-solubilized nuclear fractions of the uterus were analysed by thin layer chromatography (Borgna and Rochefort, 1979). We found that polar metabolites of tamoxifen were present in all fractions analysed (Fig. 2). Two of these polar metabolites (fraction numbers 2 and 5) represented the major part of the radioactivity of the uterine extracts, conversely tamoxifen became negligible. These two polar metabolites appeared to occupy the uterine oestrogen receptor sites on the basis of the following three observations: (i) a progressive enrichment from plasma to cytosol and nuclear fractions; (ii) a saturable accumulation in uterine fractions; (iii) a resistance to charcoal which was higher for polar metabolites than for tamoxifen.

The concentrations of these metabolites in uterine fractions varied according to time (Fig. 3). During the day following injection of tamoxifen a monohydroxy derivative of tamoxifen (OH tamoxifen) in TLC fraction 5 was predominant. This metabolite has been identified by co-crystallization with authentic non-radioactive 4-monohydroxytamoxifen until constant specific activity. During the following two days, the uterine content of OH tamoxifen decreased while an unidentified (but probably hydroxylated) more polar compound (metabolite M_2 in fraction 2) became predominant.

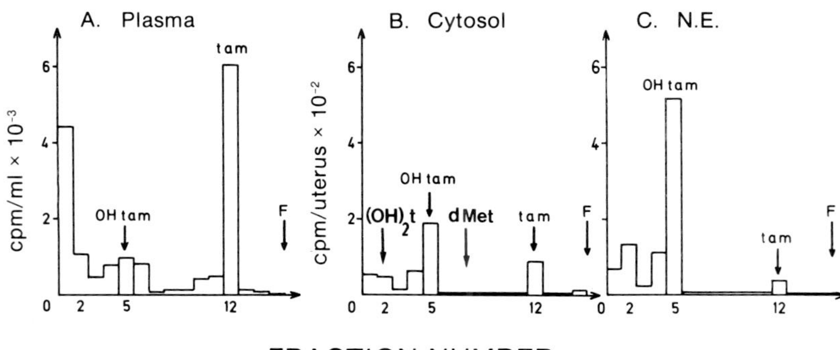

Fig. 2. Radiochromatograms of plasma, cytosol and nuclear fractions of rat uterus, after [^{3}H]tamoxifen administration. Three immature female Wistar rats, 20 days old, received a single subcutaneous injection of 15 μg of [^{3}H]tamoxifen (S.A. = 2.8 Ci/mmole). Eight hours later, the plasma, the cytosol and the KCl-solubilized nuclear fraction (NE) of pooled uteri were prepared. The ethyl acetate-extracted radioactive compounds from plasma and charcoal-treated (1 hour at 0°C) uterine fractions were analysed by thin layer chromatography on silica gel plates. Fraction 1 = deposit; fraction 15 = solvent front (F). From Borgna and Rochefort (1979).

Similar results were obtained in male chicken liver. High levels of polar metabolites were found after *in vivo* injection, or *in vitro* incubation of liver, with [^{3}H]tamoxifen. The OH tamoxifen formed *in vitro* appeared the main compound bound to the oestrogen receptor in the liver nuclear fraction. The presence of OH tamoxifen in chick liver was not definite proof that OH tamoxifen was concentrated in target tissues. In fact, the liver is mostly a metabolic organ and OH tamoxifen could be secreted into the bile and not appear in plasma (Binart *et al.*, 1979).

We have thus tried to identify the metabolites accumulated after *in vivo* administration of [^{3}H]tamoxifen in a pure oestrogen target tissue, the chicken oviduct, and found that OH tamoxifen was the major compound in the nuclear extract. Moreover, the chick oviduct was shown to transform tamoxifen *in vitro* to OH tamoxifen as was also found for the lamb uterus but not for the rat uterus (Borgna and Rochefort, 1981). We therefore conclude

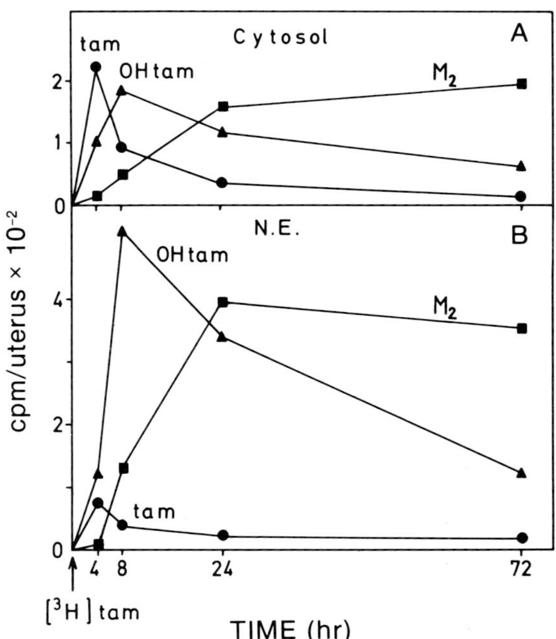

Fig. 3. Time-dependent variation of the charcoal-resistant concentrations of tamoxifen and of its main metabolites in uterine fractions. The experiment described in Fig. 2 was performed at different periods of time after [^{3}H]tamoxifen administration. The radioactivity from uterine cytosol and nuclear extracts (NE) found in fractions 2 (■); 5 (▲) and 12 (●) of the thin layer plates is presented. From Borgna and Rochefort. (1979).

that OH tamoxifen is actually formed *in vivo* and retained at the oestrogen receptor sites both in rat uterus, where it is a partial agonist-antagonist, and in chicken oviduct, where it is a full antagonist.

The site of formation of the hydroxylated metabolites *in vivo* is most likely the liver in all species, including the human. However, to our surprise, we found that some of the oestrogen target tissues, such as lamb uterus and chicken oviduct, activate tamoxifen into hydroxylated derivatives, suggesting that aryl hydroxylases might also regulate *in situ* the efficiency of antioestrogen drugs.

IV. *IN VITRO* BINDING OF MONOHYDROXYTAMOXIFEN TO OESTROGEN RECEPTORS

The binding characteristics of OH tamoxifen to the oestrogen receptor were also studied. We used competitive experiments with [^{3}H]oestradiol and direct studies with [^{3}H]monohydroxytamoxifen which was prepared biologically by hydroxylation of [^{3}H]tamoxifen in chick oviduct or liver followed by a TLC purification step (Borgna and Rochefort, 1980). The affinity of OH tamoxifen was as high as that of oestradiol and its dissociation rate from the oestrogen receptor was as slow as that of oestradiol both at 0°C and 20°C. A similar competitive efficiency of OH tamoxifen and oestradiol was found by Jordan *et al.* (1977) and Wakeling and Slater (1980). Monohydroxytamoxifen was found to bind to the 8S form of the cytosol, i.e. oestrogen receptor, and the resulting complex bound to DNA. Finally the 8S receptor-OH tamoxifen complex was displaced into an 11S complex after its interaction with specific oestrogen receptor antibodies (Garcia *et al.*, 1979). However its affinity for the oestrogen receptor was not modified by the antibodies. This finding confirmed that a non-steroidal antioestrogen like OH tamoxifen was binding to the oestrogen receptor. However, no difference could be detected between the binding of OH tamoxifen and that of oestradiol. A similar high affinity binding of OH tamoxifen has also been observed for the chick oviduct (Binart *et al.*, 1979).

V. CONCLUSIONS

The mechanism of action of synthetic antioestrogens remains unknown. It is easy to understand why these compounds prevent oestrogen action since they compete with oestrogen for binding to the oestrogen receptor. In this respect, it is logical that the high affinity metabolite OH tamoxifen is a more potent antioestrogen *in vitro* than tamoxifen. However, it is more difficult to explain why the oestrogen receptor-antioestrogen complexes are less efficient than the oestrogen receptor-oestradiol complex in inducing effects such as growth stimulation or synthesis of proteins.

Actually, all antioestrogens tested are able to translocate cytoplasmic oestrogen receptor into the nucleus with the efficiency roughly parallel to their affinity for the receptor (Rochefort *et al.*, 1972). This has been determined in the rat uterus, and was also found in MCF 7 cells (Horwitz and McGuire, 1978) and in chick oviduct (Sutherland *et al.*, 1977) where antioestrogens behave as full antagonists. The reasons for the relative inefficiency of the antioestrogen-oestrogen receptor complex have been investigated both before and after the nuclear translocation step. It has been proposed that the *in vitro* binding characteristics of antioestrogens to the oestrogen receptor would allow anticipation of their biological activity since most of these drugs have a very rapid dissociation rate (Bouton and Raynaud, 1978). However this can be excluded, since OH tamoxifen, which is a fully active antioestrogen devoid of any oestrogenic activity, as shown in MCF 7 cells, binds to the oestrogen receptor with the same affinity and the same dissociation rate as oestradiol (Rochefort *et al.*, 1979). Even though discrete differences concerning interactions with the receptor binding site but not detectable by present techniques cannot be excluded, it is more likely that the reason for the relative inefficiency of the antioestrogen–oestrogen receptor complex should be searched for beyond the nuclear translocation step. The antioestrogen–oestrogen receptor complexes are able to bind *in vitro* to double stranded DNA (Capony and Rochefort, 1978). It is possible, however, that they would not bind to productive sites in the chromatin. In this respect, it has been proposed by Baudendistel and Ruh (1976) that the way in which the oestrogen receptor–antioestrogen complex interacts with chromatin acceptor sites differs from that of the oestrogen receptor–oestradiol complex. Obviously, further studies are needed to understand the mechanisms of antagonism by antioestrogens which are currently used to treat breast cancer, and to obtain other classes of antioestrogens which would be more active and devoid of any oestrogenic activity *in vivo*.

ACKNOWLEDGEMENTS

We are grateful to Dr Patterson and I.C.I. Laboratories for providing us with [^{3}H]tamoxifen and hydroxytamoxifen. We thank Mrs S. Ladrech for her excellent technical assistance and E. Barrié and H. Spowart for preparing the manuscript.

This work was supported by the Institut National de la Santé et de la Recherche Médicale (French–US cooperation), and the Centre National de la Recherche Scientifique (ATP n° 41-61).

REFERENCES

Adam, H. K., Douglas, E. J., and Kemp, J. V. (1979). *Biochem. Pharmacol.* **27**, 145–147.

André, J. (1977). Ph. D. Thesis, University of Sciences and Technics of Montpellier (France).

Baudendistel, L. J., and Ruh, T. S. (1976). *Steroids* **28**, 233–237.

Binart, N., Catelli, M. G., Geynet, C., Puri, B., Hahnel, R., Mester, J., and Baulieu, E. E. (1979). *Biochem. Biophys. Res. Commun.* **91**, 812–818.

Borgna, J. L., and Rochefort, H. (1979). *C. R. Acad. Sci.* **287**, 1141–1144.

Borgna, J. L., and Rochefort, H. (1980). *Mol. Cell. Endocr.* **20**, 71–85.

Borgna, J. L., and Rochefort, H. (1981). *J. Biol. Chem.* **256**, 859-868.

Bouton, M. M., and Raynaud, J. P. (1978). *J. Steroid Biochem.* **1**, 9–15.

Capony, F., and Rochefort, H. (1977). *Mol. Cell. Endocr.* **8**, 47–64.

Capony, F., and Rochefort, H. (1978). *Mol. Cell. Endocr.* **11**, 181–198.

Clark, J. H., Baulieu, E. E., Baxter, J. H., de Crombrugghe, B., Jorgenson, E. C., Katzenellenbogen, B. S., Katzenellenbogen, J. A., Luebke, K., Moran, J., Rochefort, H., Sherman, M. R., and Tupert, M. (1976). *In* "Hormones and Antihormone Action at the Target Cell" (J. H. Clark, W. Klee, A. Levitzki, and J. Wolff, eds), pp. 147–169. Life Science Research Report 3, Dahlem Konferenzen Abakon Verlaqsquesellschaft, Berlin.

Daniel, C. P., Gaskell, S. J., and Nicholson, R. I. (1979). *J. Endocr.* **81**, 148P–149P.

Fromson, J. M., Pearson, S., and Brahman, S. (1973). *Xenobiotica* **3**, 693–709.

Garcia, M., Greene, G. L., Rochefort, H., and Jensen, E. V. (1979). *Cancer Treat. Rep.* **63**, 1162.

Greene, G. L., Closs, L. E., Fleming, H., DeSombre, E. R., and Jensen, E. V. (1977). *Proc. Natl Acad. Sci. U.S.A.* **74**, 3681–3685.

Gschwendt, M. (1975). *Biochim. Biophys. Acta* **399**, 395–402.

Horwitz, K. B., and McGuire, W. L. (1978). *J. Biol. Chem.* **253**, 8185–8191.

Jordan, V. C., Collins, M. M., Rowsby, L., and Prestwich, G. (1977). *J. Endocr.* **75**, 305–316.

Korenman, S. G. (1970). *Endocrinology* **87**, 1119–1123.

Rochefort, H., and Capony, F. (1972). *FEBS Letters* **20**, 11–15.

Rochefort, H., and Capony, F. (1977). *Biochem. Biophys. Res. Commun.* **75**, 277–285.

Rochefort, H., and Garcia, M. (1976). *Steroids* **28**, 549–560.

Rochefort, H., Lignon, F., and Capony, F. (1972). *Biochem. Biophys. Res. Commun.* **47**, 662–670.

Rochefort, H., Garcia, M., and Borgna, J. L. (1977). *Biochem. Biophys. Res. Commun.* **75**, 277–285.

Sutherland, R., Mester, J., and Baulieu, E. E. (1977). *Nature* **267**, 434–435.

Wakeling, A. E., and Slater, S. R. (1980). *Cancer Treat. Rep.* **64**, 741-744.

7

Antioestrogen Action in Uterus: Receptor Interactions and Antioestrogen Metabolism

BENITA S. KATZENELLENBOGEN, JOHN A. KATZENELLENBOGEN, EVAN R. FERGUSON, JAMES R. HAYES, NANCY C. LAN, DAVID W. ROBERTSON AND TOCHIRO TATEE

I. INTRODUCTION: POTENTIAL SITES OF ANTIOESTROGEN ACTION

There has long been an interest in the development of compounds capable of interfering with the actions of oestrogens. Antioestrogens are compounds which prevent oestrogens from expressing their full effects on oestrogen target tissues and, as such, they antagonize a variety of oestrogen-dependent processes, including uterine growth and the growth of hormone-dependent mammary tumours. They also act to stimulate pituitary gonadotrophin output and subsequent ovulation in certain women by antagonism of oestrogen feedback at the level of the hypothalamus and pituitary. It should be noted, however, that these compounds are not pure antagonists in some species and in some tissues, and they usually show some oestrogenicity themselves (Clark *et al.*, 1973; Horwitz and McGuire, 1978a; Jordan *et al.*,

NON-STEROIDAL ANTIOESTROGENS
ISBN 0 12 677880 9

1978a; Katzenellenbogen *et al.*, 1979). Hence these compounds are of particular interest because of their present and potential clinical importance (Horwitz and McGuire, 1978b) and because of the variety of possible mechanisms by which they might antagonize biochemical and physiological responses to oestrogens.

The compounds that we have used in some of our studies, CI 628, U 11,100A and U 23,469 have a characteristic triphenylethylene structure (Fig. 1). They are structurally related to the better known antioestrogens clomiphene and tamoxifen and to the potent oestrogen diethylstilboestrol. Our main interest in working with these compounds has been to try to elucidate some of the molecular aspects of their mode of action. Our studies have endeavoured to analyse both the cellular (target tissue) interaction of these compounds, as well as their pharmacokinetic behaviour and metabolism which may markedly modulate their efficacy *in vivo*.

Conceivably, the antagonistic action of an antioestrogen could take place at any of the stages of oestrogen interaction with the receptor mechanism of target cells or at hypothetical control points post-receptor. An antioestrogen might (a) interfere with the cellular uptake of oestradiol; (b) compete for cytoplasmic complex formation; (c) interfere with the transformation of the oestrogen receptor to an active form; (d) interfere with the transfer of the receptor complex to the nucleus or with its proper association with nuclear sites; (e) interfere with nuclear turnover or release of receptor and regeneration of cytoplasmic receptor; (f) exert a post-receptor block (such as at the level of transcription).

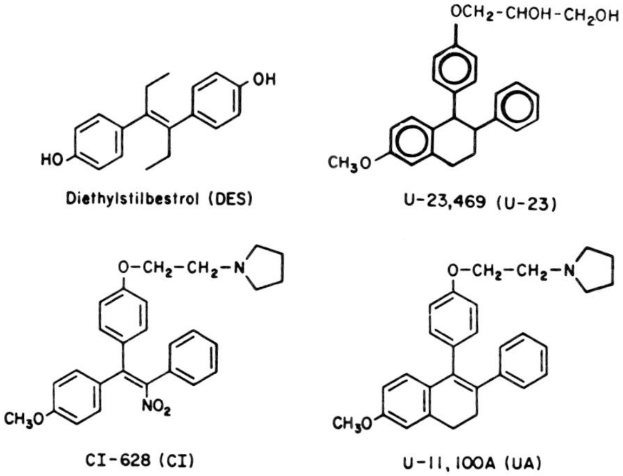

Diethylstilbestrol (DES)

U-23,469 (U-23)

CI-628 (CI)

U-11,100A (UA)

Fig. 1. Structures of the antioestrogens CI 628, U 11,100A and U 23,469. Note their structural similarity to diethylstilboestrol (DES).

There is evidence from the studies to be described here and from the studies of other laboratories (reviewed in part in Horwitz and McGuire, 1978b; Jordan *et al.*, 1978a; Katzenellenbogen *et al.*, 1979; and see below) indicating that antioestrogens have some effects at levels b, d, and e. That is, they compete for cytoplasmic complex formation; they appear to alter the association of the receptor complex and the nuclear binding sites; and, under some conditions, particularly at high doses, they alter the regeneration of the cytoplasmic receptor.

II. EFFECTS OF ANTIOESTROGENS IN UTERUS

Figure 2 shows typical uterotrophic assays utilized to demonstrate the agonist and antagonist character of antioestrogens. Although antioestrogens alone do increase uterine weight, the stimulation seen after 3 days is less than that elicited by a low (0.125 μg) dose of oestradiol. Concomitant administration of antioestrogen with oestradiol significantly diminishes the uterine response to oestradiol, and on the basis of such assays, these compounds are considered to be partial agonists and partial antagonists of oestrogen action in rat uterus.

In some early studies (Katzenellenbogen and Ferguson, 1975; Ferguson and Katzenellenbogen, 1977), we examined the effects of antioestrogens on the subcellular distribution of oestrogen receptors in the immature (day 20–23) rat uterus (Fig. 3). We found that, like oestradiol, a variety of antioestrogens moved cytoplasmic receptor sites into the nucleus. However, while the oestradiol-receptor complex was lost from the nucleus rather rapidly and cytoplasmic receptor levels were replenished soon thereafter, the antioestrogens retained some receptor in the nucleus for a prolonged period of time, and cytoplasmic receptor levels remain depleted for a long period. These findings confirmed the earlier reports of Clark *et al.* (1973) and Rochefort and Capony (1973), demonstrating prolonged nuclear retention and cytoplasmic depletion of receptor following administration of high doses of nafoxidine (U 11,100A).

We wanted to explore what the state of the uterus was in terms of its responsiveness to oestrogen, during this period when antioestrogen had depleted the cytoplasmic receptor. Further studies (Katzenellenbogen and Ferguson, 1975) showed that during the period in which antioestrogen has depleted the cytoplasmic receptor, the uterus is incapable of responding to oestradiol as monitored by the synthesis of the oestrogen-induced protein (Fig. 4) or by uterine weight gain (Katzenellenbogen and Ferguson, 1975). However, after oestradiol, the more rapid return of uterine responsiveness to oestrogen parallels the return of the cytoplasmic receptor.

In other studies we were doing, aimed at delineating the relationship between nuclear receptor occupancy and biological responses in the uterus, we found that long-acting oestrogens, which are very potent stimulators of uterine growth, also evoked a protracted retention of nuclear receptor and a prolonged depletion of the cytoplasmic receptor, much like that seen after antioestrogen treatment (Lan and Katzenellenbogen, 1976). Likewise, our study of structure–activity relationships among antioestrogens (Ferguson and Katzenellenbogen, 1977) indicated that some antioestrogens might be pro-drugs, which might account, at least in part, for their prolonged action on the uterus. This caused us to investigate whether some of the effects ascribed to antioestrogens might be due to the fact that they are long-acting compounds and that pharmacokinetic differences between the most commonly studied antioestrogens and oestradiol might be obscuring basic differences between these two classes of compounds. Therefore, we decided to compare in detail differences in the actions of long-acting oestrogens and antioestrogens on the uterus.

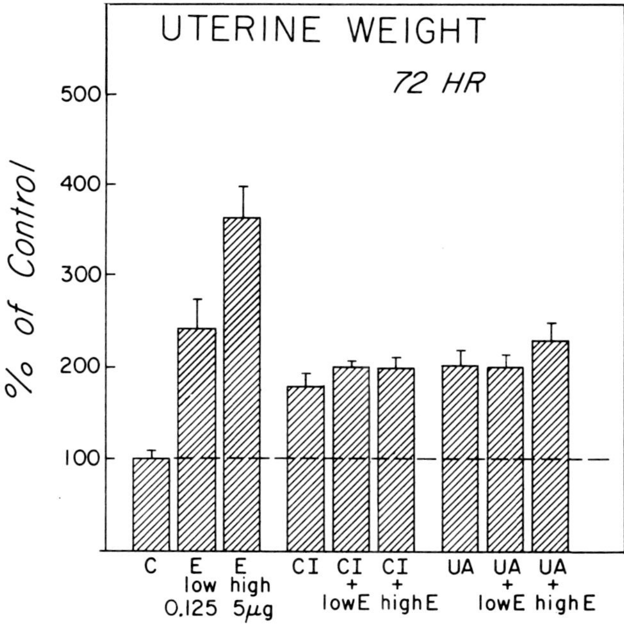

Fig. 2. The effect of administration of oestradiol or antioestrogen alone, or oestradiol plus antioestrogen, on uterine weight. Oestradiol (low dose, 0.125 μg or high dose, 5 μg) or antioestrogen (50 μg) or a combination thereof was injected once daily at 24 hour intervals on 3 successive days and uterine wet weight was determined at 24 hours after the last, third injection. Each determination employed 5 or 6 immature rat uteri. Values represent the mean ± S.E.M. From Katzenellenbogen and Ferguson (1975).

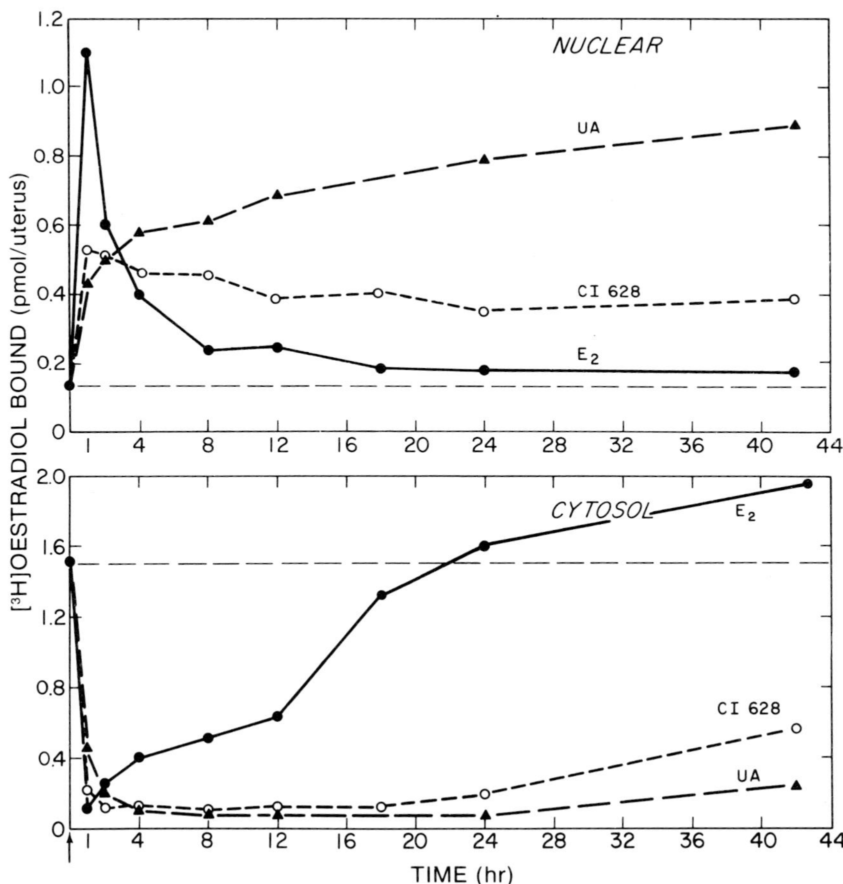

Fig. 3. Content of specific oestrogen binding sites present in nuclear (upper panel) and cytosol (lower panel) fractions of the immature rat uterus as a function of time after a single injection of oestradiol-17β (5 μg s.c./rat) or antioestrogen (50 μg s.c./rat) as determined by the nuclear and cytosol exchange assays. Each point represents the mean of two closely corresponding determinations in duplicate per point (3 uteri/group) and is corrected for nonspecific binding. Cytosol exchange data is after 24 hours of exchange and hence represents "total cytosol sites". In the upper and lower panels, values on the ordinate connected to lightly dashed lines are those obtained for the control (saline injected) uteri. From Katzenellenbogen and Ferguson (1975).

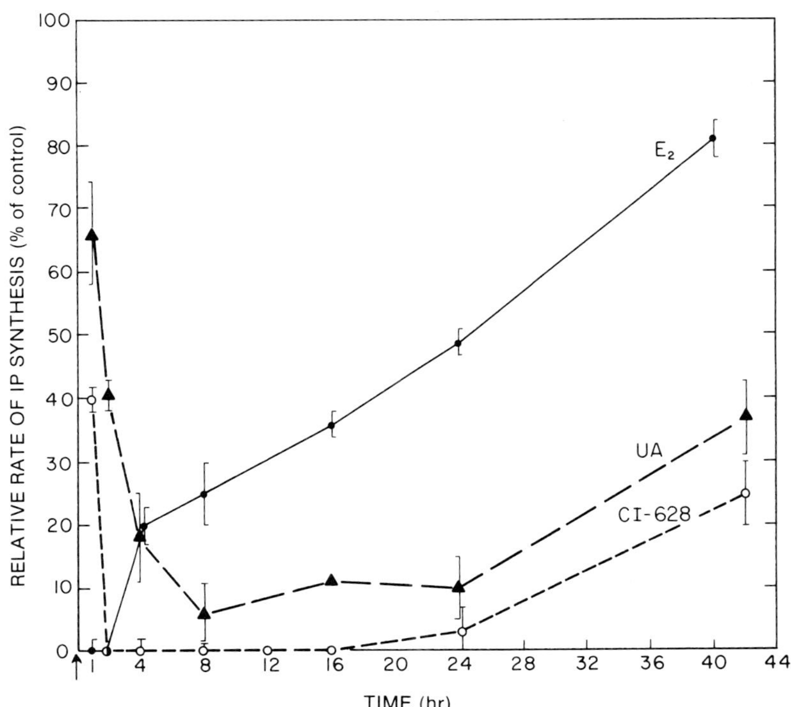

Fig. 4. The effect of a prior injection of antioestrogen or oestradiol on the subsequent ability of oestradiol to stimulate induced protein (IP) synthesis. Note that this figure represents the relative rate of IP synthesis that results from the second injection (5 μg oestradiol) given at the indicated time after an initial injection of oestradiol or antioestrogen at zero time. Immature rats (6 per group) were injected with oestradiol (5 μg s.c.) or antioestrogen (50 μg s.c.) at zero time, and at the indicated times thereafter (beginning at 1 hour) rats received an injection of either oestradiol (5 μg s.c.) or saline alone. At 1 hour after the second injection, uteri were excised and allowed to incorporate labelled leucine (^3H for experimentals and ^{14}C for controls) into protein for 2 hours at 37°C. Control and oestradiol-treated uteri in each set were homogenized together. Following centifugation, the supernatant fraction was separated by polyacrylamide gel electrophoresis and the relative rate of IP synthesis (experimental/control) was determined by gel analysis. 100% is set as the relative rate of IP synthesis seen in the immature rat uterus at one hour after a s.c. injection of 5 μg oestradiol. Each point represents the mean ± S.E.M. of two to three determinations employing three experimental and three control rat uteri per determination. Arrow indicates the time of the first injection (oestradiol and antioestrogen). From Katzenellenbogen and Ferguson (1975).

As seen in Figure 5, we compared the action of a long-acting oestrogen, 17α-ethinyl oestriol-3-cyclopentyl ether (abbreviated EE_3CPE), and a long-acting antioestrogen, U 11,100A, and have analysed single and multiple injection regimens in studying the effects of these compounds on uterine growth and on oestrogen receptor distribution between nuclear and cytoplasmic compartments. Following a single injection (solid line), both compounds show relatively similar effects on receptor distribution and uterine

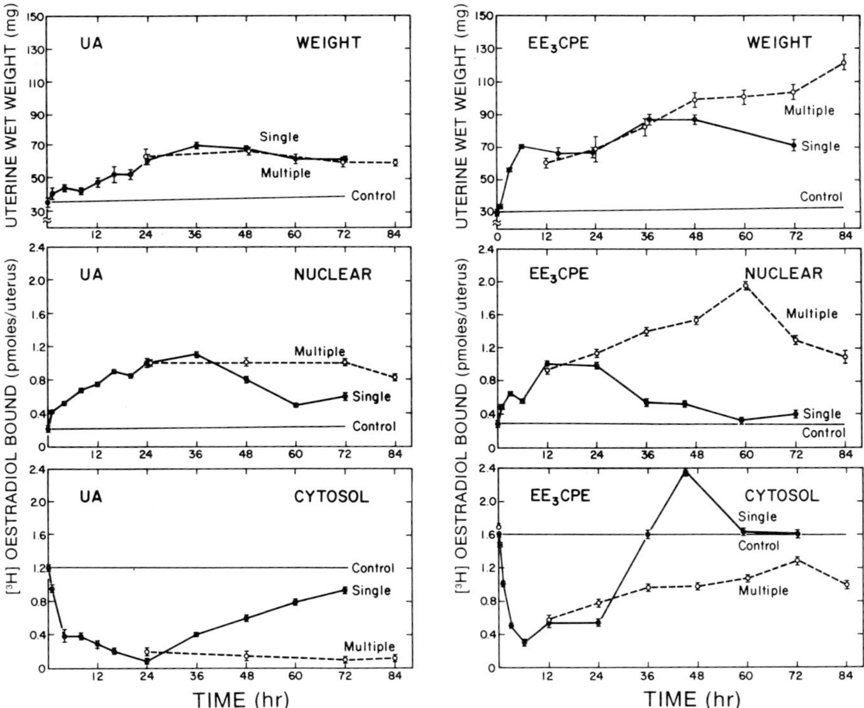

Fig. 5. Temporal effects of single or multiple injections of U 11,100A (UA) (left panels) or 17α-ethinyl oestriol-3-cyclopentyl ether (EE_3CPE) (right panels) on uterine weight and uterine content of specific oestrogen binding sites in the nuclear and cytosol fractions. Immature rats received either (a) a single injection of UA (50 μg) or EE_3CPE (5 μg) at zero time or (b) multiple injections of UA (50 μg every 24 hours) or EE_3CPE (5 μg every 12 hours) and were sacrificed at the indicated times. Uteri were weighed and the content of specific oestrogen binding sites present in the nuclear (middle panel) and cytosol (lower panel) fractions of uteri were determined by the nuclear and cytosol exchange assays. Multiple injections of UA (50 μg) every 12 hours showed receptor and weight patterns similar to those seen after 24 hour injections. Uterine weight values (upper panel) are the mean ± S.E.M. with 6 uteri per point. For nuclear and cytosol receptor content, each value is the mean ± S.E.M. of three determinations per point (3 uteri/group) and is corrected for nonspecific binding. From Katzenellenbogen *et al.* (1977).

weight gain. They both show a gradual movement of receptor to the nucleus (Fig. 5, middle panels) and maintenance of elevated levels of nuclear receptor for 24-48 hours. Both compounds also show a gradual depletion of cytoplasmic receptor sites, and receptor levels remain low for 24 hours after which time they increase. Both compounds also evoke similar uterine weight increases after a single injection.

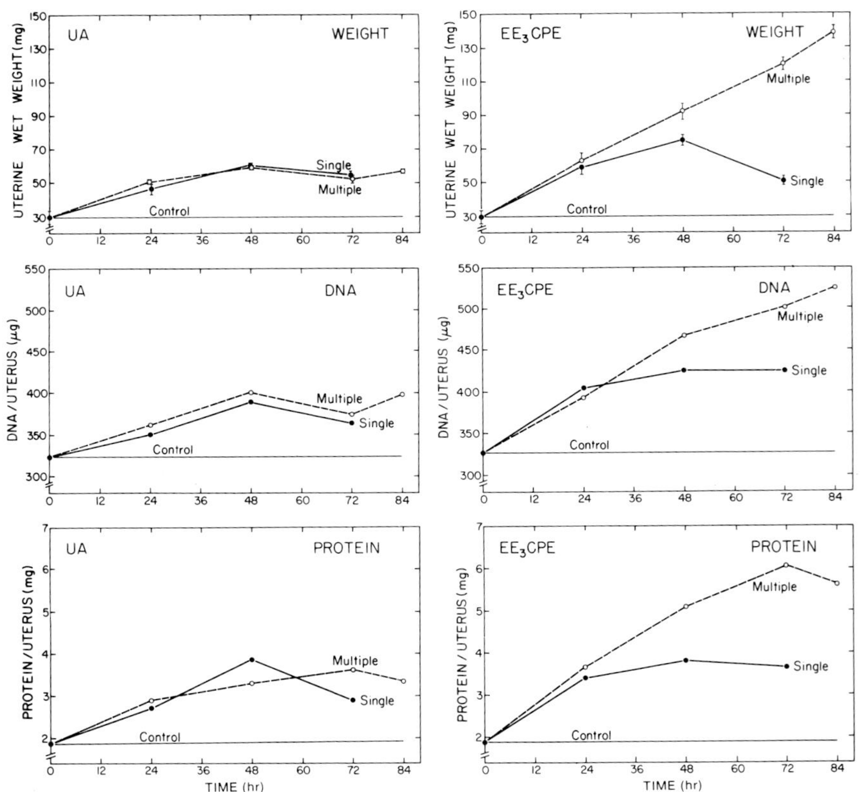

Fig. 6. Temporal effects of single or multiple injections of U 11,100A (UA) (left panels) or 17α-ethinyl oestriol-3-cyclopentyl ether (EE$_3$CPE) (right panels) on uterine weight and uterine DNA and protein content. Immature rats received either (a) a single injection of UA (50 μg) or EE$_3$CPE (5 μg) at zero time or (b) multiple injections of UA (50 μg every 24 hours) or EE$_3$CPE (5 μg every 12 hours) and were sacrificed at the indicated times. Uterine wet weight (upper panel) was determined and uteri were then homogenized; DNA content of the 800 × g × 20 minute nuclear pellet (middle panel) and protein content of the 180,000 × g × 60 minute cytosol (lower panel) were determined. Uterine weight values are the mean ± S.E.M. of 4 determinations per point. DNA and protein values are the means of 2 closely corresponding values employing replicate determinations on 4 uteri. From Katzenellenbogen *et al.* (1977).

Differences between the two compounds, however, become evident following multiple injections. With the antioestrogen (dashed line; 50 μg every 24 hours), there is prolonged maintenance of elevated levels of nuclear receptor and a depletion of cytoplasmic receptor, but there is no further increase in uterine wet weight or DNA or protein content (Figs 5 and 6) above that elicited by a single injection. In contrast, with multiple injections of EE_3CPE, nuclear receptor levels continue to increase beyond the levels seen at 12 hours, and cytosol receptor levels are never fully depleted; there is also a continued rise in uterine weight and DNA and protein content to levels considerably above those evoked by a single injection.

At the doses used in this study, the distribution of receptor that develops after multiple injections of the two compounds is different: after antioestrogen (UA), over 90 % of receptor is in the nucleus, while in the case of the oestrogen (EE_3CPE), 35–50 % of the total receptor remains in the cytoplasm. Thus, these studies suggested that some of the antagonistic actions of antioestrogens are derived from their ability to effect a marked perturbation in the subcellular distribution of receptor whereby very little (approximately 10 %) of receptor is cytoplasmic and further oestrogen receptor accumulation is blocked.

Nuclear maintenance and cytoplasmic depletion of oestrogen receptors are dose-related events, and there is evidence (Gardner *et al.*, 1978; Jordan *et al.*, 1978b; Koseki *et al.*, 1977; Hayes *et al.*, 1981) that antioestrogens can antagonize oestrogen-stimulated uterine growth at lower doses that cause only partial cytoplasmic receptor depletion. Hence, even low doses of antioestrogen may interfere with oestrogen sensitivity in a more direct way than by affecting cytoplasmic receptor depletion.

III. RECEPTOR INTERACTIONS AND METABOLISM STUDIES WITH RADIOLABELLED ANTIOESTROGENS

With the hope of looking directly at the interaction of antioestrogens with receptor, and at possible antioestrogen metabolism, we have prepared two of the antioestrogens (CI 628 and U 23,469) in high specific activity tritium labelled form. In studies presented below, we have found that the interaction of radiolabelled antioestrogen with the oestrogen receptor parallels that of oestradiol in many respects. In addition, both of the antioestrogens are metabolized *in vivo* to more polar forms that have a higher affinity for receptor. These antioestrogen metabolites are found associated with the nuclear oestrogen receptor, and we believe that they may be the true agents active *in vivo*.

Studies with [^{3}H]CI 628 revealed high affinity oestrogen specific binding of [^{3}H]CI 628 in uterine cytosol ($K_d = 1.7 \times 10^{-9}$ M) corresponding to an affinity approximately 6 % that of oestradiol (Katzenellenbogen *et al.*, 1978).

Sucrose density gradient analyses of antioestrogen cytoplasmic receptor complexes on low salt gradients indicated that over 90% of the antioestrogen-receptor complexes sedimented at 8S, as did oestradiol-receptor complexes (Katzenellenbogen *et al.*, 1979).

After administration of tritiated CI 628 *in vivo*, radioactivity can be found associated with specific oestrogen receptor sites in uterine nuclei, and salt extracted nuclear receptor-antioestrogen complexes sediment at 5.4S on high salt containing sucrose gradients, as do [^{3}H]oestradiol nuclear receptor complexes (Fig. 7). In dimethylbenzanthracene-induced mammary tumours, nuclear antioestrogen receptor complexes and oestradiol-receptor complexes are likewise indistinguishable by sucrose density gradient analysis (T. L. Tsai and B. S. Katzenellenbogen, unpublished).

Studies we had carried out with a series of structurally modified antioestrogens (Ferguson and Katzenellenbogen, 1977) suggested that some antioestrogens (such as CI 628) possessing a methyl ether group might undergo metabolism to form a compound with a higher affinity for receptor

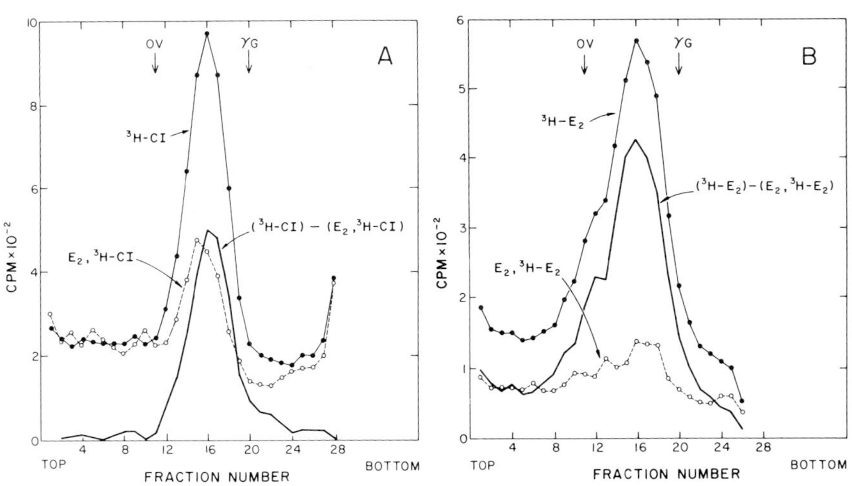

Fig. 7. High salt sucrose density gradient centrifugation profiles of salt-extracted nuclear receptor complexes after exposure to [^{3}H]CI 628 (panel A) or [^{3}H]oestradiol (panel B) *in vivo*. Groups of rats were pretreated for one hour *in vivo* with 5 μg unlabelled E_2 or with vehicle saline alone, and then received a subcutaneous injection of 50 μg [^{3}H]CI 628 or 3 μg [^{3}H]oestradiol (containing 0.9 μg [^{3}H]oestradiol plus 2.1 μg unlabelled oestradiol). At one hour after injection, uteri were excised and the three-times washed 800 × g nuclear pellet was extracted with buffer containing 0.4 M KCl for one hour at 0°C. Extracts were treated with 10% charcoal-dextran prior to addition of [^{14}C]labelled marker proteins, and 300 μl aliquots (containing 1.6 uterine equivalents, panel A; 1.0 uterine equivalents, panel B) were layered onto gradients. Centrifugation was for 16 hours at 4°C at 270,000 × g. From Katzenellenbogen *et al.* (1978).

and a faster onset of action. Therefore, we investigated the chemical nature of the antioestrogen associated with the nuclear receptor. Analyses of ethyl acetate extracts of the nuclear receptor peak fractions from sucrose gradients showed that a polar metabolite of CI 628 was selectively bound to the 5S nuclear receptor (Katzenellenbogen *et al.*, 1978).

This polar metabolite co-chromatographs with the demethylated form of CI 628 in a variety of solvent systems. Further confirmation of its identity with the demethylated CI 628 was indicated by experiments employing diazomethane. Treatment of the metabolite with diazomethane, a reagent that selectively methylates phenolic hydroxyl groups, completely converts the metabolite back to CI 628 (Katzenellenbogen *et al.*, 1981).

Pharmacokinetic studies (Fig. 8) reveal that high levels of antioestrogen persist in serum and uterus for long periods of time (half cleared in 18–24 hours), whereas oestradiol is much more rapidly cleared (half cleared in 30 minutes). Hence, it is likely that the prolonged *in vivo* activity of this antioestrogen derives, at least in part, from its slow rate of clearance, and that the active agent *in vivo* may be a metabolite of CI 628.

Studies with another antioestrogen, U 23,469, indicate that it is also rapidly converted to a more polar metabolite that selectively accumulates in the target cell nucleus (Fig. 9). By one hour after the *in vivo* administration of [^{3}H]U 23,469, there is already some metabolite present in the nucleus, and by 13 hours it accounts for almost all of the nuclear radioactivity. In dimethylbenzanthracene-induced mammary tumours, a similar situation is seen (B. S. Katzenellenbogen and T. L. Tsai, unpublished).

U 23,469 itself has a low affinity for the cytoplasmic oestrogen receptor (approximately 0.1 % that of oestradiol; Ferguson and Katzenellenbogen, 1977). Preliminary characterization indicates that the metabolite is the demethylated material which has an affinity for receptor more than 100 times that of the parent compound (Tatee *et al.*, 1979). In addition, specific nuclear antioestrogen-receptor complexes can be detected after administration of [^{3}H]U 23,469 *in vivo* (Fig. 10). Salt-extractable nuclear receptor complexes sediment at 5S on high salt sucrose gradients, as do oestradiol-receptor complexes (Fig. 10A), and chromatographic analysis (Fig. 10B) reveals that it is only the metabolite that accumulates in the nuclear receptor fraction.

We have now synthesized the presumed antioestrogen metabolites, and we are beginning to examine their interactions with oestrogen receptors. Figure 11 shows competitive binding assays using rat uterine cytosol receptor. It can be seen that the metabolites have a much higher affinity for oestrogen receptor than the parent compounds do. In the case of U 23,469, the demethylated form (U 23,469 M) has an affinity for receptor approximately 300 times that of the parent compound, while there is a 10-fold increased affinity of the CI 628 metabolite, resulting in an affinity for receptor greater than that of oestradiol.

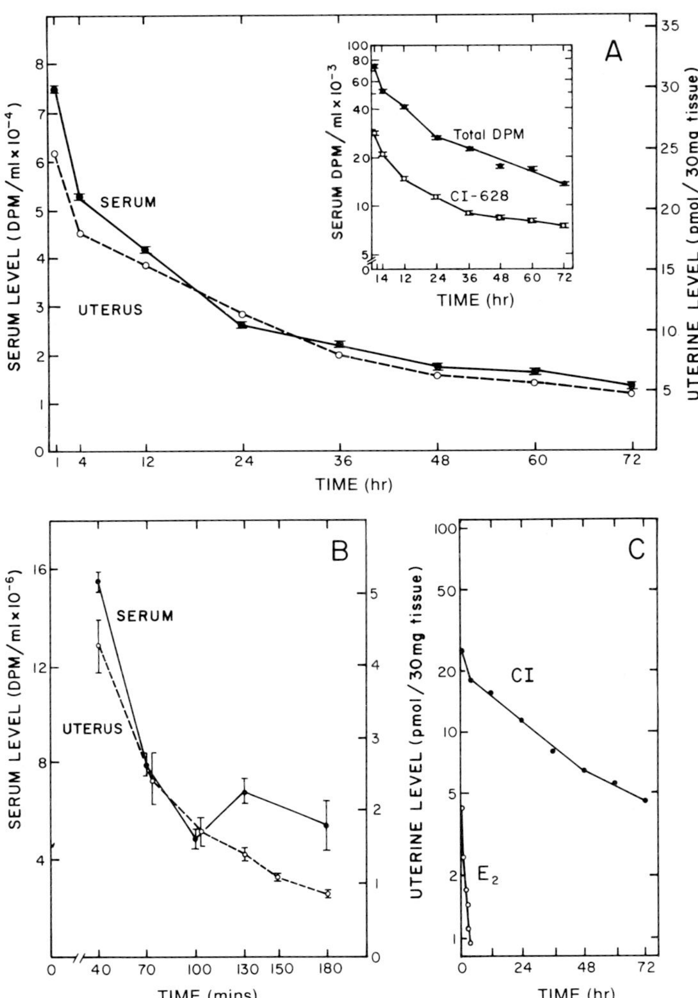

Fig. 8. Rates of clearance of [^{3}H]CI 628 and [^{3}H]oestradiol from uterus and serum. Immature rats (2 or 3 per group) were injected at zero time with 48.6 μg CI 628 per rat containing 0.7 μg (25 μCi) of [^{3}H]CI 628, and serum and uterine radioactivity were determined at 1–72 hours after injection. For serum radioactivity, each point is the mean $\pm$ S.E.M. of three determinations from the pooled serum samples (3 rats per group). For uterine content, each point is the mean of two determinations. The inset is a semilogarithmic plot of total serum dpm and dpm which co-migrated with CI 628 on thin-layer chromatography. (B) Immature rats (2 per group) were injected at zero time with 3 μg oestradiol containing 0.5 μg [^{3}H]oestradiol (88 μCi) and serum and uterine radioactivity were determined. Error bars indicate the range of the determinations. (C) Semilogarithmic plot comparing rates of clearance of CI 628 and oestradiol from uterus. Data are taken from panels A and B (dashed lines). From Katzenellenbogen *et al.* (1978).

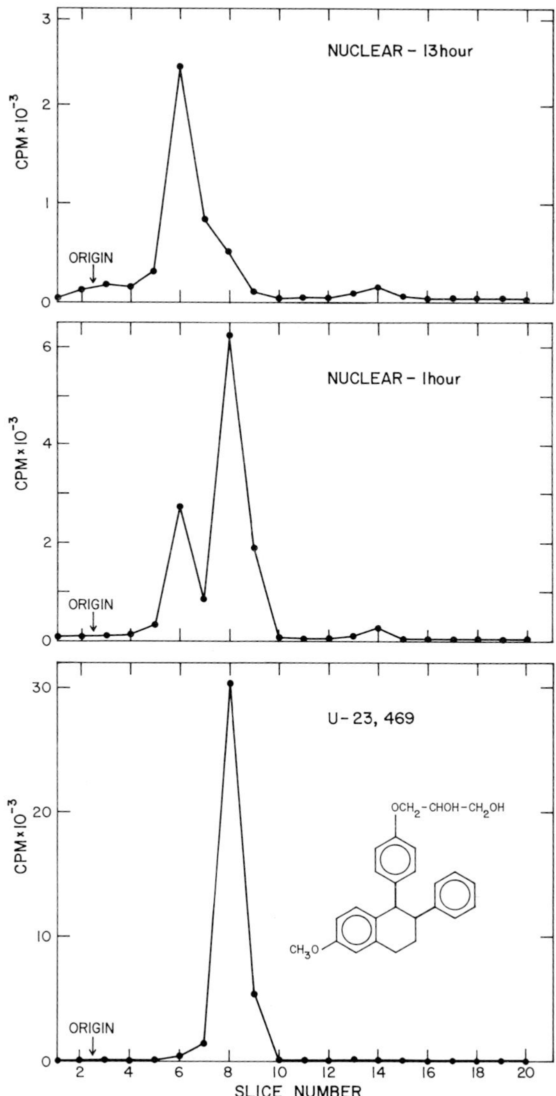

Fig. 9. Thin-layer chromatographic profiles of authentic [^{3}H]U 23,469 (lower panel) and of uterine nuclear radioactivity after *in vivo* injection of [^{3}H]U 23,469. Immature rats were injected with [^{3}H]U 23,469 (25 μg s.c./rat) and at one hour and 13 hours after injection uteri were excised and homogenized, and the three-times washed nuclear pellet was then ethanol extracted. Ethanol extracts were then analysed on thin-layer silica gel plates developed in anaesthetic ether:ethanol (98:2 v/v). From Katzenellenbogen *et al.* (1979).

Since biological potency obviously depends upon many factors in addition to receptor affinity, our present studies have focused on assessing the biological effectiveness of these *in vivo* metabolites as oestrogen antagonists. These studies document that the demethylated metabolites of the anti-oestrogens have a higher affinity for receptor and a greater biological potency *in vitro*. However, *in vivo*, where the parent compounds are rapidly and efficiently converted to the metabolites, both forms have comparable potency (Hayes, *et al.*, 1981). In addition, the high affinity of these antioestrogen metabolites for receptors should enable detailed analyses of the receptor

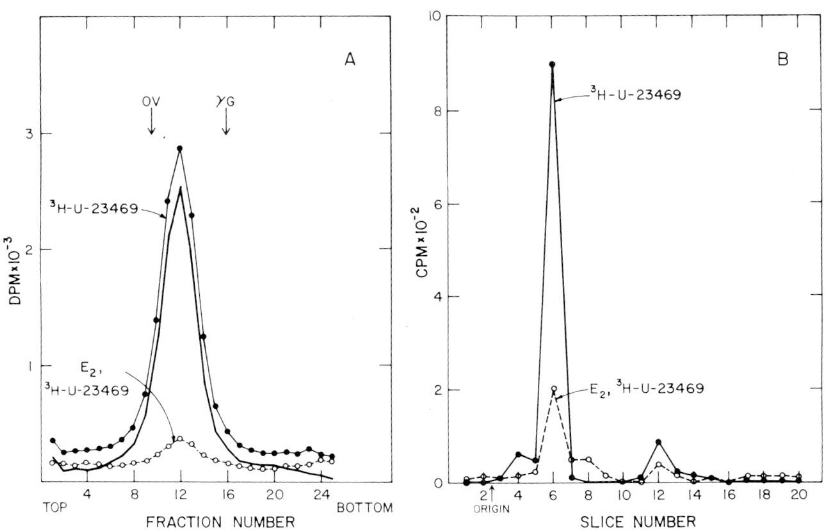

Fig. 10. High salt sucrose density gradient analysis of salt-extracted nuclear receptor complexes after exposure to [^{3}H]U 23,469 *in vivo* (A) and thin-layer chromatographic analysis of 5S oestrogen receptor complexes purified on sucrose gradients (B). Groups of rats were pretreated for one hour *in vivo* with 5 μg unlabelled oestradiol or with vehicle, saline alone, and each then received a subcutaneous injection of 25 μg [^{3}H]U 23,469. At 2 hours after injection, uteri were excised and the three-times washed nuclear pellet was extracted with buffer containing 0.4 M KCl for one hour at 0°C. (A) Extracts were treated with charcoal-dextran prior to addition of [^{14}C]labelled marker proteins (ovalbumin, OV, and gamma globulin, γG), and a 350 μl aliquot (containing 1.2 uterine equivalents) was layered onto gradients. Centrifugation was for 17 hours at 4°C at 270,000 × g. (B) The peak region of the gradient (fractions 9–15, Panel A) was extracted with ethyl acetate and analysed by thin-layer chromatography. The profile of material from animals treated with [^{3}H]U 23,469 alone is indicated by the solid curve and that of [^{3}H]U 23,469 after unlabelled oestradiol pretreatment is indicated by the dashed curve. The difference between these two profiles represents radioactivity associated with oestrogen-specific nuclear binding sites. Authentic [^{3}H]U 23,469 chromatographs at slice 8. From Tatee *et al.* (1979).

interactions that may serve to characterize their agonist and antagonist activities. Of interest here are related studies that have documented *in vivo* metabolism of tamoxifen and the enhanced activity of monohydroxytamoxifen (Fromson *et al.*, 1973a, 1973b; Jordan *et al.*, 1977, 1978a; Borgna and Rochefort, 1979).

IV. CONCLUSION

We do not yet have sufficient information to propose a definitive model to explain the molecular mechanism of antioestrogen action, but Figure 12 may serve to summarize some of the experiments discussed.

The top portion of Figure 12 presents the standard picture of oestrogen action. After exposure to oestrogen, the steroid binds to the cytoplasmic receptor present in the target cell. The cytoplasmic receptor becomes localized in the nucleus and the nuclear receptor interacts with chromatin in a manner in which a whole series of biochemical and physiological responses are elicited, including replenishment of cytoplasmic receptor (Mester and Baulieu, 1975; Sarff and Gorski, 1971).

When antioestrogen or a more active metabolite of the antioestrogen enters the target cell, it also binds to the cytoplasmic receptor. By the criteria

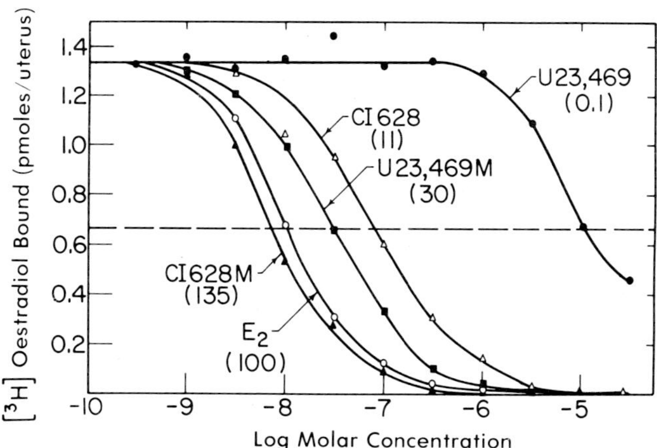

Fig. 11. Competitive binding assay of the parent antioestrogens and antioestrogen metabolites with rat uterine cytosol. Cytosol from immature rat uteri was incubated for 6 hours at 0° with 10^{-8} M [^{3}H]oestradiol and the indicated concentrations of unlabelled competitor. Bound [^{3}H]oestradiol was then determined by charcoal-dextran adsorption. Numbers in parentheses indicate the binding affinity of each compound relative to oestradiol which is set at 100%.

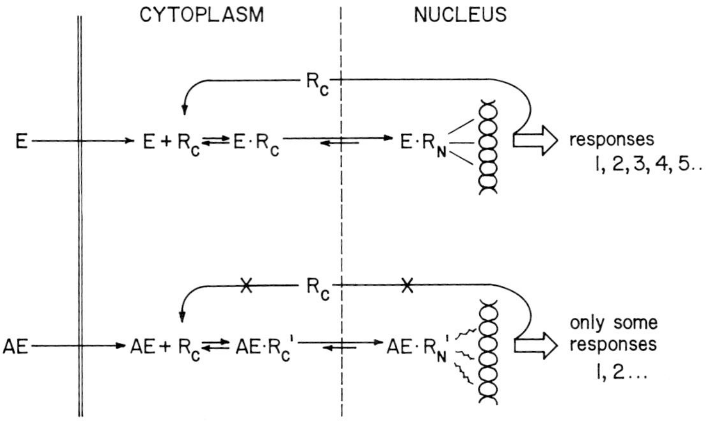

Fig. 12. Model for antioestrogen action, indicating our present state of knowledge about how oestrogens (E) and antioestrogens (AE) interact with the oestrogen receptor system in target cells. R_C, cytoplasmic receptor; R_N, nuclear receptor. From Katzenellenbogen *et al.* (1979).

we have used thus far, the interaction of antioestrogen with cytoplasmic receptor does not appear to be different from the interaction of oestrogen with this receptor, but we have indicated R_C and R_C' here to indicate that the receptor complex with antioestrogen may be different. The antioestrogen-receptor complex does move into the nucleus and binds to chromatin, but its nuclear interaction must be different because it initiates only some responses, and in some tissues, such as the chick oviduct, it does not appear to evoke any oestrogen-like responses (Sutherland *et al.*, 1977), although receptor does localize in the nucleus. Differences in the salt extractability of nuclear receptor-oestrogen complexes versus nuclear receptor-antioestrogen complexes (Katzenellenbogen *et al.*, 1978; Ruh and Baudendistel, 1977) and in the processing of such nuclear receptor complexes (Horwitz and McGuire, 1978a) may be manifiestations of genuine differences in the chromatin interaction of these compounds.

At high doses, antioestrogens influence cytoplasmic receptor replenishment resulting in depletion of cytoplasmic receptor levels. This may account for the antagonistic effects of antioestrogens in terms of certain responses (Katzenellenbogen *et al.*, 1979). However, antioestrogens can be antagonists of some responses such as uterine growth under conditions where there is only partial depletion of cytoplasmic receptor (Gardner *et al.*, 1978; Jordan *et al.*, 1978b; Koseki *et al.*, 1977), suggesting a more direct or active role of the antioestrogen-receptor complex in blocking or interfering with the action of the nuclear oestrogen-receptor complex. Additional studies should provide further refinement of a molecular model of antioestrogen action.

ACKNOWLEDGEMENTS

Research from our laboratories discussed in this chapter was supported in part by National Institutes of Health research grants CA 18119 and HD 06726 (to B. S. Katzenellenbogen) and AM 15556 (to J. A. Katzenellenbogen) from the United States Public Health Service, American Cancer Society grant BC-223 and a Camille and Henry Dreyfus Foundation award (to J. A. Katzenellenbogen). We are very grateful to the Parke-Davis and Upjohn Companies for providing us with antioestrogens.

REFERENCES

Borgna, J. L., and Rochefort, H. (1979). *C. R. Acad. Sci.* **289**, 1141–1144.

Clark, J. H., Anderson, J. N., and Peck, E. J., Jr. (1973). *Steroids* **22**, 707–718.

Ferguson, E. R., and Katzenellenbogen, B. S. (1977). *Endocrinology* **100**, 1242–1251.

Fromson, J. M., Pearson, S., and Bramah, S. (1973a). *Xenobiotica* **3**, 693–710.

Fromson, J. M., Pearson, S., and Bramah, S. (1973b). *Xenobiotica* **3**, 711–716.

Gardner, R. M., Kirkland, J. L., and Stancel, G. M. (1978). *Endocrinology* **103**, 1583–1589.

Hayes, J. R., Rorke, E. A., Robertson, D. W., Katzenellenbogen, B. S., and Katzenellenbogen, J. A. (1981). *Endocrinology* **108**, 164–172.

Horwitz, K. B., and McGuire, W. L. (1978a). *J. Biol. Chem.* **253**, 8185–8191.

Horwitz, K. B., and McGuire, W. L. (1978b). *In* "Breast Cancer 2" (W. L. McGuire, Ed.), pp. 155–204. Plenum Press, New York.

Jordan, V. C., Collins, M. M., Rowsby, L., and Prestwich, G. (1977). *J. Endocr.* **75**, 305–316.

Jordan, V. C., Dix, C. J., Naylor, K. E., Prestwich, G., and Rowsby, L. (1978a). *J. Toxicol. Envir. Health* **4**, 363–390.

Jordan, V. C., Rowsby, L., Dix, C. J., and Prestwich, G. (1978b). *J. Endocr.* **78**, 71–81.

Katzenellenbogen, B. S., and Ferguson, E. R. (1975). *Endocrinology* **97**, 1–12.

Katzenellenbogen, B. S., Ferguson, E. R., and Lan, N. C. (1977). *Endocrinology* **100**, 1252–1259.

Katzenellenbogen, B. S., Katzenellenbogen, J. A., Ferguson, E. R., and Krauthammer, N. (1978). *J. Biol. Chem.* **253**, 697–707.

Katzenellenbogen, B. S., Bhakoo, H. S., Ferguson, E. R., Lan, N. C., Tatee, T., Tsai, T. L., and Katzenellenbogen, J. A. (1979). *Recent Progr. Horm. Res.* **35**, 259–300.

Katzenellenbogen, B. S., Pavlik, E. J., Robertson, D. W., and Katzenellenbogen, J. A. (1981). *J. Biol. Chem.* **256**, 2908-2915.

Koseki, Y., Zava, D. T., Chamness, G. C., and McGuire, W. L. (1977). *Endocrinology* **101**, 1104–1109.

Lan, N. C., and Katzenellenbogen, B. S. (1976). *Endocrinology* **98**, 220–227.

Mester, J., and Baulieu, E. E. (1975). *Biochem. J.* **146**, 617–623.

Rochefort, H., and Capony, F. (1973). *C. R. Acad. Sci.* **276**, 2321–2325.

Ruh, T. S., and Baudendistel, L. J. (1977). *Endocrinology* **100**, 420–426.
Sarff, M., and Gorski, J. (1971). *Biochemistry* **10**, 2557–2563.
Sutherland, R., Mester, J., and Baulieu, E. E. (1977). *Nature* **267**, 434–435.
Tatee, T., Carlson, K. E., Katzenellenbogen, J. A., Robertson, D. W., and Katzenellenbogen, B. S. (1979). *J. Med. Chem.* **22**, 1509–1517.

8

Oestrogen Stimulation of Uterine Growth: Effects of Steroidal and Non-Steroidal Oestrogen Antagonists

BARRY M. MARKAVERICH, SUSAN UPCHURCH, STANLEY R. GLASSER, SHIRLEY A. McCORMACK AND JAMES H. CLARK

I. INTRODUCTION

Two classes of binding sites for oestradiol have recently been described for the immature rat uterus (Eriksson *et al.*, 1978). Type I sites represent the "classical" oestrogen receptor which binds oestradiol with high affinity ($K_d \sim 1$ nM) and low capacity (~ 1 pmole/uterus). Following oestrogen administration, type I receptor sites are translocated from the cytoplasm to the nucleus (Jensen *et al.*, 1971; Shyamala and Gorski, 1967) where the receptor oestrogen complex presumably interacts with nuclear acceptor sites

NON-STEROIDAL ANTIOESTROGENS
ISBN 0 12 677880 9

(Means and O'Malley, 1972; O'Malley and Means, 1974) prior to the initiation of transcriptional events associated with oestrogen stimulation of uterine growth (Hamilton, 1968; Glasser *et al.*, 1972; Hardin *et al.*, 1976; Markaverich *et al.*, 1978). In contrast, the cytoplasmic type II sites bind oestradiol with a higher capacity (1–4 pmoles/uterus) and lower affinity ($K_d \sim 30$ nM) than the "classical" oestrogen receptor (J. H. Clark *et al.*, 1978; Eriksson *et al.*, 1978), and these sites do not appear to be translocated from the cytoplasm to the nucleus (J. H. Clark *et al.*, 1978). Thus, type II sites remain in the cytoplasm following oestrogen administration even through the levels of nuclear type II sites are increased by the hormone. While the physiological significance of these cytoplasmic and nuclear type II oestrogen binding sites remains speculative, it is apparent from studies in the immature rat that elevated uterine levels of nuclear type II sites can result in erroneous estimates of the oestrogen receptor (Eriksson *et al.*, 1978).

The purpose of this chapter is to demonstrate that nuclear type II sites exist in the mature rat uterus and that they are stimulated by oestrogen treatment under circumstances which produce true uterine growth. In addition, we have examined the effects of steroidal (progesterone and dexamethasone) and non-steroidal (triphenylethylene derivatives, nafoxidine and clomiphene) oestrogen antagonists on the stimulation of nuclear type II sites and uterine growth. This was done with whole uterine homogenates and with purified preparations of epithelium, stroma and myometrium. Purified cell preparations were used because we (Clark and Peck, 1979), as well as others (E. R. Clark *et al.*, 1978), had noted that triphenylethylene derivatives cause differential cell stimulation. Thus, in order to examine the effects of these drugs on the oestrogen receptor and nuclear type II binding sites, it was necessary to measure them in the three tissue layers of the uterus.

II. MEASUREMENT OF TYPE I AND TYPE II OESTROGEN BINDING SITES BY [^{3}H]OESTRADIOL EXCHANGE

To examine uterine nuclei for type II-oestradiol binding sites and to evaluate the influence of this second class of sites on estimates of the classical oestrogen receptor (type I), mature ovariectomized rats were injected with 10 μg of oestradiol (80 μg/kg body weight). One hour following treatment, saturation analysis was performed on the uterine nuclear fractions by the [^{3}H]oestradiol exchange assay (Anderson *et al.*, 1972a). Analysis of these data revealed that these nuclear fractions contained two specific binding components for [^{3}H]oestradiol (Fig. 1A). The high affinity, low capacity [^{3}H]oestradiol binding component (approximately 0.5 pmoles/ml; 1.0 pmole/uterus) represents the type I sites which are translocated from the

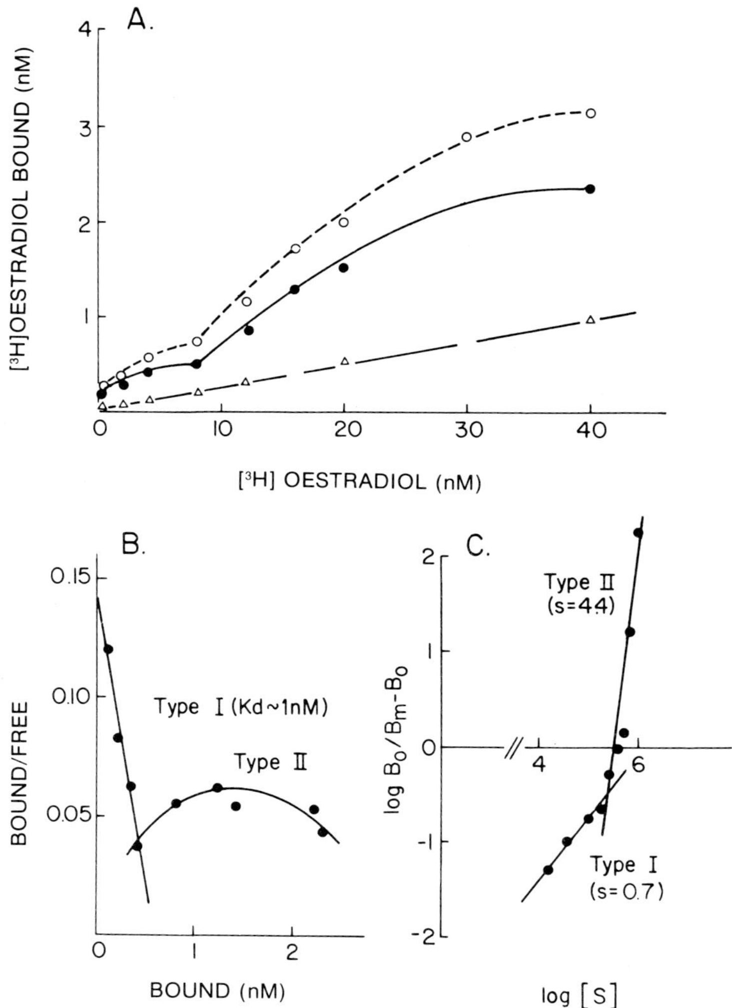

Fig. 1. Saturation analysis of oestrogen binding sites in rat uterine nuclear fractions. (A) The quantity of specifically bound [^{3}H]oestradiol (●) was determined by incubating nuclei with [^{3}H]oestradiol (○) or [^{3}H]oestradiol plus 100-fold molar excess of diethylstilboestrol (△) at 37°C for 30 minutes. Mature ovariectomized rats were injected with 10 μg oestradiol 1 hour prior to sacrifice. (B) Scatchard analysis of specific binding in Fig. 1A. (C) Hill analysis of specific binding in Fig. 1A.

cytoplasm to the nucleus. Scatchard and Hill analyses of these data, respectively, yielded a $K_d \sim 1$ nM (Fig. 1B) and a Hill coefficient of 1 for the type I sites (Fig. 1C). In addition, high levels (>2.0 pmoles/ml; >4 pmoles/uterus) of the second oestrogen binding component (type II) were also observed (Fig. 1A). While not conclusive, the sigmoidal nature of the saturation curve at higher [^{3}H]oestradiol concentrations and the Hill coefficient of 4 (Fig. 1C) suggest that the nuclear type II component may have multiple binding sites for [^{3}H]oestradiol which display positive co-operativity. As predicted from the sigmoidal nature of the saturation curve, a hyperbolic Scatchard plot for nuclear type II sites was obtained (Fig. 1B). Consequently, the K_d for the nuclear type II-[^{3}H]oestradiol complex and the concentration of these sites in uterine nuclei could not be accurately determined by Scatchard analysis. Reasonable estimates of these parameters were obtained from the saturation curve. The dissociation constant for the nuclear type II-[^{3}H]oestradiol complex as determined from the concentration of [^{3}H]oestradiol required to half saturate these type II sites was in the range of 16–20 nM.

While the physiological significance of the nuclear type II oestrogen binding site will be discussed in the subsequent sections of this chapter, it is apparent from the data presented in Figure 1A that nuclear type II sites can interfere with the measurement of oestrogen receptors. Quantitative resolution of type I and type II sites can be accomplished by temperature or by saturation analysis (Eriksson *et al.*, 1978; Fig. 1A) using a wide range of [^{3}H]oestradiol concentrations. The use of single point exchange assays with [^{3}H]oestradiol concentrations in excess of 10 nM has undoubtedly led to erroneous estimates of oestrogen receptors in earlier studies by this laboratory and others.

III. RELATIONSHIP OF TYPE I AND TYPE II OESTROGEN BINDING SITES TO UTERINE GROWTH

We have previously demonstrated that the analysis of differential growth response patterns of the uterus to treatment with oestradiol or oestriol are useful in analysing important events that control uterine growth (Anderson *et al.*, 1974; 1975). The results of such analyses are shown in Figure 2. Oestradiol and oestriol are of equal potency with respect to all events that occur within the first 3–4 hours after an injection of the hormone. However, after this time the effects of oestriol decline rapidly while those of estradiol are sustained for long periods of time. The ability of oestradiol to maintain uterotrophic responses and to cause uterine growth is correlated with its capacity to cause long-term nuclear retention of the oestrogen receptor. Likewise, the inability

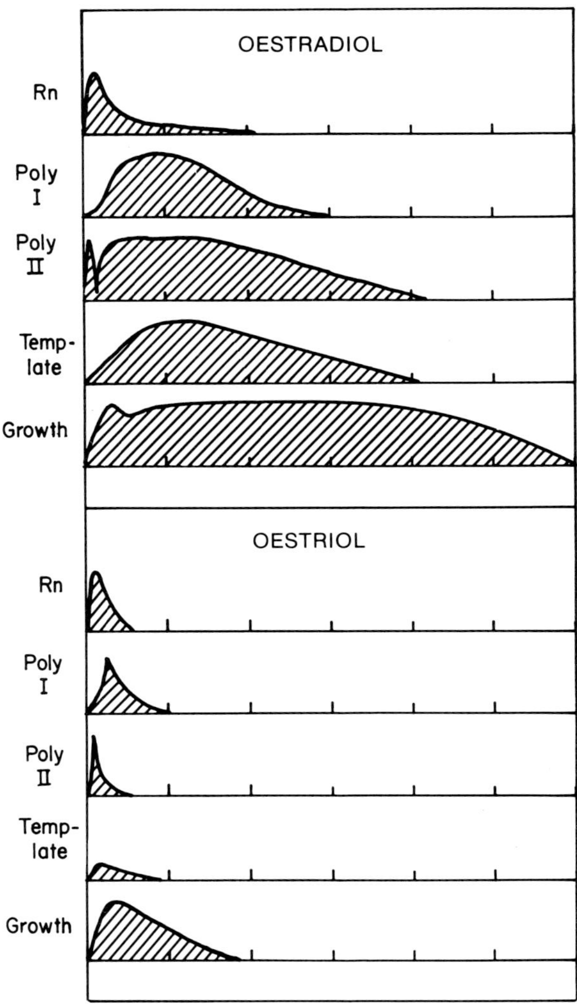

Fig. 2. Effects of oestradiol and oestriol on several uterotropic responses. Immature rats were injected with 1.0 μg oestradiol or oestriol and the following responses were measured as a function of time: oestrogen receptor in the nucleus (R_n), RNA polymerase I activity (Poly I), RNA polymerase II activity (Poly II), RNA polymerase initiation sites (template) and uterine wet weight (growth).

of oestriol to cause uterine growth is due to short-term residency in the nucleus. These data have important implications for certain concepts which have been proposed to explain the mechanism of action of oestrogens, e.g. the cascade hypothesis (Baulieu *et al.*, 1972) and the oestriol protection theory of breast cancer (Wotiz *et al.*, 1978). Such implications have been discussed elsewhere (Clark and Peck, 1979) and hence will not be presented here. Instead, the differential uterotrophic response pattern will be used to ask whether type II sites are also influenced differently by oestradiol or oestriol.

Mature ovariectomized rats were treated with 10 μg oestradiol or oestriol and sacrificed at various times following injection. The nuclear levels of type I and II oestrogen binding sites were determined by saturation analysis as described in Figure 1A. The data demonstrate that the patterns of nuclear retention of type I sites and elevations of nuclear type II oestradiol binding sites are very similar (Fig. 3A). Maximal levels of type I and type II sites were reached by one hour after an injection of oestradiol. The quantity of type I sites then declined gradually to control levels by 72 hours. The quantity of type II sites declined gradually, but was maintained 2–3 fold above controls at 24, 48 and 72 hours. Oestriol treatment also elevated the quantity of type I sites one hour after the injection (compare Fig. 3A and B) and caused a corresponding increase in uterine wet weight at 4 hours (Fig. 3C). However, only oestradiol induced long-term nuclear retention of the type I site (4–6 hours), sustained elevations of nuclear type II sites (4–48 hours) and stimulated true uterine growth (uterine wet weight at 24–48 hours). Failure of an injection of oestriol to stimulate true uterine growth (Fig. 3C) correlated with the inability of this hormone to induce long-term (4–6 hours) nuclear retention of type I sites or to increase the levels of nuclear type II oestrogen binding sites above control levels (Fig. 3B).

To examine the relationship between nuclear type II sites and oestrogen stimulation of true uterine growth, mature ovariectomized rats were treated with paraffin pellets containing either oestradiol or oestriol and sacrified 48 hours following hormone administration. Under these conditions, oestriol treatment results in the sustained elevation of nuclear type I sites and the stimulation of true uterine growth in the immature rat (Clark *et al.*, 1977b; Martucci and Fishman, 1977). If elevated levels of nuclear type II sites are related to oestrogen stimulation of true uterine growth (either causally or as a secondary response), then increased quantities of this second nuclear oestrogen binding component should be observed in animals treated with an oestriol implant. The data presented in Figure 4B support this hypothesis and are compared to results obtained by injection (Fig. 4A). Saturation analysis of nuclear fractions by the [^{3}H]oestradiol exchange assay demonstrated that, while not as effective as the oestradiol implant, the oestriol implant resulted in the sustained elevation of occupied type I sites (0.4 pmole/uterus) and a 6–8

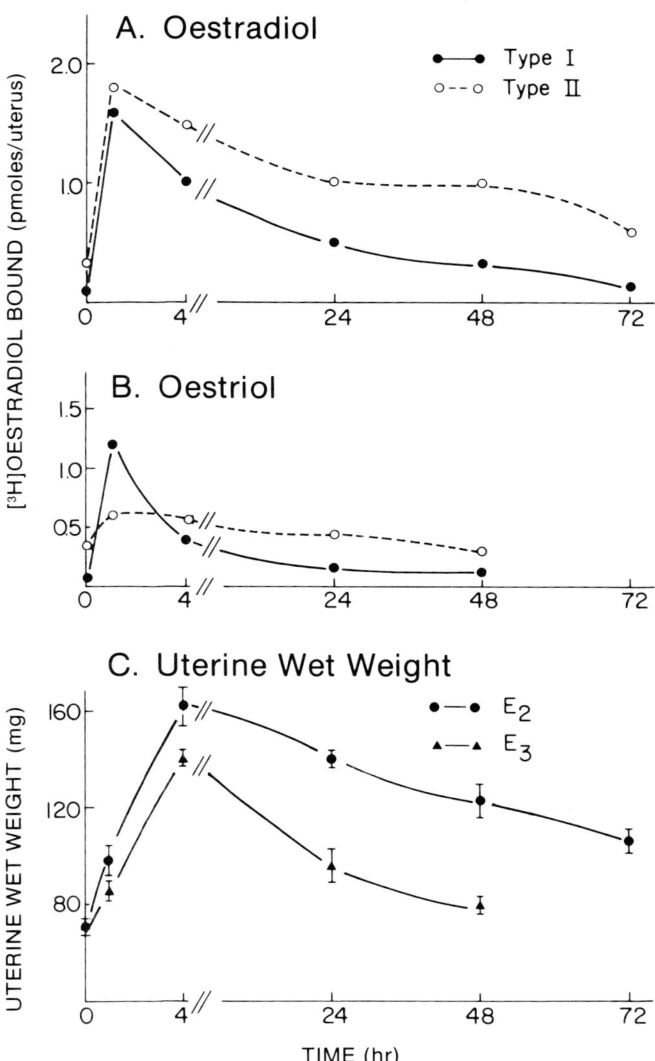

Fig. 3. Temporal effects of oestradiol (A) and oestriol (B) injection on uterine wet weights (C) and nuclear type I (●) and type II (○) oestrogen binding sites. Mature ovariectomized rats were treated with 10 μg of oestradiol or oestriol and sacrificed at the indicated times following injection. The quantity of specifically bound [³H]oestradiol was determined by saturation analysis of uterine nuclear fractions at 37°C for 30 minutes.

fold increase in the numbers of nuclear type II sites compared to the paraffin controls. Elevation of nuclear type II sites also correlated with the ability of oestradiol or oestriol to stimulate true uterine growth (Figs 3 and 4).

These results demonstrate that a positive correlation exists between elevated levels of nuclear type II sites and the stimulation of true uterine growth. This correlation is better than that observed for the classical oestrogen receptor (type I site). Type I sites accumulate rapidly in the nucleus after an injection of oestradiol; however, they decline to low levels by 24 hours. In contrast, the level of type II remains elevated for 24–48 hours and true growth of the uterus is observed during this time. An injection of oestriol also

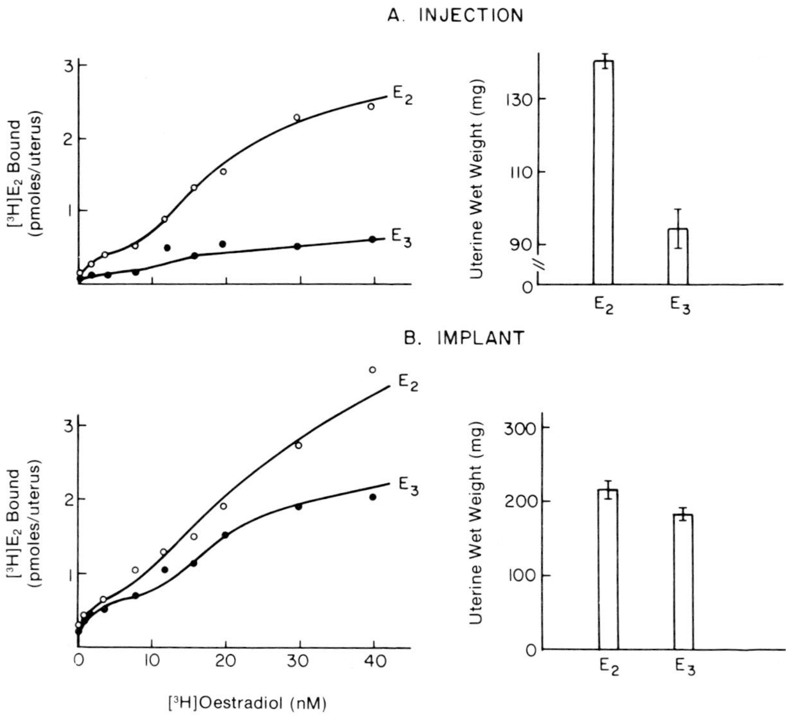

Fig. 4. Saturation analysis of nuclear oestrogen binding sites and uterine wet weight response to oestradiol (E_2; ○) and oestriol (E_3; ●) when administered by injection (A) or paraffin implant (B). Mature ovariectomized rats received a single subcutaneous injection (10 μg) of oestradiol or oestriol, or were implanted with paraffin pellets containing the oestrogen (~ 2 mg). Animals were sacrificed by cervical dislocation 24 hours following the injection or 48 hours following implant administration. Nuclear fractions were assayed for oestrogen binding sites by the [^{3}H]oestradiol exchange assay as described in Fig. 1.

causes nuclear accumulation of type I, but these sites rapidly disappear from the nucleus and, in addition, neither stimulation of type II sites nor true uterine growth occurs. We have shown previously that a single injection of oestradiol stimulated sustained RNA polymerase activity, increased chromatin template activity over long periods of time, and elevated DNA synthesis. In contrast, a single injection of oestriol failed to cause these long-term uterotropic responses (Fig. 2) (Hardin *et al.*, 1976; Markaverich *et al.*, 1978). We have suggested that these events relate to the ability of oestradiol to maintain receptor occupancy in the nucleus for a period of time that is sufficient to stimulate the nuclear mediated events which are obligatory for the production of true growth. One of these obligatory events may be the elevation of type II sites. The failure of an oestriol injection to cause true growth results from its inability to maintain type I sites in the nucleus for a sufficient period of time. That type II sites at least attend, if not cause, true growth appears to be the case since implants of oestriol, which sustain occupancy of type I sites, cause the elevation of type II sites and true uterine growth (Fig. 4). Thus, oestrogen stimulation of true uterine growth appears to result from nuclear retention of type I sites and to be attended by the rapid and sustained elevation of the level of the nuclear type II oestrogen binding site.

In contrast to the above observations, elevations of the nuclear type II site do not correlate with the ability of oestradiol or oestriol to stimulate early uterotropic responses (1–4 hours) in the rat uterus (Figs 2 and 3). A single injection of oestriol was equivalent to oestradiol in stimulating uterine wet weight at 1–4 hours even though oestriol treatment failed to elevate nuclear levels of type II sites. We have suggested that early uterotropic events are not obligatory for the stimulation of true growth and that these early responses do not produce a cascade effect which culminates in growth (Anderson *et al.*, 1972b, 1975; Markaverich and Clark, 1979). Our present results support this concept. The elevated levels of nuclear type II sites do not appear to result from a nuclear translocation process as seen for type I sites (Clark *et al.*, 1977b; Jensen *et al.*, 1971; Shyamala and Gorski, 1967). Type II sites may represent components which are always present in the nuclear compartment and which are activated by oestradiol and/or the receptor oestradiol complex.

The precise requirements for oestrogenic stimulation of the nuclear type II site remain to be resolved. The ability of oestriol when administered by paraffin implant (Fig. 4) to increase nuclear type II sites and to stimulate true uterine growth suggests that one requirement for the elevation in nuclear type II sites may be sustained nuclear occupancy by receptor hormone complexes. In addition, the specificity of the interaction between receptor hormone complexes and nuclear sites which results in the increase in type II sites must also be considered. This conclusion is supported by the observation that, while a single injection of either oestradiol or oestriol resulted in an equivalent accumulation of receptor hormone complexes at 1–4 hours post-injection, only the receptor oestradiol complexes were associated with rapid and sustained elevations of nuclear type II sites between one and 48 hours after treatment. Whether the increase in nuclear type II sites in oestriol-implanted animals was due to long-term nuclear occupancy by receptor oestriol complexes or to saturation of specific nuclear binding sites through a lower affinity interaction with receptor oestriol complexes remains to be established.

In conclusion, these data indicate that two oestrogen binding sites may be involved in the response of the rat uterus to oestrogenic hormones. Whereas responses may be mediated through the interaction of oestrogen with type I sites (Anderson *et al.*, 1975; Gorski *et al.*, 1968; O'Malley and Means, 1974), nuclear events with true uterine growth (Glasser *et al.*, 1972; Hardin *et al.*, 1976; Harris and Gorski, 1978; Markaverich *et al.*, 1978; Stormshak *et al.*, 1976) may require not only long-term nuclear retention of type I sites, but also the sustained elevation of the level of nuclear type II sites.

IV. PROGESTERONE AND DEXAMETHASONE ANTAGONISM OF TYPE II SITES AND UTERINE GROWTH

As discussed above, the elevation of nuclear type II sites is closely correlated with the stimulation of true uterine growth (Markaverich and Clark, 1979) and, therefore, it is conceivable that these sites might be involved in the mechanism by which oestrogens cause uterotropic stimulation. One way to test this hypothesis is to block the stimulation of nuclear type II sites and examine the uterotropic response pattern. Since progesterone and glucocorticoids have been used to block uterotropic responses in various ways (Campbell, 1978; Clark *et al.*, 1977a; Huggins and Jensen, 1955; Lerner, 1964; Szego and Roberts, 1953; Velardo *et al.*, 1956), it seemed possible that these hormones could be used for this purpose.

Mature ovariectomized rats were given two daily injections of oestradiol or a single injection of oestradiol on day 1 and an injection of either oestradiol plus dexamethasone or oestradiol plus progesterone on day 2. All animals were sacrificed 24 hours following the second injection. Pretreatment with oestradiol (day 1) was to increase the uterine response to progesterone, presumably by increasing the level of progesterone receptor (Leavitt *et al.*, 1974; Milgrom *et al.*, 1973; Walters and Clark, 1978). Saturation analysis of specific nuclear binding sites by the [^{3}H]oestradiol exchange assay (Fig. 5A) revealed that uterine nuclei from oestradiol-treated controls contained approximately 0.2 and 6.0 pmol/uterus of type I and type II sites, respectively. It should be noted that nuclear type II sites are not saturated by 40 nM

[^{3}H]oestradiol, and thus the levels of this second oestrogen binding component were somewhat underestimated.

Dexamethasone treatment completely blocked the oestrogen stimulated increase in the nuclear type II site (Fig. 5A) and in uterine wet weight (Fig. 5B; $p<.01$) normally observed 24 hours following a second injection of oestradiol. Nuclear levels of the type I site were very similar (0.2 pmol/uterus) in the oestradiol and oestradiol plus dexamethasone treatment groups, suggesting that this antagonist failed to alter nuclear oestrogen receptor levels at 24 hours. While not as effective as dexamethasone, administration of progesterone to mature ovariectomized rats reduced levels of the nuclear type II site and decreased ($p<.05$) the uterine wet weight response to oestradiol but failed to influence nuclear levels of the type I site.

These results suggest that the antagonistic properties of dexamethasone and progesterone on oestradiol-induced uterine growth reside in the ability of these compounds to reduce the numbers of nuclear type II sites while not altering nuclear levels of type I oestrogen binding sites. However, these compounds may interfere with nuclear translocation and "processing" of type I sites, thereby reducing the availability of oestrogen receptor. To examine this possibility in detail, we measured cytoplasmic and nuclear levels of oestrogen receptor at 1, 4 and 24 hours following dexamethasone or progesterone administration to mature ovariectomized rats (Fig. 6). The levels of cytoplasmic type I sites were identical in animals treated with oestradiol, oestradiol plus dexamethasone, or oestradiol plus progesterone at 1 and 4 hours post-injection. By 24 hours, the level of cytoplasmic type I was increased above control (2.0 pmol/uterus) in oestradiol (3.6 pmol/uterus) and oestradiol plus dexamethasone (3.0 pmol/uterus) treated animals. The lower level of type I sites in the cytosol of progesterone treated rats (2.0 pmol/uterus) as compared to the oestradiol treatment group (3.6 pmol/uterus) is consistent with previous reports from this laboratory, demonstrating that progesterone blocks the oestrogen-induced synthesis of cytoplasmic oestrogen receptors 8–24 hours post-injection (Hseuh *et al.*, 1976). Apparently, dexamethasone treatment does not inhibit this phase of cytoplasmic receptor synthesis (Fig. 6A; compare E_2 *vs* E_2 plus DEX, 24 hours). Similarly, the antagonistic effects of dexamethasone and progesterone on nuclear type II sites and uterine growth do not appear to be the result of alterations in nuclear retention patterns of type I sites since nuclear levels of oestrogen receptor were identical at 1, 4 and 24 hours following injection of oestradiol, oestradiol plus dexamethasone or oestradiol plus progesterone (Fig. 6B).

These data suggest that the nature of dexamethasone and progesterone antagonism of uterotropic responses to oestradiol are due to an inhibition of the expression of nuclear type II sites rather than an impedance of receptor/nuclear interactions, "processing" and/or cytoplasmic receptor

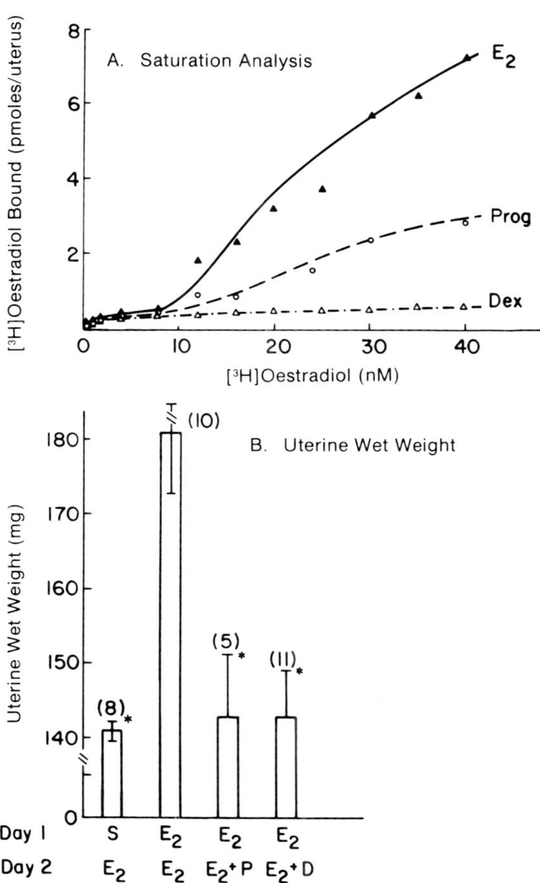

Fig. 5. Saturation analysis of nuclear oestrogen binding sites in rat uterine fractions. (A) The quantity of specifically bound [^{3}H]oestradiol (pmol/uterus) for each oestradiol concentration was determined as described. Mature ovariectomized rats were primed with an injection of oestradiol (10 μg) 24 hours prior to receiving a second injection of oestradiol (▲), oestradiol + progesterone (○), or oestradiol + dexamethasone (△). Animals were sacrificed 24 hours following the second injection. Oestradiol (10 μg), progesterone (2.5 mg) and dexamethasone (5 mg) were injected subcutaneously in 30% ethanol in 0.9% NaCl (v/v). (B) Effects of progesterone and dexamethasone on uterine wet weight. Animals received a priming injection of vehicle (30% ethanol in 0.9% saline v/v) or oestradiol (10 μg) on day 1 and a second injection of oestradiol, oestradiol + progesterone, or oestradiol + dexamethasone on day 2 and were sacrificed 24 hours later. Values represent the mean ± SEM for the numbers of observations indicated in parentheses. *Significantly different from animals receiving two daily injections of oestradiol ($p < .01$).

replenishment. This concept is supported by the observation that a single injection of dexamethasone 24 hours prior to oestradiol administration inhibited oestrogen stimulation of uterine growth and nuclear type II sites (Table I) even though effects on type I sites do not appear to be involved in this inhibition (Fig. 6A and 6B). Apparently, antagonistic effects of progesterone on nuclear type II sites and uterine growth are dependent upon oestrogen pretreatment since progesterone failed to antagonize either of these parameters in the unprimed rat uterus (Table I; compare E_2 *vs* E_2 + P; primed *vs* unprimed rats).

Progesterone and dexamethasone were clearly antagonistic when the oestrogen was administered acutely (injection). However, antagonism of nuclear type II sites and uterine growth may not be observed if nuclear sites

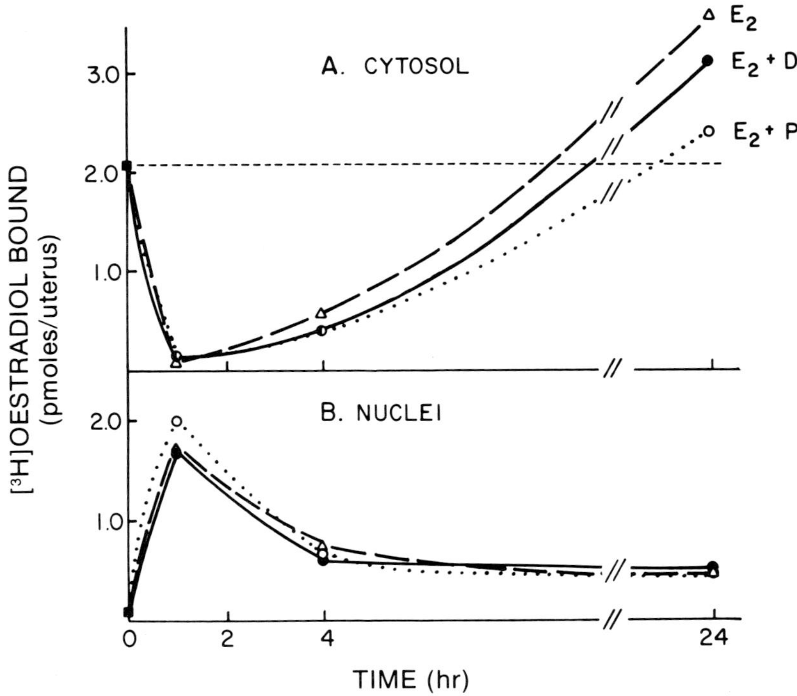

Fig. 6. Temporal effects of progesterone and dexamethasone on cytoplasmic (A) and nuclear (B) levels of nuclear type I sites determined by saturation analysis. Mature ovariectomized rats were treated exactly as described in Fig. 5A and were sacrificed 1, 4 and 24 hours following the second injection of oestradiol (△), oestradiol + progesterone (○), or oestradiol + dexamethasone (●).

TABLE I
Progesterone and Dexamethasone Antagonism of Oestradiol Stimulation of Uterine Growth in Unprimed and Oestradiol-Primed Ovariectomized Rats

Injection[a] Day 1 (0900 hr)	Day 2 (0900 hr)	N[b]	Uterine wet weight (mg)	Type II sites (pmoles/uterus)
S	S	19	80 ± 2.6	0.4
S	E_2	9	141 ± 5.6[c]	2.0
D	$E_2 + D$	10	101 ± 4.1	0.5
P	$E_2 + P$	11	154 ± 4.1[c]	1.6
E_2	E_2	14	178 ± 7.8	8.0
E_2	$E_2 + D$	14	136 ± 5.5[d]	1.0
E_2	$E_2 + D$	9	142 ± 5.3[d]	3.0

[a] Oestradiol (E; 10 μg), dexamethasone (D; 5 mg) and progesterone (P; 2.5 mg) were injected in 30% ethanol:saline vehicle. Animals were sacrificed 24 hours following the second injection.
[b] Number of animals in the treatment group.
[c] Significantly different from saline injected controls ($p < .01$).
[d] Significantly different from $E_2 + E_2$ treatment group ($p < .01$).

are continually occupied by the receptor oestrogen complexes. To examine this possibility, the effects of dexamethasone and progesterone on nuclear type II sites and uterine growth were examined in animals treated with an oestradiol-containing paraffin implant. Under these experimental conditions, nuclear sites are continually occupied by type I-oestradiol complexes (Clark *et al.*, 1977b; Markaverich and Clark, 1979; Martucci and Fishman, 1977), and serum levels of oestradiol are maintained at 700 pg/ml (data not shown). As illustrated in Figure 7, an injection of dexamethasone or progesterone in animals with an oestradiol implant results in a 4–5 fold reduction in nuclear levels of type II sites 24 hours after injection. These reductions in nuclear type II sites in dexamethasone or progesterone treated rats were accompanied by significant decreases in uterine wet ($p < .01$) and dry ($p < .05$) weight (Table II). In fact, under these experimental conditions, a single injection of dexamethasone antagonized uterine wet weight and nuclear type II sites for at least 8 days (data not shown), and this response was dose-dependent. Doses of dexamethasone ranging from 0.6–5 mg reduced levels of type II sites (Fig. 8) and uterine wet weight (Fig. 9) in stepwise fashion with maximum inhibition being achieved with 2.5–5 mg of dexamethasone.

Differential effects of dexamethasone and progesterone were observed on luminal fluid volume (Table II), suggesting that these two antagonists may be acting through separate mechanisms. Whereas progesterone treatment significantly reduced ($p < .01$) fluid inbibition 3-fold below controls, dexamethasone administration did not alter this uterine response to oestradiol.

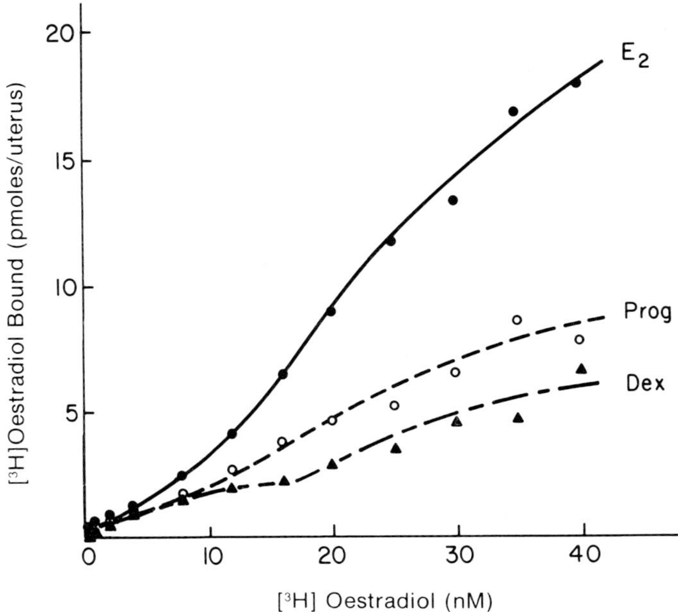

Fig. 7. Saturation analysis of nuclear oestrogen binding sites in rat uterine fractions. Specific [^{3}H]oestradiol binding is expressed in pmoles bound/uterus and was determined as described in Fig. 1A. Mature ovariectomized rats received a paraffin implant containing oestradiol (~ 2 mg) 72 hours prior to an injection of vehicle (oestradiol controls) (●), progesterone (○), or dexamethasone (▲). Hormones were diluted and injected as described in Fig. 5A. Animals were sacrificed 24 hours following injection.

These results clearly indicate that, in addition to the oestrogen receptor (type I site), the mature ovariectomized rat uterus contains a second nuclear oestrogen binding component which may be directly involved in hormone action. As discussed earlier, we have demonstrated that long-term nuclear retention of a limited number (~ 2000 sites/cell) of the type I sites is necessary for oestrogen stimulation of transcriptional events required for true uterine growth (Anderson *et al.*, 1972b, 1973; Clark and Peck, 1976; Hardin *et al.*, 1976; Markaverich *et al.*, 1978). The results in this section suggest that elevated levels of nuclear type II site may also be required for these responses. This concept is supported, but not proven, by the observation that dexamethasone or progesterone antagonism of uterine growth was attended by substantial or complete inhibition of nuclear type II sites without measurable effects on nuclear levels of oestrogen receptors (Figs 5 and 7, Table I and II). In fact, dexamethasone administration 24 hours prior to an injection of oestradiol (Table I) inhibited uterine growth (E_2 *vs* D + E_2)

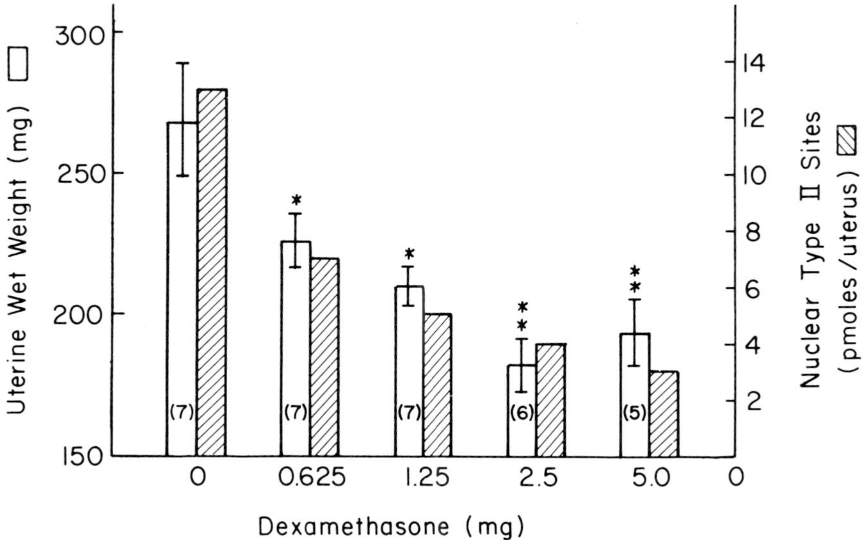

Fig. 8. Effect of increasing doses of dexamethasone on uterine wet weight and nuclear levels of type II sites. Mature ovariectomized rats were implanted with paraffin pellets containing ~2 mg oestradiol 72 hours prior to an injection of vehicle or dexamethasone (0.6–5.0 mg). Uterine wet weights and levels of nuclear type II sites were determined 24 hours post-injection. *Significantly different from vehicle control ($p < .05$). **Significantly different from vehicle control ($p < .01$).

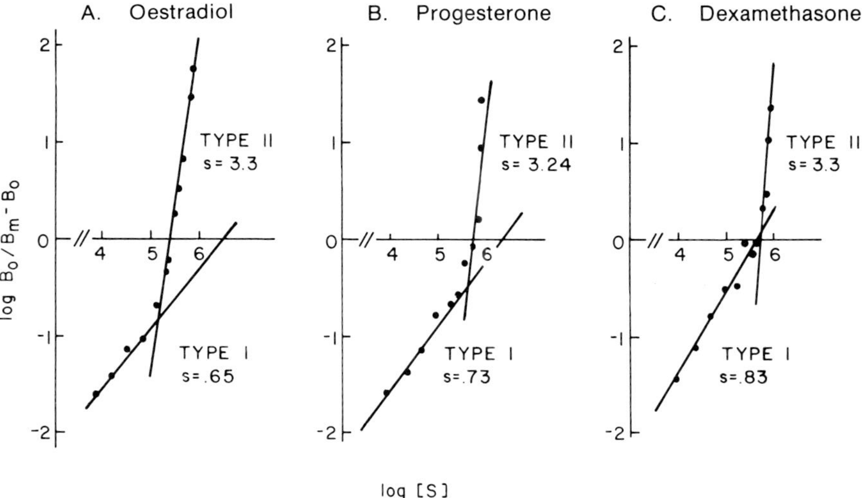

Fig. 9. Hill analysis of specific binding in Fig. 7 for (A) vehicle (oestradiol) controls, (B) progesterone, and (C) dexamethasone treated animals.

without altering the cytoplasmic depletion/replenishment (Fig. 6A) or nuclear accumulation/retention patterns (Fig. 6B) of type I sites. These findings and previous reports from this laboratory have demonstrated that, in addition to long-term nuclear retention of oestrogen receptors, the elevation of nuclear type II oestrogen binding sites may be required for uterine growth (Markaverich and Clark, 1979).

In contrast to our results, which show no significant effect of progesterone or dexamethasone on the total level of the nuclear type I sites, it has been suggested that these hormones decrease the quantity of type I receptor sites in rat uterine nuclei (Campbell, 1978; Hseuh *et al.*, 1976). These experiments employed one point assays with 10 nM (or greater) [^{3}H]oestradiol and the data were not corrected for the presence of type II sites. Since low levels of type II sites will be measured at this concentration of [^{3}H]oestradiol (Figs 6 and 8), these results probably reflect the effects of dexamethasone on type II sites. As demonstrated in the present study and in previous reports from this laboratory (Eriksson *et al.*, 1978, Clark *et al.*, 1979), quantitative resolution of type I and type II sites is difficult and can only be obtained by saturation analysis (Figs 5 and 7) using a wide range of [^{3}H]oestradiol concentrations.

While the present studies have clearly demonstrated the antagonism of oestradiol-induced nuclear type II sites and uterine growth by dexamethasone and progesterone, the mechanism of this antagonism remains to be resolved. Cytoplasmic and nuclear receptors for progesterone (Walters and Clark, 1977, 1978) and glucocorticoids (King and Mainwaring, 1974) have been identified and characterized in the mature ovariectomized rat uterus, and these steroid binding proteins are probably involved in the antagonism of nuclear type II oestrogen binding sites and uterine growth. Although

TABLE II
Effects of Progesterone and Dexamethasone on Luminal Fluid Volume and Uterine Wet and Dry Weights in Oestradiol-Implanted Rats

Injection[a]	Luminal fluid volume (ml)	Uterine wet weight (mg)	Uterine dry weight (mg)
Saline (10)[b]	0.75 ± 0.13	288 ± 8.5	45.4 ± 2.1
Progesterone (10)	0.25 ± 0.04[c]	230 ± 7.4[c]	40.0 ± 2.9[d]
Dexamethasone (11)	0.66 ± 0.09	219 ± 9.6[c]	40.2 ± 3.0[d]

[a] Mature ovariectomized rats were implanted with 2 mg oestradiol 72 hours prior to receiving an injection of vehicle (30 % ethanol in saline), progesterone (2.5 mg) or dexamethasone (5 mg) and sacrificed 24 hours post-injection.
[b] Number in parenthesis is the number of observations in the treatment group.
[c] Significantly different from saline controls ($p < .01$).
[d] Significantly different from saline controls ($p < .05$).

progesterone and naturally occurring glucocorticoids have been shown to interact with both progesterone and glucocorticoid receptors (King and Mainwaring, 1974; Feil *et al.*, 1972), dexamethasone binds to the progesterone receptor only to a very limited extent (Panko *et al.*, 1980). Therefore, dexamethasone antagonism of nuclear type II sites uterine growth is probably a specific event mediated through the glucocorticoid receptor. Similarly, although progesterone binds to a limited extent to the glucocorticoid receptor, data presented in these studies suggest progesterone antagonism of uterotropic responses to oestradiol is mediated primarily through the progesterone receptor, not the glucocorticoid receptor. This was demonstrated by the failure of progesterone, but not dexamethasone, to inhibit oestradiol stimulation of nuclear type II sites and uterine growth in the unprimed rat uterus (Table I; compare unprimed *vs* oestradiol primed, treatment groups). If progesterone were acting to a significant degree through the glucocorticoid receptor, inhibition of these uterotropic responses by this progestin would not have been totally dependent upon oestrogen priming. This dependency on oestradiol priming probably results from the ability of oestradiol to elevate the quantity of progesterone receptors and thus create a progesterone sensitive uterus (Leavitt *et al.*, 1974; Hseuh *et al.*, 1976).

In addition, the ability of progesterone but not dexamethasone to decrease the replenishment of the cytoplasmic oestrogen receptor (Fig.6) and uterine fluid imbibition (Table II) argues for different mechanisms of action. Although dexamethasone (Szego and Roberts, 1953; Huggins and Jensen, 1955; Velardo *et al.*, 1956; Campbell, 1978) and a number of glucocorticoids have been demonstrated to inhibit oestrogen stimulation of uterine fluid imbibition (uterine wet weight 3–4 hours post-injection), apparently this antagonism is not long lasting in the presence of continuous oestrogen. This conclusion is supported by the observation that dexamethasone treatment failed to block fluid imbibition in the presence of an oestradiol implant (Table II).

The observed inhibition of nuclear type II sites by dexamethasone and progesterone appears to be due to a decrease in numbers of sites and not to changes in their oestradiol binding properties. Hill coefficients for [^{3}H]oestradiol binding to type II sites in nuclear fractions from oestradiol, progesterone and dexamethasone treated rats (Fig. 9) were 3.3., 3.2, and 3.3, respectively, suggesting the antagonism did not alter the hormone binding characteristics of this second nuclear component for [^{3}H]oestradiol. Furthermore, dexamethasone or progesterone administration did not change the binding specificity of nuclear type II sites for oestrogens (data not shown). Only diethylstilboestriol, oestradiol and oestriol, but not progesterone, R5020, cortisol, testosterone or dexamethasone effectively competed with [^{3}H]oestradiol for nuclear type II sites. The level of this competition was not substantially influenced by type I sites since these nuclear preparations were labelled with 40 nM [^{3}H]oestradiol $\pm$ 100 or 1000 (data not shown) fold excess of competitor, and the levels of type I sites (~ 0.5 pmoles/uterus) were 10–40 times lower than type II (6–20 pmoles/uterus) oestrogen binding sites (Fig. 7).

The nature of the interaction of progesterone and dexamethasone with the uterine genome and subsequent inhibition of nuclear type II oestrogen binding sites remains to be resolved. However, this effect is long lasting following a single injection of progesterone (48 hours) and dexamethasone (8 days) and is not influenced by acute (injection; Fig. 5) or continuous (paraffin implant; Fig. 7) oestrogen administration. While only indirect, these observations suggest that dexamethasone or progesterone do not block nuclear type II sites by competing with the oestradiol receptor hormone complexes for identical sites in the nucleus. If this had been the case, the continued nuclear occupancy by type I sites in oestradiol implanted animals (Markaverich and Clark, 1979; Martucci and Fishman, 1977; Fig. 7) should have resulted in a diminished response to dexamethasone or progesterone. That the nuclear retention patterns of type I sites and presumable interactions with nuclear acceptor sites (O'Malley and Means, 1974) were not altered by dexamethasone or progesterone administration (Fig. 3) also supports this hypothesis.

In summary, these data demonstrate that dexamethasone and progesterone inhibit the ability of oestradiol to elevate nuclear type II oestrogen binding sites in the rat uterus, and this is correlated with an antagonism of uterine growth. Since the nuclear binding and cytoplasmic replenishment of type I receptors is normal under these circumstances, we propose that the estrogen induced elevation of nuclear type II sites may be involved in the mechanism by which oestrogen causes uterine growth.

V. TRIPHENYLETHYLENE DERIVATIVES AND OESTROGEN ANTAGONISM: DIFFERENTIAL CELLULAR RESPONSE

As stated in the preceding section of this chapter, the antagonistic properties of dexamethasone and progesterone on uterine growth may reside in the ability of these compounds to block oestradiol stimulation of nuclear type II sites (Figs 5 and 7). Neither compound has demonstrable effects on cytoplasmic depletion/replenishment or nuclear retention patterns of oestrogen receptors (Fig. 6). These results are in sharp contrast to those obtained with the triphenylethylene derivatives such as nafoxidine, tamoxifen, clomiphene and MER-25 which have been shown to possess both agonistic and antagonistic properties (Emmens, 1970).

We have proposed that triphenylethylene derivatives antagonize oestrogen-induced uterine growth as a result of their failure to stimulate the replenishment of the cytoplasmic oestrogen receptor (Clark *et al.*, 1973, 1974; Fig. 10). However, such a mechanism does not explain how antagonism is observed when large quantities of oestrogen receptor are being retained for long periods of time in the nucleus. This should cause continued stimulation of uterine growth. Instead, nafoxidine, when administered as a single or as multiple injections, causes the uterus to double in size, whereas serial injections of oestradiol result in a 5-fold increase in uterine weight (Fig. 11). One explanation for this effect is that the receptor–nafoxidine complex has a reduced intrinsic activity when compared to the receptor–oestradiol complex, and consequently the level of stimulation is reduced. Histological examination of the uterus reveals that this is not the case in all cell types. An injection of nafoxidine causes full oestrogenic stimulation in the luminal epithelial cells of the uterus while having only intermediate effects on the stroma and myometrium in the immature rat uterus (Clark and Peck, 1979). Similar histological data were obtained in mature ovariectomized rats which were implanted with high levels (2 mg) of oestradiol, clomiphene, or nafoxidine for 96 hours (data not shown). Continuous administration of oestradiol stimulated extensive growth of the epithelial, stromal, and myometrial layers of the uterus. In contrast, nafoxidine and clomiphene implants caused extensive stimulation of the luminal epithelium while having only intermediate effects on the stroma and myometrium. This differential cell response to these triphenylethylene derivatives correlated with the intermediate stimulation of uterine growth obtained with nafoxidine or clomiphene as compared to oestradiol (Fig. 12).

To study the biochemical basis for this differential cellular response to oestradiol and the triphenylethylene derivatives, we measured nuclear levels of type I and type II oestrogen binding sites by [^{3}H]oestradiol exchange in highly purified preparations of epithelium, stroma and myometrium from oestradiol, nafoxidine and clomiphene implanted rats. The procedures for enzymatic separation, purification and culture of these cells have been described in detail and will not be presented here (McCormack and Glasser, 1980). The saturation analysis for oestrogen binding sites in uterine epithelium is presented in Figure 13. These data clearly demonstrate that uterine epithelial cells contain both type I and type II oestrogen binding sites, and that sustained nuclear occupancy of type I sites and the elevation in nuclear type II sites are correlated to a certain degree with the growth of the epithelium observed histologically (data not shown). Surprisingly, oestradiol stimulation of nuclear type II sites in the uterine epithelium was approximately 2-fold greater than that obtained with nafoxidine and clomiphene even though, histologically, the triphenylethylenes were more

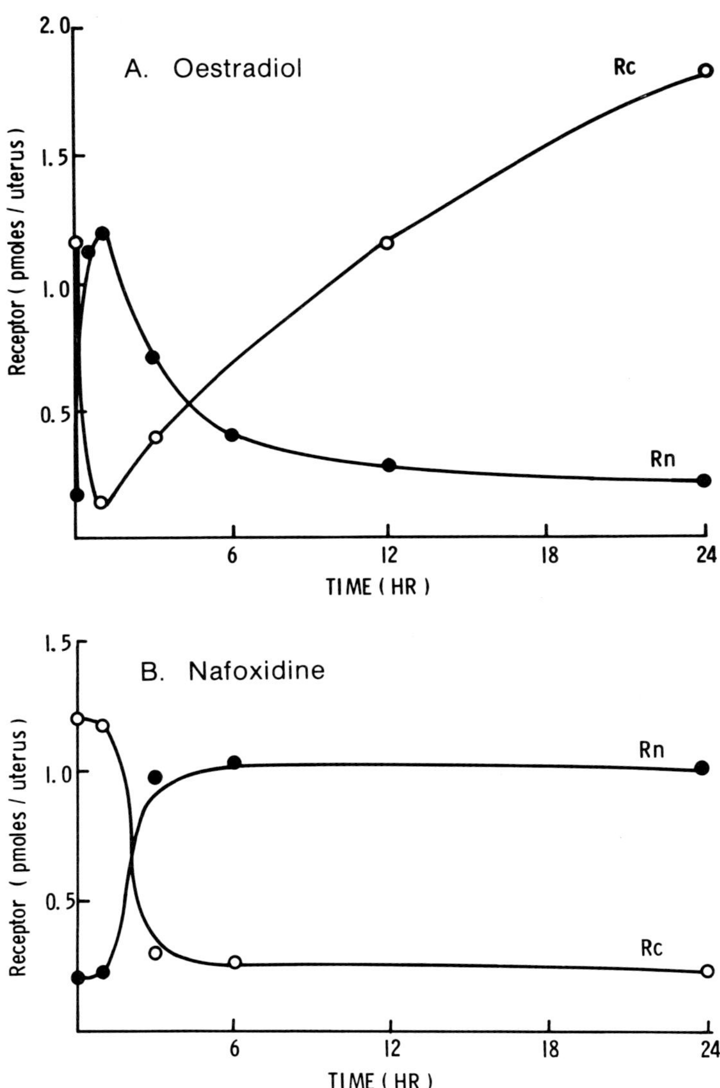

Fig. 10. Effects of oestradiol and nafoxidine on nuclear retention and cytoplasmic replenishment of the oestrogen receptor. Immature rats were injected with oestradiol (2.5 μg) or nafoxidine (50 μg) and the quantities of oestrogen receptor in the nuclear (R_n; ●) and cytoplasmic fractions (R_c; ○) were determined by the [^{3}H]oestradiol exchange assay.

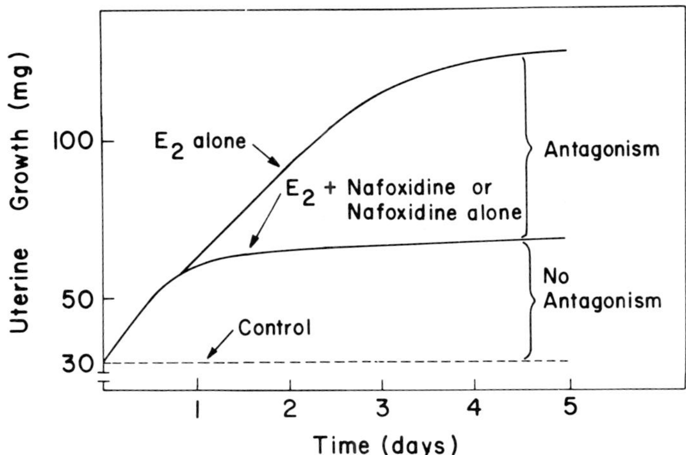

Fig. 11. Effect of oestradiol and nafoxidine on uterine growth. Immature rats were injected with either 1.0 μg of oestradiol, 50 μg of nafoxidine, a combination of the two hormones or saline. At 24 hour intervals, a portion of each group of animals was sacrificed and uterine weights determined while the remaining animals were reinjected.

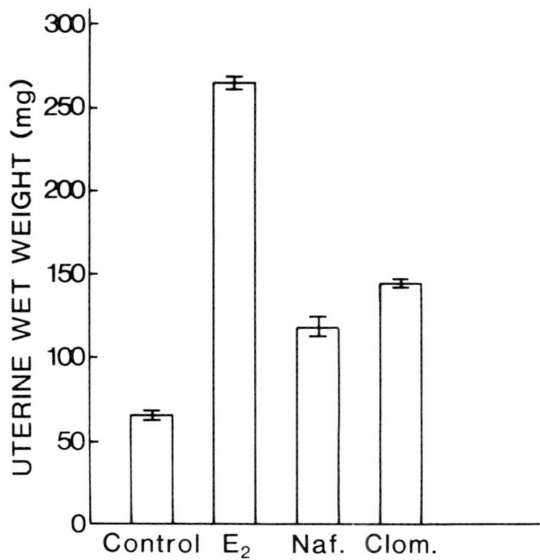

Fig. 12. Effects of oestradiol (E_2), nafoxidine (Naf) and clomiphene (Clom) on uterine growth. Mature ovariectomized rats were implanted with paraffin pellets containing 2 mg (w/w) oestradiol, clomiphene or nafoxidine. Uterine weights were determined 96 hours following hormone administration.

potent in this regard (Clark and Peck, 1979). Thus, whether elevations in this second nuclear binding site for oestradiol are proportionately correlated with the epithelial growth response remains to be established. Likewise, nuclear levels of the type I site were not directly correlated with luminal epithelial growth. Both oestradiol and clomiphene treatment stimulated uterine growth to the greatest extent, both histologically (Clark and Peck, 1979; data not shown) and on a weight basis (Fig. 12), yet elevated nuclear type I sites were only slightly above controls (Fig. 13). Conversely, nafoxidine caused maximal accumulation of type I sites (Fig. 13) and was equally effective in stimulating epithelial growth (Clark and Peck, 1979), but was the least effective of the three compounds in increasing uterine wet weight (Fig. 12). Although it could be argued that nuclear levels of type I sites are not different from controls in the clomiphene and oestradiol treated rats (Fig. 13), this is probably due to a "repartitioning" of cytoplasmic sites to the nucleus which has been observed following both enzymatic (McCormack and Glasser, 1980) and mechanical (Martel and Psychoyos, 1978) methods of cell separation.

Nuclear levels of both oestrogen binding sites in nuclei from uterine stromal cells more closely correlated with the uterotropic responses to oestradiol and the triphenylethylene derivatives (Fig. 14). The ability of nafoxidine, clomiphene, and oestradiol in stimulating uterine growth (Fig. 12)

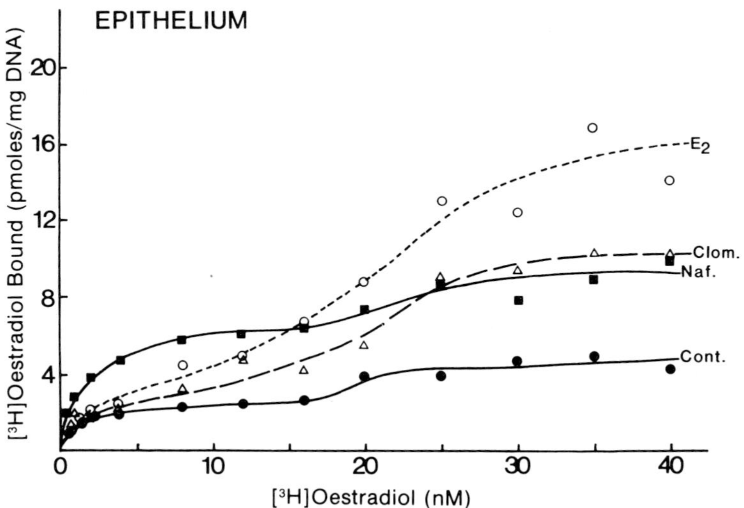

Fig. 13. Saturation analysis for nuclear oestrogen binding sites in uterine epithelial cells from controls (●), oestradiol (○), nafoxidine (■), and clomiphene (△) treated rats. Hormones (2 mg) were administered in paraffin pellets 96 hours prior to sacrifice. Uterine epithelial cells were isolated exactly as described by McCormack and Glasser (1980).

correlated with corresponding increases in nuclear accumulation of type I sites and the stimulation of type II oestrogen binding sites. Similar, but more pronounced effects were observed in cellular preparations of myometrium (Fig. 15). In this tissue oestradiol elevated the level of type II sites 30-fold above controls, while nafoxidine and clomiphene had little effect on type II in the myometrium. This ability of oestradiol and the inability of nafoxidine and clomiphene to cause elevations in type II sites is highly correlated with their differential capacities to stimulate growth in the myometrium (Clark and Peck, 1979; data not shown). Nuclear levels of type I sites in oestradiol, clomiphene and nafoxidine treated rats were not significantly elevated above controls (Fig. 15), perhaps because of a "repartitioning" of sites between the cytoplasm and nucleus following cell isolation as described earlier.

Due to the potential for "artifactual" redistribution of type I sites during the cellular preparations, accurate correlations between nuclear levels of these sites and oestrogenic response are not possible at this time. These studies, however, do show positive correlations between elevated levels of nuclear type II sites and the differential cellular response to oestradiol and the triphenylethylene derivatives. These results are summarized in Figure 16. With the exception of the discrepancies previously noted for the uterine

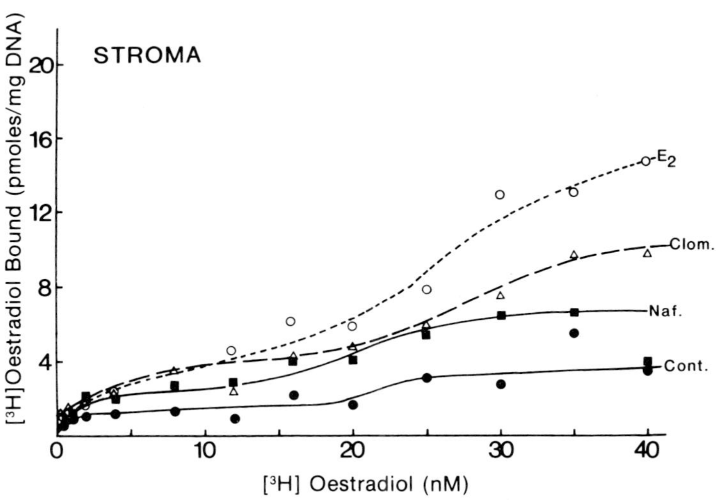

Fig. 14. Saturation analysis for nuclear oestrogen binding sites in purified stromal cells from paraffin controls (●), oestradiol (○), nafoxidine (■), and clomiphene (△) implanted rats. Stromal cells were isolated enzymatically as described by McCormack and Glasser (1980).

epithelium (Fig. 16A), there appears to be a direct correlation between the differential stimulation of uterine growth (Fig. 16) and nuclear levels of type II sites. The more pronounced the oestrogenic properties of the compound (oestradiol < clomiphene < nafoxidine), the more dramatic the uterine growth response (Fig. 16).

From these studies, we conclude that oestradiol, clomiphene and nafoxidine cause accumulation of type I sites in the epithelium, stroma, and myometrium of the rat uterus. Likewise, nuclear type II sites are elevated to some degree in all three tissues; however, the ability of oestradiol to stimulate these sites in the myometrium greatly exceeds that of nafoxidine or clomiphene. This stimulation of nuclear type II sites is correlated with the agonistic properties of oestradiol, while the reduced responses observed with clomiphene and nafoxidine are correlated with their antagonistic properties.

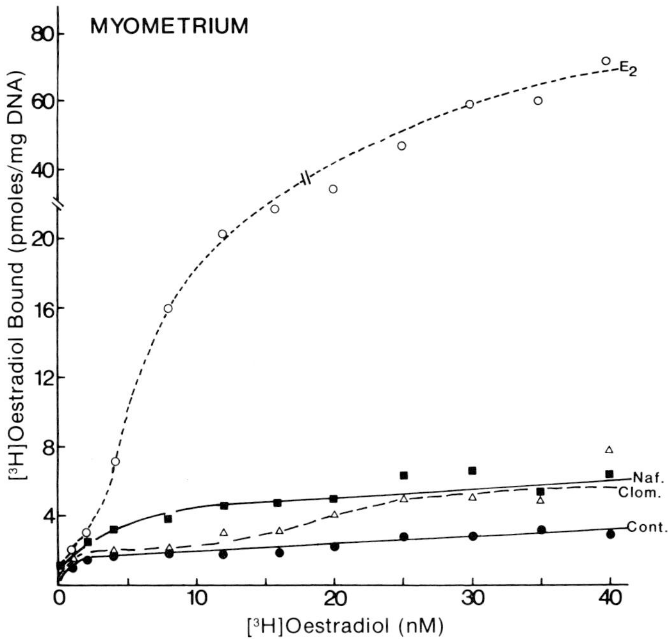

Fig. 15. Saturation analysis for nuclear oestrogen binding sites in purified myometrial cell preparations (McCormack and Glasser, 1980) from paraffin controls (●), oestradiol (○), nafoxidine (■), and clomiphene (△) implanted rats 96 hours following hormone (2 mg) administration.

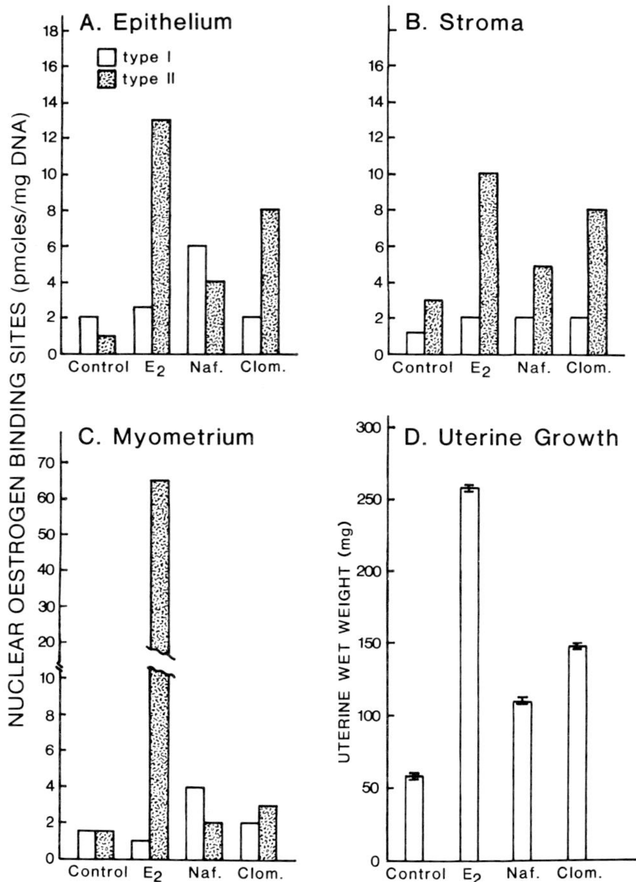

Fig. 16. Summary of data from Figs 13, 14, and 15. Type I and type II sites were quantitated graphically as described in detail (J.H. Clark *et al.*, 1978). Uterine wet weights were determined 96 hours following hormone administration (2 mg) by paraffin implant.

VI. CONCLUSIONS

These studies have demonstrated that, in addition to the oestrogen receptor, nuclear type II sites may be involved in the mechanism by which oestrogens and antagonists stimulate and inhibit the growth of the rat uterus. The interaction of an oestrogen or antagonist with cytoplasmic type I sites and subsequent nuclear retention of receptor oestrogen ligand complexes is undoubtably a primary event in steroid hormone action (O'Malley and

Means, 1974). However, elevations in nuclear type II sites precede and persist throughout the entire duration of true uterine growth (Fig. 3). This relationship is extended by the observations that were made with the short acting oestrogen, oestriol. The inability of oestriol to stimulate true uterine growth when administered by injection is correlated with the short-term nuclear residency of the oestrogen receptor–oestriol complex (Fig. 3), and its failure to elevate nuclear type II sites. Under conditions where nuclei are continually occupied by type I oestradiol complexes (hormone implant), nuclear type II sites are elevated by oestriol and uterine growth is observed (Fig. 4).

In further support of this concept is the observation that oestrogen antagonists such as dexamethasone and progesterone antagonize the growth response to oestradiol by mechanisms which may involve the inhibition of nuclear type II sites (Figs 5, 7 and 8). Surprisingly, this antagonism apparently does not involve the oestrogen receptor directly. These sites (type I) undergo normal cytoplasmic depletion/replenishment and nuclear retention in dexamethasone-treated and progesterone-treated animals (Fig 6). Thus, the primary mechanism by which dexamethasone and progesterone antagonize uterotropic responses appears to occur through an inhibition of nuclear type II sites.

These results with dexamethasone and progesterone are in sharp contrast with studies on the mechanism of action of the triphenylethylene derivatives (Clark *et al.*, 1973; Katzenellenbogen and Ferguson, 1975; Katzenellenbogen *et al.*, 1977). These compounds probably interfere with the cytoplasmic replenishment of the oestrogen receptor (Fig. 11) so that, when administered by multiple injection (Fig. 10) or paraffin implant, the uterus is insensitive to subsequent oestrogen administration. Failure to replenish cytoplasmic type I sites following nafoxidine or clomiphene treatment is apparently related to an atypical interaction of the oestrogen receptor–antagonist complex with the genome, since oestradiol or oestriol, even when administered continuously by paraffin implant, facilitate cytoplasmic receptor replenishment (data not shown). If this were not the case, one might predict oestradiol or oestriol implants to cause only a doubling in uterine weight (24–48 hours), as is the case for nafoxidine or clomiphene, instead of the 5-fold increases which were observed with these oestrogens (Fig. 12).

In addition to effects on cytoplasmic receptor replenishment, the mechanism of action of triphenylethylene derivatives may also involve a differential cell response in the uterus. The basis for this response is not well understood. The uterine epithelium, stroma and myometrium all contain oestrogen receptors which accumulate in the nucleus following nafoxidine or clomiphene treatment (Figs 13–16), yet these compounds primarily stimulate the luminal epithelium (Clark and Peck, 1979). The basis for the differential cell response cannot be solely attributed to a deficiency in the oestrogen receptor–antagonist complex or its interaction with nuclear sites. The present studies, particularly in uterine myometrial cells, suggest that the antagonistic properties of nafoxidine and clomiphene may reside in their inability to stimulate nuclear type II sites. Oestradiol increased these sites 30-fold in uterine myometrium, whereas nafoxidine and clomiphene were only slightly stimulatory (Fig. 16). The inability of these drugs to stimulate nuclear type II sites could be related to their failure to cause replenishment of type I sites; however, this does not seem likely. Both dexamethasone and progesterone block oestrogen stimulation of nuclear type II sites and uterine growth (Fig. 5) without having any effects on the nuclear retention or cytoplasmic depletion/replenishment patterns of type I sites (Fig. 6). Thus, it is unlikely that the failure of the triphenylethylenes to cause cytoplasmic receptor replenishment is a direct result of their inability to stimulate nuclear type II sites.

The implications of these studies regarding the differential stimulation of uterine cells by oestrogen agonists/antagonists are far reaching. Triphenylethylene derivatives are generally considered to be weakly oestrogenic, and they are primarily used as antioestrogens. It is clear from the studies presented here and elsewhere (Clark and Peck, 1979) that these designations require reassessment. Triphenylethylene derivatives are fully oestrogenic in the luminal epithelium of the rat uterus, and their potency is near that of oestradiol (unpublished observations). In contrast, these drugs display mixed agonist/antagonist functions in the stroma and myometrium. Therefore, a proper evaluation of their relative agonist/antagonist properties must take into consideration the cell or tissue type being studied.

Differential cell stimulation may explain the paradoxical effects that triphenylethylene derivatives have on the stimulation of inhibition of ovulation (Holtkamp, *et al.*, 1960; Ross, *et al.*, 1973). These drugs are known to bind oestrogen receptors in the hypothalamus and pituitary (Clark and Peck, 1979). By analogy to the effects on the uterus, they may have a positive effect on some hypothalamic and/or pituitary cells, while in other cell types negative effects may predominate.

Differential cell stimulation of the uterine epithelium during the perinatal period in rats is known to be associated with the subsequent development of reproductive tract abnormalities (Clark and McCormack, 1977; McCormack and Clark, 1979). Thus, exposure to drugs such as clomiphene, which is routinely used for the induction of ovulation in infertile women, could have profound effects in the human. We have recently demonstrated that clomiphene can stimulate endometrial proliferation in the castrated baboon (Clark, *et al.*, 1980), and evidence from the literature indicates that this can occur in humans. Since treatment with clomiphene can result in a situation which resembles continuous oestrogen exposure, the potential danger should be obvious.

REFERENCES

Anderson, J. N., Clark, J. H., and Peck, E. J., Jr. (1972a). *Biochem. J.* **126**, 561–567.

Anderson, J. N., Clark, J. H., and Peck, E. J., Jr. (1972b). *Biochem. Biophys. Res. Commun.* **48**, 1460–1468.

Anderson, J. N., Peck, E. J., Jr., and Clark, J. H. (1973). *Endocrinology* **92**, 1488–1495.

Anderson, J. N., Peck, E. J., Jr., and Clark, J. H. (1974). *Endocrinology* **95**, 174–178.

Anderson, J. N., Peck, E. J., Jr., and Clark, J. H. (1975). *Endocrinology* **96**, 160–167.

Baulieu, E. E., Wira, C. R., Milgrom, E., and Raynaud-Jammett, C. (1972). *In* "Karolinska Symposia on Research Methods in Reproductive Endocrinology: Protein Synthesis in Reproductive Tissue" (E. Dicsfausy, ed.), pp. 396–419. Karolinska Institutet, Stockholm.

Campbell, P. S. (1978). *Endocrinology* **103**, 716–723.

Clark, E. R., Dix, C. J., Jordan, V. C., Prestwich, G., and Sexton, S. (1978). *Br. J. Pharmacol.* **62**, 442P–443P.

Clark, J. H., and McCormack, S. A. (1977). *Science* **197**, 164–165.

Clark, J. H., and Peck, E. J., Jr. (1976). *Nature* **260**, 635–637.

Clark, J. H., and Peck, E. J., Jr. (1979). *In* "Female Sex Steroids: Receptors and Function" pp. 1–102. Springer-Verlag, Berlin.

Clark, J. H., Anderson, J. N., and Peck, E. J., Jr. (1973). *Steroids* **22**, 707–718.

Clark, J. H., Anderson, J. N., and Peck, E. J., Jr. (1974). *Nature* **251**, 446–448.

Clark, J. H., Hseuh, A. J. W., and Peck, E. J., Jr. (1977a). *Ann. N. Y. Acad Sci.* **286**, 161–179.

Clark, J. H., Paszko, Z., and Peck, E. J., Jr. (1977b). *Endocrinology* **100**, 91–96.

Clark, J. H., Hardin, J. W., Upchurch, S., and Eriksson, H. (1978). *J. Biol. Chem.* **253**, 7630–7634.

Clark, J. H., Markaverich, B. M., Upchurch, S., Eriksson, H., and Hardin, J. W. (1979). *In* "Steroid Hormone Receptor Systems" (W. W. Leavitt and J. H. Clark, eds.) pp. 17–46. Plenum Press, New York.

Clark, J. H., McCormack, S. A., Kling, R., Hodges, D., and Hardin, J. W. (1980) *In* "Hormones and Cancer " (S. Iacobelli, ed.), pp. 295–307. Raven Press, New York.

Emmens, C. W. (1970). *Ann. Rev. Pharmacol.* **4**, 237–254.

Eriksson, H., Upchurch, S., Hardin, J. W., Peck, E. J., Jr., and Clark. J. H. (1978). *Biochem. Biophys. Res. Commun.* **81**, 1–7.

Feil, D., Glasser, S. R., Toft, D. O., and O'Malley, B. W. (1972). *Endocrinology* **91**, 738–746.

Glasser, S. R., Chytil, F., and Spelsberg, T. C. (1972). *Biochem. J.* **130**, 947–957.

Gorski, J., Toft, D., Shyamala, G., Smith, D., and Notides, A. (1968) *Recent Progr. Horm. Res.* **24**, 45–80.

Hamilton, T. H. (1968). *Science* **161**, 649–660.

Hardin, J. W., Clark, J. H., Glasser, S. R., and Peck, E. J., Jr. (1976). *Biochemistry* **15**, 1370–1374.

Harris, J., and Gorski, J. (1978). *Endocrinology* **103**, 240–245.

Holtkamp, D. E., Greslin, J. G., Rout, C. A., and Lerner, L. J. (1960). *Proc. Soc. Exp. Biol. Med.* **105**, 197–201.

Hsueh, A. J. W., Clark, J. H., and Peck, E. J., Jr. (1976). *Endocrinology* **98**, 438–444.

Huggins, C., and Jensen, E. V. (1955). *J. Exper. Med.* **102**, 335–346.

Jensen, E. V., Numata, M., Brecher, P. I., and DeSombre, E. R. (1971). *In* "The Biochemistry of Steroid Hormone Action" (R. M. S. Smellie, ed.), pp. 133–159. Academic Press, London.

Katzenellenbogen, B. S., and Ferguson, E. R. (1975). *Endocrinology* **97**, 1–12.

Katzenellenbogen, B. S., Ferguson, E. R., and Lan, N. C. (1977). *Endocrinology* **100**, 1252–1259.

King, R. J. B., and Mainwaring, W. I. P. (1974). *In* "Steroid-Cell Interactions" pp. 288–316. University Park Press, Baltimore.

Leavitt, W. W., Toft, D. O., Strott, C. A., and O'Malley, B. W. (1974). *Endocrinology* **94**, 1041–1053.

Lerner, L. J. (1964). *Recent Progr. Horm. Res.* **20**, 435–490.

Markaverich, B. M., and Clark, J. H. (1979). *Endocrinology* **104**, 1458–1462.
Markaverich, B. M., Clark, J. H., and Hardin, J. W. (1978). *Biochemistry* **17**, 3146–3152.
Martel, D., and Psychoyos, A. (1978). *J. Endocr.* **76**, 145–151.
McCormack, S. A., and Clark, J. H. (1979). *Science* **204**, 629–631.
McCormack, S. A., and Glasser, S. R. (1980). *Endocrinology* **106**, 1634–1649.
Martucci, C., and Fishman, J. (1977). *Endocrinology* **101**, 1709–1715.
Means, A. R., and O'Malley, B. W. (1972) *Progr. Endocr. Metab.* **21**, 357–370.
Milgrom, E., Thi, L., Atger, M., and Baulieu, E. E. (1973). *J. Biol. Chem.* **248**, 6366–6347.
O'Malley, B. W., and Means, A. R. (1974). *Science* **183**, 610–620.
Panko, W. B., Clark, J. H., and Walters, M. R. **(1981)**. *Endocrinology* (in press).
Ross, J. W., Shryne, J., Gorski, R. A., and Marshall, J. R. (1973). *Endocrinology* **92**, 1079–1083.
Shyamala, G., and Gorski, J. (1967). *J. Biol. Chem.* **244**, 1094–1103.
Stormshak, F., Leake, R., Wertz, N., and Gorski, J. (1976). *Endocrinology* **99**, 1501–1511.
Szego, C. M., and Roberts, S. (1953). *Recent Progr. Horm, Res.* **8**, 419–469.
Velardo, J. T., Hisaw, F. L., and Bever, A. T. (1956). *Endocrinology* **59**, 165–169.
Walters, M. R., and Clark. J. H. (1977). *J. Steroid Biochem.* **8**, 1137–1144.
Walters, M. R., and Clark. J. H. (1978). *Endocrinology* **103**, 601–609.
Wotiz, H. H., Shane, J. A., Vigersky, R., and Brecher, P. I. (1968). *In* "Prognostic Factors in Breast Cancer" (A. P. M. Forest and P. B. Kunkler, eds), pp. 368–376. Churchill-Livingstone, Edinburgh.

9

Effects of Antioestrogens on Cell Proliferation in the Rodent Reproductive Tract

L. MARTIN

I. INTRODUCTION

An ideal antihormone would inhibit all effects of the hormone, in all circumstances, specifically, and not by other hormonal, anti-hormonal, pharmacological or toxic actions; it would be devoid of agonist activity. Such inhibitors of sex hormones would produce complete chronic chemical castration. Some anti-androgens approach the ideal, no antioestrogens do. Progestins, the classical non-competitive antioestrogens, are hormonally active in other ways, and antagonize or synergize with oestrogen, depending on species and tissue (Courrier, 1950; Martin and Finn, 1971). Competitors like dimethylstilboestrol and oestriol are only antagonists in short-term tests, or when applied locally; if their levels are maintained in the target organ they are complete agonists (Martin, 1969; Miller, 1969).

NON-STEROIDAL ANTIOESTROGENS
ISBN 0 12 677880 9

These limitations do not apply to non-steroidal antioestrogens like nafoxidine, CI 628 or tamoxifen, which are effective when given systemically and continuously. However, none of them fulfils the ideal completely; all are to some extent oestrogenic, though this varies greatly between species. Even in the rat uterus (from which so many ideas of antioestrogen action derive) they are only partial antagonists, since they inhibit oestrogen-induced weight increases by no more than 50%, and at these maximum inhibitory doses induce significant weight increases themselves (Duncan *et al.*, 1963; Callantine *et al.*, 1966; Harper and Walpole, 1967). It is surprising, therefore, that there is so little information on their effects on cell proliferation. Oestrogens themselves, often described as mitogenic, are not equally so in all uterine tissues. Thus the mixed properties of the antagonists could arise from different effects in different subsets of target cells.

II. PARAMETERS OF PROLIFERATION

In vivo, cell populations in the female reproductive tract turn over, i.e. cells are continuously produced by mitosis and lost by death. The relative magnitude of the two processes determines whether populations expand, decline, or remain constant. Antioestrogens could affect either or both. Measurement of whole organ DNA does not discriminate between alternatives, and one is forced to use histological methods.

Overall effects can be monitored by counting cells: in uteri fixed at the same length the number per transverse section is a measure of the whole population. Birth-rates can be estimated from the proportion of mitotic cells (mitotic index). After mitosis there is an interval (G_1) before a cell enters the period of DNA synthesis (S) and a further interval (G_2) precedes mitosis. Cells in S can be detected auto-radiographically after brief exposure of the population to [^{3}H]thymidine. As cells in S normally proceed to mitosis, the [^{3}H]thymidine pulse-labelling index gives another estimate of the birthrate. Since this depends on the average time taken by cells to pass through the whole sequence of G_1–S–G_2–M, and antioestrogens might lengthen any one phase, the duration of each must be known for precise analysis. However, the methods involved (e.g. labelled mitosis curves), are tedious and are valid only in steady-state conditions, which rarely occur in experiments involving hormonal stimulation. It appears that proliferation in normal cells is usually regulated in G_1, because its duration varies widely between populations growing at different rates, whereas S and G_2 remain relatively constant (Smith and Martin, 1973). This is true for tissues of the reproductive tract (Das, 1972). In practice, therefore, one can gain much information by combined measurements of cell number, mitotic index, [^{3}H]thymidine labelling index and dead cell index.

It is important to determine whether growth elicited by an antagonist which is a partial agonist differs in quality or only in degree from that induced by oestrogen, for there are many examples, including tumours, in which growth is stimulated by small doses of oestrogen but inhibited by high ones.

III. OESTROGEN-INDUCED CELL PROLIFERATION

In ovariectomized rodents the vaginal epithelium comprises one or two basal layers plus a superficial mucified layer of cells (Fig. 1). Proliferation is confined to the former and the rate is low, but it involves the whole population. The rate of entry of cells into S increases 8–18 hours after administration of oestrogen, followed by increases in mitotic rate. Increased

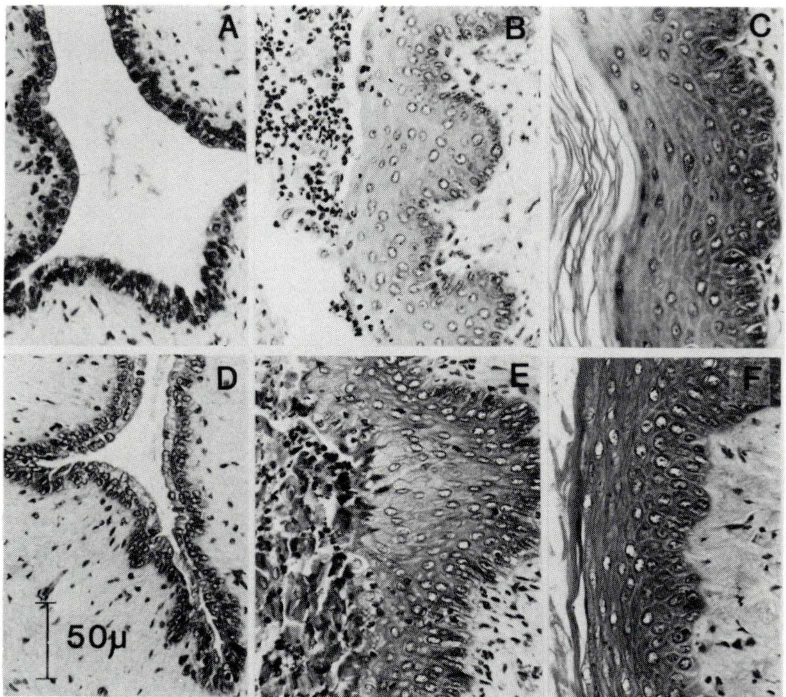

Fig. 1. Transverse sections (5 μ H and E) of vaginae from adult ovariectomized QS mice (body weight approx. 30 g) (upper), and Sprague-Dawley rats (body weight approx. 300 g) (lower): A, D, untreated; B, E, 4 weeks after 2 s.c. injections, given 24 hours apart, of 1.5 or 5 mg, respectively, of tamoxifen in arachis oil; C, F, after 4 weeks with 100 or 800 ng/ml respectively of oestradiol in the drinking water. From Martin (1980).

proliferation rate arises mainly from shortening of G_1 (Thrasher *et al.*, 1967). As the number of cell layers increases, the surface ones stratify, cornify and finally desquamate. With continuous oestrogen treatment labelling indices and epithelial thickness correlate almost perfectly with each other, suggesting that thickness simply reflects proliferation rate (Peckham *et al.*, 1963). Essentially then, the cornification response is one of increased proliferation rate; if the rate is high the epithelium thickens enough to cornify, if not it becomes hyperplastic but not cornified.

Oestrogen stimulates proliferation in all tissues of the immature (Kaye *et al.*, 1972), but not the adult uterus (Clark, 1971). In the latter, the myometrium reacts to oestrogen by hypertrophy and increased contractility but with little proliferation. The highly vascular connective tissue stroma (Fig. 2) comprises fibroblasts, mast cells and wandering cells, including lymphocytes, macrophages, polymorphs and eosinophils. The content of eosinophils increases substantially after oestrogen stimulation (Tchernitchin *et al.*, 1976). While this involves migration, not proliferation, such population shifts presumably contribute to changes in uterine DNA content.

Oestrogen alone induces small increases in stromal cell proliferation which in mice appear to be confined to endothelial cells (Martin *et al.*, 1973). Substantial proliferation of fibroblasts is induced by oestrogen in animals pretreated with progestins (Martin and Finn, 1968; Clark, 1971), and this proliferation normally occurs in pregnancy as a precursor to ovum implantation.

Simple columnar epithelia constitute some 5–10% of the total uterine tissues in ovariectomized rodents (Fig. 2). Despite morphological similarity, the luminal and gland populations respond differently to oestrogens. In untreated animals, proliferation rates are low in both. Estimates of turnover times vary between laboratories, with disagreement about whether all or part of the population turns over (Martin, 1980). Histologically, one always sees signs of turnover; i.e. mitotic, labelled and dead cells. Whereas vaginal cells are lost by desquamation, uterine epithelial cells die *in situ* by karyorrhexis, the products being phagocytosed by adjoining cells. This debris is an index of the rate and timing of cell death (Martin *et al.*, 1973). After oestrogen injection there is a lag of 6–12 hours in which cell debris disappears. Cells then enter S at an increased rate; the [^{3}H]thymidine pulse labelling index rises, then falls as cells enter G_2 and divide. Increased proliferation rate results from a shortening of G_1 (probably by recruitment from A state; Smith and Martin, 1973), plus some shortening of S-phase. In mice all luminal cells divide, doubling their numbers by 24 hours. Throughout this period cell death is minimal, but if oestrogen treatment is not continued mitotic rate falls, cell death increases from 30 hours onwards, and cell numbers plummet. A short-acting oestrogen like oestriol stimulates cells to enter DNA synthesis and mitosis, but they die prematurely and numbers do not rise (Martin *et al.*, 1976). With continued

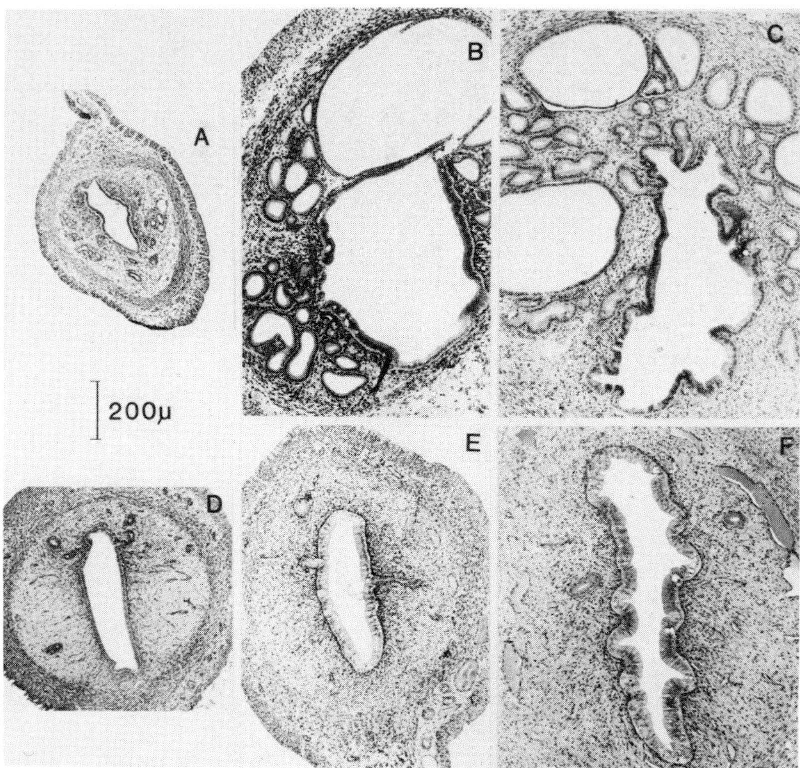

Fig. 2. Transverse sections (5 μ H and E) of uteri from QS mice (upper) and Sprague-Dawley rats (lower). Details as for Figure 1. From Martin (1980).

stimulation luminal numbers rise at increasingly slower rates; birth-rate falls, due to lengthening of G_1 in the stem cell compartment (Lee *et al.*, 1974); and death rate rises as differentiated cells reach the end of their life. After 3–4 days numbers reach a maximum at which they remain indefinitely, even though proliferation rates oscillate for some time thereafter (Lee, 1972).

In the glands oestrogen stimulates a sequence of DNA synthesis and mitosis like that in the lumen, but peak indices are lower, cell death rate rises earlier and (in mice) no more than 50% of cells enter S. With continuous stimulation proliferation rates rise and fall as in the lumen. Nevertheless, numbers continue to increase, and all strains of mice tested rapidly develop endometrial adenomatous hyperplasias (Fig. 2). Rats, in contrast, do not (Martin, 1980).

IV. ANTIOESTROGENS AND CELL PROLIFERATION IN THE MOUSE REPRODUCTIVE TRACT

Harper and Walpole (1967) described tamoxifen as an oestrogen in mice. Emmens and Martin (1965) found that nafoxidine was oestrogenic in mouse vaginal smear and tetrazolium tests, but its dose response lines turned down at high doses and at these levels it weakly inhibited oestrogen. It did not reduce oestrogen-induced uterine weight gain at any dose, but produced maximal increases itself. Terenius (1970, 1971) also found that tamoxifen and nafoxidine were oestrogenic in mouse vaginal smear and uterine weight tests. Tamoxifen was not antagonistic in the latter, but nafoxidine was weakly so.

In the short-term nafoxidine reduces uterine luminal cell death and induces as much epithelial proliferation as oestradiol, when given alone, and as much stromal proliferation when given to progesterone-treated mice (Fig. 3). Lee (1974) found that over several days neither tamoxifen nor nafoxidine inhibited uterine proliferation induced by oestrogen, but induced comparable increases themselves. Despite tamoxifen's short-term oestrogenicity, Emmens (1971) and Jordan (1975) found large doses had prolonged effects which were later antioestrogenic in smear tests: it seemed that here tamoxifen might be inhibiting proliferation. We therefore treated adult ovariectomized mice with tamoxifen in the same way as Jordan, but examined the histology and rates of target cell proliferation up to 60 days later (Martin and Middleton, 1978).

Vaginal weights increase rapidly after treatment and remain higher than the controls throughout the experiment. Smears are cornified at 48–96 hours, but thereafter increasing numbers become negative with leucocytes. These results resemble Jordan's. However, sections show that from 48 hours epithelia of treated mice are multi-layered with stratified or cornified layers, whereas controls are atrophic (Fig. 1). Basal mitotic indices quadruple within 24 hours; thereafter they fluctuate but always remain 2–3 times higher than control values. Previously we argued (Martin and Middleton, 1978) that antioestrogenicity in long-term smear tests arises artefactually because evaluation of positive smears places prime importance on the absence of leucocytes and since continuous oestrogen treatment can induce uterine leucocytosis it might affect the vagina in a similar manner. Subsequently we have found that oestradiol maintains leucocyte-free cornified smears for up to 8 weeks. Presumably, therefore, tamoxifen cannot maintain *maximal* rates of cell proliferation and prevents oestrogen from doing so by saturating the receptor system. How then does it induce full cornification in the short-term? Possibly this arises from the kinetics of proliferation. Initially most cells are in G_1, so stimulation leads to their quasi-synchronous entry into S-phase. The resultant transient high birth-rate increases the number of cell layers rapidly, enabling the surface ones to cornify. Thereafter, as proliferation rate drops

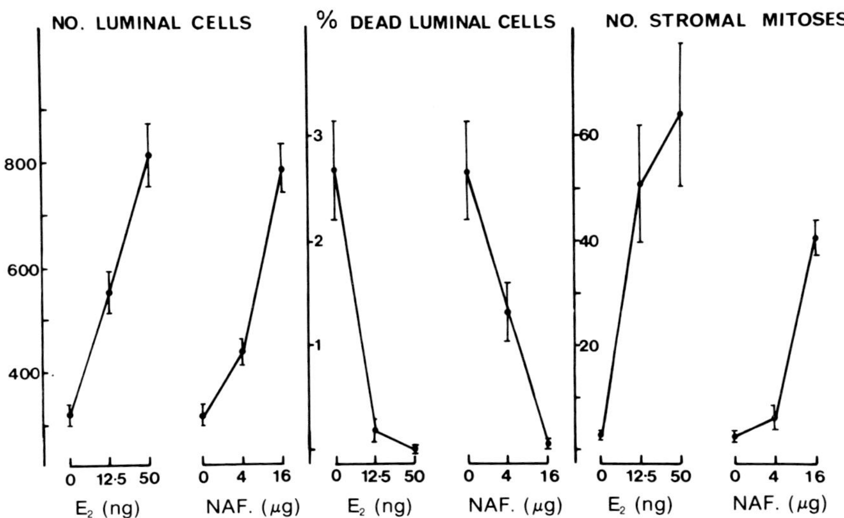

Fig. 3. Effects of nafoxidine on cell proliferation in mouse uterus. Luminal cell numbers and proportion of dead cells (means ± S.E.M., n = 10). Ovariectomized mice primed by 3 daily injections of 100 ng oestradiol, 5 days later received 2 injections 24 hours apart of oestradiol or nafoxidine and were killed 6 hours after the second. Counts made as described by Martin *et al.* (1973). Stromal mitoses (means ± S.E.M., n = 5); ovariectomized mice primed as above were left untreated for 2 days, then given 4 daily injections of 1.0 mg progesterone, and with the last a single injection of oestradiol or nafoxidine. They were killed 24 hours later, 2 hours after an i.p. injection of 0.1 mg colcemid. Counts made as described by Martin and Finn (1968).

(Fig. 6) due to desynchronization arising from inherent variability of the cell cycle, the epithelium no longer maintains a thickness permitting cornification. Alternatively, tamoxifen might limit receptor replenishment as postulated for rat uterus, antagonistic metabolites might slowly accumulate, or non-receptor-mediated effects on metabolism might gradually slow growth (Desphande *et al.*, 1978). Interestingly tamoxifen's *cis*-isomer, which is otherwise a weak but complete agonist in both rat and mouse, also induced long-term vaginal refractoriness (Emmens, 1973).

Uterine weights triple after injection of tamoxifen and are still double those of controls at 60 days. The pattern of luminal proliferation resembles that induced by oestradiol — disappearance of dead cells and a rapidly increased mitotic index. As cell numbers reach a maximum at 48 hours, the mitotic index falls and the dead cell index rises. By day 60 turnover rates are still elevated, with mitotic and dead cell indices respectively 4 and 16 times greater than in controls.

Uteri from treated mice autopsied at 28 days onwards contain cystic glands (Fig. 2) a development preceded by a steady increase in cell numbers and fluctuations in mitotic and dead cell indices, as produced by oestradiol (Finn and Martin, 1973; Lee, 1972). Turnover rates remain elevated throughout the experiment. At 60 days, numbers, mitotic indices and dead cell indices are respectively 3, 9 and 21 times higher than in controls. Some uteri still contain cysts.

These effects are identical to those of oestradiol, including the induction of cysts. Other triarylalkenes do this (Emmens and Carr, 1973). CI 628 is also oestrogenic but not significantly antioestrogenic in mice (Emmens, 1973). As a general rule, therefore, compounds of this type appear to be partial antagonists in rats but virtually complete agonists in mice.

V. ANTIOESTROGENS AND CELL PROLIFERATION IN THE RAT REPRODUCTIVE TRACT

Kang *et al.* (1975) found that CI 628 induced proliferation in the uterine stroma, but suppressed it in the epithelia where it induced hypertrophy. They described it as a progestin! Jordan and co-workers (Jordan, 1976a; Jordan *et al.*, 1977) found that tamoxifen did not induce consistent increases in uterine DNA of ovariectomized adult or intact immature rats, and suggested (Clark *et al.*, 1978) that weight increases induced by tamoxifen result from hypertrophy without hyperplasia. There seem to be no reports on vaginal cell proliferation though Marois and Marois (1977) found tamoxifen to induce a multilayered epithelium.

I have used adult (6–8 weeks old; 250–300 g body weight) female Sprague-Dawley rats, ovariectomized 2 weeks before treatment, and primed one week later with two injections, 24 hours apart, of 1.0 μg oestradiol-17β s.c. in 0.1 ml arachis oil. They were then given oestradiol, tamoxifen or combinations thereof for periods up to 28 days; controls received vehicle. Animals were killed by CO_2 asphyxiation, usually receiving 1.0 μCi/g body weight of [^{3}H]thymidine s.c. in 0.25 ml H_2O one hour beforehand. Organs were dissected, weighed and fixed in Bouin's fluid. Histological procedures, methods of estimating cell numbers, mitotic indices, labelling indices and dead cell indices were as described by Martin *et al.* (1973, 1976).

Two oestradiol regimes were used: (a) daily injections of 0.5 μg s.c. in 0.1 arachis oil for up to 5 days; and (b) drinking water containing 800 ng/ml. Two tamoxifen regimes were used: (a) daily injections of 250 μg s.c. in 0.1 ml arachis oil for up to 5 days; and (b) two s.c. injections, 24 hours apart, of 5 mg in 0.5 ml arachis oil. The latter produces prolonged inhibition of the growth of DMBA-induced rat mammary tumors (Jordan, 1976b). In our rats it induces prolonged increases in uterine weight but also prolonged decreases in body weight (Fig. 4). Some animals received up to 4 daily injections of 250 μg of nafoxidine s.c. in 0.1 ml arachis oil, or of lower doses of tamoxifen.

Figure 5 compares the effects of these regimes on uterine and vaginal growth. The high doses of antagonists always inhibit oestradiol maximally, but lower doses also achieve substantial inhibition. Uterine weight was not suppressed completely and higher doses of antagonists increased it themselves. Extensive data show that typical control wet weights are about 100 mg, oestrogen treated around 350 mg, and tamoxifen treated around 200 mg falling, over 2–4 weeks, to 160 mg. Uteri treated with oestradiol and tamoxifen are usually no heavier than those treated with tamoxifen alone. Tamoxifen reduces luminal mitotic indices below control values whether oestrogen is given or not, but only reduces cell numbers below control values in the long term, increasing them slightly in the short term.

In contrast, vaginal mitotic indices are increased above control values in both long-term and short-term tests, even though tamoxifen suppresses the increases induced by oestradiol. More extensive data (Fig. 6) confirms that tamoxifen always stimulates vaginal proliferation, though not as much as oestrogen, and the epithelium becomes multilayered and hyperplastic, but not cornified (Fig. 1). Mitotic indices are also increased, being higher than those induced by oestradiol at early times, but lower from day 4 on. Anomalies between early mitotic and labelling indices probably arise because of the

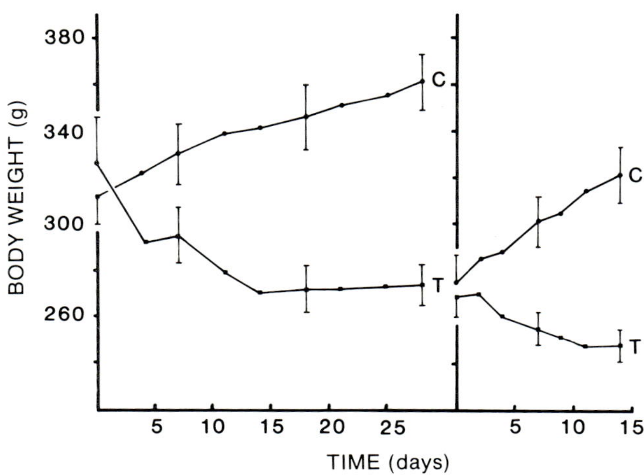

Fig. 4. Body weights of control (C) and tamoxifen-treated (T; 5 mg s.c. in oil on days 1 and 2) adult ovariectomized rats. Results are means ± S.E.M., n = 4 from two experiments.

synchrony of proliferation during initial stimulation. After this, the labelling and mitotic indices induced by even massive doses of tamoxifen equilibrate at values substantially below those induced by oestradiol, i.e. tamoxifen *cannot* induce maximum proliferation. Interestingly, the maximal mitotic indices attained are approximately equal in rat and mouse.

Neither oestrogen nor tamoxifen induce significant myometrial proliferation. At dissection, oestrogen and tamoxifen treated uteri are haemorrhagic, but the latter are limp and flaccid even if oestrogen has also been given. This suggests tamoxifen might inhibit myometrial contractility as CI 628 does (Callantine *et al.*, 1966).

Both oestradiol and tamoxifen induce initial hypertrophy of the stromal cells and increase the number incorporating [^{3}H]thymidine (Fig. 7). The logistics of counting all stromal cells per section precluded the estimation of

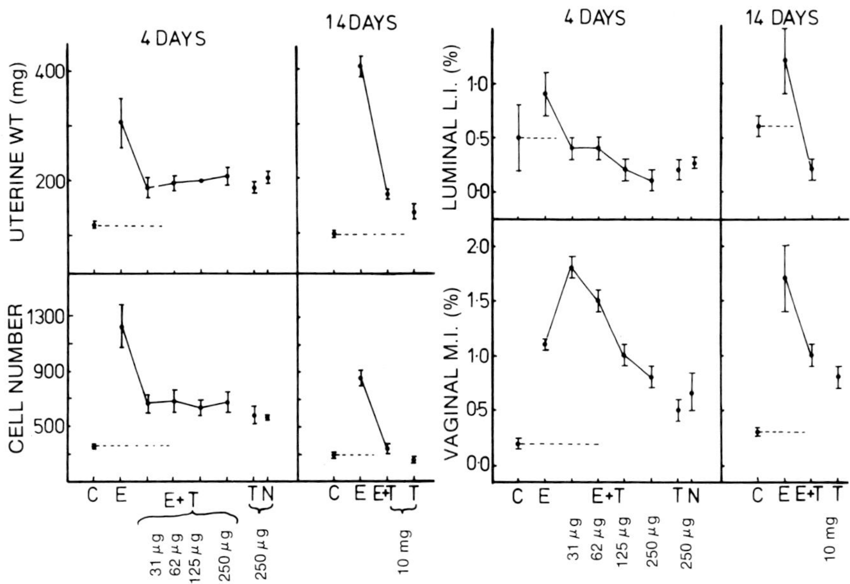

Fig. 5. Effects of tamoxifen and oestrogen on uterine and vaginal growth in the rat. Results are means ± S.E.M., n = 4; C = untreated controls. 4 days: ovariectomized rats killed 24 hours after the last of 4 daily injections of 0.5 μg oestradiol given alone (E), or with various doses of tamoxifen (E + T), or after tamoxifen (T) or nafoxidine (N) alone. 14 days: rats were killed after 14 days on drinking water containing 800 ng/ml oestradiol (E) or after 2 s.c. injections of 5 mg of tamoxifen (T), or both treatments (E + T). Counts were made as described by Martin *et al.* (1973) and Martin and Middleton (1978). Data are uterine wet weights, uterine luminal epithelial cell numbers and labelling indices (L.I.) and vaginal basal cell mitotic indices (M.I.).

labelling indices, but the impression was gained that they are probably of the same order as in the mouse (i.e. 1–3%). Tamoxifen induces more stromal labelling than oestradiol, and this is true for animals pretreated with progesterone, in which labelled stromal cells appear much earlier. It is not clear how many go on to divide, or whether they are arrested in G_2 since mitotic cells are rare. The number of labelled cells decreases as treatment continues; with tamoxifen the stromal cells become densely packed and shrunken, particularly in the subepithelial layers (Fig. 2). This atrophy may account for some of the long-term inhibitory effects of tamoxifen on the epithelia, but the early stromal responses make it unlikely that the acute inhibition of epithelial proliferation (see below) is due to any deficiency in stromal stimulation on the part of tamoxifen. It follows that such inhibition probably involves a direct action of the inhibitor on the epithelium.

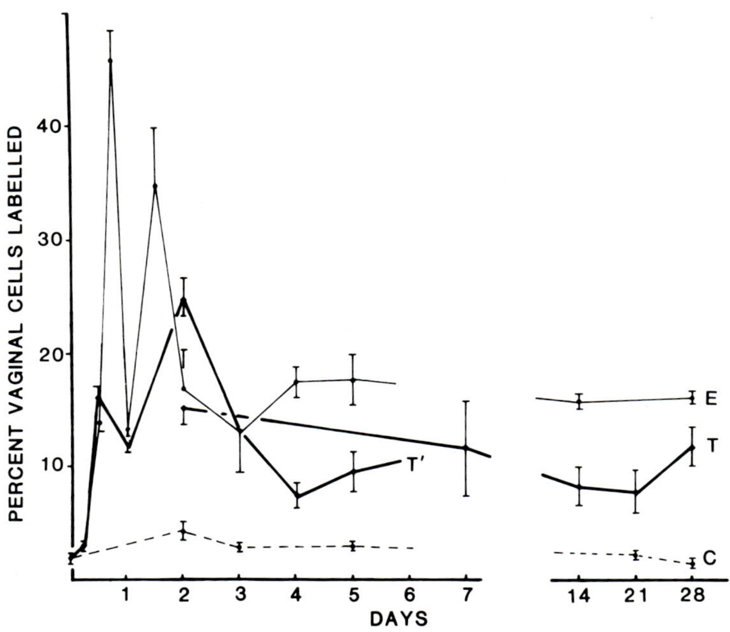

Fig. 6. Vaginal basal cell labelling indices; adult ovariectomized rats; [^{3}H]thymidine given one hour before sacrifice; C, controls; T′, 250 μg tamoxifen daily; T, 2 × 5 mg tamoxifen days 0 and 1; E, 0.5 μg oestradiol daily s.c. (points to day 5) or 800 ng/ml in drinking water (day 14 points on). Results are means ± S.E.M. based on counts of 2,000 cells per organ with the following numbers of rats per group (reading from left to right): C, 4, 8, 4, 4, 4, 4; T, all 4; T′, 4, 4, 4, 4, 4, 8, 4; E, 4, 4, 3, 14, 4, 4, 8, 8, 4, 4, 4. Redrawn from Martin (1980).

In the luminal epithelium, oestradiol induces hypertrophy and rapidly increases labelling index, mitotic index (not shown) and cell numbers (Fig. 8). Cell death rates remain low until day 3 when they rise to remain above control values thereafter, i.e. the population turns over.

Tamoxifen induces prolonged hypertrophy of the luminal cells (Fig. 2) but only small increases in labelling index and cell numbers (Fig. 8). Mitotic index and cell death rates do not increase significantly (data not shown) and numbers fluctuate slightly above control values in the early part of the experiments only falling below after 28 days. However tamoxifen completely inhibits the increase in cell numbers induced by continuous oestradiol treatment (Fig. 8.).

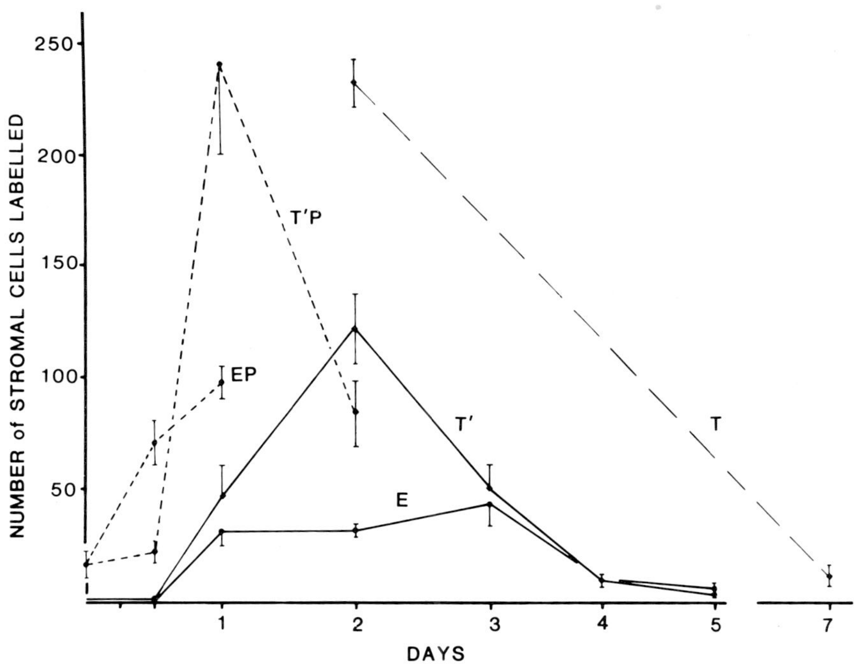

Fig. 7. Number of stromal cells per section in the uteri of ovariectomized rats labelled by [^{3}H]thymidine given one hour before death. E, T and T′ are as in Figure 6. EP and T′P are results from rats pretreated with 3 daily s.c. injections of 2 mg progesterone before receiving respectively one s.c. injection of 0.5 μg oestradiol (day 0) or 2 s.c. injections of 250 μg tamoxifen (days 0, 1). Counts made on one section selected at random from the mid-region of each horn. The results are means ± S.E.M., n = 4. Part redrawn from Martin (1980).

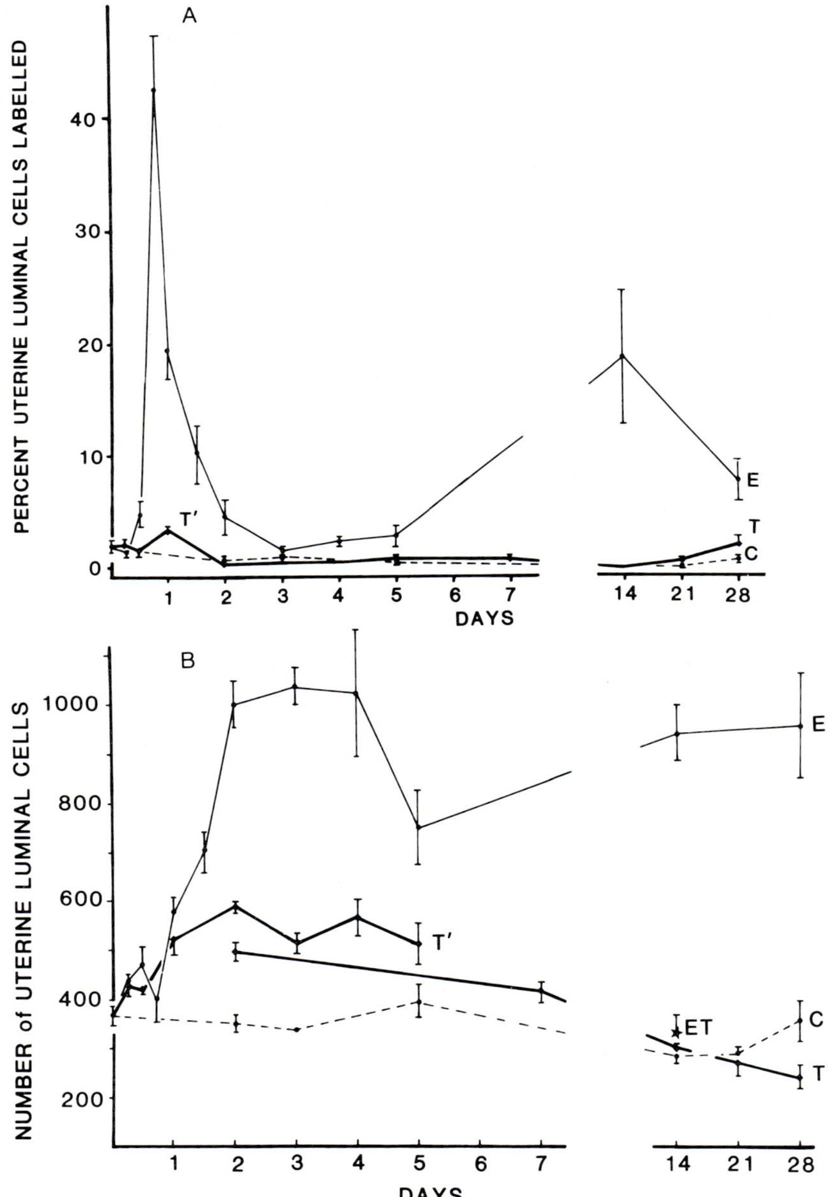

Fig. 8. (A) [^{3}H]thymidine pulse-labelling indices and (B) number of cells in uterine luminal epithelium of ovariectomized rats. [^{3}H]thymidine as before; C, T, T′ and E, as in Figure 6, ET as in Figure 5. Results are means ± S.E.M. with number per group as in Figure 6 except for day 14 numbers: C, n = 16; T, n = 16; ET, n = 4. Part redrawn from Martin (1980).

Oestradiol induces hypertrophy of the glands (Fig. 2) and transient increases in labelling index (Fig. 9), followed in quick succession by peaks of cell death after which labelling and dead cell indices remain above control values. In the long term, numbers show little increase over controls. Tamoxifen also induces hypertrophy, but only small transient increases in labelling index. However, it also induces a peak in cell death as large as that appearing after oestradiol, and though values then fall they remain higher than controls. The net result is that, within two weeks, gland cell numbers fall six-fold below controls (Fig. 9). This decrease is *not* reversed by continuous oestrogen treatment and in this respect differs from the effects of tamoxifen on cultured MCF 7 cells (Lippman *et al.*, 1976). The rise in labelling index from 14 to 28 days probably reflects falling tamoxifen levels and the start of gland regeneration. There are signs that cell death rate is dropping at this time. However, cell numbers remain low.

VI. ARE INHIBITORY EFFECTS RECEPTOR MEDIATED?

Clearly, tamoxifen induces an overall pattern of uterine growth in the rat which differs qualitatively from that induced by oestradiol, yet it exhibits a remarkable diversity of actions in individual tissues. It stimulates vaginal proliferation, causes more uterine stromal DNA synthesis than oestradiol, but virtually no epithelial proliferation, and inhibits that induced by oestradiol. It induces hypertrophy of both luminal and glandular epithelial cells yet only

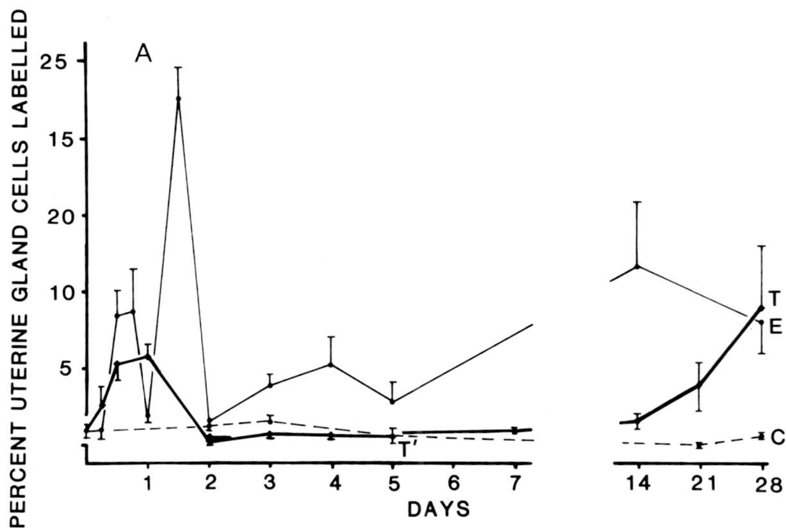

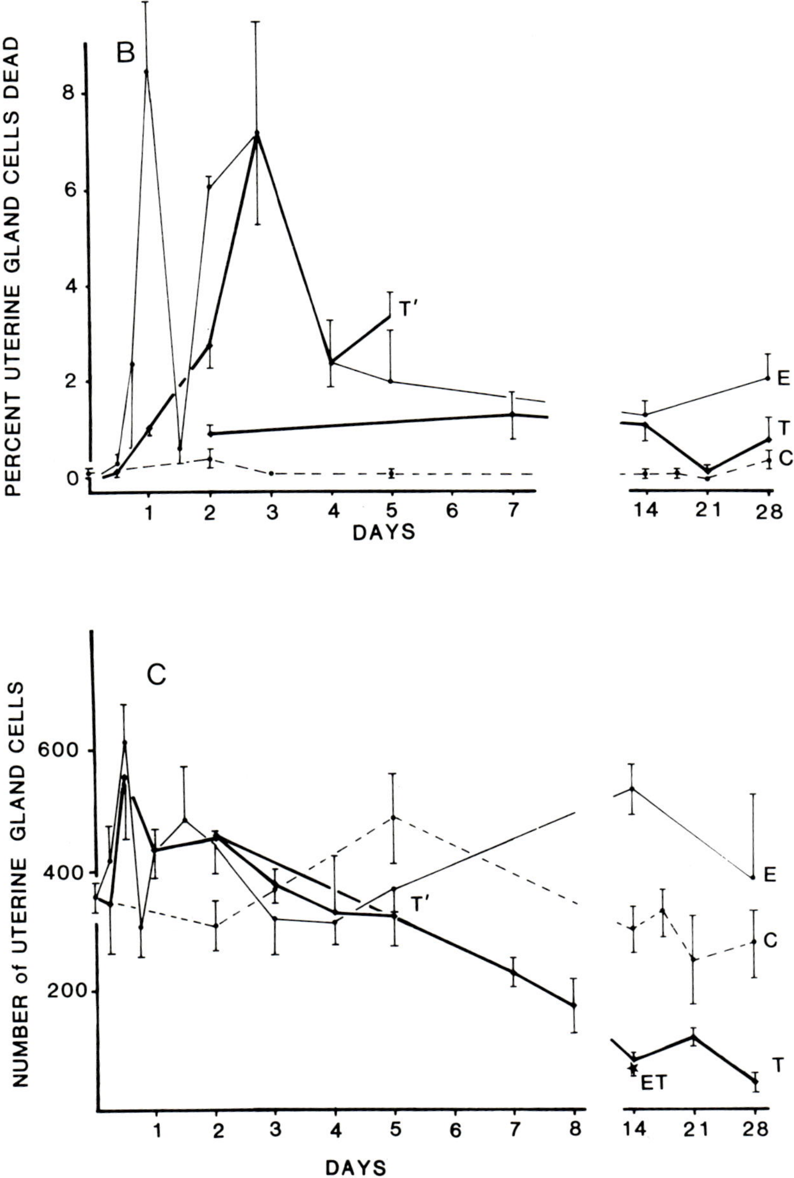

Fig. 9. The proportion of uterine gland cells, (A) labelled by [^{3}H]thymidine or (B) dead, and (C) the number per section, in the uteri of ovariectomized rats; results are means ± S.E.M. with numbers and symbols as in Figure 8. From Martin (1980).

kills the latter. This last effect may hold important clues to the mechanism whereby tamoxifen induces tumor regression: many mammary and uterine carcinomas are adenocarcinomas, i.e. cancers of glands or gland-like cancers. The current view is that tamoxifen suppresses growth via the oestrogen-receptor pathway. It is difficult, however, to explain tamoxifen's diverse actions by a *single* receptor-mediated pathway, particularly when one also considers its strikingly different effects in rat and mouse. Mechanisms apart, these differences are puzzling because the two species are reproductively and endocrinologically so close. They have similar oestrous cycles, modes of ovum implantation, placentation, gestation and parturition, with uteri and vaginae of comparable morphology.

Quirks of metabolism might account for some species differences but would not easily accommodate, in both species, similar actions in one organ, dissimilar actions in another, or diverse actions within the one organ. In terms of receptor pathways one must postulate that the oestrogen receptors differ or that their ligand complexes act differently (e.g. binding to different chromatin sites), not only in different cell types, but also within the same cell type in different species. As yet, however, receptor studies have not detected significant differences. The oestrogen receptors of rat and mouse share many attributes including the same ranking of binding affinities for non-steroidal antagonists (Skidmore *et al.*, 1972); tamoxifen and its oestrogenic *cis*-isomer induce comparable depletion of cytoplasmic receptor and augmentation of nuclear levels in both species (Jordan *et al.*, 1978).

High doses of oestrogen inhibit growth responses stimulated by low ones. The inhibitory doses are often so far above those saturating receptors that mechanisms involving the latter seem unlikely. Tamoxifen in high doses inhibits body weight increase in female rats (Fig. 4; Jordan, 1976b), some glycolytic enzymes of rat liver and muscle (Deshpande *et al.*, 1978), and prostaglandin synthesis in various tissues (Furr *et al.*, 1979), though generally it seems to have low toxicity. Clearly its oestrogenic action involves the receptor pathway, but its inhibitory ones might not, though they could be enhanced in target tissues where the drug accumulates by virtue of its affinity for receptors. Is tamoxifen a "site directed" cytotoxin?

To check this possibility I compared the effects of tamoxifen on luminal proliferation induced by luminal dilation (Leroy *et al.*, 1976). In the "oestrogenic" compartment of this experiment rats were killed one hour after a s.c. injection of [^{3}H]thymidine and 24 hours after a s.c. injection of 0.5 μg oestradiol or vehicle (0.1 ml arachis oil) given alone, at the same time as one injection of 250 μg tamoxifen or the last of three such daily injections, or 8 days after two daily injections of 5 mg tamoxifen (Fig. 10, left). Oestradiol stimulates a large increase in labelling index; this is completely blocked by all three tamoxifen regimes, including the single 250 μg dose which itself induces a small but significant increase in the 24 hour labelling index.

The "dilation" experiment was carried out in two replicates. In the first, rats were killed one hour after [^{3}H]thymidine and 17 hours after dilating one uterine horn by ligation and instillation of 20–30 μl isotonic saline via a 26 gauge hypodermic needle inserted 2 mm into the lumen, 1.0 cm anterior to the cervix. This was done via a midventral incision using "Avertin" anaesthesia (0.1 ml/g body weight i.p. of 2.5% tribromoethanol; 1.25% 2-methylbutan-2-ol in water). The contralateral horn was left untouched as a control. Dilation induces a large increase in labelling index. This is suppressed in animals given 2 × 5 mg tamoxifen 8 days previously, suggesting that the drug has some non-specific antimitotic effects. In contrast, the single 250 μg dose augments rather than inhibits, strongly suggesting that short-term suppression of oestrogen-induced proliferation is a specific antioestrogenic effect. However, this dose of tamoxifen induces much higher labelling indices in the contralateral horns,

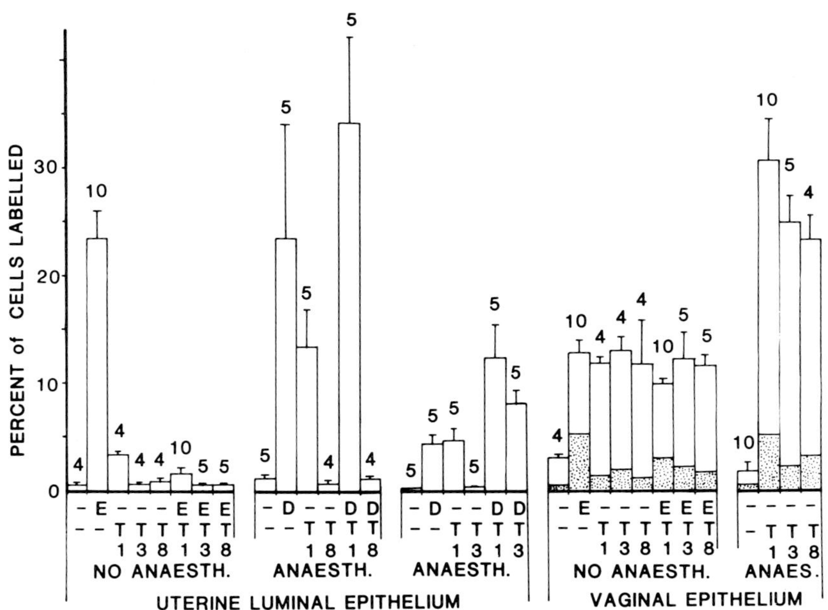

Fig. 10. The proportion of uterine luminal and vaginal basal cells labelled by [^{3}H]thymidine given one hour before death. Results are means ± S.E.M. (n above each histogram). In the first block, rats received 0.5 μg oestradiol (E) or vehicle (–) at the same time as one injection of 250 μg tamoxifen (T1) or the last of three such injections (T3), or 8 days after 2 injections of 5 mg tamoxifen (T8). They were killed 24 hours later. In the second and third blocks uteri were left untouched (–) or were dilated (D) as described in the text, tamoxifen being given as before (T1, T3, T8). Rats were killed respectively 17 and 24 hours after dilation. The fourth and fifth blocks show the corresponding vaginal data plus mitotic indices (hatched areas).

than in the experiment of Figure 8. Since initial proliferation may be highly synchronized, the anomaly could be a consequence of earlier sampling.

Accordingly, in the second experiment rats were killed 24 hours after dilation. The labelling index again increases though less than before. Both 1 and 3 injections of 250 μg of tamoxifen augment the response — neither inhibit, and similar effects are seen on mitotic index. This appears to confirm the specificity of the short-term inhibition of oestrogen-induced proliferation. Luminal labelling indices are low in the contralateral horns after 3 days treatment with tamoxifen, but after the single injection are still somewhat higher than previously. Vaginal labelling indices show striking increases in tamoxifen treated organs from animals undergoing uterine distension. These increases are not simply a result of prolongation of S-phase, since mitotic indices are also increased, nor do they stem from quirks of sampling and synchrony, because they occur in the 8-day high-dose group. Since basal levels of proliferation are not significantly altered in animals undergoing uterine distension, the effect is specifically a modulation of the response to tamoxifen: submaximal is converted to maximal stimulation, the partial is converted to the full agonist. Have we in some way produced an anti-antioestrogen? Might this be why tamoxifen doesn't suppress distension-induced proliferation? Is the "specific" inhibition of oestrogen-induced proliferation so specific after all? A further experiment with control and oestrogen-treated rats ± tamoxifen and sham-operated is now under way to test these possibilities.

VII. DISCUSSION

The trauma of anaesthesia and surgery could modulate the biological effects of tamoxifen by many mechanisms. The cell membrane is a possible point of interaction. Regulation of proliferation of cells in culture has repeatedly been shown to be mediated at the membrane, but to vary from cell type to cell type. Anaesthetics themselves are membrane active agents (Richards, 1978). Remembering the acute inhibition of myometrial contractility by CI 628 (Callantine *et al.*, 1966) and the flaccidity of uteri exposed to tamoxifen, one wonders to what extent all antagonists of this type might be active at the membrane and whether some of the tissue diversity discussed above might involve tissue-specific regulation at the membrane level. Is there in fact any evidence that tamoxifen binds to membranes?

I have purposely emphasized non-receptor mediated pathways of antioestrogen action, because there are so many anomalies regarding tamoxifen's anti-tumour activity. For example, it suppresses mammary tumour growth in mice (Sluyser, 1979; Matsuyawa and Tamamoto, 1979). In women it induces remission of mammary tumours without the side effects of high dose oestrogen therapy (Furr *et al.*, 1979), and was thought to be a pure antagonist, but a recent report (Ferrazi *et al.*, 1977) indicates that therapeutic doses induce oestrogenic changes in the vagina; another described two cases in which tamoxifen stimulates human mammary tumour growth (McIntosh and Thynne, 1977). In breast cancer patients, therapeutically effective doses produce blood levels of 250 ng/ml or more (Nicholson *et al.*, 1979), values far above those which saturate the oestrogen receptor pathway.

As a further complication, many responses stimulated by low doses of oestrogen are inhibited by high ones. This includes embryo implantation (Martin *et al.*, 1960) and mammary growth in mice (Gardner, 1941), and the growth of human mammary tumor cells *in vitro* (Lippman *et al.*, 1976). High oestrogen doses inhibit various enzymes, including the oestrogen-sensitive human placental transhydrogenase (Hagerman and Villee, 1957). Low doses accelerate mammary tumour appearance in mice with pituitary isografts, but high doses retard (Röpke and Boot, 1972). Quite low doses of oestrogen inhibit the growth of oestrogen-sensitive rat mammary tumours (Kledzik *et al.*, 1976). Massive doses induce regression of human mammary tumours (Stoll, 1973), but have unpleasant side effects. Apparently the therapeutic usefulness of lower doses has not been investigated. Where the same effect can be achieved by an agonist or an antagonist, and where compounds are partial agonists and partial antagonists, one must be cautious in attributing a given end point to one or other mode of action. Reversing the effect of a putative antioestrogen with oestrogen indicates an antagonist origin; failure to do so does not necessarily indicate an oestrogenic origin — the underlying antagonism may not involve competition. For compounds like tamoxifen, the questions remain. Do they inhibit cancer growth because of their oestrogenic properties, their antioestrogenic properties or because they possess some other growth inhibiting action enhanced by accumulation in the tumour because they bind to oestrogen receptors?

ACKNOWLEDGEMENTS

My thanks to Rosemary Jeffery for the histology, Ewan Middleton for so much counting, Audrey Lee and Len Rogers for assorted help and discussion, Margaret Barker for the typing and my wife, Kay, for invaluable advice, criticism and patience. The tamoxifen used in these studies was a gift from I.C.I. via the good offices of Barry Furr. Finally, my thanks to the editors for the opportunity to participate in this volume.

REFERENCES

Callantine, M. R., Humphrey, R. R., Lee, S. L., Windsor, B. L., Schottin, N. H., and O'Brien, O. P. (1966). *Endocrinology* **79**, 153–167.

Clark, B. F. (1971). *J. Endocr.* **50**, 527–528.

Clark, E. R., Dix, C. J., Jordan, V. C., Prestwick, G., and Sexton, S. (1978). *Br. J. Pharmacol.* **62**, 442–443.

Courrier, R. (1950). *Vitam. Horm.* **8**, 179–214.

Das, R. M. (1972). *J. Endocr.* **55**, 21–30.

Deshpande, N., Mitchell, I., and Martin, L. (1978). *J. Steroid Biochem.* **9**, 995–999.

Duncan, G. W., Lyster, S. C., Clark, J. J., and Lednicer, D. (1963). *Proc. Soc. Exp. Biol. Med.* **112**, 439–442.

Emmens, C. W. (1971). *J. Reprod. Fert.* **26**, 175–182.

Emmens, C. W. (1973). *J. Reprod. Fert.* **34**, 23–28.

Emmens, C. W., and Carr, W. L. (1973). *J. Reprod. Fert.* **34**, 29–40.

Emmens, C. W., and Martin, L. (1965). *J. Reprod. Fert.* **9**, 269–275.

Ferrazi, E., Cartei, G., Mattarazzo, R., and Fiorintino, H. (1977). *Brit. Med. J.* **9**, 1351–1352.

Finn, C. A., and Martin, L. (1973). *Biol. Reprod.* **8**, 585–588.

Furr, B. J., Patterson, J. S., Richardson, D. N., Slater, S. R., and Wakeling, A. E. (1979). *In* "Pharmacological and Biochemical Properties of Drug Substances" (M. E. Goldberg, ed.), Vol II, pp. 355–399. American Pharmacological Association, Washington.

Gardner, W. U. (1941). *Endocrinology* **28**, 53–61.

Hagerman, D. D., and Villee, C. A. (1957). *J. Biol. Chem.* **229**, 589–592.

Harper, M. J. K., and Walpole, A. L. (1967). *J. Reprod. Fert.* **13**, 101–119.

Jordan, V. C. (1975). *J. Reprod. Fert.* **42**, 251–258.

Jordan, V. C. (1976a). *Cancer Treat. Rep.* **60**, 1409–1419.

Jordan, V. C. (1976b). *Eur. J. Cancer* **12**, 419–424.

Jordan, V. C., Dix, C. J., Rowsby, L., and Prestwich, G. (1977). *Mol. Cell. Endocr.* **7**, 177–192.

Jordan, V. C., Rowsby, L., Dix, C. J., and Prestwich, G. (1978). *J. Endocr.* **78**, 71–81.

Kang, Y. H., Anderson, W. A., and DeSombre, E. R. (1975). *J. Cell Biol.* **64**, 682–691.

Kaye, A. M., Sheratzky, D., and Lindner, H. R. (1972). *Biochim. Biophys. Acta* **261**, 474–486.

Kledzik, S., Bradley, C. J., Marshall, S., Campbell, G. A., and Meites, J. (1976). *Cancer Res.* **36**, 3265–3268.

Lee, A. E. (1972). *J. Endocr.* **55**, 507–513.

Lee, A. E. (1974). *J. Endocr.* **60**, 167–174.

Lee, A. E., Rogers, L., and Trinder, G. (1974). *J. Endocr.* **61**, 117–121.

Leroy, F., Bogart, C., and Van Hoeck, J. (1976). *J. Endocr.* **45**, 441–447.

Lippman, M., Bolan, G., and Huff, K. (1976). *Cancer Treat. Rep.* **60**, 1421–1429.

McIntosh, I. H., and Thynne, G. S. (1977). *Brit. J. Surg.* **64**, 900–901.

Marois, M., and Marois, G. (1977). *C. R. Soc. Biol.* **171**, 280–286.

Martin, L. (1969). *Steroids* **13**, 1–10.

Martin, L. (1980). *In* "Estrogens in the Environment" (J. A. McLachlan, ed.), pp. 103–129. Elsevier/North Holland, New York.

Martin, L., and Finn, C. A. (1968). *J. Endocr.* **41**, 363–371.

Martin, L., and Finn, C. A. (1971). *In* "Basic Actions of Sex Steroids on Target Organs" (P. O. Hubinont, F. Leroy and P. Galand, eds), pp. 172–188. Karger, Basle.

Martin, L., and Middleton, E. (1978). *J. Endocr.* **78**, 125–129.

Martin, L., Emmens, C. W., and Cox, R. I. (1960). *J. Endocr.* **20**, 299–306.

Martin, L., Finn, C. A., and Trinder, G. (1973). *J. Endocr.* **56**, 133–144.

Martin, L., Pollard, J., and Fagg, B. (1976). *J. Endocr.* **69**, 103–115.

Matsuyawa, A., and Tamamoto, T. (1979). *Gann* **70**, 387–388.

Miller, B. G. (1969). *J. Endocr.* **43**, 563–570.

Nicholson, R. I., Daniel, P., Gaskell, S. J., Syne, J. S., Davies, P., and Griffiths, K. (1979). *In* "Antihormones" (M. K. Agarwal, ed.), pp. 253–267. North Holland, Amsterdam.

Peckham, B., Barash, H., Emlen, J., Kiekhofer, W., and Ladinsky, J. (1963). *Expl. Cell Res.* **30**, 339–343.

Richards, C. D. (1978). *Int. Rev. Biochem.* **19**, 157–220.

Röpke, G., and Boot, L. M. (1972). *Excerpta Med. Int. Congr. Ser.* **273**, 1232–1236.

Skidmore, J. R., Walpole, A. L., and Woodburn, J. (1972). *J. Endocr.* **52**, 289–298.

Sluyser, M. (1979). *Cancer Treat. Rep.* **63**, 1170.

Smith, J. A., and Martin, L. (1973). *Proc. Natl Acad. Sci. U.S.A.* **70**, 1263–1267.

Stoll, B. A. (1973). *Clin. Obstet. Gynecol.* **16**, 130–148.

Tchernitchin, A., Tchernitchin, X., and Galand, P. (1976). *Differentiation* **5**, 145–150.

Terenius, L. (1970). *Acta Endocr.* **64**, 47–58.

Terenius, L. (1971). *Acta Endocr.* **66**, 431–447.

Thrasher, J. D., Clark, F. I., and Clarke, D. R. (1967). *Expl. Cell Res.* **45**, 232–236.

10

Antioestrogen and Progestin Action in Diethylstilboestrol-Induced Endometrial Abnormalities in the Syrian Hamster

WENDELL W. LEAVITT, RAWDEN W. EVANS,
WILLIAM J. HENDRY III AND KENNETH I. H. WILLIAMS

I. INTRODUCTION

The non-steroidal oestrogen diethylstilboestrol (DES) has been shown to induce congenital abnormalities and neoplasia of the female reproductive tract when administered during critical stages of development. The DES syndrome of women occurs in the female progeny of mothers who have taken DES for threatened abortion, and such women characteristically have a high incidence of vaginal adenosis, dysplasia and a possible predisposition to clear cell carcinoma of the vagina and cervix (Herbst *et al.*, 1979). Newborn rodents exposed to DES develop symptoms akin to those observed in women with the

NON-STEROIDAL ANTIOESTROGENS
ISBN 0 12 677880 9

DES-syndrome (Forsberg, 1973; McLachlan, 1979). These include alteration of Müllerian duct development with the Müllerian epithelium growing down beyond the cervix into the upper vagina. In addition to this teratogenic action of DES on Müllerian duct development, it is likely that DES itself has carcinogenic potential. However, it is neither clear whether DES acts as an initiator or promoter of carcinogenesis nor is it certain whether DES is carcinogenic by virtue of its oestrogenic activity.

Experimental model systems are needed for the study of hormone-dependent tumours of the reproductive system. While there are several systems available for work on breast cancer, an experimental paradigm of endometrial cancer is lacking. While studying DES-induced developmental changes in female hamster reproductive organs it came to our attention that there was a high incidence of endometrial hyperplasia and endometrial adenocarcinoma (CA) in animals that had been treated on the day of birth with DES. We report here on our studies of endometrial tumour induction, oestrogen and progesterone receptor systems, and the influence of oestrogen, progestin and antioestrogen therapy.

II. TUMOURIGENESIS

Rustia (1979) found a high percentage (28–50%) of reproductive tract neoplasms in the female progeny of hamster mothers given 20 or 40 mg DES/kg during late pregnancy. Similar reproductive abnormalities are produced in mice after DES exposure during the neonatal period (McLachlan, 1979). When female hamsters were treated subcutaneously on the day of birth (day 1) with corn oil vehicle (control) or 100 µg DES (40 mg/kg) in 50µl oil, there was a high (100%) incidence of endometrial hyperplasia and endometrial CA in DES animals compared to no such problems in controls (Table I). Other DES-induced abnormalities included anovulatory ovaries with cystic follicles, metaplasia and inflammation of oviducts, squamous cell metaplasia and fibromuscular development of the cervix, and hyperplasia of the vaginal epithelium. Endometrial hyperplasia was found in 28/28 DES animals at 4–7 months of age, whereas endometrial CA occurred in animals with intact ovaries or in ovariectomized animals exposed chronically to oestrogen implants (Table I). These results support the hypothesis that exposure of the DES-altered uterus to oestrogen in later life increases the growth and/or incidence of endometrial tumours. Extrapolation of these findings to the human would suggest that women with the DES-syndrome should be watched carefully for endometrial abnormalities when exposed to protracted oestrogen stimulation from either endogenous or exogenous sources.

TABLE I
Incidence of Endometrial Hyperplasia (H) and Adenocarcinoma (CA) in Adult Hamsters Exposed to DES during Development[a]

	Oil (Control)		DES	
	H	CA	H	CA
Intact ovaries	0/7	0/7	9/9	9/9
Ovariectomized	0/5	0/5	5/5	0/5
Ovariectomized + E pellet for ~ 100 days	7/10	1/10	14/14	12/14

[a] Animals were treated on the day of birth with either 50 μl corn oil (oil control) or 100 μg DES in 50 μl oil. Animals were 4–7 months old at autopsy. H = endometrial hyperplasia. CA = endometrial adenocarcinoma. E pellet = Silastic tube filled with crystalline oestradiol-17β.

III. ONTOGENY OF DIETHYLSTILBOESTROL-INDUCED ABNORMALITIES

A. Uterine Growth

To determine whether ovarian steroid production contributes to DES-induced uterine growth during postnatal development, 3-day-old control and DES-treated hamsters were ovariectomized (ovex) or subjected to sham surgery (intact) and studied at 9, 15, and 21 days of age (Fig. 1). Neonatal DES treatment produced a 6-fold increase in uterine weight at day 9 and a 2-fold elevation in uterine mass at day 15 in both intact and ovariectomized animals. Therefore, it can be concluded that DES-induced uterine growth up to day 15 was mediated by direct action of DES on the uterus as opposed to an indirect effect mediated by alteration of ovarian steroid secretion. Serum oestradiol, progesterone and testosterone were not changed up to day 21 after DES treatment on day 1 (Table II), confirming the idea that DES did not stimulate ovarian steroid production during postnatal development. Additionally, no differences in serum oestradiol and progesterone levels were observed between intact and ovariectomized animals, demonstrating that the ovaries were relatively inactive during the first 3 weeks of life. However, differences between the uterine weights of intact and ovariectomized hamsters became apparent at day 21, indicating that ovarian steroid hormones may begin to modify DES-induced uterine changes at this time and beyond.

B. Oestrogen and Progesterone Receptors

The ontogeny of cytosol oestrogen receptor (Re) and progesterone receptor (Rp) in uterus and vagina of DES-treated and control hamsters was studied at 10, 20 and 30 days of age (Figs 2–4). In the control animal, cytosol Rp remained low in uterus and vagina until day 20; then levels rose between day 20 and day 30 in response to the prepubertal increase in ovarian oestrogen secretion (Fig. 2). In the DES-treated animal, cytosol Rp was increased at day 10 in both uterus and vagina, and uterine Rp but not vaginal Rp remained elevated on days 20 and 30. Cytosol Re was increased in uterus but not vagina

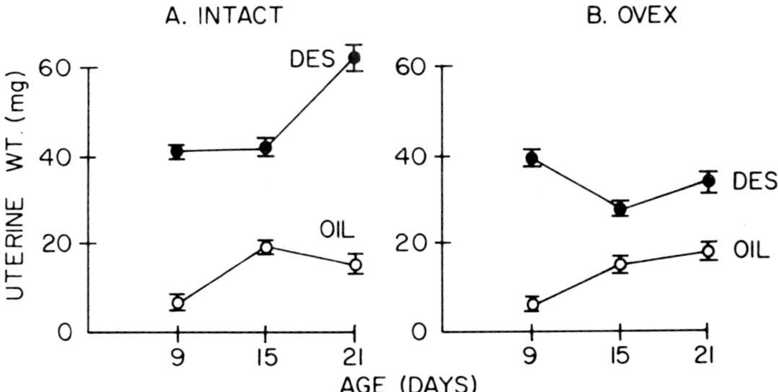

Fig. 1. Uterine development in hamsters treated on the day of birth (day 1) with DES or oil vehicle. At day 3, animals were either subjected to a sham surgical procedure (intact, panel A) or ovariectomized (ovex, panel B). Each point represents the mean ± S.E.M. (n = 8 or more). DES = 100 μg DES/animal (40 mg/kg) administered in 50 μl oil. OIL = corn oil vehicle (control).

TABLE II
Comparison of Serum Steroid Levels in Intact and Neonatally Ovariectomized Animals[a]

Steroid	Age (days)	Intact		Ovariectomized	
		Oil	DES	Oil	DES
Oestradiol	9	21 ± 3.1	23 ± 2.5	29 ± 5.2	26 ± 3.1
(pg/ml)	15	29 ± 4.9	19 ± 4.2	16 ± 1.0	20 ± 1.5
	21	10 ± 1.9	16 ± 3.2	13 ± 2.3	10 ± 3.1
Progesterone	9	< 0.3	< 0.3	< 0.3	< 0.3
(ng/ml)	15	< 0.3	< 0.3	< 0.3	< 0.3
	21	1.4 ± 0.2	0.3	0.4 ± .02	0.3 ± .02
Testosterone	9	79 ± 51	64 ± 34	39 ± 36	5 ± 2
(pg/ml)	15	15 ± 4	34 ± 15	< 6	< 6
	21	24 ± 11	4 ± 1	< 6	9 ± 6

[a] Assay sensitivity was oestradiol (6 pg/ml); progesterone (0.3 ng/ml); and testosterone (6 pg/ml). Animals were given 100 μg DES or 50 μl oil vehicle at birth (day 1) and on day 3 either were ovariectomized or subjected to a sham surgical procedure (intact).

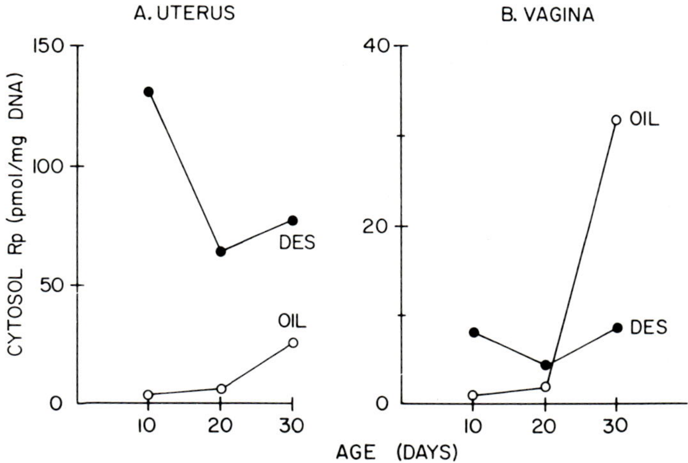

Fig. 2. Cytosol progesterone receptor (Rp) concentration in uterus and vagina of hamsters treated at one day old with DES or oil vehicle. Rp was measured as described by Leavitt *et al.* (1978). Each point represents the mean of duplicate assays performed on a pool of cytosol.

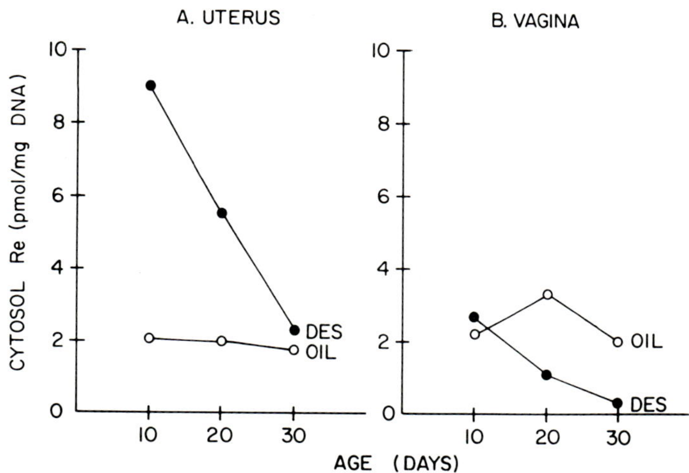

Fig. 3. Cytosol oestrogen receptor (Re) concentration in uterus and vagina of hamsters treated at one day old with DES or oil vehicle. Re was measured as described by Leavitt *et al.* (1979). Each point represents the mean of duplicate assays performed on the cytosol pool used for Figure 2.

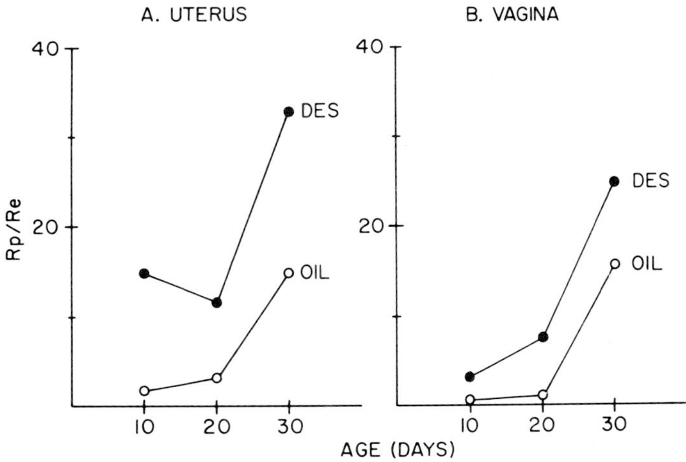

Fig. 4. Ratio of progesterone receptor (Rp) to oestrogen receptor (Re) in uterine and vaginal cytosol following neonatal treatment with DES or oil vehicle. The Rp and Re values used to calculate the Rp/Re ratio are depicted in Figures 2 and 3.

at day 10 after DES exposure on day 1, and thereafter uterine Re levels dropped to control values between day 10 and day 30 (Fig. 3). The ratio of cytosol Rp to cytosol Re was higher in the uterus and vagina of the DES animal at all times studied (Fig. 4). This suggests the hypothesis that neonatal DES treatment may permanently increase Rp numbers relative to Re in oestrogen target cells.

To determine whether neonatal DES treatment had induced permanent changes in receptor numbers, control and DES-treated hamsters were ovariectomized beginning on day 21 and compared at various intervals thereafter. At 9–15 days after ovariectomy, uterine weight, but not vaginal weight, was significantly higher in the DES animal than in the control, and this weight difference was correlated with a significant increase in uterine Rp content (pmol/uterus) and concentration (pmol/g tissue and pmol/mg DNA). Nuclear Re levels in the vagina and uterus of the ovariectomized DES animal were significantly elevated when expressed either per organ (pmol/uterus) or on a tissue weight basis (pmol/g tissue). However, when nuclear Re was expressed on a cellular basis (pmol/mg DNA), there was no difference between DES and control animals. These results demonstrate permanent, ovarian-independent changes in uterine Rp numbers as early as day 30 following DES treatment on day 1 of life. Although nuclear Re concentration is higher in the DES uterus when expressed on a tissue weight basis, this difference cannot be attributed to differences in the numbers of receptors per cell. Rather, these results support the conclusion that the cellular composition of the uterus is modified by neonatal DES treatment with an attendant permanent change in the cellular Rp content.

IV. RESPONSIVENESS TO OESTROGEN, PROGESTIN AND ANTIOESTROGEN ACTION

A. Oestrogen Action

Uterine weight, DNA and cytosol Rp responses to oestrogen action were measured using ovariectomized control (oil vehicle) and DES animals. After 3 days of oestradiol treatment (0, 0.1, 1, and 10 μg/animal/day), similar patterns of uterine weight response were observed in DES and control animals (Fig. 5). However, DES uteri weighed more than controls at each dose of oestradiol, resulting in an upward shift in the dose-response curve of DES uteri. The uterine DNA content (μg DNA/uterus) was higher in DES animals than in oil controls at each dose of oestradiol, but uterine DNA concentration (mg DNA/g tissue) was not different in control and DES animals. These results show that the DES uterus contains significantly more cells, and this difference in cellularity is maintained during oestrogen stimulation. Cytosol Rp content (pmol/uterus) was higher in the DES uterus than in the control, and oestrogen priming increased Rp levels in both preparations (Fig. 5). However, it should be noted that the cellular Rp concentration of unprimed uteri was higher for DES (7 pmol/mg DNA) than control (2 pmol/mg DNA) groups, and that oestrogen priming raised the cellular Rp concentration to the same maximum value (20 pmol/mg DNA). Since the difference observed in cellular Rp content of DES and control uteri disappeared upon oestrogen stimulation, the higher baseline Rp level in the DES uterus may represent a persistent oestrogen-like effect of neonatal DES exposure.

B. Progestin Action

We recently discovered that progesterone rapidly reduces nuclear Re levels in hamster uterus (Evans *et al.*, 1980; Leavitt *et al.*, 1979). Thus, it was of interest to determine whether DES and control uteri differed in terms of nuclear Re response to progesterone action. Uterine Re response to progesterone action and to oestrogen withdrawal was studied using ovariectomized DES and control animals bearing Silastic oestradiol implants. Oestrogen withdrawal was accomplished by removing the oestradiol implant, and within 4 hours nuclear Re levels were reduced by about 20 % in DES and control groups (Fig. 6). Combined oestrogen withdrawal and progesterone (2.5 mg/animal) treatment resulted in about a 50% decrease in nuclear Re in each group. Thus, the nuclear Re responses of the DES uterus to oestrogen withdrawal and progestin action appear to be normal.

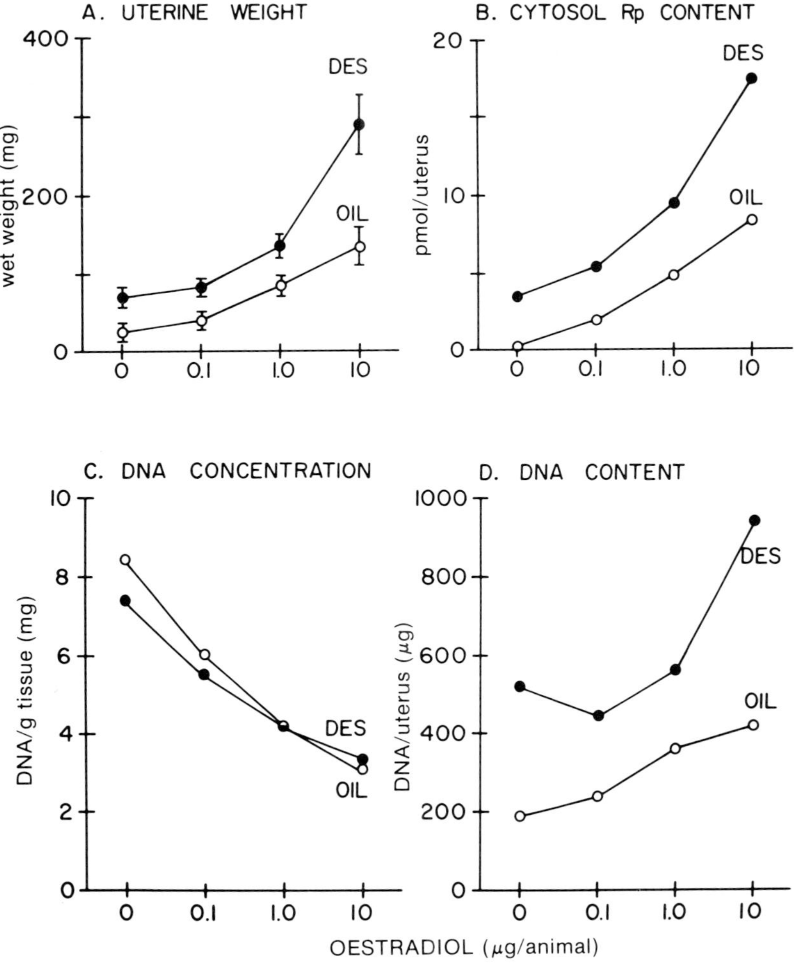

Fig. 5. Uterine response to oestrogen action. DES-treated and control (OIL) animals were ovariectomized at day 25 and treated with 0, 0.1, 1, and 10 μg oestradiol/animal/day for 3 days beginning on day 35. Animals were sacrificed 24 hours after the last injection and uterine weight, DNA (diphenylamine procedure) and cytosol Rp determined.

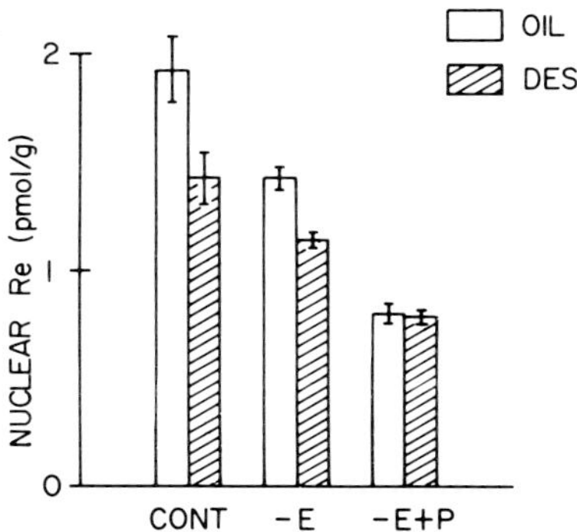

Fig. 6. Uterine nuclear Re response to oestrogen withdrawal (−E) and oestrogen withdrawal plus progesterone treatment (−E+P). Animals were treated with DES or oil vehicle on the day of birth and ovariectomized at day 25. Silastic tubes containing crystalline oestradiol (E implants) were placed subcutaneously at the time of ovariectomy. Ten days later (day 35), the animals were given the following treatments: control (CONT) = E implant left in place; −E = E implant removed for 4 hours; −E + P = E implant removed and progesterone (2.5 mg/animal) treatment for 4 hours. Nuclear Re was measured as described by Leavitt *et al.* (1979). Each bar represents the mean ± S.E.M. (n = 4).

C. Antioestrogen and Progestin Action

Our previous studies established that a variety of oestrogenic compounds could induce Rp synthesis in hamster uterus (Leavitt *et al.*, 1977). Several antioestrogens were found to be weak or partial agonists which induced Rp synthesis more effectively than they stimulated uterine growth. These and other findings suggested that regulation of Rp relative to Re availability might be an important aspect of antioestrogen action in the uterine target cell (Leavitt *et al.*, 1978). Thus we tested the responsiveness of control and DES uteri to the antioestrogen enclomiphene (formerly called *cis*-clomiphene) when combined with oestrogen and progestin therapy.

Three notable findings stemmed from this experiment. First, enclomiphene did not selectively inhibit oestrogen-induced responses in the DES-modified uterus compared to the control uterus (Figs 7 and 8). Second, enclomiphene behaved as an agonist which stimulated Rp production and uterine growth (Figs 7 and 8). Third, enclomiphene was a poor antagonist in that it failed to block oestradiol-induced uterotrophic response and Rp synthesis, and it did not prevent Rp and uterine weight response to combined oestradiol and progesterone treatment. Thus, it would appear that enclomiphene is not particularly effective as an inhibitor of oestrogen action

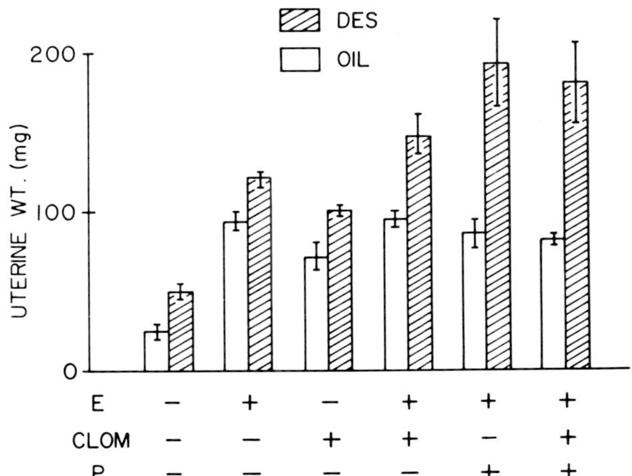

Fig. 7. Uterine weight response to oestradiol (E), enclomiphene (CLOM) and progesterone (P). DES-treated and oil-treated animals were ovariectomized on day 25 and treated with oestradiol (1 μg/day), enclomiphene (300 μg/day), progesterone (1 mg/day), or combinations of these for 3 days beginning on day 35. A plus below the bar designates the treatments which were given to that group. Each bar represents the mean ± S.E.M. (n = 5 or more).

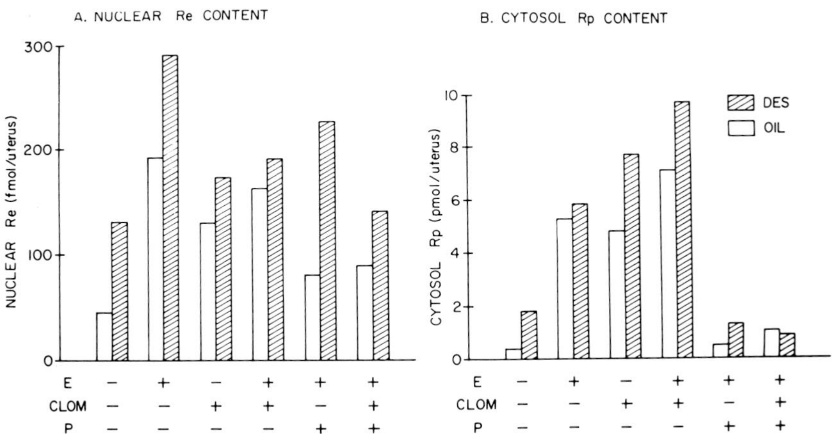

Fig. 8. Nuclear oestrogen receptor (Re) and cytosol progesterone receptor (Rp) content of the uterus following 3 day treatment with oestradiol (E), enclomiphene (CLOM), progesterone (P), or combinations thereof. Other conditions are as described in the legend of Figure 7.

in the DES uterus. However other regimens of enclomiphene may be more effective in this regard, and additional study is required to evaluate the long-term effect of antioestrogen treatment on DES-induced uterine lesions.

V. SUMMARY AND CONCLUSIONS

We have described a new experimental model system for the induction of endometrial hyperplasia and endometrial tumours in hamster uterus after neonatal DES treatment. Exposure of the DES-altered uterus to oestrogen later in life increased the growth and/or incidence of endometrial tumours. Thus, this system can be used to prepare oestrogen-sensitive endometrial tumours in a highly reproducible manner.

Our preliminary work with the DES-modified uterus has revealed permanent, hormone-independent changes in uterine morphology, cell composition and Rp levels. Alteration of the uterine target cells occurs by direct action of DES during the first two weeks of life. The DES-altered uterus is responsive to oestrogen and progesterone action suggesting that DES-induced lesions may be modified by antioestrogen and/or progestin therapy. The antioestrogen, enclomiphene, was not particularly effective in preventing oestrogen-induced responses in the DES uterus. However, the efficacy of enclomiphene and other antioestrogens in regulating the growth and development of DES-induced uterine lesions remains to be evaluated.

ACKNOWLEDGEMENTS

This work was supported by NIH grants CA 23362, CA 23693, CA 25614 and a grant from the Upjohn Co., Kalamazoo, Michigan. Enclomiphene was generously supplied by Merrell National Laboratories, Cincinnati, Ohio.

REFERENCES

Evans, R. W., Chen, T. J., Hendry, W. J. III, and Leavitt, W. W. (1980). *Endocrinology* **107**, 383–390.

Forsberg, J. -G. (1973). *Am. J. Obstet. Gynecol.* **115**, 1025–1043.

Herbst, A. L., Scully, R. E., and Robboy, S. J. (1979). *Natl Cancer Inst. Monograph* **51**, 25–35.

Leavitt, W. W., Chen, T. J., Allen, T. C., and Johnston, J. O. (1977). *Ann. N. Y. Acad. Sci.* **286**, 210–225.

Leavitt, W. W., Chen, T. J., Do, Y. S., Carlton, B. D., and Allen, T. C. (1978). *In* "Receptors and Hormone Action" (B. W. O'Malley and L. Birnbaumer, eds), Vol. II, pp. 157–188. Academic Press, New York.

Leavitt, W. W., Chen, T. J., and Evans, R. W. (1979). *Adv. Exp. Med. Biol.* **117**, 197–222.
McLachlan, J. A. (1979). *Natl Cancer Inst. Monograph* **51**, 67–72.
Rustia, M. (1979). *Natl Cancer Inst. Monograph* **51**, 77–87.

11

Mechanisms of Oestrogen Antagonism by Tamoxifen and Monohydroxytamoxifen in Chick Oviduct

J. MEŠTER, N. BINART, M. G. CATELLI, C. GEYNET, R. HÄHNEL, V. PURI, D. SEELEY, R. L. SUTHERLAND AND E. E. BAULIEU

I. INTRODUCTION

The discovery of intracellular receptors (Jensen and DeSombre, 1972; Baulieu *et al.*, 1975; Gorski and Gannon, 1976) which appear necessary for mediating oestrogen action in target tissues has led to attempts to construct antagonist molecules which compete with the agonist for the receptor binding sites and form a receptor-antagonist complex incapable of inducing oestrogenic responses. Certain triphenylethylene derivatives, such as tamoxifen (*trans*-1-(p-β-dimethylaminoethoxyphenyl)-1,2-diphenylbut-1-ene), have been shown to antagonize, but never completely abolish, some of the actions of oestrogen in the rat uterus when administered together with, or prior to, oestradiol. Like other antioestrogens in this system, tamoxifen itself is a weak inducer of uterine growth and a good inducer of some uterine proteins, e.g. progesterone receptor. The antagonistic, as well as agonistic,

NON-STEROIDAL ANTIOESTROGENS
ISBN 0 12 677880 9

properties of the antioestrogens are generally correlated with their affinities for the oestrogen receptor, suggesting that their action indeed results from competition with oestradiol for the binding to the oestrogen receptor (Katzenellenbogen and Ferguson, 1975; Jordan *et al.*, 1978; Rochefort *et al.*, 1979). Their use in studying hormone action in mammalian systems is, however, severely complicated by the fact that these compounds form partially active complexes with the oestrogen receptor.

While testing the action of various compounds in the chick oviduct, we found, in the case of tamoxifen, a striking lack of any oestrogenic activity even at high doses of the compound (Sutherland *et al.*, 1977a). Subsequent studies, summarized here, were undertaken in order to better understand the mechanisms of oestrogen and antioestrogen action in the chick oviduct.

II. RECEPTOR BINDING PROPERTIES

For the experiments on antioestrogen binding described here, a high salt (0.5 M NaCl) extract of purified nuclei from laying hen oviduct was used as the source of receptor. Endogenous ligand was removed by incubation with charcoal for 2 hours at 30°C (Best-Belpomme *et al.*, 1975; Sutherland and Baulieu, 1976). Both tamoxifen and its monohydroxylated derivative, 4-hydroxytamoxifen (OH-tamoxifen), showed competitive inhibition of oestradiol binding to the receptor (Fig. 1), the apparent affinity constants of these compounds being about 0.3 nM for oestradiol, 2 nM for tamoxifen and 0.2 nM for OH-tamoxifen. In the case of tamoxifen, where the radioactive form of the compound was available, estimation of affinity by direct binding yielded the same value as by competition (Mester *et al.*, 1979). The relatively high affinity of tamoxifen for the oestrogen receptor, as assessed by inhibition studies and direct binding experiments, was in contrast to the data obtained by studying the kinetics of dissociation (Fig. 1B). Dissociation of the [^{3}H]oestradiol-receptor complex proceeded in two stages characterized by half-lives of 4 hours ("fast" component) and 160 hours ("slow" component) respectively, with the majority of the ligand bound at zero time to the slow component (cf. Best-Belpomme *et al.*, 1975). In the case of tamoxifen, 85% of the receptor-bound ligand dissociated very rapidly (half-time of dissociation $>$ 5 hours). It is possible that the existence of the slowly dissociating component is necessary for the agonistic properties of the receptor-ligand complex. To test this hypothesis, experiments with other non-agonistic antioestrogens, available in a radiolabelled form, are necessary.

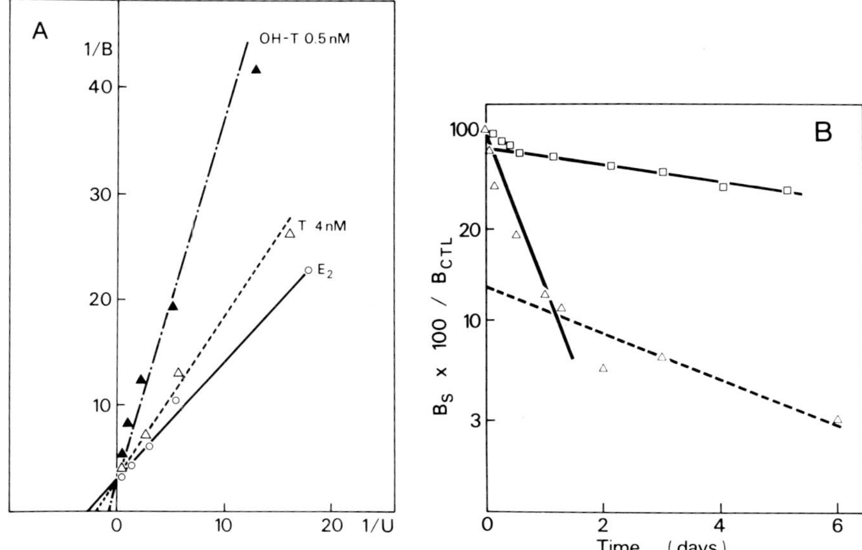

Fig. 1. Interaction of tamoxifen and monohydroxytamoxifen with oviduct nuclear oestrogen receptor.

(A) Competition of tamoxifen and OH-tamoxifen for [^{3}H]oestradiol binding to the oestrogen receptor. The 0.5 M NaCl extract of purified laying hen oviduct nuclei was treated with charcoal (0.5%) for 2 hours at 30°C; after centrifugation, portions (0.1 ml) of the supernatant were incubated with [^{3}H]oestradiol (0.1–2.5 nM) in the absence (○) or presence of competitors (4 nM tamoxifen, △; or 0.5 nM OH-tamoxifen, ▲). After 24 hours at 0°C the bound (B) and unbound (U) hormone were separated by charcoal absorption (cf. Best-Belpomme *et al.*, 1975).

(B) Dissociation kinetics. The complexes between laying hen oviduct nuclear receptor and 2.5 nM [^{3}H]oestradiol (□) or 10 nM [^{3}H]tamoxifen (△) were formed by 40 hours preincubation at 0°C. Their dissociation was measured after addition of unlabelled ligand (2.5 μM). B_s = concentration of the specifically bound [^{3}H]labelled ligand; B_{CTL} = concentration of the specifically bound [^{3}H]labelled ligand in the control solution to which the unlabelled ligand was not added. Adapted from Mester *et al.* (1979).

III. EFFECTS ON SUBCELLULAR RECEPTOR DISTRIBUTION

In the oestrogen withdrawn chick oviduct,* most of the oestrogen receptors are found in the cytoplasmic fraction of the tissue homogenate (Sutherland and Baulieu, 1976). Treatment with oestradiol or oestradiol

* Unless otherwise stated all experiments *in vivo* employed chicks which had been primed by 10 injections of 1 mg of oestradiol benzoate per chick over two weeks, and subsequently left without treatment (withdrawal) for 4–6 weeks. This treatment leads to differentiation of tubular gland cells which are ready to respond rapidly to secondary hormonal stimulation (Oka and Schimke, 1969; Kohler *et al.*, 1969).

benzoate leads to a rapid reversal of this situation, and within one hour maximum shift ("translocation") of the receptor molecules to the nuclear compartment has taken place. If the dose administered was ⩾ 0.1 mg/kg, 70% of the total cellular oestrogen receptor content was found in the nuclear fraction at one hour post-injection. The elevated nuclear receptor levels persisted for a length of time which was a function of the dose administered, and presumably of the concentration of oestrogen in the blood. With sufficiently high doses (1 mg/kg or more) the nuclear receptor level exhibits a second increase from 6 hours onwards, most likely as a result of the oestrogen-induced receptor synthesis *de novo* and continued translocation due to the persistence of oestradiol in the plasma (Fig. 2). As in the rat uterus (Anderson *et al.*, 1973; Clark *et al.*, 1973), the time of retention of the oestrogen receptor in the nucleus was correlated with the magnitude of oestrogenic response accumulated by 24 hours (Mester *et al.*, 1979).

Tamoxifen, in a similar way to oestradiol caused a rapid redistribution of the oestrogen receptor, with 80% of the binding sites present in the "crude"

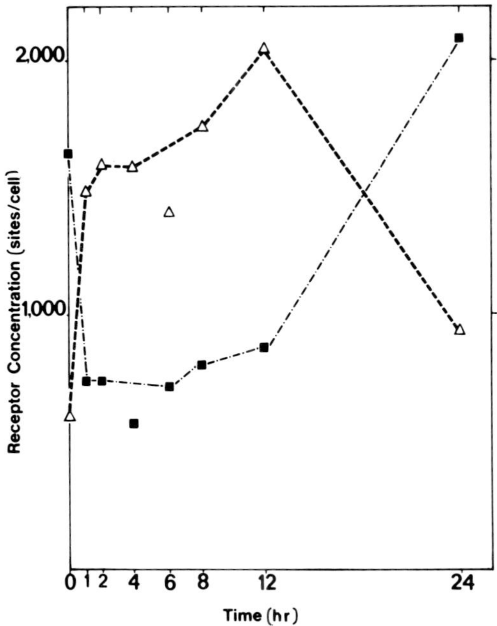

Fig. 2. Effect of oestradiol benzoate injection on oestrogen receptor subcellular distribution. Withdrawn chicks received a single intramuscular injection of 1 mg/kg of oestradiol benzoate in propylene glycol. Groups of 3 chicks were sacrificed at various periods of time afterwards and the oestrogen receptor concentration determined in the cytoplasmic (■) and nuclear (△) fractions of the magnum tissue as described by Sutherland and Baulieu (1976). From Sutherland *et al.* (1977a).

nuclear fraction one hour after administration (Fig. 3). This "nuclear" receptor, however, was not tightly bound to the chromatin, according to the work of Lebeau *et al.* (1981). The tamoxifen-induced translocation persisted for at least 24 hours when the dose of the drug was large (10 mg/kg). Contrary to the effects of oestrogen, and in agreement with the general lack of oestrogenic action of tamoxifen in the chick, no additional increase in nuclear receptor concentration was noted after one hour (Fig. 3).

Like tamoxifen, OH-tamoxifen also caused translocation and prolonged retention of the receptor in the nuclear fraction without changing the total cellular receptor (cytoplasmic plus nuclear) content. When administered together with oestradiol benzoate, OH-tamoxifen inhibited, in a dose-dependent manner, the oestrogen-induced increase in the total oestrogen receptor concentration (Table I).

The implications of these results are that the action of oestrogens (on the expression of the genes under their control) in the chick oviduct is probably dependent on binding of the steroid to the cytoplasmic receptor and on the translocation of the receptor-ligand complex to the nuclear compartment, as has been suggested by Jensen and co-workers for the mammalian uterus

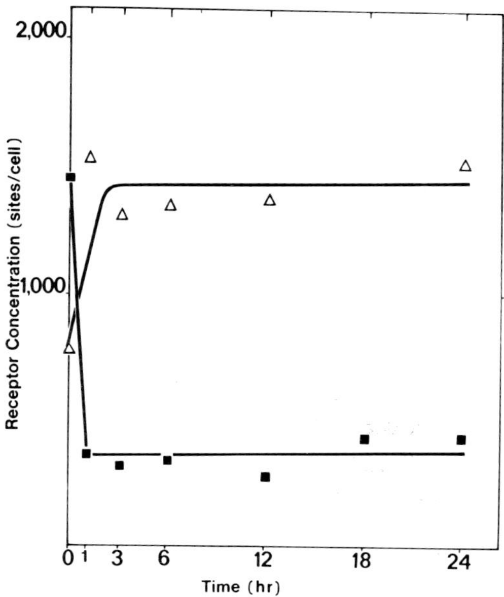

Fig. 3. Effect of tamoxifen injection on oestrogen receptor subcellular distribution. Withdrawn chicks received a single intramuscular injection of 10 mg/kg of tamoxifen in propylene glycol. Groups of 3 chicks were sacrificed at various periods of time afterwards and the oestrogen receptor concentration measured in the cytoplasmic (■) and nuclear (△) fractions of the magnum tissue as described by Sutherland and Baulieu (1976). From Sutherland *et al.* (1977a).

(Jensen and DeSombre, 1972). However, the translocation which also takes place with the receptor–antagonist complex is not sufficient to trigger further action, indicating that certain characteristics of the ligand are indispensable for its agonist properties.

TABLE I
Effects of Oestradiol Benzoate and Monohydroxytamoxifen on Cytoplasmic and Nuclear Oestrogen Receptor Levels in Chick Oviduct[a]

Compound injected	Magnum wet weight (mg)	Oestrogen receptor content		
		Cytoplasm	Nuclei	Total (cytoplasm plus nuclei)
None	87	970	240	1,210
E_2B	260	1,820	1,020	2,840
E_2B + OH-T 0.5 mg/kg	140	1,460	1,400	2,860
E_2B + OH-T 1 mg/kg	113	1,380	1,140	2,520
E_2B + OH-T 10 mg/kg	97	580	680	1,260
OH-T 10 mg/kg	93	560	620	1,180

[a] Withdrawn chicks (groups of 3) were injected with 1 mg/kg of oestradiol benzoate (E_2B) and with varying doses of monohydroxytamoxifen (OH-T). They were killed 24 hours later and the oestrogen receptor concentration measured in cytoplasmic and nuclear fractions of the magnum (Sutherland and Baulieu, 1976). Results are expressed as fmol [^{3}H]oestradiol bound per mg of DNA. From Binart *et al.* (1979).

IV. ANTIOESTROGENIC ACTIVITY OF TAMOXIFEN AND MONOHYDROXYTAMOXIFEN

When administered *in vivo* with oestradiol benzoate, tamoxifen is a potent antagonist of oestrogenic responses. As can be seen in Table II and Figure 4, an equal dose of tamoxifen was sufficient to diminish by 50 % the response to 1 mg/kg of oestradiol benzoate. When the dose of tamoxifen was 10 times that of the oestrogen, virtually no response was detected in terms of weight increase, progesterone receptor induction, ovalbumin and conalbumin synthesis (Figs 4 and 5). These conclusions are valid for short (1 day) as well as for prolonged treatments (3–10 days). Tamoxifen alone elicited no change in these and several other oestrogen controlled parameters such as oestrogen receptor content (see above), ornithine decarboxylase activity, DNA content of the oviduct, and cell differentiation (as assessed by histological examination) in the immature (non-hormone primed) as well as oestrogen-withdrawn chick oviduct.

TABLE II
Effects of Oestradiol Benzoate and Tamoxifen on Magnum Wet Weight and Cytoplasmic Progesterone Receptor Concentration[a]

	Treatment					
	Control	E_2B	E_2B + Tam(1)	E_2B + Tam(5)	E_2B + Tam(10)	Tam(10)
Magnum weight (mg)	115	670	265	120	115	113
PR_c (% control)	100	290	180	140	110	97

[a] Groups of 3 chicks were treated for 3 days with 1 mg/kg oestradiol benzoate (E_2B) and/or tamoxifen (Tam) at the dose indicated in parenthesis (in mg/kg), and sacrificed 24 hours after the last injection. Magnum weight and cytoplasmic progesterone receptor (PR_c) concentrations (Mester and Baulieu, 1977) were recorded. From Sutherland *et al.* (1977b).

The antioestrogenic activity of tamoxifen was greater than would be predicted on the basis of its affinity for the oestrogen receptor. This apparent paradox could result from either "metabolic activation" of the drug by hydroxylation in the 4 position, as was suggested in the rat by Rochefort *et al.* (1979), since the product, OH-tamoxifen, is an excellent binder, or from a longer half-life of elimination of tamoxifen from the circulation. To distinguish between these possibilities we have carried out experiments aimed at assessing the antioestrogenic properties of OH-tamoxifen, the metabolic clearance rates of oestradiol benzoate and tamoxifen, and the metabolic formation of OH-tamoxifen from tamoxifen.

The action of OH-tamoxifen *in vivo* is illustrated in Figure 6 and Table I. In spite of its 10 times greater affinity for the oestrogen receptor this compound was no more potent as an antioestrogen than tamoxifen. It is to be noted that, as with tamoxifen, no oestrogenic activity could be detected with OH-tamoxifen in the chick oviduct.

The metabolic clearance rate of tamoxifen in the chick was studied by injecting [^{3}H]tamoxifen (250 μCi/kg) together with unlabelled tamoxifen (10 mg/kg) intramuscularly in propylene glycol (conditions under which the action *in vivo* was tested) and measuring the amount of [^{3}H]tamoxifen remaining in the plasma between one and 24 hours afterwards. The elimination of tamoxifen was slow, the estimated half-life being 20 hours (Fig. 7). Thin layer chromatography on silica gel of ether extracts of plasma confirmed that practically all the radioactive material migrated as tamoxifen, and formation of OH-tamoxifen could not be detected under these conditions. However, when a sample of the bile, taken at 24 hours after the injection of [^{3}H]tamoxifen, was extracted and run on thin layer plates, about 20% of the

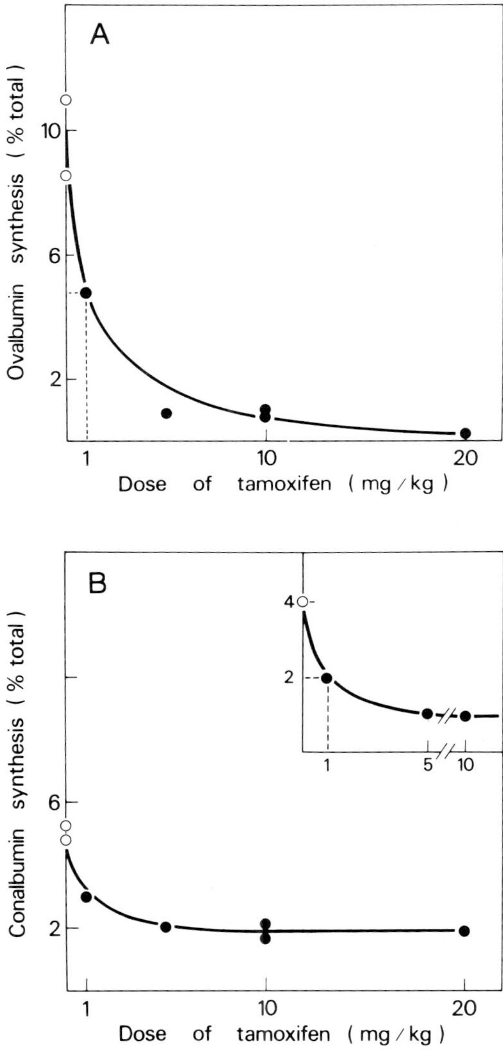

Fig. 4. Effect of various doses of tamoxifen on (A) ovalbumin and (B) conalbumin induction by a single injection of oestradiol benzoate. Withdrawn chicks were given oestradiol benzoate (1 mg/kg) (○) or oestradiol benzoate plus tamoxifen (●) at the doses indicated. The animals were killed 16 hours after each treatment, and the relative rate of synthesis of the two proteins measured. The dotted line represents the dose of tamoxifen necessary for a 50 % inhibition of the oestrogen effect. In the case of conalbumin (insert) the values obtained for the rate of synthesis were corrected by subtracting the control value of 1 % measured in non-hormone exposed animals. From Catelli *et al.* (1980).

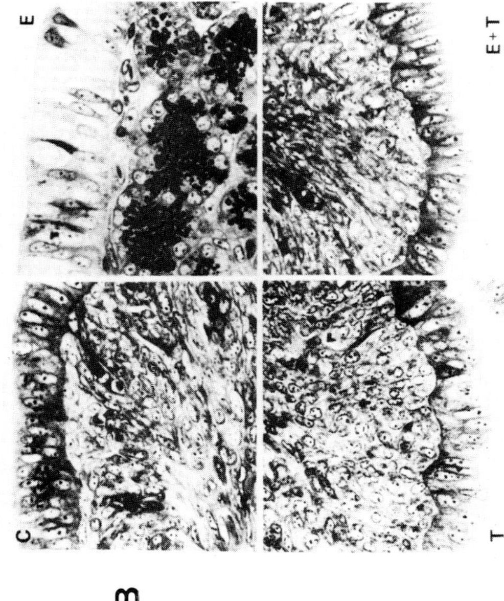

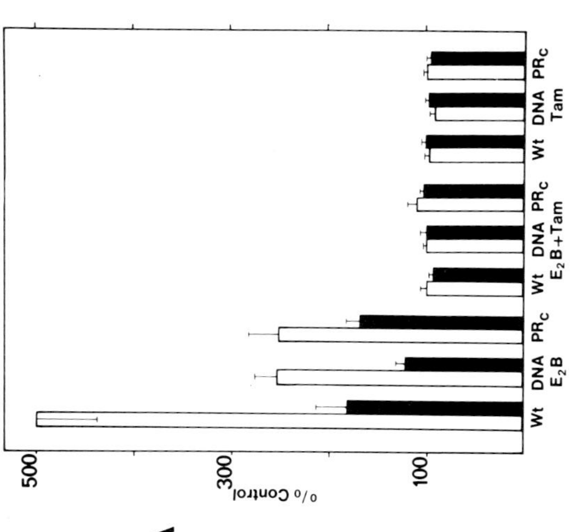

Fig. 5. Long term effects of oestradiol benzoate and tamoxifen.

(A) Groups of oestrogen withdrawn chicks (4–6 animals/group) received either 3 injections at 24 hour intervals (open bars) or a single injection (full bars) of the following compounds: 1 mg/kg oestradiol benzoate (E_2B); 10 mg/kg tamoxifen (Tam); or both drugs simultaneously (E_2B + Tam). 24 hours after the final injection, animals were sacrificed and magnum wet weight (Wt), DNA content (DNA) and cytoplasmic progesterone receptor concentration (PR_c) assessed. From Sutherland *et al.* (1977a).

(B) 7-week-old chicks, without prior hormonal treatment, were injected for 10 days with 1 mg/kg of oestradiol benzoate (E), 10 mg/kg of tamoxifen (T), or both (E + T). Control animals (C) received no treatment. Sections of mid-oviduct were glutaraldehyde fixed and stained as described by Boisvieux-Ulrich *et al.* (1977).

radioactive material migrated in the position of OH-tamoxifen, suggesting that as in the rat tamoxifen does get metabolized to its monohydroxylated derivative in the chick. This metabolite appears to be predominantly excreted and not reabsorbed into the circulation.

To study the rate of elimination of oestradiol benzoate from the plasma, 1 mg/kg of the compound was injected intramuscularly in propylene glycol, and blood samples were collected at time intervals between one and 24 hours. Plasma was extracted with ethylacetate and radioimmunoassay of oestradiol was carried out as described by Abraham (1969). The data obtained represented predominantly the oestradiol liberated by progressive hydrolysis of the ester bond, since the cross-reactivity of the antibody with oestradiol benzoate was very low (1 ng of oestradiol benzoate equivalent to 3.5 pg of oestradiol). The elimination of immunoreactive oestrogen from the plasma was rapid when compared to that of tamoxifen and proceeded in two stages characterized by half-lives of one and 6 hours, respectively (Fig. 7). It appears, therefore, that the powerful antioestrogenic activity of tamoxifen is due largely to its long persistence in the circulation.

That both tamoxifen and OH-tamoxifen were active as antioestrogens in the chick was confirmed with experiments *in vitro* where their effect on ornithine decarboxylase induction by oestradiol was examined. In this system,

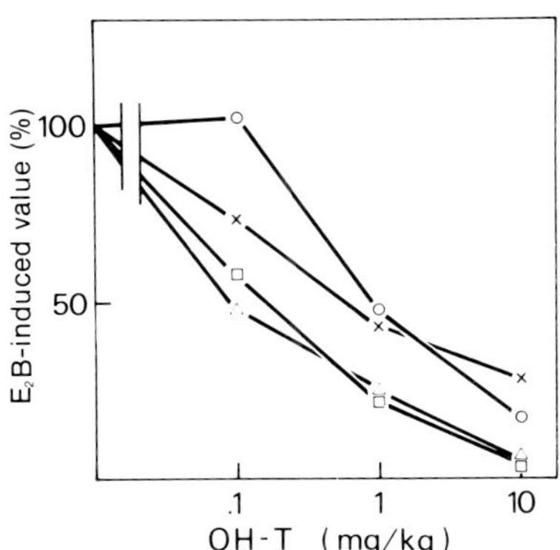

Fig. 6. Inhibition of oestrogen effects *in vivo* by monohydroxytamoxifen: dose dependence. Chicks (groups of 3) were given 1 mg of oestradiol benzoate (E_2B) together with various doses (0, 0.1, 1 or 10 mg/kg) of monohydroxytamoxifen (OH-T). The induction of conalbumin synthesis (×) at 4 hours (determined according to Palmiter *et al.* 1971), ornithine decarboxylase activity (□) at 4 hours (Pegg and Williams-Ashman, 1968), ovalbumin synthesis (△) at 16 hours (Palmiter *et al.*, 1971) and progesterone receptor levels (○) at 16 hours were determined. The values obtained in the untreated chick (identical to those in chick given OH-tamoxifen alone) have been subtracted. From Binart *et al.* (1979).

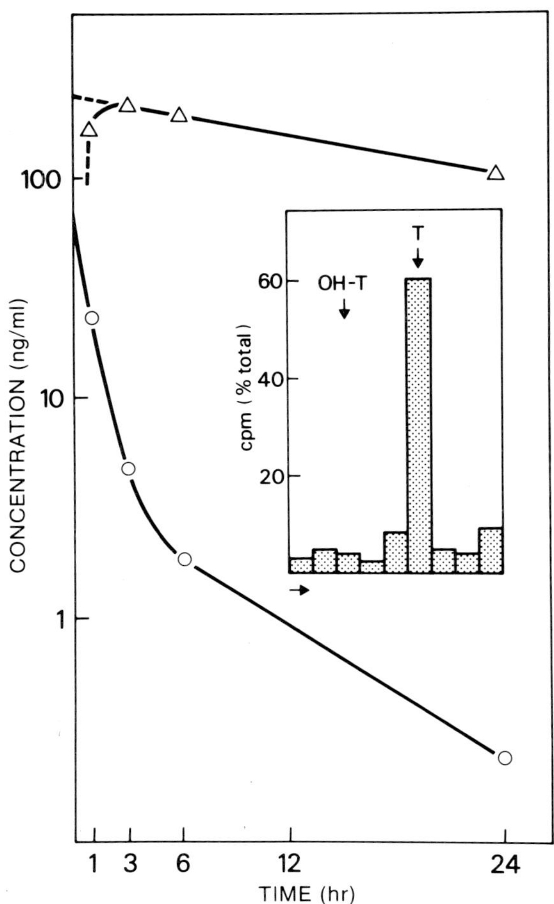

Fig. 7. Plasma clearence rate of [^{3}H]tamoxifen and oestradiol benzoate in the chick. Chicks were given a single intramuscular injection of a mixture of [^{3}H]tamoxifen (0.25 mCi/kg) and unlabelled tamoxifen (10 mg/kg); blood samples were taken from the wing vein at 1, 3, 6, and 24 hours; serum radioactivity was determined; and the concentration of tamoxifen was calculated on the basis of specific activity of the injected mixture (△). An aliquot (0.5 ml) of a serum sample taken at 6 hours was extracted with ether (2 × 5 ml), dried and chromatographed on a silica gel thin layer plate in benzene: triethylamine mixture (9:1). Sections (1 cm) of the track were scraped and counted (inset).

Another group of chicks received a single intramuscular injection of 1 mg oestradiol benzoate/kg and blood samples were taken from the wing vein at 0, 1, 3, 6 and 24 hours, serum was extracted with ethylacetate (2 × 5 ml) and oestradiol was determined by radioimmunoassay. The data (○) represent the means of 2 chicks. From Binart *et al.* (1979).

OH-tamoxifen demonstrated more potent antioestrogenic activity than tamoxifen, in correlation with the affinities for the oestrogen receptor (Table III). However, in both cases, relatively high concentrations were necessary in order to observe their antagonistic properties; this may result from either their relative instability (formation of the inactive *cis*-isomer, for instance) or to preferential uptake of oestradiol by the oviduct tissue *in vitro*. The possibility that OH-tamoxifen might be formed from tamoxifen directly in the target cells was also tested. No formation of OH-tamoxifen from [^{3}H]tamoxifen could be detected in either the incubation medium or the subcellular fractions of the oviduct under tissue incubation conditions identical to those used in the ornithine decarboxylase induction studies *in vitro* (Binart *et al.*, 1979).

TABLE III
***In vitro* Inhibition of Oestradiol Induced Ornithine Decarboxylase Activity by Tamoxifen and Monohydroxytamoxifen**[a]

Compounds added	Ornithine decarboxylase activity (% E_2 alone)
E_2 + OH-T (200nM)	74
E_2 + OH-T (2μM)	0
OH-T (2μM)	0
E_2 + Tam (200nM)	102
E_2 + Tam (2μM)	23
Tam (2μM)	0

[a] Pieces of magnum tissue from withdrawn chicks were randomized and incubated in Eagles Minimal Essential Medium (2 ml per vial contained about 50 mg tissue) for 2 hours at 37°C. Tissue was then homogenized and the ornithine decarboxylase activity measured in the high speed supernatant fraction according to the method of Pegg and Williams-Ashman (1968). The data represented means of 3 independent experiments. The mean value induced by 20 nM oestradiol was 42 pmol CO_2 liberated per hour/μg DNA, and the results are expressed as percentages of oestradiol-induced activity. From Binart *et al.* (1979).

V. REVERSIBILITY OF OESTROGEN AND ANTIOESTROGEN ACTION

Experiments in which a large dose of tamoxifen (10 mg/kg) was administered simultaneously with, or at various time intervals after, oestradiol benzoate (1 mg/kg), and the induction of ovalbumin and conalbumin synthesis measured are shown in Figures 8 and 9. It has been shown that the relative rate of synthesis of these proteins is proportional to the cellular concentration of their respective mRNAs (Palmiter *et al.*, 1976). When injected up to 2 hours after oestrogen, tamoxifen's inhibitory action on the rate of synthesis of both ovalbumin and conalbumin was observed throughout the entire period of study. However, when tamoxifen treatment was delayed for 4 hours, the inhibitory effect was immediate for conalbumin but the induction of ovalbumin synthesis was little affected during the following 3 hours although it declined thereafter (Fig. 9). To explain these observations, we propose that tamoxifen can enter the target cells even if injected during a period of time when the majority of oestrogen receptors are localized in the nucleus, as a result of prior exposure to oestradiol benzoate. A rapid exchange of oestradiol for tamoxifen then takes place, leading to cessation of unidentified processes dependent on the presence of the receptor-agonist complex. The fact that the formation of ovalbumin mRNA, once fully induced (past the "lag period" of 3 hours; cf. Schimke *et al.*, 1975), continues for several hours after tamoxifen treatment would support the existence of short-lived intermediary products or structures capable of carrying on the process even in the absence of the receptor–agonist complex (Baulieu *et al.*, 1972; Palmiter *et al.*, 1976; Mester *et al.*, 1979).

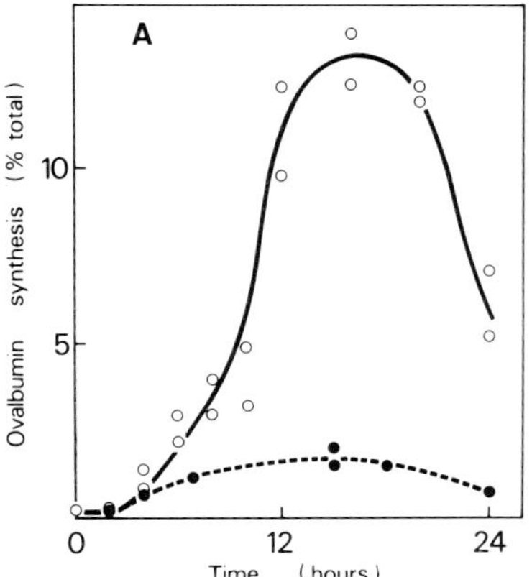

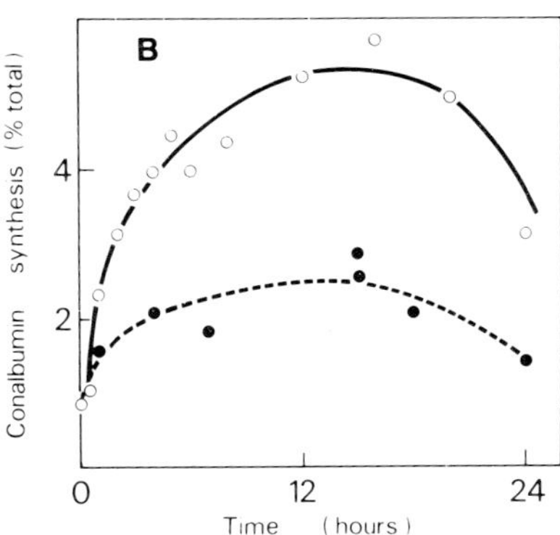

Fig. 8. Relative rates of ovalbumin and conalbumin synthesis during secondary stimulation with a single injection of oestradiol benzoate or oestradiol benzoate plus tamoxifen. Chicks (four per group) were given a secondary injection of 1 mg/kg oestradiol benzoate (○) or 1 mg/kg oestradiol benzoate plus 10 mg/kg tamoxifen (●). At the indicated times chicks were sacrificed and pieces of the magnum incubated with a mixture of [^{3}H]amino acids, homogenized and centrifuged. Aliquots of the cytosol were immunoprecipitated with anti-ovalbumin (A) or anti-conalbumin (B) antibody and the relative rates of synthesis determined as described by Palmiter *et al.* (1971). From Catelli *et al.* (1980).

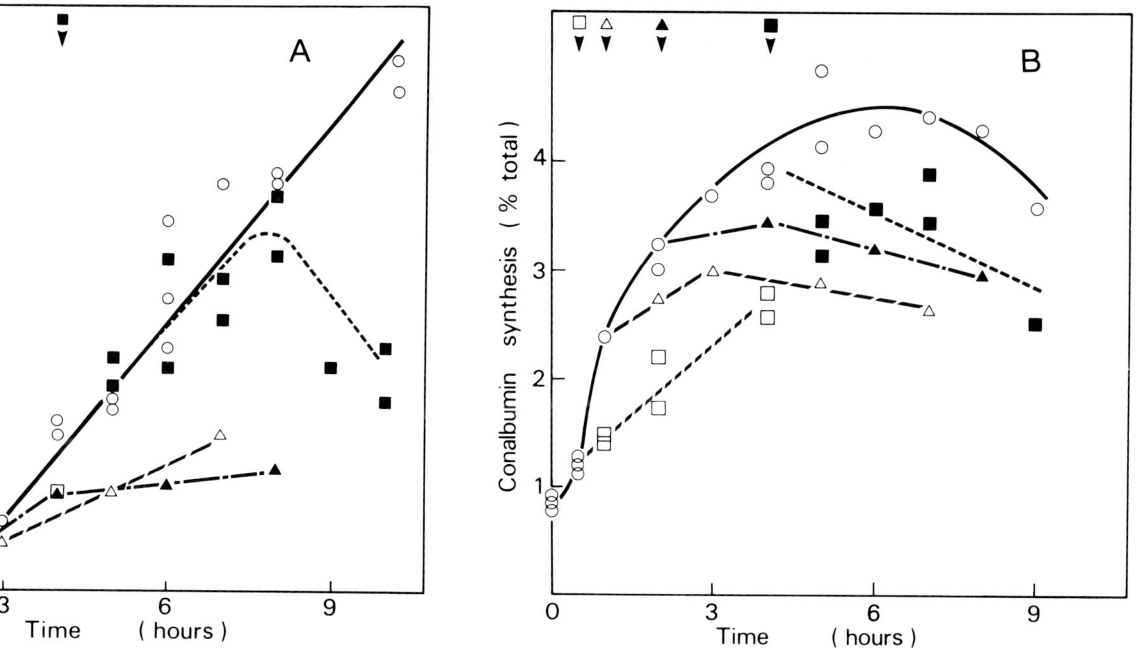

Fig. 9. Effect of delayed administration of tamoxifen on the early induction of ovalbumin and conalbumin synthesis by oestradiol benzoate. All chicks received 1 mg/kg oestradiol benzoate as secondary stimulation. Tamoxifen (10 mg/kg) was injected at the times indicated by arrows, and the relative rates of ovalbumin (A) and conalbumin (B) synthesis were measured. Treatment with oestradiol benzoate alone (○), or by tamoxifen injected: $\frac{1}{2}$ (□), 1 (△), 2 (▲) or 4 hours (■) after the oestradiol benzoate are shown. From Catelli *et al.* (1980).

The reversal of oestrogen action by tamoxifen administered up to 6 hours after oestradiol benzoate was also observed for other parameters, namely tissue weight, DNA content and induction of progesterone and oestrogen receptor synthesis (Mester *et al.*, 1977).

When oestrogen was administered 4 hours after tamoxifen the induction of ovalbumin and conalbumin synthesis was observed. The kinetics of induction were the same as in the absence of pretreatment with the antagonist, and the amplitude of induction was similar to that seen with simultaneous administration of the two compounds (Fig. 10; cf. Palmiter *et al.* 1977). Apparently, the entry of oestrogen molecules can also occur in the situation where the receptor has been occupied by tamoxifen and is located predominantly in the nucleus. Exchange between the agonist and antagonist ligands at the nuclear receptor sites establishes rapidly and at equilibrium is probably a function of their respective concentrations in the circulation and their relative affinities for the receptor.

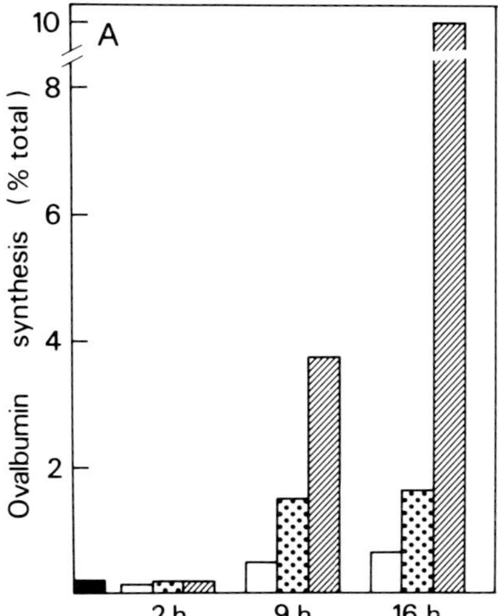

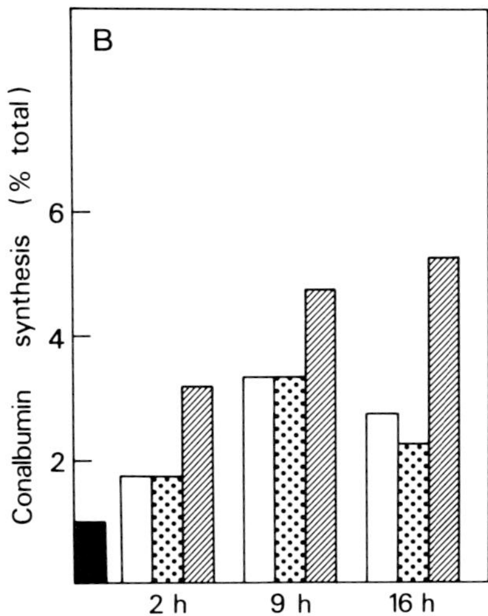

Fig. 10. Comparison of tamoxifen effects on ovalbumin (A) and conalbumin (B) synthesis when injected 4 hours before, simultaneous with, or 6 hours after oestradiol benzoate. Chicks were injected with 1 mg/kg oestradiol benzoate and 10 mg/kg tamoxifen as follows: tamoxifen 4 hours before oestradiol benzoate (open bars), tamoxifen and oestradiol benzoate at the same time (dotted bars), oestradiol benzoate alone (hatched bars), controls (solid bars). The chicks were killed at various times after oestradiol benzoate administration as indicated on the abscissa and the rates of ovalbumin and conalbumin synthesis were measured. From Catelli *et al.* (1980).

VI. EFFECTS OF TAMOXIFEN ON THE PROGESTERONE-INDUCED RESPONSES

In the withdrawn chick oviduct progesterone induces several "oestrogenic" effects, although to a different extent and with different kinetics than in the case of oestrogens. Amongst these effects are induction of tissue growth and egg white protein synthesis (Palmiter *et al.*, 1976; Schimke *et al.*, 1975). The action of progesterone could be partly or totally due to the presence of oestrogen formed directly by, or as a consequence of, progesterone stimulation of the pituitary and subsequent gonadotrophin secretion. To check on this possibility, we treated withdrawn chicks with tamoxifen and progesterone. Not only did tamoxifen have no inhibitory activity under these circumstances, but, surprisingly, certain of the progesterone-induced responses were enhanced by administration of tamoxifen together with progesterone. In particular, conalbumin synthesis, tissue growth and DNA content were significantly augmented (Table IV).

TABLE IV
Effect of Tamoxifen on the Induction of Tissue Growth and Ovalbumin and Conalbumin Synthesis by Oestradiol Benzoate and Progesterone[a]

Treatment	Magnum weight (mg)	DNA / magnum (mg)	Relative rate of synthesis (% total)	
			Ovalbumin	Conalbumin
Control	76	0.70	0.16	0.74
E_2B	1,187	5.46	46.8	8.04
P	203	1.02	38.3	8.22
E_2B + Tam	94	0.71	0.22	1.9
P + Tam	467	1.52	39.0	19.3

[a] Withdrawn chicks (groups of 3) were given 4 daily injections of oestradiol benzoate (E_2B; 1 mg/kg) or progesterone (P; 3 mg/kg) alone or in combination with tamoxifen (Tam; 10 mg/kg). Animals were sacrificed 24 hours after the last injection. The relative rates of synthesis of ovalbumin and conalbumin were measured according to Palmiter *et al.* (1971) and DNA content of the tissue was assessed by the method of Burton (1956).

The mechanisms by which these phenomena are induced are not clear at present. It could be that tamoxifen induces certain processes which alone are insufficient for provoking complete expression at any hormone-controlled gene(s), but which may augment such expression once induced by progesterone. The amplification of progesterone action by tamoxifen illustrates once more the complexity of hormone action *in vivo* and should be taken as a warning against predictions of results of multiple hormone and antagonist treatments.

ACKNOWLEDGEMENTS

We thank J. Langlois for performing the radioimmunoassay of oestradiol, M. Gouezou for preparing the histology, J. C. Lambert for preparing the illustration, and I.C.I. for their gifts of the antioestrogens. This work was supported in part by INSERM (contract no. 78.5.220.4).

REFERENCES

Abraham, G. E. (1969). *J. Clin. Endocr.* **29**, 866–870.

Anderson, J. N., Peck, E. J., and Clark, J. H. (1973). *Endocrinology* **92**, 1488–1495.

Baulieu, E. E., Alberga, A., Raynaud-Jammet, C., and Wira, C. R. (1972). *Nature, New Biol.* **236**, 236–239.

Baulieu, E. E., Atger, M., Best-Belpomme, M., Corvol, P., Courvalin, J. C., Mester, J., Milgrom, E., Robel, P., Rochefort, H., and De Catalogne, D. (1975). *Vitamins and Hormones* **33**, 649–731.

Best-Belpomme, M., Mester, J., Weintraub, H., and Baulieu, E. E. (1975). *Eur. J. Biochem.* **57**, 537–547.

Binart, N., Catelli, M. G., Geynet, C., Puri, V., Hahnel, R., Mester, J., and Baulieu, E. E. (1979). *Biochem. Biophys. Res. Commun.* **91**, 812–818.

Boisvieux-Ulrich, E., Sandoz, D., and Chailley, B. (1977). *Biol. Cell.* **30**, 245–252.

Burton, K. (1956). *Biochem. J.* **62**, 315–323.

Catelli, M. G., Binart, N., Elkik, F., and Baulieu, E. E. (1980). *Eur. J. Biochem.* **107**, 165–172.

Clark, J. H., Anderson, J. N., and Peck, E. J. Jr. (1973). *In* "Receptors for Reproductive Hormones" (B. W. O'Malley and A. R. Means, eds), pp. 15–59. Plenum Press, New York.

Gorski, J., and Gannon, F. (1976). *Ann. Rev. Physiol.* **38**, 425–456.

Jensen, E. W., and DeSombre, E. R. (1972). *Ann. Rev. Biochem.* **41**, 203–230.

Jordan, V. C., Dix, C. J., Naylor, K. E., Prestwich, G., and Rowsby, L. (1978). *J. Toxicol. Environ. Health* **4**, 363–390.

Katzenellenbogen, B. S., and Ferguson, E. R. (1975). *Endocrinology* **97**, 1–12.

Kohler, P. O., Grimley, P. M., and O'Malley, B. W. (1969). *J. Cell. Biol.* **40**, 8–27.

Lebeau, M. C., Massol, N., and Baulieu, E. E. (1981). This volume, pp. 249-260.

Mester, J., and Baulieu, E. E. (1977). *Eur. J. Biochem.* **72**, 405–414.

Mester, J., Geynet, C., Binart, N., and Baulieu, E. E. (1977). *Biochem. Biophys. Res. Commun.* **79**, 112–118.

Mester, J., Seeley, D., Catelli, M. G., Binart, N., Geynet, C., Sutherland, R., and Baulieu, E. E. (1979). *J. Steroid Biochem.* **11**, 307–313.

Oka, T., and Schimke, R. T. (1969). *J. Cell Biol.* **41**, 816–831.

Palmiter, R. D., Oka, T., and Schimke, R. T. (1971). *J. Biol. Chem.* **246**, 727–737.

Palmiter, R. D., Moore, P. B., Mulvihill, E. K., and Emtage, S. (1976). *Cell* **8**, 557–572.

Palmiter, R. D., Mulvihill, E. R., McKnight, G. S., and Senear, A. W. (1977). *Cold Spring Harbor Symp. Quant. Biol.* **42**, 639–647.

Pegg, A. E., and Williams-Ashman, H. G. (1968). *Biochem. J.* **72**, 405–414.

Rochefort, H., Garcia, M., and Borgna, J. L. (1979). *Biochem. Biophys. Res. Commun.* **88**, 351–357.

Schimke, R. T., McKnight, G. S., Shapiro, D. J., Sullivan, D., and Palacios, R. (1975). *Recent Progr. Horm. Res.* **31**, 175–211.

Sutherland, R. L., and Baulieu, E. E. (1976). *Eur. J. Biochem.* **70**, 531–541.
Sutherland, R. L., Mester, J., and Baulieu, E. E. (1977a). *Nature* **267**, 434–435.
Sutherland, R. L., Mester, J., and Baulieu, E. E. (1977b). *In* "Hormones and Cell Regulation" (J. Dumont and J. Nunez, eds), Vol I, pp. 31–48. Elsevier/North Holland, Amsterdam.

12

Synthetic Oestrogen Antagonists in Chick Oviduct: Antagonist Activity and Interactions with High-Affinity Cytoplasmic Binding Sites

R. L. SUTHERLAND AND M. S. FOO

I. INTRODUCTION

The oestrogen-withdrawn immature chick oviduct has become a popular experimental model for studies on the biochemical events leading to the action of sex steroid hormones, i.e. androgens, oestrogens and progestins. Such studies have not been confined to steroid receptors but have included data on the effects of sex steroids on cytodifferentiation and eukaryotic genetic expression (O'Malley and Means, 1974; O'Malley *et al.*, 1977; Schimke *et al.*, 1975, 1977). In view of these well documented effects of sex steroids, especially

NON-STEROIDAL ANTIOESTROGENS
ISBN 0 12 677880 9

oestrogens, we thought the chick oviduct might have advantages over other oestrogen target tissues for studies on the modes of action of the synthetic non-steroidal oestrogen antagonists. Our prejudice for the oviduct was heightened by the observation that one of the non-steroidal antioestrogens, tamoxifen, was a pure oestrogen antagonist in this tissue, i.e. it was capable of completely antagonizing the effects of oestradiol without exerting any weak oestrogenic activity of its own (Sutherland *et al.*, 1977b). This was in sharp contrast to the behaviour of non-steroidal antioestrogens in rat uterus, the most widely studied oestrogen target tissue, where they were all partial agonists–partial antagonists. It was therefore important to test if these pure antagonist properties were confined to tamoxifen or shared by other non-steroidal antioestrogens. In view of the narrow concentration range of tamoxifen employed by Sutherland *et al.* (1977b) it also seemed important to test the properties of these drugs over a wide concentration range, especially as in other systems some of them are known to have dose-dependent agonist then antagonist activity (Horwitz *et al.*, 1978). In this paper we document the agonist–antagonist activity of eight structurally related synthetic compounds in the oestrogen-withdrawn chick oviduct and quantitate their interactions with high-affinity saturable binding sites in oviduct cytosol.

II. AGONIST ACTIVITY

The oestrogen agonist activity of the eight synthetic non-steroidal compounds (illustrated in Fig. 1) was assessed in the oestrogen-withdrawn chick oviduct by determining their ability to increase oviduct wet weight, DNA content, protein content, and progesterone receptor concentration following 1 or 3 daily injections of each compound at doses ranging from 0.1–100 mg/kg body weight. All experimental procedures were as previously described (Sutherland and Baulieu, 1976; Vu Hai and Milgrom, 1978).

Figure 2A illustrates the oviduct wet weight dose-response curve for nafoxidine and compares it with that for oestradiol benzoate. The comparable data for changes in oviduct DNA content, protein content and progesterone receptor concentration are presented in Figures 2B and 2C.

Single injections of oestradiol benzoate to chicks withdrawn from primary oestrogen stimulation for 6 weeks resulted in dose-dependent changes in all the measured parameters at 24 hours (Fig. 2). By contrast nafoxidine was unable to elicit a significant increase in any of the measured parameters over the wide concentration range tested (Fig. 2). Indeed, none of the compounds under study showed any measurable response following 1 or 3 days administration. It was therefore concluded that in this experimental system non-steroidal antioestrogens show no oestrogenic activity at the target tissue level.

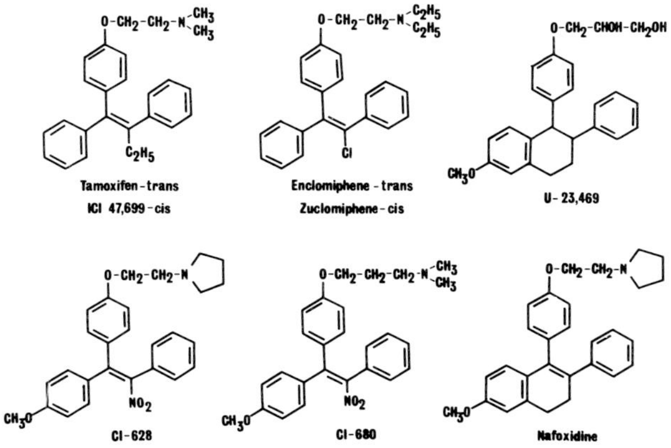

Fig. 1. Structures of the 8 synthetic non-steroidal compounds studied.

III. ANTAGONIST ACTIVITY

The ability of the same eight compounds to antagonize the oestrogenic response was assessed by administering 5 mg/kg oestradiol benzoate with or without varying doses of the antagonists and measuring any reduction in oviduct weight, DNA, protein and progesterone receptor concentration 24 hours after administration. The wet weight and protein concentration data are illustrated in Figure 3 where it can be seen that enclomiphene, nafoxidine, tamoxifen, CI 628 and CI 680 were potent antagonists when administered at 25 mg/kg. Enclomiphene was clearly the most potent antagonist since it completely obliterated the oestrogenic response at this dose. At higher doses (i.e. 50–100 mg/kg) nafoxidine, tamoxifen, CI 628 and CI 680 were also complete antagonists. By contrast zuclomiphene, U 23,469 and ICI 47,699 showed little or no antagonism at 25 mg/kg. Similar results were obtained when progesterone receptor concentration was used as the response parameter (Fig. 4). When the dose of the three compounds showing no antagonist activity was increased to 125 mg/kg (i.e. to an agonist:antagonist ratio of 1:25), zuclomiphene showed significant inhibition of the oestradiol benzoate induced increase in oviduct wet weight and protein content while U 23,469 and ICI 47,699 demonstrated small but nonsignificant reductions in these parameters (Fig. 3).

Because it was considered important to establish whether or not the *cis*-isomers of clomiphene (zuclomiphene) and tamoxifen (ICI 47,699) were antioestrogenic in the chick while being full agonists in rodent systems, further experiments were performed. Groups of 4 chicks received four daily injections

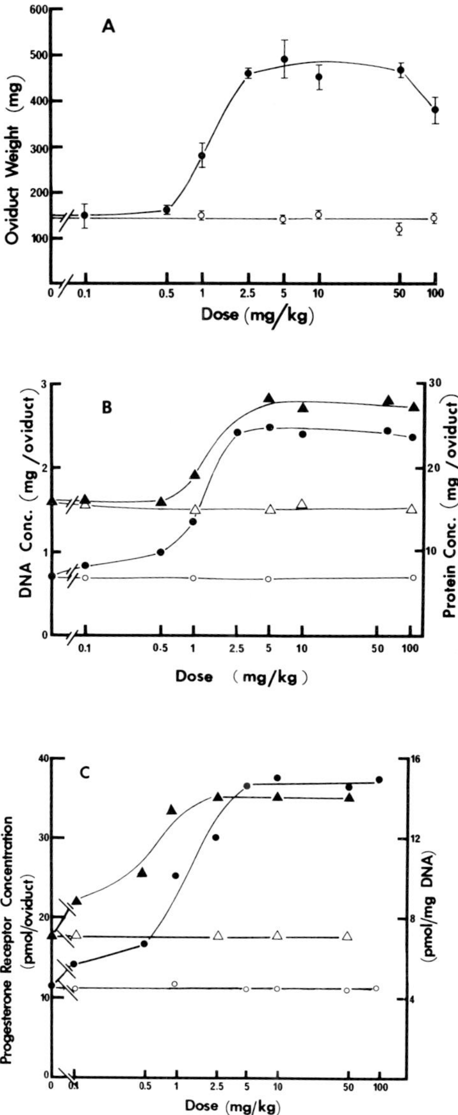

Fig. 2. Changes in oviduct wet weight, DNA content, protein content and progesterone receptor concentration 24 hours after administration of a single dose of oestradiol benzoate or nafoxidine to oestrogen-withdrawn chickens. Groups of 4 chickens received single intramuscular injections of various doses of oestradiol benzoate (closed symbols) or nafoxidine (open symbols) 24 hours before sacrifice. The following parameters were measured: (A) oviduct wet weight; (B) oviduct DNA (triangles) and protein content (circles); (C) progesterone receptor concentration expressed as either pmol/oviduct (circles) or pmol/mg DNA (triangles). Similar experiments with tamoxifen also failed to induce any significant increase in these parameters (Sutherland, 1981).

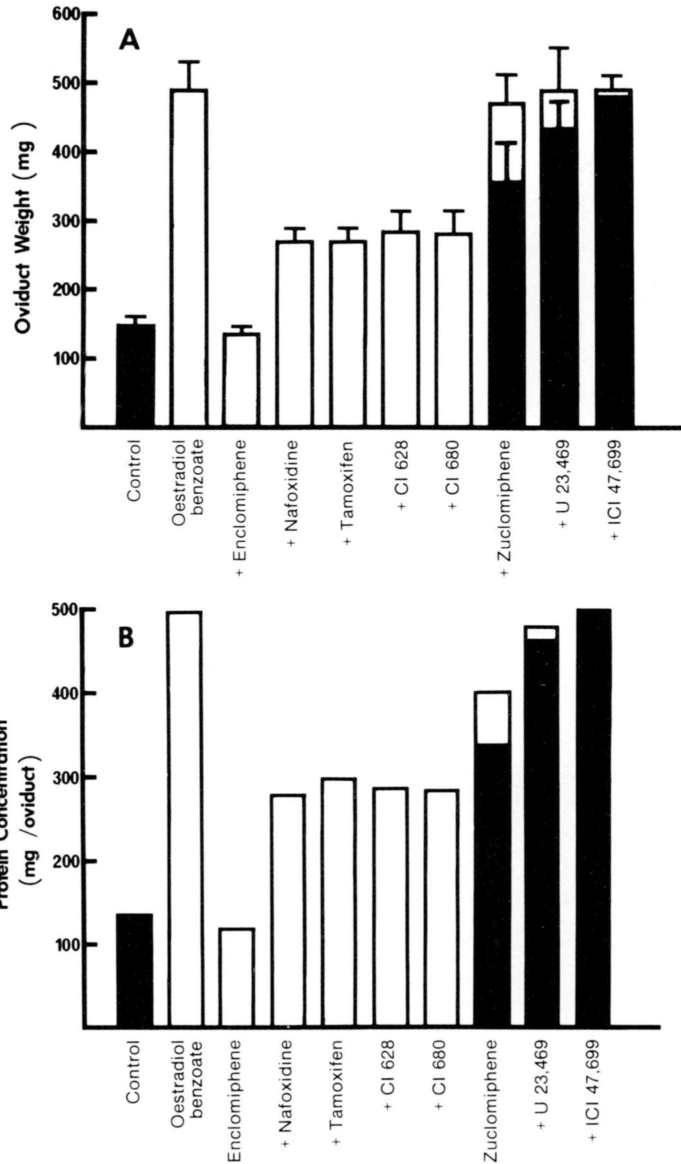

Fig. 3. Antagonism of oestrogen-induced increases in oviduct wet weight and protein content by 8 synthetic non-steroidal compounds. Groups of 4 chickens received a single intramuscular injection of 5 mg/kg oestradiol benzoate with or without a single injection of the test compound at either 25 mg/kg (open bars) or 125 mg/kg (solid bars). Chickens were sacrificed 24 hours post-injection and oviduct wet weights (A) and protein concentration (B) measured.

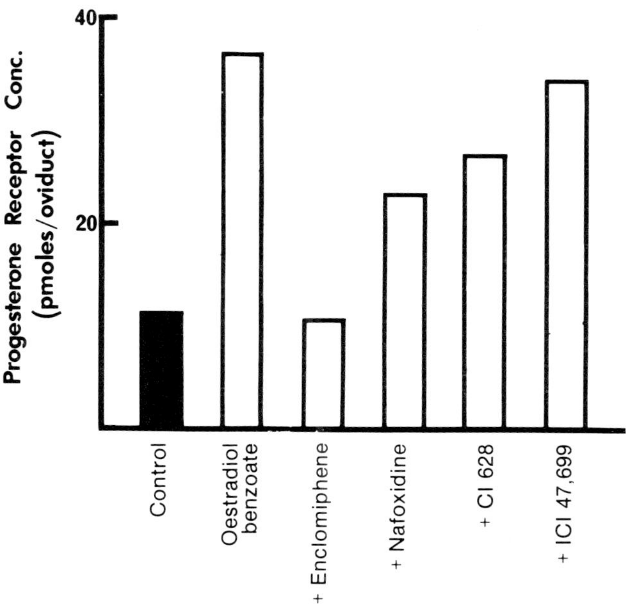

Fig. 4. Antagonism of oestrogen-induced increases in oviduct progesterone receptor concentration by four synthetic non-steroidal compounds. The experimental design is described in Figure 3.

of either oestradiol benzoate (1 mg/kg), ICI 47,699 (25 mg/kg), or both compounds together. Animals were sacrificed 24 hours after the last injection, the oviducts removed and weighed, and the concentration of DNA, protein and progesterone receptor measured. The data are presented in Figure 5 where it can be seen that under these experimental conditions ICI 47,699 caused a large and significant reduction in the oestradiol benzoate induced responses without having any measurable oestrogenic activity of its own. It was concluded that both the *cis*- and *trans*-isomers of clomiphene and tamoxifen are antioestrogens in the chick oviduct.

IV. COMPETITION FOR OESTROGEN RECEPTOR SITES IN OVIDUCT CYTOPLASM AND NUCLEUS

The relative ability (cf. oestradiol) of the eight non-steroidal anti-oestrogens to inhibit the binding of tritiated oestradiol to specific oestrogen receptor sites was investigated in oviduct cytosol from oestrogen-withdrawn chicks and in KCl extracts of oviduct nuclei from oestrogen-stimulated chicks.

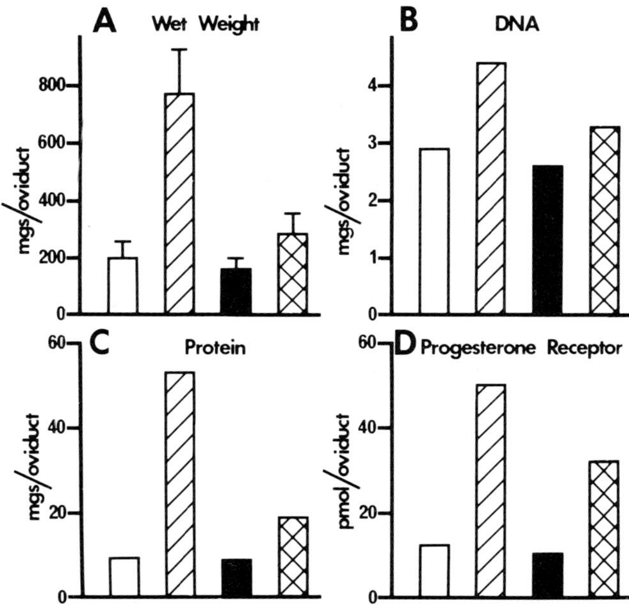

Fig. 5. Antagonism of oestrogen-induced increases in oviduct wet weight, DNA content, protein content and progesterone receptor concentration by ICI 47,699. Groups of four chickens received four daily injections of propylene glycol (open bars), 1 mg/kg oestradiol benzoate (hatched bars), 25 mg/kg ICI 47,699 (solid bars), or oestradiol benzoate plus ICI 47,699 (cross hatched bars). Animals were sacrificed 24 hours after the last injection and the following parameters measured: (A) oviduct wet weight; (B) oviduct DNA content; (C) oviduct protein content; and (D) oviduct progesterone receptor concentration.

The data are presented in Figure 6 and summarized in Table I where it is shown that all the compounds tested are able to compete with oestradiol for binding to the oestrogen receptor. The three compounds which had previously been shown to have weak antioestrogenic activity (i.e. zuclomiphene, U 23,469 and ICI 47,699) also demonstrated low relative affinities for the oestrogen receptor (i.e. 0.2–1.4 % that of oestradiol). By contrast the other five compounds, which were potent antagonists, had relatively high affinities for the oestrogen receptor. Interestingly, the relative affinities differed between the cytosol and the nuclear extract. Competition for binding to the cytoplasmic oestrogen receptor was in the order CI 680 < CI 628 < nafoxidine < tamoxifen < enclomiphene < U 23,469 < ICI 47,699 < zuclomiphene, whilst in the nuclear extract the order was nafoxidine < CI 628 < tamoxifen < CI 680 < enclomiphene < U 23,469 < ICI 47,699 <

zuclomiphene. The relative binding affinities of these compounds for rat uterine cytosol are included in Table 1 for comparison. It is interesting that the order of potencies for inhibition of tritiated oestradiol binding are almost identical for the immature rat uterine cytosol and the chick oviduct nuclear extract.

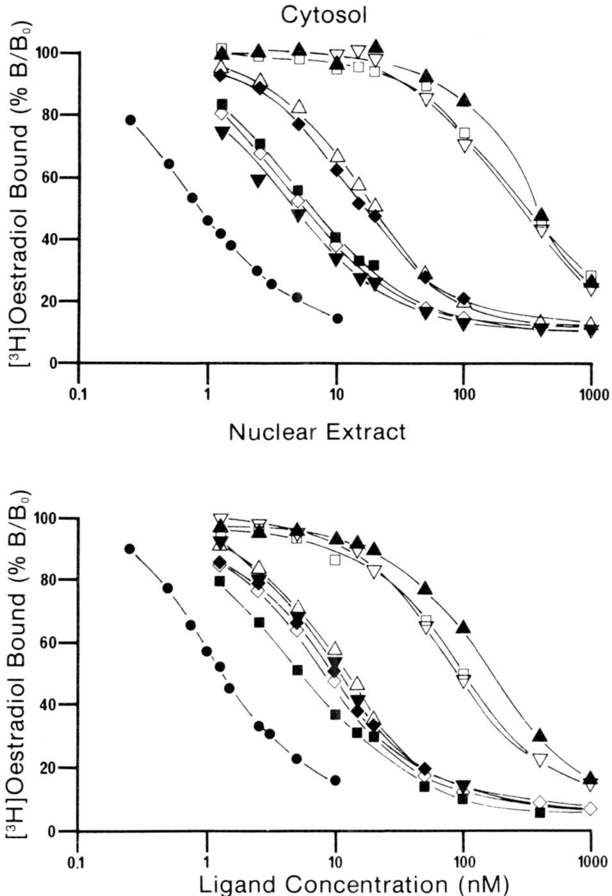

Fig. 6. Antioestrogen inhibition of tritiated oestradiol binding to oestrogen receptors in oestrogen-withdrawn chick oviduct cytosol and 0.5 M KCl extracts of oestrogen-stimulated chick oviduct nuclei. Oviduct nuclear extracts free of endogenous steroids were prepared as described by Best-Belpomme *et al.* (1975). The following ligands were tested: oestradiol (●); tamoxifen (◆); ICI 47,699 (□); enclomiphene (△); zuclomiphene (▲); CI 628 (◇); CI 680 (▼); nafoxidine (■); and U 23,469 (▽).

TABLE I
Relative Binding Affinities for Oestrogen Receptors[a]

Ligand	Relative binding affinity		
	Rat uterine cytosol	Chick oviduct cytosol	Chick oviduct nuclear extract
Oestradiol-17β	100	100	100
Tamoxifen (trans)	12.8	5.1	13.4
ICI 47,699 (cis)	0.94	0.27	1.3
Enclomiphene (trans)	7.4	4.4	10.2
Zuclomiphene (cis)	0.55	0.24	0.98
CI 628	14.8	15.9	15.0
CI 680	14.4	19.9	11.6
Nafoxidine	17.7	13.5	23.6
U 23,469	0.10	0.37	1.4

[a] The relative binding affinities (oestradiol-17β = 100) for the eight synthetic compounds were calculated according to Korenman (1970).

V. BINDING STUDIES WITH TRITIATED ANTIOESTROGENS

The experiments illustrated in Figure 6 demonstrated that all eight test compounds were able to completely inhibit the binding of tritiated oestradiol to its saturable binding sites in chick oviduct cytoplasm and nuclei. Such data suggest that these compounds bind to the oestrogen binding site of the oestrogen receptor molecule. Evidence that antioestrogens and oestrogens bind to the same site has been obtained from experiments with immature rat uterine cytosol (Katzenellenbogen *et al.*, 1978; Capony and Rochefort, 1978). In these experiments, where tritiated antioestrogens were employed, oestradiol and the antioestrogens CI 628 and tamoxifen were bound to the same number of saturable binding sites. In addition oestradiol could completely inhibit the binding of tritiated antioestrogen to its saturable binding site, indicating that oestradiol and antioestrogens were probably bound to the same site. Experiments were therefore conducted to test if similar results could be obtained with chick oviduct cytosol.

A. Direct Binding Studies

In order to measure the concentration of saturable antioestrogen binding sites in chick oviduct cytosol, direct binding studies were performed using tracer concentrations of tritiated CI 628 or tamoxifen and increasing concentrations of the same unlabelled ligands. Oestrogen-withdrawn chick oviducts were homogenized in 10 volumes (w/v) of buffer (10 mM Tris-HCl, 1.5 mM EDTA buffer, pH 7.4 containing 0.5 mM dithiothreitol) and a cytosol was prepared (see Sutherland and Foo, 1979). Aliquots of cytosol were incubated for 16 hours at 4°C with 1.25 nM tritiated antioestrogen and unlabelled antioestrogen in the range of 1.25 nM to 1.0 μM. Following incubation protein-bound and unbound ligands were separated by charcoal adsorption and the molar concentrations of protein-bound and unbound antioestrogens were calculated. Data were plotted according to Scatchard (Scatchard, 1949) and compared with those for oestradiol measured on the same samples. Typical data illustrating the binding of oestradiol and CI 628 to the same oviduct cytosol preparation are shown in Figures 7 and 8. The Scatchard plots were curvilinear prior to correction for non-specific binding. However, when a correction for non-specific binding was made using the graphical method of Rosenthal (1967), as modified by Chamness and McGuire (1976), a single straight line Scatchard plot was obtained for both ligands. When the intercepts of these straight lines on the abscissa were compared, the number of saturable high-affinity binding sites for CI 628 was three-fold greater than that for oestradiol (Figs 7 and 8).

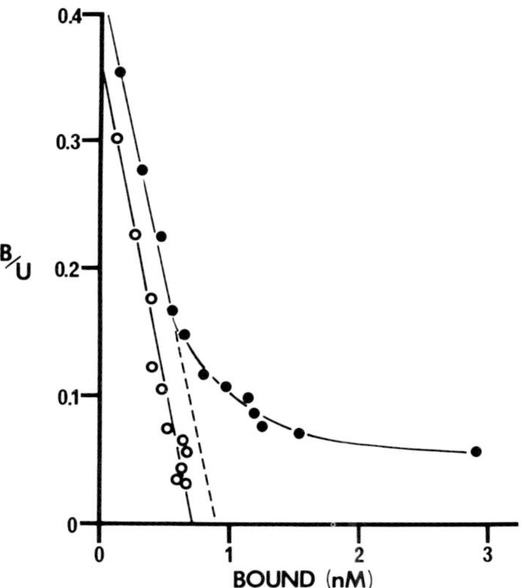

Fig. 7. Scatchard plot of CI 628 binding to chick oviduct cytosol. The closed circles represent the binding data uncorrected for non-specific binding while the open circles represent the same data corrected for non-specific binding by the method of Chamness and McGuire (1976).

In this laboratory we have preferred to analyse binding data by a previously described non-linear, least squares regression technique (Sutherland and Simpson-Morgan, 1975). When the measured protein-bound and unbound ligand concentrations for oestradiol, CI 628 and tamoxifen binding to oviduct cytosol were analysed in this way, the data for all three ligands were best fitted by a model consisting of one saturable binding component and non-specific binding (cf. Sutherland and Simpson-Morgan, 1975; Sutherland and Brandon, 1976). Replicate estimates on several different cytosol preparations demonstrated that both tamoxifen and CI 628 were bound to a similar number of saturable binding sites, but these sites were present at approximately three times the concentration of the oestrogen receptor sites (Table II). CI 628 had a five-fold higher affinity for the saturable binding sites than tamoxifen did (Table II). These data indicated that antioestrogens were bound to saturable cytoplasmic binding sites in addition to the oestrogen binding site.

B. Competition Studies

In an attempt to investigate the specificity of the saturable antioestrogen binding sites, competition studies were performed. Tracer concentrations (1.25 nM) of tritiated CI 628 and tamoxifen were incubated for 16 hours at 4°C with cytosol and increasing concentrations of oestradiol or antioestrogen.

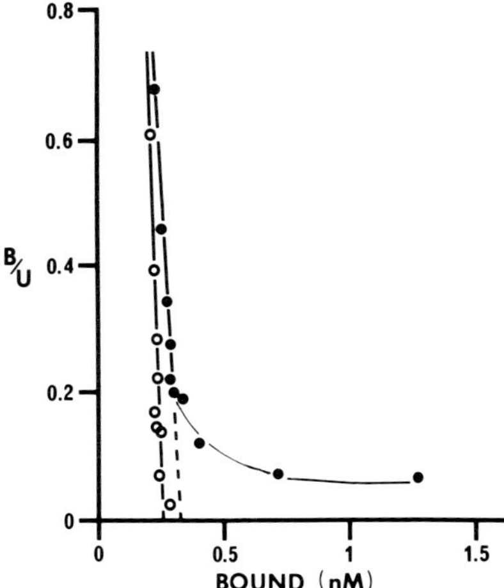

Fig. 8. Scatchard plot of oestradiol binding to the same chick oviduct cytosol illustrated in Figure 7.

The protein-bound radioactivity was determined following charcoal adsorption and plotted against the concentration of competing ligand. Data for CI 628 are illustrated in Figure 9. Similar data were obtained when tritiated tamoxifen was the radio-ligand (Sutherland and Foo, 1979). In both cases oestradiol could only partially inhibit the binding of tritiated antioestrogen to its saturable binding site, indicating that a significant portion of the saturable antioestrogen binding capacity was due to a site other than the oestrogen binding site of the oestrogen receptor.

TABLE II
Binding Parameters for Oestrogen and Antioestrogen Interactions with Chick Oviduct Cytosol[a]

Ligand	Kd (nM)	C (nM)
Oestradiol	0.07 ± 0.02	0.19 ± 0.01
Tamoxifen	9.82 ± 1.96	0.66 ± 0.24
CI 628	1.90 ± 0.72	0.61 ± 0.17

[a] The mean ± S.E.M. binding parameters; i.e. the apparent equilibrium dissociation constant, Kd, and the binding capacity, C, were calculated as described in the text. Binding capacity is expressed as nmole/litre of reaction medium which is a two-fold dilution of the cytosol preparation. Data from Sutherland and Foo (1979).

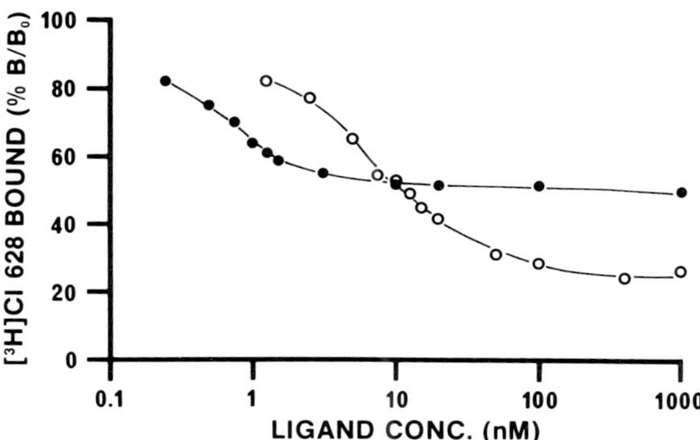

Fig. 9. Competition of oestradiol (●) and CI 628 (○) for saturable CI 628 binding sites in chick oviduct cytosol.

VI. EFFECT OF ANTIOESTROGENS ON CYTOPLASMIC AND NUCLEAR OESTROGEN RECEPTOR LEVELS

We have previously demonstrated that administration of a single injection of tamoxifen to the oestrogen-withdrawn chicken causes translocation of oestrogen receptors from the cytoplasm to the cell nucleus (Sutherland *et al.*, 1977b). When administered at 10 mg/kg, cytoplasmic oestrogen receptor levels were depleted and nuclear receptors were elevated for at least 24 hours. Additional preliminary experiments have demonstrated that all the compounds illustrated in Figure 1 are capable of inducing time and dose-dependent translocation of cytoplasmic receptors to the nucleus.

The effect of simultaneous administration of oestradiol and antioestrogens on oestrogen receptor levels in the chick oviduct has not been extensively investigated (see Mester *et al.*, 1977). We therefore designed an experiment to measure changes in oestrogen receptor levels and the oestrogenic response, following administration of oestradiol benzoate and various concentrations of tamoxifen. Groups of 3 chickens received three daily injections of vehicle alone (propylene glycol), oestradiol benzoate alone (1 mg/kg), or oestradiol benzoate (1 mg/kg) plus 1, 5 or 10 mg/kg tamoxifen. Chickens were killed 24 hours after the final injection and the following parameters were measured as previously described (Sutherland and Baulieu, 1976; Mester and Baulieu, 1977): oviduct wet weight, progesterone receptor concentration, cytoplasmic and nuclear oestrogen receptor concentration. As can be seen in Figure 10 the simultaneous administration of tamoxifen with oestradiol benzoate caused a dose-dependent inhibition of the increases in oviduct wet weight and progesterone receptor concentration induced by oestradiol. The highest dose of tamoxifen (i.e. 10 mg/kg) completely inhibited the oestrogenic response (Fig. 10).

Administration of three daily injections of oestradiol benzoate resulted in significant increases in both cytoplasmic and nuclear oestrogen receptor levels (Fig. 11). Simultaneous administration of tamoxifen caused a dose-dependent decrease in cytoplasmic and total oestrogen receptor concentrations. Nuclear oestrogen receptor levels following tamoxifen treatment were equivalent to, or higher than, those in oestradiol treated chickens despite a significant reduction in the oestrogenic response (cf. Figs 10 and 11).

These data also demonstrate that administration of tamoxifen in combination with oestradiol benzoate results in the majority of oestrogen receptors being located in the cell nucleus (Fig. 11). This is similar to the pattern seen following injection of tamoxifen alone (Sutherland *et al.*, 1977b, 1977c). In addition tamoxifen inhibits oestrogen-induced increases in total cellular oestrogen receptor levels. At the highest dose of tamoxifen the

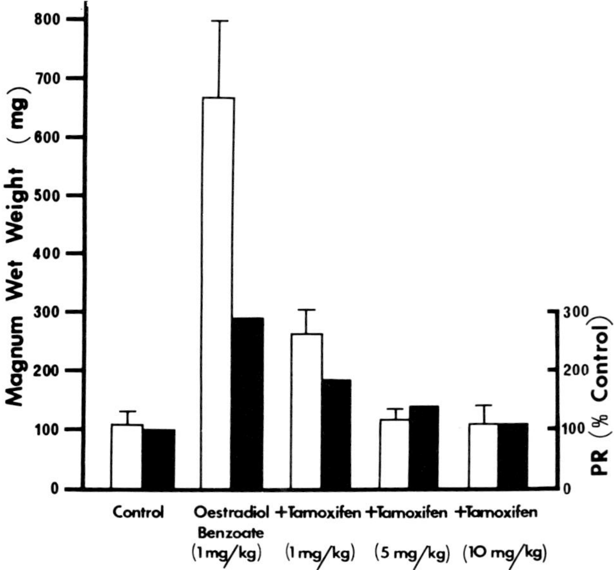

Fig. 10. Tamoxifen inhibition of oestradiol benzoate induced increases in oviduct (magnum) wet weight and progesterone receptor (PR) concentration. Dose-response relationship. The experimental design is described in the text.

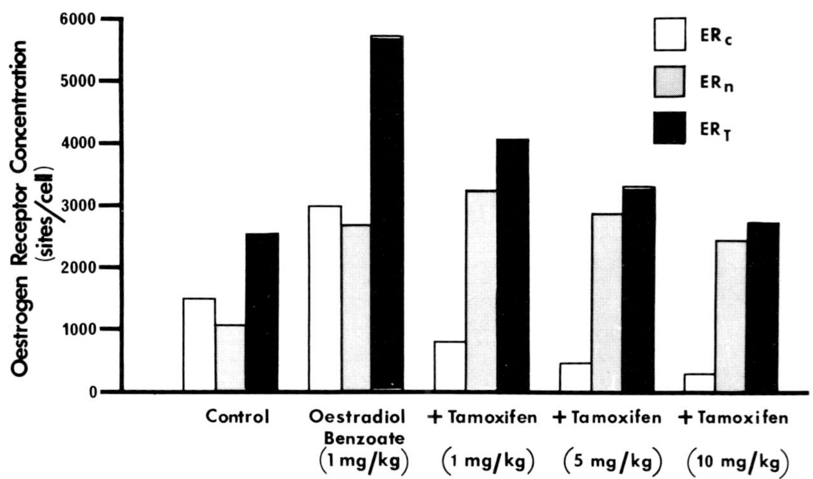

Fig. 11. Tamoxifen inhibition of oestradiol benzoate induced changes in cytoplasmic (ER_c), nuclear (ER_n), and total (ER_t) cellular oestrogen receptor levels. Dose-response relationship. Data are from the same experiment depicted in Figure 10.

concentration of total cellular oestrogen receptors was not significantly greater than control and approximately half that seen in chickens receiving oestrogen alone (Fig. 11).

VII. DISCUSSION

None of the eight structurally related non-steroidal oestrogen antagonists used in this study were capable of inducing measurable oestrogenic responses in the chick oviduct under the present experimental conditions. This lack of oestrogenic activity in an avian system is strongly contrasted with their biological properties in the immature rat uterus where they are all partial agonists (Harper and Walpole, 1966, 1967; Clark *et al.*, 1974; Katzenellenbogen and Ferguson, 1975). or in the case of the *cis*-isomer, ICI 47,699, a full agonist (Harper and Walpole, 1966, 1967).

It is of interest that some of these compounds have been tested in another avian oestrogen target tissue, the chick liver, where they also failed to demonstrate measurable oestrogenic activity (Gschwendt, 1975; Lazier *et al.*, 1981). Such species differences in the biological properties of non-steroidal antioestrogens are not unprecedented since tamoxifen has different biological activities in the rat and mouse (Harper and Walpole, 1966; Jordan *et al.*, 1978).

In terms of their antagonist activity, the eight compounds tested could be divided into two distinct groups, i.e. potent antagonists, e.g. enclomiphene, nafoxidine, tamoxifen, CI 628 and CI 680, and compounds which demonstrated little or no antagonism following a single injection, e.g zuclomiphene, U 23,469 and ICI 47,699. Under the experimental conditions described in Figure 3 enclomiphene was the most potent oestrogen antagonist, but all five compounds in the former group were complete antagonists when administered at higher doses. This illustrated that the previously reported property of pure oestrogen antagonism in chick oviduct (Sutherland *et al.*, 1977b) is not confined to tamoxifen alone. The *cis*-isomer of clomiphene (zuclomiphene) was also antioestrogenic following a single injection when the dose was elevated from 25 mg/kg to 125 mg/kg, indicating that the lack of potent antagonism by the latter group of weak antagonists may be purely dose related. Antioestrogenic properties of another *cis*-isomer, ICI 47,699, in the chick were confirmed in experiments where this compound and oestradiol were administered at a ratio of 25:1 on 4 consecutive days (Fig. 5). The possibility that these results could be due to contamination of zuclomiphene and ICI 47,699 with the corresponding *trans*-isomers cannot, as yet, be discarded. The weak antioestrogenic activity of U 23,469 in chick oviduct may be related to an inability of the chick to metabolize this compound to a more active metabolite, a process which is known to occur in the rat (Katzenellenbogen *et al.*, 1979).

All eight compounds inhibited the binding of oestradiol to its cytoplasmic and nuclear high affinity receptor sites (Fig. 6). The three compounds which showed weak oestrogen antagonism following a single dose also had relatively low affinities for oestrogen receptors, i.e. 0.2–1.4% that of oestradiol. However, the degree of antioestrogenic potency of the other five compounds was not correlated with their relative affinities for oestrogen receptor sites. Indeed amongst these compounds, the most potent antagonist, enclomiphene, was the weakest competitor for oestradiol binding in both the cytoplasm and nucleus. Thus, antioestrogenic potency is not solely a function of affinity for the oestrogen receptor but must also be influenced by a number of other parameters including absorption, plasma clearance rate, tissue uptake, metabolism and tissue retention.

In addition to confirming earlier observations that synthetic non-steroidal antioestrogens bind to cytoplasmic and nuclear oestrogen receptor sites in oestrogen target tissues our data also demonstrate the existence of an additional high affinity, saturable antioestrogen binding site in chick oviduct which does not bind oestradiol. Evidence for the existence of such a site is strong and is based on two different pieces of information. First, direct binding studies with tritiated CI 628 and tamoxifen revealed that these antioestrogens were bound to a significantly greater number of saturable binding sites in chick oviduct cytosol than oestradiol was (Figs 7 and 8, Table II). Secondly, competition experiments in which unlabelled oestradiol could only partially inhibit the binding of tritiated antioestrogens to their saturable binding sites (Fig. 9) support the existence of a population of saturable antioestrogen binding sites distinct from the classical oestrogen receptor site.

At present we have no information on the role of this novel, specific antioestrogen binding site in the modulation of antioestrogenic action in the chick oviduct. However, its affinity and concentration are such that it binds significant amounts of the drug *in vitro* and presumably *in vivo*. This may partially explain the differences in the relative binding affinities of antioestrogens in chick oviduct cytosol; cf. rat uterine cytosol and chick oviduct nuclear extracts (Table I) where relatively less antioestrogen binding sites are present. A more detailed study of this specific antioestrogen binding site is presented in a later chapter (Murphy *et al.*, 1981).

Since all the antioestrogens utilized in this study were capable of binding to the oviduct cytoplasmic oestrogen receptor it was not surprising that they were also able to translocate this receptor to the cell nucleus. As yet the dose and time dependence of this phenomenon have not been completely characterized for each compound due to the need to optimize *in vitro* exchange conditions for each ligand under study. In view of the differential rates of dissociation of antioestrogens and oestradiol from the oestrogen receptor

(Katzenellenbogen *et al.*, 1978; Capony and Rochefort, 1978; Mester *et al.*, 1979) and differential degrees of protection against thermal inactivation by various oestrogenic and antioestrogenic ligands (Capony and Rochefort, 1978), it may not be valid to assume that *in vitro* exchange conditions developed for oestradiol will be suitable for other ligands. For this reason further comments will be confined to tamoxifen, which is the only ligand studied in detail to date.

Our previously published data (Sutherland *et al.*, 1977b, 1977c) illustrated that administration of a single dose of tamoxifen to the oestrogen-withdrawn chick induced translocation of the cytoplasmic oestrogen receptor to the nucleus and long-term retention of the antagonist–receptor complex in the nuclear compartment. At this dose (10 mg/kg) the cytoplasmic oestrogen receptor levels remained depleted for at least 24 hours (the longest time interval studied). Similar results have been obtained with a single injection of monohydroxytamoxifen (Binart *et al.*, 1979). Following prolonged (3 days) administration of tamoxifen alone and in combination with oestradiol benzoate a number of interesting changes in the oestrogen receptor profile were observed (Fig. 11). Simultaneous administration of a fixed dose of oestradiol benzoate and increasing concentrations of tamoxifen resulted in a dose-dependent decrease in cytoplasmic and total cellular oestrogen receptor levels. However, the nuclear oestrogen receptor levels differed little between the treatment groups despite large differences in the oestrogenic response (Figs 10 and 11). Thus, following simultaneous administration of oestradiol and tamoxifen, the magnitude of the oestrogenic response was not highly correlated with the level of nuclear oestrogen receptors. This is in marked contrast to the situation seen following administration of several oestrogen agonists and following treatment with oestrogen and progesterone (Sutherland *et al.*, 1977a, 1980; Mester *et al.*, 1979). These results are likely to be explained by the fact that, as the tamoxifen dose was increased, a greater proportion of the nuclear sites were occupied by the antagonist, and such sites do not induce any measurable response (Sutherland *et al.*, 1977b, 1977c).

Unlike the situation in the rat, tamoxifen was antagonistic following a single injection of oestradiol benzoate and tamoxifen to the chick (Fig. 3 and Sutherland *et al.*, 1977b, 1977c). Under these conditions low cytoplasmic receptor levels could not be a limiting factor in the ability of the oviduct to respond to oestrogen, shedding doubt on the earlier suggestion that inhibition of cytoplasmic oestrogen receptor replenishment was the primary event in oestrogen antagonism by non-steroidal antioestrogens (Clark *et al.*, 1974). This was not purely a species difference since more recent data, using lower concentrations of antagonist, have illustrated that non-steroidal anti-oestrogens are antagonists in the rat at doses which cause only minor depletions of cytoplasmic oestrogen receptor levels (Gardner *et al.*, 1978; Jordan *et al.*, 1978).

Further evidence that reduced cytoplasmic receptor levels are not the major event controlling antioestrogenic action, at least in the chick, is supplied by the experimental data of Mester *et al.*, (1977) and Catelli *et al.*, (1980) which are reviewed in Chapter 11. These results illustrate that the effects of oestradiol benzoate or tamoxifen in chick oviduct can be reversed by subsequent administration of the other ligand. The administration regimes in these experiments were such that in both cases (i.e. when oestradiol benzoate was administered subsequent to tamoxifen or *vice versa*) the cytoplasmic oestrogen receptor levels were at their nadir (Sutherland *et al.*, 1977b, 1977c). Thus, despite depletion of cytoplasmic receptor levels, the compound which was administered some hours later was able to attain access to the nuclear oestrogen receptor sites, bind to these sites and induce a response characteristic of that following administration of this ligand alone. This result is likely to be explained in one of two ways. Either cytoplasmic receptor synthesis and turnover is so rapid in the chick that the ligand binds to newly synthesized cytoplasmic receptor and is carried into the nucleus or, more likely, the ligand is freely diffusable into the nucleus where it can readily exchange at physiological temperature with the ligand already attached to the nuclear oestrogen receptor. The final ratio of agonist-receptor and antagonist-receptor complexes in the nucleus, which presumably governs the magnitude of the oestrogenic response, would then depend upon the relative affinities of the ligands for the receptor and their relative concentrations in the nucleus.

It is now only four years since it was first reported that tamoxifen was a pure oestrogen antagonist in the chicken oviduct (Sutherland *et al.*, 1977b) and already considerable progress has been made in elucidating the biochemical events leading to its mechanism of action. Following intramuscular administration in propylene glycol, tamoxifen rapidly enters the circulation from which it is cleared very slowly (cf. oestradiol; Binart *et al.*, 1979). There is some debate about whether tamoxifen or its metabolite, monohydroxytamoxifen, is the active compound *in vivo* (Binart *et al.*, 1979; Borgna and Rochefort, 1979). However, it seems likely that metabolism may help but is not essential for the antioestrogenic action of tamoxifen in the chick (Binart *et al.*, 1979). Whilst the drug has a relatively high affinity for the cytoplasmic oestrogen receptor, i.e. about 5% that of oestradiol (Table I, Sutherland and Foo, 1979), its antagonistic potency is markedly greater than would be predicted from its relative binding affinity. This is presumably due to its slow plasma clearance rate.

On entering the oviduct, tamoxifen binds to the cytoplasmic oestrogen receptor and translocates it to the nucleus, but this tamoxifen-nuclear receptor complex must be impaired in some way (cf. the oestrogen-nuclear receptor complex) since no measurable biological response is observed (Sutherland *et al.*, 1977b, 1977c). The question that then arises is what nuclear events can the antagonist-receptor complex elicit. This has not been studied in detail, but, whilst the quantity of nuclear receptor is equivalent to that seen following oestrogen administration, the nuclear receptor following tamoxifen treatment does not form the characteristic 13–14S form seen after micrococcal nuclease digestion of nuclei from oestrogen treated oviduct (Lebeau *et al.*, 1981). Thus the antagonist-nuclear oestrogen receptor complex differs in some way from the agonist-nuclear receptor complex. The recent intriguing observation that tamoxifen and progesterone act synergistically in the chick oviduct (Catelli *et al.*, 1980) suggests that the tamoxifen-nuclear receptor complex may induce some oestrogen-like effects in the nucleus facilitating and augmenting the action of the progesterone-receptor complex.

Clearly, the fact that non-steroidal antioestrogens are pure antagonists in the chick oviduct makes it an extremely useful model for studying the molecular modes of action of synthetic non-steroidal oestrogen antagonists. Future research is likely to concentrate on understanding the impairment in tamoxifen–nuclear oestrogen receptor function and extending these types of studies to other ligands in the hope of better understanding structure–function relationships within this group of compounds.

ACKNOWLEDGEMENTS

We thank the following companies for their generous gifts of the compounds used in this study: I.C.I., Upjohn, Parke-Davis and Merrel.

REFERENCES

Best-Belpomme, M, Mester, J., Weintraub, H., and Baulieu, E. E. (1975). *Eur. J. Biochem.* **57**, 537–547.

Binart, N., Catelli, M. G., Geynet, C., Puri, B., Hahnel, R., Mester, J., and Baulieu, E. E. (1979). *Biochem. Biophys. Res. Commun.* **91**, 812–818.

Borgna, J. L., and Rochefort, H. (1979). *C. R. Acad. Sci.* **287**, 1141–1144.

Capony, F., and Rochefort, H. (1978). *Mol. Cell. Endocr.* **11**, 181–198.

Catelli, M. G., Binart, N., Elkik, F., and Baulieu, E. E. (1980). *Eur. J. Biochem.* **107**, 165–172.

Chamness, G. C., and McGuire, W. L. (1976). *Steroids* **26**, 538–542.

Clark, J. H., Peck, E. J., and Anderson, J. N. (1974). *Nature* **251**, 446–448.

Gardner, R. M., Kirkland, J. L., and Stancel, G. M. (1978). *Endocrinology* **103**, 1583–1589.

Gschwendt, M. (1975). *Biochim. Biophys. Acta* **399**, 395–402.

Harper, M. J. K., and Walpole, A. L. (1966). *Nature*. **212**, 87.

Harper, M. H. K., and Walpole, A. L. (1967). *J. Reprod. Fert.* **13**, 101–119.

Horwitz, K. B., Koseki, Y., and McGuire, W. L. (1978). *Endocrinology* **103**, 1742–1751.

Jordan, V. C., Rowsby, L., Dix, C. J., and Prestwich, G. (1978). *J. Endocr.* **78**, 71–81.

Katzenellenbogen, B. S., and Ferguson, E. R. (1975). *Endocrinology* **97**, 1–12.

Katzenellenbogen, B. S., Katzenellenbogen, J. A., Ferguson, E. R., and Krauthammer, N. (1978). *J. Biol. Chem.* **253**, 697–707.

Katzenellenbogen, B. S., Bhakoo, H. S., Ferguson, F. R., Lan, N. C., Tatee, T., Tsai, T.S., and Katzenellenbogen, J. A. (1979). *Recent Progr. Horm. Res.* **35**, 259–300.

Korenman, S. G. (1970). *Endocrinology* **87**, 1119–1123.

Lazier, C. B., Capony, F., and Williams, D. L. (1981). This volume, pp. 215-230.

Lebeau, M. C., Massol, N., and Baulieu, E. E. (1981). This volume, pp. 249-260.

Mester, J., and Baulieu, E. E. (1977). *Eur. J. Biochem.* **72**, 405–414.

Mester, J., Geynet, C., Binart, N., and Baulieu, E. E. (1977). *Biochem. Biophys. Res. Commun.* **79**, 112–118.

Mester, J., Seeley, D., Catelli, M. G., Binart, N., Geynet, C., Sutherland, R., and Baulieu, E. E. (1979). *J. Steroid Biochem.* **11**, 307–313.

Murphy, L. C., Foo, M. S., Green, M. D., Milthorpe, B. K., Whybourne, A. M., Krozowski, Z. S., and Sutherland, R. L. (1981). This volume, pp. 317-337.

O'Malley, B. W., and Means, A. R. (1974). *Science* **183**, 610–620.

O'Malley, B. W., Tsai, M. J., and Towle, H. C. (1977). *In* "Receptors and Hormone Action" (B. W. O'Malley and L. Birnbaumer, eds), vol. I, pp. 359–381. Academic Press, New York.

Rosenthal, H. E. (1967). *Anal. Biochem.* **20**, 525–532.

Scatchard, G. (1949). *Ann. N. Y. Acad. Sci.* **51**, 660–672.

Schimke, R. T., McKnight, G. S., Shapiro, D. J., Sullivan, D., and Palacios, R. (1975). *Recent Progr. Horm. Res.* **31**, 175–211.

Schimke, R. T., Pennequin, P., Robins, D., and McKnight, G. S. (1977). *In* "Hormones and Cell Regulation" (J. Dumont and J. Nunez, eds), Vol. I, pp. 209–221. North Holland, Amsterdam.

Sutherland, R. L. (1981). *Endocrinology* (In Press).

Sutherland, R. L., and Brandon, M. R. (1976). *Endocrinology* **98**, 91–98.

Sutherland, R. L., and Baulieu, E. E. (1976). *Eur. J. Biochem.* **70**, 531–541.

Sutherland, R. L., and Foo, M. S. (1979). *Biochem. Biophys. Res. Commun.* **91**, 183–191.

Sutherland, R. L., and Simpson-Morgan, M. W. (1975). *J. Endocr.* **65**, 319–322.

Sutherland, R. L., Lebeau, M. C., Schmelck, P. J., and Baulieu, E. E. (1977a). *FEBS Letters* **79**, 253–257.

Sutherland, R. L., Mester, J., and Baulieu, E. E. (1977b). *Nature* **267**, 434–435.

Sutherland, R. L., Mester, J., and Baulieu, E. E. (1977c). *In* "Hormones and Cell Regulation" (J. Dumont and J. Nunez, eds), Vol. I, pp. 31–48. North Holland, Amsterdam.

Sutherland, R. L., Geynet, C., Binart, N., Catelli, M. G., Schmelck, P. H., Mester, J., Lebeau, M. C., and Baulieu, E. E. (1980). *Eur. J. Biochem.* **107**, 155–164.

Vu Hai, M. T., and Milgrom, E. (1978). *J. Endocr.* **76**, 21–31.

13

Antioestrogen Action in Chick Liver: Effects on Oestrogen Receptors and Oestrogen-Induced Proteins

CATHERINE B. LAZIER, FRANCOISE CAPONY AND DAVID L. WILLIAMS

I. INTRODUCTION

In female oviparous vertebrates, oestrogens exert striking control over certain hepatic metabolic activities as part of the process generally termed vitellogenesis. This is characterized by the synthesis of specific proteins and lipids destined for deposition in the developing egg yolk. In males oestrogen treatment influences the same range of hepatic activities, but the yolk precursors accumulate in large quantities in the blood (Clemens, 1974; Deeley and Goldberger, 1979; Tata and Smith, 1979). A major yolk precursor protein induced by oestradiol is vitellogenin, a large multicomponent phospholipo-

NON-STEROIDAL ANTIOESTROGENS
ISBN 0 12 677880 9

glycoprotein which is specifically cleaved on uptake by the oocyte to give the insoluble yolk proteins phosvitin and lipovitellin (Bergink *et al.*, 1974). Oestradiol also mediates substantial increases in the synthesis and plasma accumulation of lipids and of the major apoproteins of very low density lipoprotein (VLDL), the plasma carrier of large amounts of triglyceride (Chan *et al.*, 1976, 1978; Williams, 1979; Capony and Williams, 1980).

Oestrogen action in vitellogenesis, particularly in the transcriptional events in vitellogenin induction, has attracted the attention of researchers interested in its potential as a specialized model for studying the control of gene expression (Ryffel, 1978; Deeley and Goldberger, 1979; Tata and Smith, 1979).

In order to optimally exploit the system, clear understanding of the hepatic oestrogen receptor system will be essential. Studies with anti-oestrogens should provide useful insights into the relation between receptor and genomic responses. To date, only 4 papers primarily concerned with antioestrogen action in chick liver have been published (Gschwendt, 1975a, 1977; Chan *et al.*, 1977; Lazier and Alford, 1977). In order to illustrate the numerous possibilities for further investigation, we review in Section II current knowledge of oestrogenic activities in liver and in Section III deal specifically with antioestrogens.

II. THE SPECTRUM OF OESTROGENIC ACTIVITIES IN CHICK LIVER

A. Secreted Proteins

1. Vitellogenin

Native avian vitellogenin is composed of two subunits of molecular weight about 240,000 (Deeley *et al.*, 1975; Christmann *et al.*, 1977). Its high phosphorous content (about 3%) has provided a facile, although not very sensitive, method for measurement of the protein in plasma. More definitive techniques for measuring vitellogenin gene expression involve immunochemical and electrophoretic analysis of the protein and specific cDNA hybridization or translation assays for vitellogenin mRNA.

Liver from unstimulated roosters contain very little vitellogenin mRNA (0–5 molecules/cell) (Deeley *et al.*, 1977; Burns *et al.*, 1978; Jost *et al.*, 1978). A single injection of oestrogen results in the accumulation of about 6,000 molecules/cell at the peak of the response (3 days). In general, the rate of vitellogenin synthesis bears a close relationship to the hepatic content of the specific mRNA. An exception to this is during the 4–6 hour lag phase which characteristically attends the first appearance of vitellogenin molecules in plasma. It seems likely that this time is required for adaptation of the cellular mechanisms responsible for phosphorylation and other post-translational modifications of the vitellogenin apoprotein (Burns *et al.*, 1978).

2. *VLDL Apoproteins*

Two major oestrogen-induced apoproteins of VLDL have been studied in some detail. Apo VLDL-B has an apparent molecular weight of about 350,000. It is synthesized at a rate comprising about 2–3% of total protein synthesis in unstimulated roosters and at a rate of 10–15% at the peak of the oestrogen response (Williams *et al.*, 1979; Capony and Williams, 1980). The kinetics of induction of apo VLDL-B are distinctly different from those observed for vitellogenin: a maximal rate is achieved more rapidly in the former case (Williams *et al.*, 1979). This is reminiscent of the situation in oviduct for oestrogenic induction of conalbumin and ovalbumin (Palmiter *et al.*, 1976).

The apo VLDL-B protein synthesized under basal conditions appears to be the same gene product as that stimulated by oestrogen since peptide maps obtained by limited protease digestion give identical patterns in each case (Capony and Williams, unpublished data).

The major small apoprotein of VLDL from oestrogen-treated chicks, apo VLDL-II, has been sequenced and consists of two chains of 82 amino acids, linked by a single disulphide bond (Jackson *et al.*, 1977). Apo VLDL-II appears to be synthesized at a low rate under basal conditions and the kinetics of its induction after oestrogen treatment are strikingly similar to those observed for vitellogenin and contrast with the kinetics of apo VLDL-B induction (Chan *et al.*, 1978; Capony and Williams, unpublished data). The stimulation of apo VLDL-II synthesis parallels the liver concentration of specific mRNA for the apoprotein (Chan *et al.*, 1976, 1978).

3. *Other Proteins*

A riboflavin-binding protein (RBP), destined to be a minor constituent of egg yolk, is induced by oestrogen in avian liver with kinetics resembling those observed for vitellogenin (Murthy and Adiga, 1978). As with vitellogenin, there is no basal synthesis of RBP in liver of unstimulated animals, but unlike vitellogenin, the molecular weight of the protein in plasma and in yolk appears to be unchanged, i.e. 36,000.

Another protein induced to a great extent by oestrogen can as yet be referred to only as that specified by clone E-18, an 800-nucleotide segment of DNA derived from the specific oestrogen-induced mRNA population of liver from oestrogen-treated roosters (King *et al.*, 1979). The cloned fragment does not contain sequences corresponding to vitellogenin mRNA, but clearly represents an unknown protein with a very high induction ratio.

A comparatively very small, but significant oestrogenic stimulation of transferrin synthesis is seen in avian liver. This is particularly interesting since the same protein (conalbumin) is stimulated to a much greater extent in chick oviduct (Lee *et al.*, 1978). Kinetic and dose response considerations led to the suggestion that the mechanism of oestrogen action of transferrin synthesis is indirect, related to iron mobilization.

Oestrogenic regulation of specific gene expression in avian liver thus appears to fall into several distinct classes based on the presence or absence of a basal level of synthesis and on the relative kinetics of induction.

B. Intrahepatic Effects

It is not surprising that the liver of the laying hen responds to its task of synthesizing enough protein and lipid to fill an egg yolk every day by expansion of the cellular synthetic and secretory machinery (Schjeide *et al.*, 1963). Oestrogen treatment of immature birds results in increased liver weight, RNA and ribosome content (Jost *et al.*, 1973; Mäenpää, 1976; Smith *et al.*, 1976; Bast *et al.*, 1977), increases in various enzymes and factors associated with transcription and translation (Smith *et al.*, 1976; Weckler and Gschwendt, 1976; Van den Berg *et al.*, 1976), increases in polyamine synthesis (Eloranta *et al.*, 1976) and changes in the properties of microsomal membranes (Lippiello *et al.*, 1979).

Some workers have observed a small increase in liver DNA content (Jost *et al.*, 1973), but others did not (Smith *et al.*, 1976). The increase in liver weight probably represents more hypertrophy than hyperplasia. DNA synthesis does not appear to be a prerequisite for vitellogenin production (Jost *et al.*, 1973). On the other hand the co-ordinated expansion of the translational and post-translational processing apparatus may in some cases be a rate-limiting step (Burns *et al.*, 1978; Jost *et al.*, 1978).

C. Oestrogen Receptors

The properties and dynamics of oestrogen receptors in avian liver have recently been reviewed (Lazier, 1979). Briefly, the hepatic receptor system is qualitatively quite similar to that in more widely studied tissues, but there are several outstanding problems. Cytosol from cockerel liver contains a small amount of a specific high-affinity (Kd $\sim$ 1.0 nM) oestradiol-binding protein. The binder is relatively labile and has been difficult to characterize by physical-chemical techniques. However, as would be predicted from classical models for receptor behaviour, it does appear to be translocated to the nucleus after oestrogen treatment (Lazier and Haggarty, 1979). Thereafter, the nuclear receptor levels accumulate to a much greater extent than can be accounted for solely by translocation. Schneider and Gschwendt (1977) have suggested that initial transfer of cytosol receptor is followed by a phase of nuclear receptor accumulation by a mechanism involving receptor synthesis or stabilization.

Oestrogen receptor in liver nuclei of oestrogen-treated cockerels has been detected in several different forms: salt-soluble (Mester and Baulieu, 1972; Lazier, 1975); in a salt-insoluble residue (Lebeau *et al.*, 1977); chromatin-bound (Gschwendt and Kittstein, 1974); bound to the nuclear matrix (Barrack *et al.*, 1979); and associated with a Mg^{2+} soluble fraction of chromatin prepared by limited DNAase II digestion (Alberga *et al.*, 1979). The relationship between the different forms of receptor and their respective roles in specific oestrogen responses are not understood. Estimates of the fraction of salt-soluble receptor vary between 20% and 66% in different studies (Lebeau *et al.*, 1977; Schneider and Gschwendt, 1977; Snow *et al.*, 1978). The nuclear matrix fraction, which may be equivalent to the salt-insoluble form, appears to constitute 50% of total nuclear binding 24 hours after oestrogen injection (Barrack *et al.*, 1979). The Mg^{2+} soluble partially digested chromatin fraction represents 20% of chromatin-associated receptor 48 hours after oestrogen treatment. The fraction is 2-fold enriched with receptor and 4-fold enriched with vitellogenin gene sequences compared to unfractionated chromatin (Alberga *et al.*, 1979).

Detailed comparison of the kinetic and dose-response characteristics for the increases in each of the nuclear receptor forms after oestrogen treatment could give some helpful insights into their relationships and possible functions, particularly if simultaneous measurements of the specific genomic responses are carried out. As yet, kinetic studies have been reported only for the salt-soluble, insoluble, and intact-chromatin associated forms (Mester and Baulieu, 1972; Lazier, 1975; Lazier and Haggarty, 1979; Lebeau *et al.*, 1977; Gschwendt and Kittstein, 1974; Schneider and Gschwendt, 1977). In each of these cases, treatment with the usual vitellogenin-inducing doses of oestrogen (20–50 mg/kg) results in a 3–8 fold increase in nuclear receptor concentration which is maintained for a sustained period (at least 24–48 hours). Snow *et al.* (1978) found a relatively shorter time course for the increase in total exchangeable oestrogen receptor levels in purified liver nuclei from diethylstilboestrol (DES)-treated cockerels, but this could be due to the oestrogen used. Low doses of oestradiol (1.0 mg/kg) do not result in measurable serum accumulation of vitellogenin, but do provoke an early transient rise in soluble nuclear receptor concentration (Joss *et al.*, 1976; C. B.

Lazier, unpublished results). It is not known whether the small doses give a response in terms of vitellogenin synthesis or accumulation of vitellogenin mRNA sequences. Apo VLDL-B induction appears to require relatively lower doses of oestrogen (Capony and Williams, 1980), but in this case measurements were made at the level of protein synthesis and are probably much more sensitive than those used for vitellogenin. It is conceivable, however, that induction of one gene could require less input of nuclear receptor than another (Mulvihill and Palmiter, 1977). This may particularly be the case for a gene which is expressed constitutively compared to one which is not.

III. ANTIOESTROGEN ACTION

A. Agonistic Effects

Various antioestrogens have been examined for potential agonistic activities with regard to the induction of several yolk proteins. In no case has evidence of any oestrogenic response been seen. Figure 1 illustrates the lack of effect of nafoxidine at two doses on the serum vitellogenin concentration. Gschwendt (1975a) found no suggestion of vitellogenin induction by CI 628 or nafoxidine using electrophoretic analysis of serum. Further, tamoxifen does not stimulate vitellogenin synthesis measured by [^{3}H]amino acid incorporation into a vitellogenin immunoprecipitate (Capony and Williams, unpublished data). Although the latter technique is relatively sensitive, a vitellogenin synthetic rate of less than 0.5 % of total protein synthesis might not have been detected. The available data, therefore, do not preclude a small degree of agonistic action of antioestrogens with regard to vitellogenin induction. The most sensitive test, that of measuring vitellogenin mRNA sequences with a cDNA probe, has apparently not yet been applied to this problem.

Antioestrogens do not appear to induce the VLDL apoproteins either at the level of synthesis or of serum accumulation (Chan *et al.*, 1977; Capony and Williams, 1980). Figure 2 shows the effects of different times of exposure and different doses of tamoxifen on the rate of synthesis of apo VLDL-B. The synthetic rate is uniformly the same as the basal rate seen in untreated roosters. Similarly, tamoxifen does not affect the basal rate of apo VLDL-B synthesis in chick embryo liver (Nadin-Davis *et al.*, 1980).

Radioimmunoassay for serum riboflavin-binding protein failed to reveal any agonistic action of the clomiphene isomers (Murthy and Adiga, 1978). Therefore, with the reservations expressed above regarding the sensitivity of the assays, antioestrogens do not appear to have agonistic activities related to specific protein induction.

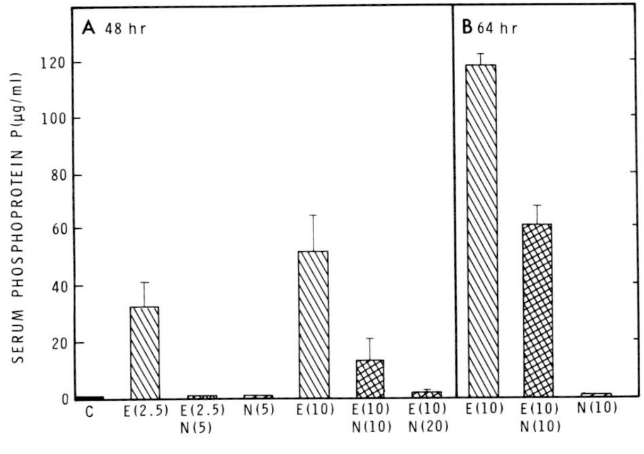

Fig. 1. Agonistic and antagonistic effects of nafoxidine on serum vitellogenin levels. Cockerels were injected with the doses of oestrogen and/or nafoxidine indicated and the serum phosphoprotein concentration was measured as described by Lazier (1975).

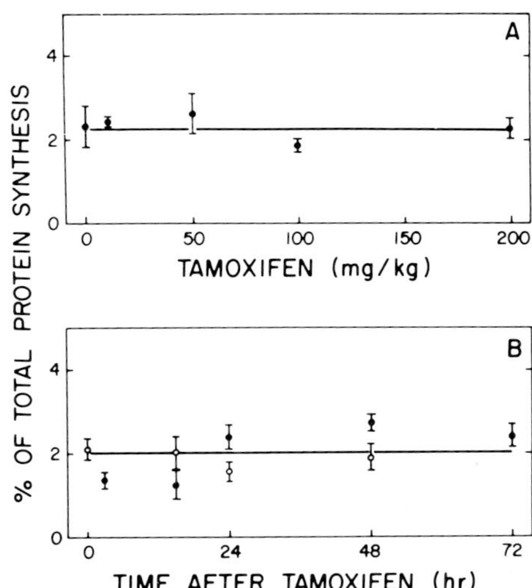

Fig. 2. The effect of tamoxifen on apo VLDL-B synthesis in the basal state. (A) The synthesis of apo VLDL-B was determined as described in the legend to Table I in liver slices from roosters which had been injected with various doses of tamoxifen citrate 15 hours earlier. (B) Tamoxifen citrate (50 mg/kg) (●) or vehicle (○) was administered to roosters at time 0 and the synthesis of apo VLDL-B was determined at the indicated times. Each point represents the mean ± S.E.M. for 3 birds per group.

More general agonistic actions of the antioestrogens in chick liver have not been widely investigated. However, Gschwendt (1977) did find that CI 628 treatment resulted in an increase of about 30% in liver weight, and in RNA and protein content. The extent of the increase was about one half that found for equal weights of oestradiol similarly injected. We do not find that exposure to tamoxifen for 18 hours significantly affects [^{3}H]leucine incorporation into liver supernatant protein (unpublished results). Chan *et al.*, (1977) however do record a small effect in this parameter for nafoxidine. Chan's group also finds a slight elevation of plasma triglycerides after nafoxidine treatment. More study is needed to determine whether or not these general effects are typical of all antioestrogens in chick liver.

Agonistic actions of antioestrogens with regard to receptor distribution and activity are discussed in Section III, C.

B. Antagonism of Specific Protein Synthesis

The antioestrogens are markedly potent inhibitors of oestrogen-induced protein synthesis in chick liver. This has been demonstrated at the level of serum accumulation for vitellogenin (Gschwendt, 1975a, 1977; Lazier, 1975; Lazier and Alford, 1977), for riboflavin-binding protein (Murthy and Adiga, 1978) and for the VLDL apoproteins (Chan *et al.*, 1977). For example, Figure 1 shows that a dose of nafoxidine of 50 mg/kg given with oestradiol (25 mg/kg) completely suppresses the vitellogenin response at 48 hours. The molar dose ratio in this case is 1.2 antioestrogen/oestrogen. A molar dose ratio of 0.6 (100 mg/kg of each compound) results in 50% inhibition of serum vitellogerin at 64 hours.

More detailed studies have recently been carried out on tamoxifen inhibition of synthesis of apo VLDL-B (Capony and Williams, 1980; and unpublished results). Figure 3 illustrates the effect of several doses of tamoxifen on the relative rate of synthesis of apo VLDL-B in liver of roosters treated with a maximal (25 mg/kg) or a suboptimal (1.0 mg/kg) dose of DES. Complete inhibition of the oestrogen-induced increment in apo VLDL-B synthesis is seen, but tamoxifen does not in either case reduce the level of synthesis below the basal rate (see also Fig. 2). We have found a similar effect of tamoxifen in embryonic chick liver where the basal rate constitutes a somewhat higher proportion of total protein synthesis (Nadin-Davis *et al.*, 1980).

Tamoxifen is an effective inhibitor of oestrogen-induced apo VLDL-B synthesis even when administered as much as 8 hours after the oestrogen (Table I). In this case, a small reduction in the relative rate of apo VLDL-B synthesis is seen 2 hours after injection of the antioestrogen, and after a further 4 hours the relative rate is reduced to 3.8% compared to 11.0% in liver from the animals given only oestradiol. This type of reversal of the oestrogen-induced synthesis has been observed in the chick oviduct (Mester *et al.*, 1977; Palmiter *et al.*, 1978). One possible explanation is that tamoxifen is able to exchange with oestrogen bound to receptor at critical nuclear sites, and by doing so disrupts the dynamic function of the complex, resulting in inhibition of transcription and destabilization of existing apo VLDL-B mRNA. The time taken to effect the inhibition could be influenced by a number of factors including the time necessary for the exchange, the time required for intermediate stages in the manifestations of the actions of the receptor complex, and the half-life of apo VLDL-B mRNA. The results underline the contention that the hormone-receptor complex must remain intact throughout a considerable portion of the phenotypic response.

Although it seems likely that, under most circumstances in oestrogen-stimulated chick liver, the rate of synthesis of an oestrogen-induced protein is a measure of the level of specific mRNA (section II, A), this has not been directly demonstrated in any experiments involving antioestrogens. The use of specific probes for particular mRNA molecules would lend a degree of precision to interpretations that is currently not possible.

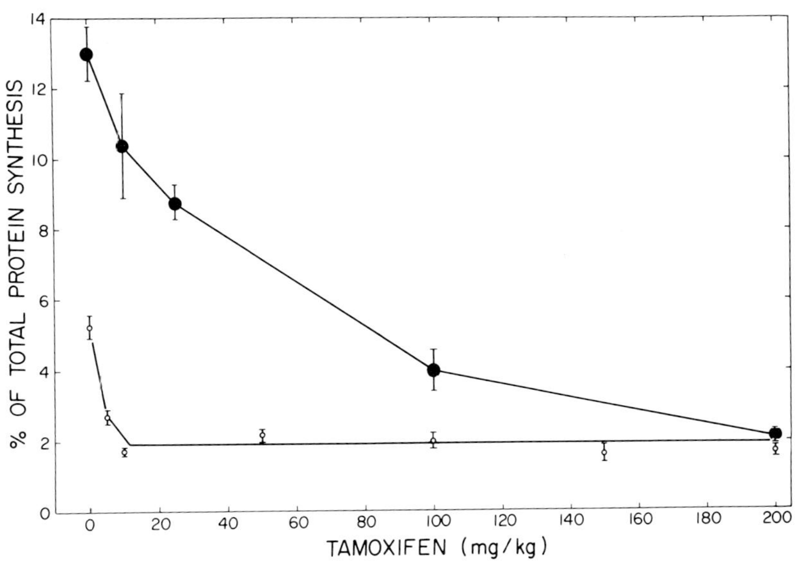

Fig. 3. Tamoxifen inhibition of DES-stimulated apo VLDL-B synthesis. Various doses of tamoxifen citrate were injected simultaneously with DES at 25 mg/kg (●) or 1 mg/kg (○). Apo VLDL-B synthesis was determined 48 hours after treatment for the higher dose of DES, and after 15 hours for the lower dose. Reproduced from Capony and Williams (1980).

TABLE I
Tamoxifen Reversal of Oestrogen-Induced Apo VLDL-B Synthesis[a]

Treatment	Time of assay	Relative rate of apo VLDL-B synthesis
1. Oestradiol	8 hr	10.0 ± 1.3
2. Oestradiol	14 hr	11.0 ± 0.8
3. Oestradiol + Tamoxifen	10 hr	7.8 ± 1.2
4. Oestradiol + Tamoxifen	14 hr	3.8 ± 0.5
5. None		2.2 ± 0.2

[a] Roosters in treatment groups 1–4 were each injected with oestradiol (3 mg/kg) at time 0. Tamoxifen (50 mg/kg) was administered 8 hours after oestradiol to groups 3 and 4. The relative rate of apo VLDL-B synthesis was determined as described by Capony and Williams (1980).

With regard to the more general effects of oestrogen and its antagonists in chick liver, it has recently been reported that nafoxidine inhibits an oestrogen-induced change in microsomal membrane properties and an increase in the activity of the stearyl-CoA desaturase (Lippiello *et al.*, 1979).

C. Interaction with Oestrogen Receptors

A few studies have been carried out on the effects of antioestrogens on the intracellular distribution of oestrogen receptor in chick liver. Nafoxidine, and to a lesser extent, CI 628, both provoke significant increases in the oestradiol-binding activity of liver chromatin (Gschwendt, 1975a, 1977). The increase (measured at 24 hours) is never more than about 40% of that seen with oestradiol alone, and is not seen with higher doses of the antioestrogen. Nafoxidine alone also stimulates the oestradiol-binding activity of the salt-soluble receptor fraction to a limited extent and with a somewhat delayed onset compared to that seen with oestradiol (Lazier and Alford, 1977). Similarly, we have recently found that tamoxifen treatment results in a small and delayed increase in total oestrogen receptor in purified nuclei and in a salt extract thereof (Table II). In the case of the nuclei from the tamoxifen-treated chicks, the proportion of total nuclear receptor that is salt-extractable is a little less than 50%. In nuclei from oestradiol treated animals, the findings are dramatically different, especially in the later stages of the response, where apparently more receptor can be assayed in salt extracts than is detected in the equivalent nuclei. Several interpretations are possible. One is that salt extraction unmasks sites which are not exchangeable in the intact purified nuclei. Another is that a receptor in intact nuclei is less stable than that in the salt extract. A further point is that the time course for the receptor increase differs in the two assays. The results underline the difficulties in comparing experiments in the literature, where different preparations and assay procedures have been used.

A common feature in our findings in this study with tamoxifen and pure nuclei, compared to our earlier work with nafoxidine and the salt-extract from crude nuclei, is that in neither case is there an increase in nuclear receptor in the early stages after treatment. This could be related to metabolism, receptor stability, or to some more fundamental feature of antioestrogen action in chick liver. In chick oviduct on the other hand, tamoxifen translocates receptor to the nucleus with a very similar initial time course to oestrogen (Sutherland *et al.*, 1977).

Administration of a single dose of antioestrogen with (or before) oestrogen results in pronounced inhibition of the rise in the liver nuclear oestrogen receptor both in the chromatin-bound and salt-soluble fractions (Gschwendt, 1975a, 1977; Lazier and Alford, 1977), Figure 4 shows the time course for total soluble receptor activity in liver after injection of chicks with oestradiol (25 mg/kg) or the same dose of oestradiol plus nafoxidine (50 mg/kg). This treatment completely inhibits serum vitellogenin accumulation (Fig. 1). By choosing a dose ratio which gives partial inhibition of serum vitellogenin, one can see partial inhibition of the soluble receptor levels, particularly at the later stages of the response (Fig. 5). The antioestrogen therefore appears to inhibit the mechanisms responsible for sustained elevation of soluble nuclear receptor.

TABLE II
Effect of Tamoxifen and Oestradiol on Total Exchangeable and Salt-Soluble Oestrogen Receptor in Purified Nuclei[a]

Time after injection (hr)	Nuclear receptor concentration (fmol/μg DNA)			
	Total receptor		Salt-soluble receptor	
	Tamoxifen	Oestradiol	Tamoxifen	Oestradiol
0	0.06 ± 0.02	0.06 ± 0.02	0.06 ± 0.04	0.06 ± 0.04
1.5	0.08 ± 0.03	0.19 ± 0.08	0.08 ± 0.06	0.29 ± 0.04
4	0.08 ± 0.03	0.73 ± 0.05	0.08 ± 0.03	0.62 ± 0.18
18	0.23 ± 0.10	0.46 ± 0.10	0.13 ± 0.03	1.16 ± 0.20
68	0.10 ± 0.07	0.38 ± 0.07	0.07 ± 0.03	1.12 ± 0.18

[a] Cockerels were injected with oestradiol (25 mg/kg) or with tamoxifen (50 mg/kg). At various times thereafter, liver nuclei were purified in glycerol and assayed for total exchangeable nuclear oestrogen receptor by the method of Snow *et al.*, (1978). A separate portion of the purified nuclei was extracted by freezing with 0.5 M KCl (Buffer B, Lazier and Haggarty, 1979) and [^{3}H]oestradiol binding was determined by exchange at 30°C. Results represent the mean ± S.D. for duplicate determinations on each of 4 animals per group.

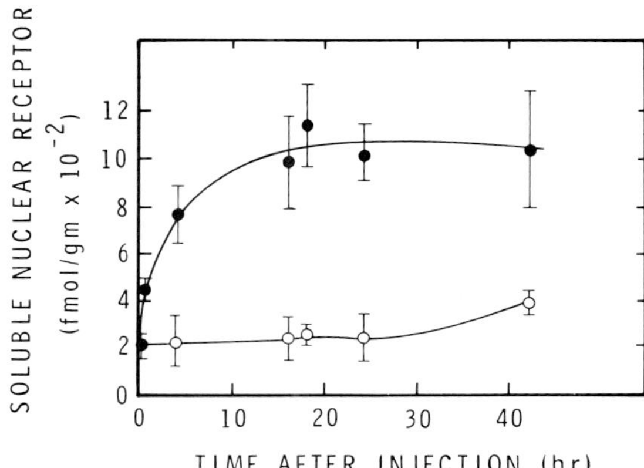

Fig. 4. Antagonistic effect of nafoxidine on the accumulation of the soluble nuclear oestrogen receptor. Oestradiol (25 mg/kg) alone (●) or with nafoxidine (50 mg/kg) (○) (molar dose ratio 1.2 antioestrogen/oestrogen) was injected into cockerels and the concentration of salt-soluble receptor in extracts of crude nuclei was determined as described by Lazier (1978). Each point is the mean ± S.D. for 4 birds per group.

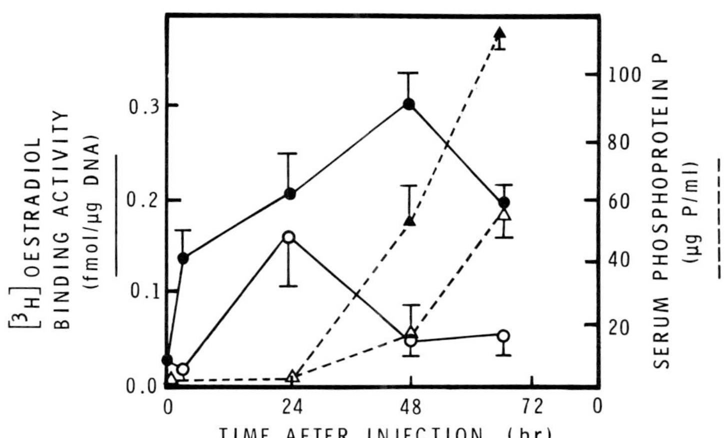

Fig. 5. The influence of nafoxidine, given with oestradiol in a molar dose ratio of 0.6, on soluble nuclear oestrogen receptor activity and on the serum vitellogenin concentration. Nafoxidine (100 mg/kg) was injected with oestradiol (100 mg/kg). Serum phosphoprotein phosphorous was determined as described by Lazier (1975). Specific binding of oestradiol in salt extracts of crude nuclei was determined using 1 nM [^{3}H]oestradiol (Lazier and Alford, 1977). Since this is not a saturating concentration, the absolute values cannot be compared to those given in Figure 4 or Table II (which were determined under conditions of [^{3}H]oestradiol saturation). (●) oestradiol; (○) nafoxidine + oestradiol.

In vitro, nafoxidine competes with oestrogen for binding to the soluble nuclear receptor with a K_i of 43 nM, representing a relative affinity of 0.04 compared to oestradiol (Lazier and Alford, 1977). The relative affinities of nafoxidine and CI 628 for the chromatin-bound receptor are 0.008 and 0.014 respectively (Gschwendt, 1975b). Binding studies with other receptor fractions have not been reported, nor has work with radio-labelled antioestrogens. Another consideration is that the antioestrogens are metabolized by liver, possibly giving rise to the actual inhibitory compounds.

The effects of nafoxidine on cytosol receptor levels have been examined to a limited extent (Fig. 6). Nafoxidine alone results in depletion of the cytoplasmic binding sites; however there is not concomitant rise in soluble nuclear receptor levels at this time (Table II; Lazier and Alford, 1977). The exchange assay used for the cytosol receptor was demonstrated to be effective for oestrogen-bound receptor (Lazier and Haggarty, 1979) and was assumed also to be adequate for nafoxidine exchange. If this is not so, the apparent depletion may not be real. On the other hand it is possible that the nafoxidine-receptor complex has become associated with a cell fraction other than that occupied by the salt-soluble nuclear oestrogen receptor.

Nafoxidine does not appear to cause a long-term depletion of cytoplasmic oestrogen binding sites in chick liver (Fig. 6). This is in contrast to the situation in oviduct (Sutherland *et al.*, 1977) and in rat uterus (Clark *et al.*, 1974). A transient inhibitory effect may prevail at 4–18 hours, but this does not appear to be sufficient to explain the striking anti-hormonal actions seen after a single injection of nafoxidine and oestradiol.

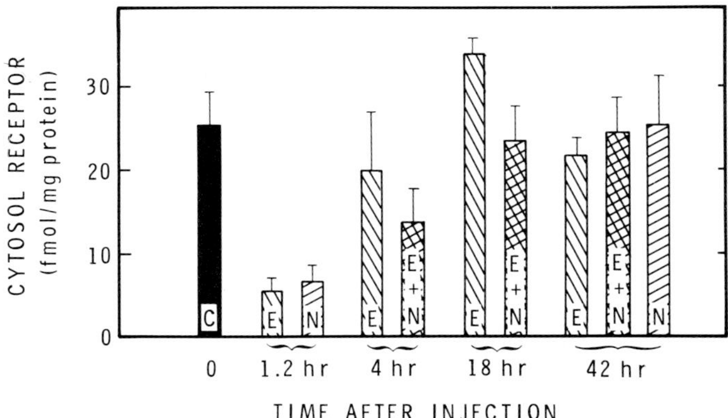

Fig. 6. The effect of nafoxidine and oestradiol on the concentration of the cytosol oestrogen receptor. Nafoxidine (50 mg/kg) and/or oestradiol (25 mg/kg) was injected into cockerels and the $(NH_4)_2SO_4$ fraction from liver cytosol was prepared at various times thereafter. [^{3}H]oestradiol binding activity was determined by exchange at 25° as described by Lazier and Haggarty (1979).

IV. SUMMARY AND CONCLUSIONS

The main points arising from the studies on antioestrogen action in chick liver can be summarized as follows:

1. No agonistic activities have been observed with regard to induction of vitellogenin, the VLDL apoproteins, or riboflavin-binding protein.
2. Profound inhibition of oestrogenic induction of the same proteins has uniformly been found.
3. Reversal of oestrogenic induction of apo VLDL-B can be accomplished by delayed administration of tamoxifen.
4. Antioestrogens injected alone result in a small and relatively delayed increase in the concentration of the nuclear oestrogen receptor.
5. The affinities of nafoxidine and CI 628 for the chromatin-bound and salt soluble forms of the nuclear receptor are less than 5% that of oestradiol.
6. Injection of antioestrogen with oestradiol results in pronounced inhibition of the increase in nuclear receptor concentration normally seen with oestradiol alone.
7. Nafoxidine treatment results in an initial depletion of cytoplasmic receptor, but without a noticeable corresponding increase in nuclear receptor at the time. A transient and small inhibition of replenishment of the cytosol receptor is observed.

An important caveat in interpretations of these data is that metabolism of the antioestrogens certainly takes place in liver and may give rise to the actual inhibitory compounds. Metabolism may explain the apparently bizarre kinetics for the increase in nuclear oestrogen receptor after antioestrogen treatment. While the affinity of the administered drugs for nuclear receptor is low, certain metabolites may compete for oestradiol binding sites with comparatively high affinity.

The uniform absence of agonistic activities of the antioestrogens is notable and suggests that the antioestrogen-oestrogen receptor complex is unable to carry out the usual functions of the agonist-receptor complex at one or more stages in the response. In particular, the mechanisms leading to nuclear receptor accumulation are disrupted. This may be a basis for the potent antagonism of oestrogen. The nature of these mechanisms is not understood.

ACKNOWLEDGEMENTS

The studies were supported by grants to C.B.L. from the Medical Research Council of Canada (MA 4880) and to D.L.W. from the National

Institutes of Health (U.S.A.) (AM 18171). F.C. was supported by the Institut National de la Santé et de la Recherche Médicale de France. The gifts of tamoxifen citrate to D.L.W. by Imperial Chemical Industries Ltd. and of nafoxidine-HCl to C.B.L. from the Upjohn Company are gratefully acknowledged.

Note added in proof — We have recently found that the 4-hydroxy derivative of tamoxifen has a very high affinity for the chick liver nuclear oestrogen receptor, and that little exchange of bound monohydroxytamoxifen for [^{3}H]oestradiol occurs during the usual incubation conditions. Thus, it is possible that the apparent inhibition of the oestradiol-induced increase in nuclear receptor on administration of antioestrogens is due to masking of oestradiol binding sites by high-affinity metabolites of the drugs (Lazier, C. B., Fraser, P. and Jordan, V. C., *Clinical Research*, 28, 673A, 1980).

REFERENCES

Alberga, A., Tran, A., and Baulieu, E. E. (1979). *Nucleic Acids Res.* **7**, 2031–2044.

Barrack, E. R., Hawkins, E. F., and Coffey, D. S. (1979). *In* "Steroid Hormone Receptor Systems" (W. W. Leavitt and J. H. Clark, eds), pp. 47–70. Plenum Press, New York.

Bast, R. E., Garfield, S. A., Gehrke, L., and Ilan, J. (1977). *Proc. Natl Acad. Sci. U.S.A.* **8**, 3133–3137.

Bergink, E. W., Wallace, R. A., Van den Berg, J. A., Bos, E. S., Gruber, M., and AB, G. (1974). *Amer. Zool.* **14**, 1177–1193.

Burns, A. T. H., Deeley, R. G., Gordon, J. I., Udell, D. S., Mullinix, K. P., and Goldberger, R. F. (1978). *Proc. Natl Acad. Sci. U.S.A.* **75**, 1815–1819.

Capony, F., and Williams, D. L. (1980). *Biochemistry* **19**, 2219–2225.

Chan, L., Jackson, R. L., O'Malley, B. W., and Means, A. R. (1976). *J. Clin. Invest.* **58**, 368–379.

Chan, L., Jackson, R. L., and Means, A. R. (1977). *Endocrinology* **100**, 1636–1643.

Chan, L., Jackson, R. L., and Means, A. R. (1978). *Circulation Res.* **43**, 209–217.

Christmann, J. L., Grayson, M. J., and Huang, R. C. C. (1977). *Biochemistry* **16**, 3250–3256.

Clark, J. H., Peck, E. J., and Anderson, J. N. (1974). *Nature* **251**, 446–448.

Clemens, M. J. (1974). *Progr. Biophys. Mol. Biol.* **28**, 69–108.

Deeley, R. G., and Goldberger, R. F. (1979). *In* "Ontogeny of Receptors and Reproductive Hormone Action" (T. H. Hamilton, J. H. Clark and W. A. Sadler, eds), pp. 291–308. Raven Press, New York.

Deeley, R. G., Mullinix, K. P., Wetekam, W., Kronenberg, H. M., Myers, M., Eldridge, J. D., and Goldberger, R. F. (1975). *J. Biol. Chem.* **250**, 9060–9066.

Deeley, R. G., Gordon, J. J., Burns, A. T., Mullinix, K. P., Binastein, M., and Goldberger, R. F. (1977). *J. Biol. Chem.* **252**, 8310–8319.

Eloranta, T. D., Mäenpää, P. H., and Raina, A. M. (1976). *Biochem. J.* **154**, 95–103.

Gschwendt, M. (1975a). *Biochim. Biophys. Acta* **399**, 395–402.

Gschwendt, M. (1975b). *J. Steroid Biochem.* **6**, vii.

Gschwendt, M. (1977). *Research on Steroids* **7**, 121–126.

Gschwendt, M., and Kittstein, W. (1974). *Biochim. Biophys. Acta* **361**, 84–96.

Jackson, R. L., Lin, M.-Y., Chan, L., and Means, A. R. (1977). *J. Biol. Chem.* **252**, 250–253.

Joss, U., Bassand, C., and Dierks-Ventling, C. (1976). *FEBS Letters* **66**, 293–298.

Jost, J. P., Keller, R., and Dierks-Ventling, C. (1973). *J. Biol. Chem.* **248**, 5262–5266.

Jost, J. P., Ohno, T., Panyim, S., and Schuerch, A. R. (1978). *Eur. J. Biochem.* **84**, 355–361.
King, C. R., Udell, D. S., and Deeley, R. G. (1979). *J. Biol. Chem.* **254**, 6781–6786.
Lazier, C. B. (1975). *Steroids* **26**, 281–298.
Lazier, C. B. (1978). *Biochem. J.* **174**, 143–152.
Lazier, C. B. (1979). *In* "Ontogeny of Receptors and Molecular Mechanism of Reproductive Hormone Action" (T. H. Hamilton, J. H. Clark and W. A. Sadler, eds), pp. 353–370. Raven Press, New York.
Lazier, C. B., and Alford, W. S. (1977). *Biochem. J.* **164**, 659–667.
Lazier, C. B., and Haggarty, A. J. (1979). *Biochem. J.* **180**, 347–353.
Lebeau, M. C., Massol, N., Lemonnier, M., Schmelck, P. H., Mester, J., and Baulieu, E. E. (1977). *In* "Hormonal Receptors in Digestive Tract Physiology" (S. Bonfils, P. Fromageot and G. Rosselin, eds), pp. 183–195. North Holland, Amsterdam.
Lee, D. D., McKnight, G. S., and Palmiter, R. D. (1987). *J. Biol. Chem.* **253**, 3494–3503.
Lippiello, P. M., Holloway, C. T., Garfield, S. A., and Holloway, P. W. (1979). *J. Biol. Chem.* **254**, 2004–2009.
Mäenpää, P. H. (1976). *Biochem. Biophys. Res. Commun.* **72**, 347–354.
Mester, J., and Baulieu, E. E. (1972). *Biochim. Biophys. Acta* **261**, 236–244.
Mester, J., Geynet, C., Binart, N., and Baulieu, E. E. (1977). *Biochem. Biophys. Res. Commun.* **79**, 112–118.
Mulvihill, E. R., and Palmiter, R. D. (1977). *J. Biol. Chem.* **252**, 2060–2068.
Murthy, U. S., and Adiga, P. R. (1978). *Biochim. Biophys. Acta* **538**, 364–375.
Nadin-Davis, S. A., Lazier, C. B., Capony, F., and Williams, D. L. (1980). *Biochem. J.* **192**, 733–740.
Palmiter, R. D., Moore, P. B., Mulvihill, E. R., and Emtage, S. (1976). *Cell* **8**, 557–572.
Palmiter, R. D., Mulvihill, E. R., McKnight, G. S., and Senear, A. W. (1978). *Cold Spring Harbor Symp. Quant. Biol.* **42**, 639–647.
Ryffel, G. U. (1978). *Mol. Cell. Endocr.* **12**, 237–248.
Schjeide, O. A., Wilkens, R., McCandless, R., Munn, R., Peterson, M., and Carlsen, G. (1963). *Amer. Zool.* **3**, 167–184.
Schneider, W., and Gschwendt, M. (1977). *Hoppe Seyler's Z. Physiol. Chem.* **358**, 1583–1589.
Smith, R. L., Baca, O., and Gordon, J. (1976). *J. Mol. Biol.* **100**, 115–126.
Snow, L. D., Erikson, H., Hardin, J. W., Chan, L., Jackson, R. L., Clark, J. H., and Means, A. R. (1978). *J. Steroid Biochem.* **9**, 1017–1026.
Sutherland, R. L., Mester, J., and Baulieu, E. E. (1977). *Nature* **267**, 434–435.
Tata, J. R., and Smith, D. F. (1979). *Recent Progr. Horm. Res.* **35**, 47–95.
Van den Berg, J. A., Kooistra, T., AB, G., and Gruber, M. (1976). *Biochem Biophys. Res. Commun.* **61**, 367–374.
Weckler, C., and Gschwendt, M. (1976). *FEBS Letters* **65**, 220–224.
Williams, D. L., (1979). *Biochemistry* **18**, 1056–1063.
Williams, D. L., Wang, S. -Y., and Capony, F. (1979). *J. Steroid Biochem.* **11**, 231–236.

14

Oestrogen–Receptor and Antioestrogen–Receptor Complex Binding to Calf Uterine Chromatin

THOMAS S. RUH, DAVID M. WOOD, PATRICK ROSS JR. AND JEFFERY L. KEENE

I. INTRODUCTION

A general model of steroid hormone action includes the following: binding by steroid to a specific receptor protein; translocation of receptor complex to the nucleus; binding of receptor complex to acceptor sites; alterations in transcription; and translation and production of specific proteins (O'Malley and Means, 1974; Gorski and Gannon, 1976). Thus, interaction of the steroid hormone molecule with its receptor is the first step in a process which leads ultimately to alteration in gene expression. Despite a vast accumulation of data and extensive investigation by numerous

NON-STEROIDAL ANTIOESTROGENS
ISBN 0 12 677880 9

laboratories, the details of the mechanism by which the receptor complex modulates gene activity remain obscure.

The initial binding by oestrogen to its receptor is characterized by specificity, high affinity and saturability; presumably, binding to specific regions in the nucleus is regulated by similar parameters. Thus, the nucleus represents a second level of specificity (Spelsberg *et al.*, 1979). However, the nuclear site of action of steroid hormone–receptor complexes has yet to be identified. DNA (King and Gordon, 1972; Kallos and Hollander, 1978), ribonucleoprotein particles (Liang and Liao, 1974), basic non-histone proteins (Puca *et al.*, 1974), and acidic non-histone proteins (O'Malley *et al.*, 1972; Klyzsejko-Stefanowicz *et al.*, 1976; Webster *et al.*, 1976) have all been advocated. The laboratories of O'Malley and Spelsberg have proposed that the acidic non-histone proteins serve as the "acceptor" sites for steroid hormone–receptor complexes. In addition to the accumulation of evidence implicating direct interaction of receptor complexes with chromatin, studies from several laboratories provide indications that there are different species of acceptors.

Spelsberg's laboratory reported the existence of multiple acceptors for the progesterone–receptor complex in chick oviduct. Initially, in their *in vitro* studies (Spelsberg *et al.*, 1975), one region of increased receptor complex binding capability became apparent as proteins were extracted from chromatin with various concentrations of guanidine hydrochloride (GuHCl). However, recently it has been shown that the isoelectric focusing of progesterone–receptor acceptor activity in total oviduct chromosomal proteins revealed the presence of three different acceptor species (Thrall *et al.*, 1978). Thus, it is likely that multiple regions on target tissue chromatin serve as acceptors for steroid receptor complex.

Evidence has accumulated that there may be two or more distinct binding sites for oestrogen receptor in uterine nuclei. Both our laboratory (Ruh and Baudendistel, 1977) and Clark's laboratory (Clark *et al.*, 1976) have reported the existence of salt-extractable and salt-resistant nuclear binding of oestrogen–receptor complexes. In addition, Markaverich and Clark (1979) have presented evidence for additional nuclear binding sites, designated Type II. These studies may be an indication that the oestrogen–receptor complex is binding to different nuclear binding sites, possibly different species of acceptor sites on the uterine genome.

For the past several years our laboratory has been concerned with the mechanisms whereby antioestrogen–receptor complexes alter oestrogen induced gene expression. Non-steroidal antioestrogens are known to inhibit oestrogen–stimulated uterine growth. These antioestrogens have many of the same characteristics as oestrogens as they will bind specifically to the cytoplasmic oestrogen receptor (Korenman, 1970; Katzenellenbogen and

Katzenellenbogen, 1973; Ruh and Ruh, 1974) and cause the translocation of the receptor complex into the uterine nuclear compartment (Ruh and Ruh, 1974; Rochefort *et al.*, 1972; Clark *et al.*, 1973; Katzenellenbogen and Ferguson, 1975). The initial uterine responses are very similar between oestrogens and antioestrogens; however, the longer term responses necessary for true uterine growth are inhibited by non-steroidal antioestrogens (Clark *et al.*, 1973; Baudendistel *et al.*, 1978; Ruh *et al.*, 1979a). The subcellular mechanisms whereby antioestrogens inhibit the full oestrogenic response are unknown. However, a reasonable assumption would be that an important locus of inhibition would be the interaction of the receptor complexes with the uterine genome. This assumption is supported by the observation that triphenylethylene antioestrogen–receptor complexes that have been translocated to the nucleus do not exhibit salt-resistant binding but are easily extracted by buffers containing 0.4 M KCl (Ruh *et al.*, 1979a). Thus, both salt-extractable and salt-resistant receptor binding would seem to be of importance in the actions of oestrogens since both types of binding (or subfractions thereof) probably are specific to certain classes of acceptor sites.

Therefore, the following studies were initiated to explore the possibility that more than one species of oestrogen-receptor acceptor site may exist in calf uterine chromatin. By working directly with chromatin in a cell free system, a range of manipulations of the binding system, which are not possible *in vivo*, can be utilized for direct analysis. We also wished to determine whether antioestrogen–receptor complexes display different binding characteristics to some of these acceptor sites as this may further elucidate the mechanism whereby antioestrogens retard true uterine growth. The antioestrogens used in this study were: CI 628 = α-[4-pyrrolidino-ethoxy] phenyl-4-methoxy-α′-nitrostilbene; tamoxifen = trans-1-(p-β-dimethylaminoethoxyphenyl) 1,2, diphenylbut-1-ene.

II. METHODOLOGIES IN NUCLEAR ACCEPTOR STUDIES

A. Receptor Preparation

Calf uteri were collected fresh at a local slaughter house and immediately placed in ice cold Tris buffer (10 mM, pH 7.5). All procedures were performed at 4°C unless otherwise indicated. After vessels and connective tissues had been dissected free, the tissue was minced in a meat grinder and gently homogenized in a blender at 4°C in 2 volumes of 50 mM Tris-HCl, pH 7.5, 1.5 mM Na_2EDTA and 1 mM dithiothreitol (TED). The homogenate was centrifuged at 130,000 × g for 60 minutes to yield a receptor-containing supernatant; cytosol subsequently was diluted with TED to 10 mg protein/ml.

At this time cytosol was charged with a radio-labelled oestrogen or antioestrogen during a 60 minute incubation at 4°C. Ligands utilized were 20 nM [^{3}H]oestradiol (Amersham, specific activity = 46–54 Ci/mmol), 70 nM [^{3}H]CI 628 (Amersham, specific activity = 22.5 Ci/mmol) and 50 nM [^{3}H]tamoxifen (ICI, specific activity = 19.5 Ci/mmol). Charged cytosol was then either precipitated by $(NH_4)_2SO_4$ or more extensively purified by heparin-Sepharose affinity binding before $(NH_4)_2SO_4$ precipitation. To precipitate the receptor complexes, finely powdered $(NH_4)_2SO_4$ was slowly added to 25% saturation while maintaining the pH at 7.5. Upon completion of a 60 minute 4°C incubation, cytosol was centrifuged at 27,000 × g for 30 minutes. Receptor pellets were stored at −70°C. In the more extensive receptor purification step, heparin-Sepharose, which had been prepared by CNBr activation (Cuatrecasas, 1970), was incubated with charged cytosol (150 mg/ml) for 60 minutes at 4°C (Sica and Bresciani, 1979). Repeated washings with TED buffer on a Buchner funnel eliminated free protein and unbound radioligand. The bulk of proteins bound to heparin-Sepharose were removed with two 0.4 M KCl incubations; receptor was eluted batchwise with 0.9 M KCl (Molinari *et al.*, 1977). The supernatant obtained in this fashion was treated with $(NH_4)_2SO_4$ as described above; pellets were stored at −70°C until the day of the experiment. Several hours before an experiment, receptor pellets were redissolved in 10 mM Tris-HCl pH 7.5, 1 mM Na_2 EDTA, 12 mM α thioglycerol (TESH). Antioestrogen receptor pellets were recharged at this time with the concentration of ligand with which the cytosol had been incubated originally. Receptor solutions were dialysed against a minimum of 100 volumes of TESH buffer at 4°C for 3 hours; dialysed solutions were centrifuged at 10,000 × g for 10 minutes. These supernatants were assayed for protein content and radioactivity, diluted with TESH/TEKCl to the desired incubation concentrations of proteins and salt, and used in the binding activity assay.

B. Chromatin–Cellulose Preparation

The procedures for purifying nuclei and chromatin and preparing chromatin-cellulose follow the general method of Spelsberg *et al.* (1978).

1. Isolation of Nuclei

Calf uteri were minced in a meat grinder and homogenized in 2 volumes of 0.5 M sucrose, 50 mM Tris-HCl, pH 7.5, 25 mM KCl, 2 mM $MgCl_2$ (TKM). This initial homogenate was diluted with 0.5 M sucrose TKM to a buffer tissue ratio of 3:1 prior to homogenization in a Glenco glass-teflon homogenizer. After being strained through dampened cheesecloth, the homogenate was centrifuged at 27,000 × g for 5 minutes. Pellets were pooled, homogenized in 9 volumes of sucrose TKM to a final concentration of 2.3 M sucrose and recentrifuged at 27,000 × g for 60 minutes. The pellets were resuspended in 2.3 M sucrose TKM and recentrifuged at 27,000 × g for 60 minutes to yield a nuclear pellet. Nuclei were resuspended with a glass-teflon homogenizer in TKM containing 0.2% Triton X-100. After filtration through organza cloth, the nuclear solution was centrifuged at 27,000 × g for 5 minutes.

2. *Isolation of Chromatin*

Purified nuclei were suspended in 80 mM NaCl, 20 mM Na_2 EDTA, pH 6.3, with a glass-teflon homogenizer prior to homogenization in a Dounce glass-glass homogenizer. Pellets were collected from a 5 minute centrifugation (27,000 × g) and resuspended in 0.35 M NaCl. A second 5 minute centrifugation (27,000 × g) yielded pellets which subsequently were placed in 2 mM Tris-HCl, pH 7.5, 1.0 mM Na_2EDTA (CTE) and strained through organza cloth. This filtrate was allowed to stand on ice for 15 minutes before being centrifuged at 27,000 × g for 10 minutes. After this centrifugation, the chromatin pellets were combined, rehomogenized in CTE buffer, and stored at −70°C. Yields of chromatin were calculated as mg of DNA determined by the diphenylamine procedure of Burton (1956). Prior to, and after, coupling to cellulose, protein: DNA ratios were ascertained for each batch of chromatin. Total protein was determined by hydrolysis in 1.0 M NaOH at 22°C. Histones were removed with 0.2 M H_2SO_4 at 4°C; non-histone proteins were stripped with 0.1 M NaOH at 22°C (Spelsberg *et al.*, 1978). Protein was quantitated with the Bio Rad Protein Assay (Bradford, 1976).

3. *Coupling of Chromatin to Cellulose*

Cellex 410 (Bio Rad) was washed three times with boiling ethanol and once with each of the following: 0.1 M NaOH, 1.0 mM Na_2EDTA and 10 mM HCl (Spelsberg *et al.*, 1978). After extensive washes with distilled water the cellulose was air dried. Washed cellulose was hydrated at 4°C for 45 minutes in CTE buffer. Resuspended chromatin was added to the cellulose solution and mixed for 2 hours. The chromatin-cellulose slurry was adjusted to 0.1 M KCl and centrifuged at 7,500 × g for 10 minutes. Chromatin-cellulose was incubated in absolute ethanol for 15 minutes followed by two washes with absolute ethanol. The chromatin-cellulose slurry was exposed to 6×10^6 ergs/cm^2 ultraviolet light (254 nM) from a Mineralight Short Wave Lamp (Ultraviolet Products) (Spelsberg *et al.*, 1978). Coupled chromatin-cellulose was rehydrated with CTE for 15 minutes at 4°C, washed twice with CTE and filtered to dryness on a Buchner funnel.

4. Preparation of Chromatin–Cellulose Pellets

Chromatin-cellulose resin equivalent to 50 μg of DNA either was weighed into 1.5 ml microfuge tubes or dispensed as a slurry in extraction buffer (1.0 mM Tris-HCl, pH 8.5, 5 mM Na_2SO_3, 0.1 M HSEtOH). The pellets were extracted with 1.0 ml of the appropriate agent (GuHCl, urea: NaCl or GuSCN) at 22°C for 30 minutes. Following the extraction, chromatin-cellulose pellets were washed 3 times at 7,800 × g for 15 seconds with cold 2 mM Tris-HCl, pH 7.5, 1.0 mM EDTA (TE) (Webster *et al.*, 1976).

C. Assay for Receptor Complex Binding Activity

Oestrogen-receptor or antioestrogen-receptor complex solutions were added to the extracted and washed chromatin-cellulose. The mixture containing 0.15 M KCl was then incubated for 90 minutes at 4°C (Webster *et al.*, 1976). Afterwards the chromatin-cellulose pellets were washed free of unbound receptor complex by three centrifugations (7,800 × g for 15 seconds). The radioligand was then extracted in 1.0 ml of absolute ethanol. An aliquot of the extract (0.5 ml) was added to 4 ml of scintillation fluid (0.4% Omnifluor in xylene) and counted in a liquid scintillation spectrometer. DNA was hydrolysed from the chromatin-cellulose pellets by a 90°C incubation for 30 minutes in 0.5 M $HClO_4$. The hydrolysate was assayed for DNA by the diphenylamine method (Burton, 1956). The binding of [^{3}H]oestrogen-receptor or [^{3}H]antioestrogen-receptor complexes to washed cellulose was determined routinely and subtracted from binding to chromatin-cellulose.

III. ANALYSIS OF OESTROGEN–RECEPTOR AND ANTIOESTROGEN–RECEPTOR COMPLEX BINDING TO CHROMATIN-CELLULOSE

A. Extraction and Binding Characteristics of Chromatin-Cellulose

Our laboratory has been interested in differentiating the binding of oestrogen-receptor complexes and antioestrogen-receptor complexes to uterine chromatin. We have chosen to probe oestrogen-receptor acceptor sites in uterine chromatin by selectively deproteinizing chromatin with certain chaotropic agents. This has proven to serve two functions, both the unmasking of acceptor sites and the extraction or removal of these same sites. In the following discussion we will use the term "acceptor site" or "acceptor activity", which is defined as high affinity binding (i.e. in the presence of 0.15

M KCl) of steroid-receptor complexes to chromatin. The technique developed by Webster *et al.* (1976) for immobilizing chromatin on an insoluble matrix in order to unmask acceptor sites was utilized.

In Figure 1 the efficiency of extracting chromatin bound proteins from calf uterine chromatin-cellulose resins with increasing concentrations of chaotropic agents is presented. Three different agents, GuHCl, urea:NaCl and GuSCN were used in varying concentrations until their limits of solubility were reached. In Figure 1A essentially all of the histones were extracted by 2–3 M GuHCl. An additional 13% of the non-histone proteins (NHP) was removed from the chromatin by 3–8 M GuHCl. In contrast to the complete removal of the histone, GuHCl was unable to extract all of the NHP. With the use of 5 M urea:1.0 M NaCl (Fig. 1B) approximately 95% of the histones and 60% of the NHP were removed. Increasing the NaCl concentration to 4 M in the extraction media surprisingly caused a decreased dissociation of NHP from the chromatin resin while completely removing the histone fraction. However, the chaotropic agent GuSCN produced an extraction profile of histones and NHP slightly different from the GuHCl profile; GuSCN appeared to be more efficient at extracting histones and slightly less efficient at extracting NHP. As the binding data will indicate, it is doubtful that the NHP extracted with increasing concentrations of GuHCl or GuSCN are exactly the same.

The binding of the [^{3}H]oestradiol receptor complexes ([^{3}H]E_2-R) to calf uterine chromatin resins previously extracted with GuSCN or urea:NaCl is

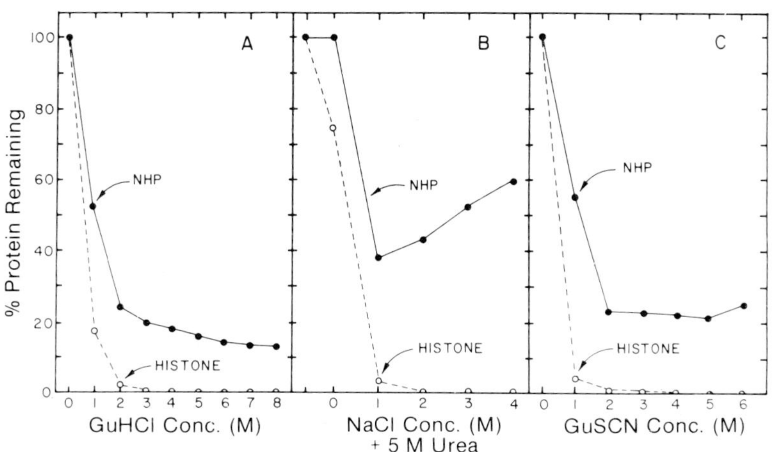

Fig. 1. Effect of various chaotropic agents on the extraction of histone and non-histone proteins from calf uterine chromatin-cellulose resins.

shown in Figure 2. Chromatin-cellulose previously extracted with GuSCN consistently displayed two regions, at 1.0 M and 5 M GuSCN, of increased high affinity binding (acceptor activity) by $[^3H]E_2$-R. Acceptor activity which was unmasked by 1.0 M and 5 M GuSCN was extracted by 3 M and 6 M GuSCN respectively. The acceptor activity peaks were most apparent using a $[^3H]E_2$-R concentration of 60 μg protein/ml in the binding assay (Fig. 2A). With higher concentrations of $[^3H]E_2$-R the peaks tended to become lost in an overall increased binding plateau until, at 1400 μg/ml no peaks were present. In contrast, experiments utilizing 5 M urea with increasing concentrations of NaCl failed to demonstrate any peaks of acceptor activity, indicating only a general increase in the binding of $[^3H]E_2$-R when the concentration of the receptor solution was 60–200 μg/ml.

Since the acceptor activity could not be extracted by higher NaCl concentrations, we pursued a more thorough analysis of the binding of $[^3H]E_2$-R to GuHCl extracted chromatin-resin. Some of the binding parameters tested are shown in Figure 3. In general, 1.0 M GuHCl extractions greatly increased acceptor activity. However, 3 M GuHCl extraction of chromatin caused this binding activity to be lost, presumably by removing acceptor sites. On occasion, 6–8 M GuHCl extraction unmasked a slight increase in acceptor activity. An additional extraction with 0–8 M GuHCl did

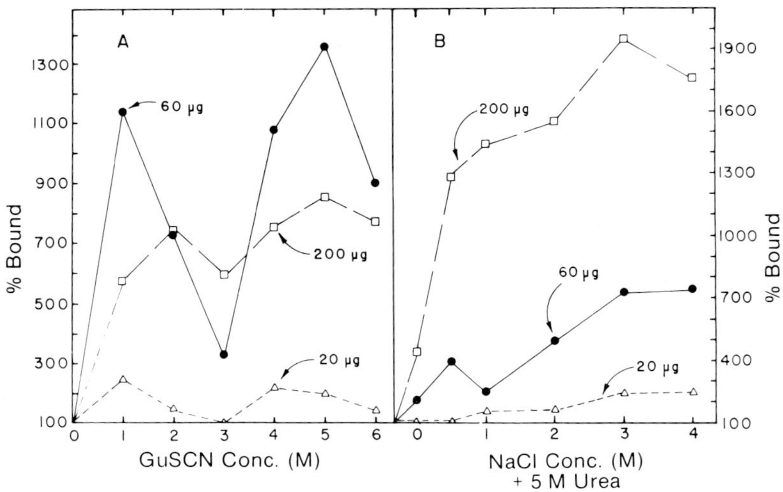

Fig. 2. Effect of varying protein concentration of the hormone-receptor preparation on binding of [^{3}H]oestradiol-receptor complexes to chromatin-cellulose previously extracted with various concentrations of GuSCN (A) or urea/NaCl (B). Protein concentration is expressed as μg per assay tube.

not alter the [^{3}H]E_2-R binding profile. Increasing the pH of the extraction buffer (Fig. 3A) caused an overall slightly depressed [^{3}H]E_2-R binding profile. In contrast, increasing the 30 minute extraction temperature from 0°C to 30°C slightly depressed the acceptor activity unmasked by higher molarities of GuHCl (Fig. 3B), while not changing the acceptor activity unmasked by 1.0 M

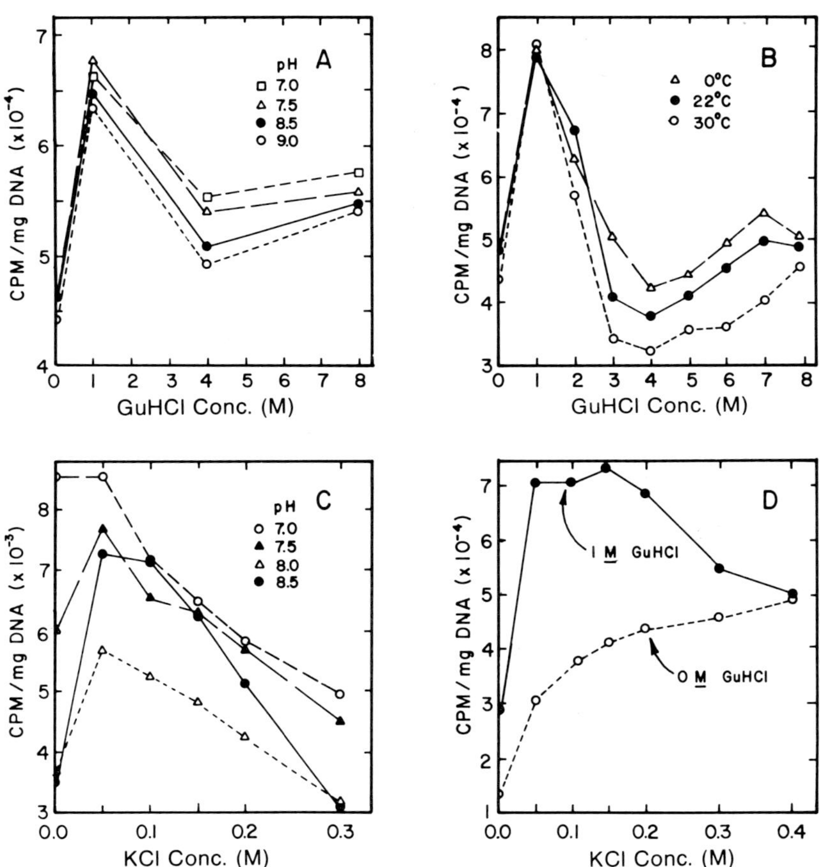

Fig. 3. The effects of various extraction and binding conditions on the interaction of [^{3}H]oestradiol-receptor complexes with calf uterine chromatin-cellulose. A = effect of varying extraction buffer pH; B = effect of varying the extraction temperature; C = effect of varying pH and KCl concentration on the binding of receptor to chromatin-cellulose previously extracted with 1.0 M GuHCl; D = effect of varying the concentration of KCl (pH 7.5) on the binding of [^{3}H]oestradiol-receptor complexes to chromatin-cellulose previously extracted with buffer or 1.0 M GuHCl.

GuHCl. In other experiments peaks of acceptor activity were lost if the chromatin cellulose resins were further extracted with 1% sodium dodecyl sulphate to deproteinize the chromatin prior to the binding assay. This would indicate that certain non-histone proteins are necessary for acceptor activity in uterine chromatin.

A further analysis of the 1.0 M binding peaks (Fig. 3C) showed that the KCl concentration and pH of the binding assay had considerable effect. At pH 7.5 binding was increased when the KCl concentration was increased to 0.05–0.15 M KCl. Higher concentrations of KCl (0.2–0.3 M) caused a decreased binding, possibly due to dissociation of $[^3H]E_2$-R from binding sites on the chromatin-resin. A further comparison of the effect of KCl on the binding of $[^3H]E_2$-R to chromatin previously extracted with buffer containing no GuHCl or with 1.0 M GuHCl is shown in Figure 3D. The $[^3H]E_2$-R binding to 1.0 M GuHC1 extracted chromatin was maximal at 0.05–0.15 M KC1 and decreased at higher (0.2–0.4 M) KCl concentrations. $[^3H]E_2$-R binding to 0 M GuHCl extracted chromatin displayed a much lower increase in receptor binding with increasing KCl concentrations. Therefore, most subsequent assays were performed at 0.15 M KCl although periodic checks have not revealed any significant difference between 0.15 M and 0.05 M KCl. An interesting finding concerning the binding of $[^3H]E_2$-R to chromatin is that the majority of the $[^3H]E_2$-R binding profile was resistant to 0.4 M KCl extraction. This is in agreement with the report of Perry and Lopez (1978) who found that oestrogen receptor binding to sheep hypothalamic chromatin was largely KCl-resistant. Obviously the relationship between this KCl-resistance and that found to occur *in vivo* (Clark *et al.*, 1976; Ruh *et al.*, 1979b) has yet to be determined.

Changing the protein concentration of $[^3H]E_2$-R preparations had a major effect on the binding assay. Two peaks of increased acceptor activity became apparent at a $[^3H]E_2$-R protein concentration of 60 μg/ml (Fig. 4). Increased protein in the receptor solution interfered with the detection of the acceptor sites unmasked by 4 M GuHCl. These experiments, therefore, suggest that there may be more than one species of acceptor sites on calf uterine chromatin.

The possibility that proteolytic activity in either the chromatin-cellulose or receptor preparations may contribute to part of the $[^3H]E_2$-R binding profile was investigated. Chromatin-cellulose preparations, incubated for 30 minutes with the proteolytic inhibitor phenylmethylsulfonyl fluoride(PMSF) showed a $[^3H]E_2$-R binding profile identical to that of chromatin-cellulose not treated with PMSF. Furthermore, chromatin-cellulose previously extracted with 0–8 M GuHCl demonstrated no protease activity, using the general proteolytic substrate Azocoll either at 4°C for 90 minutes (normal binding conditions) or at 37°C for 20 hours. Similarly, oestrogen receptor

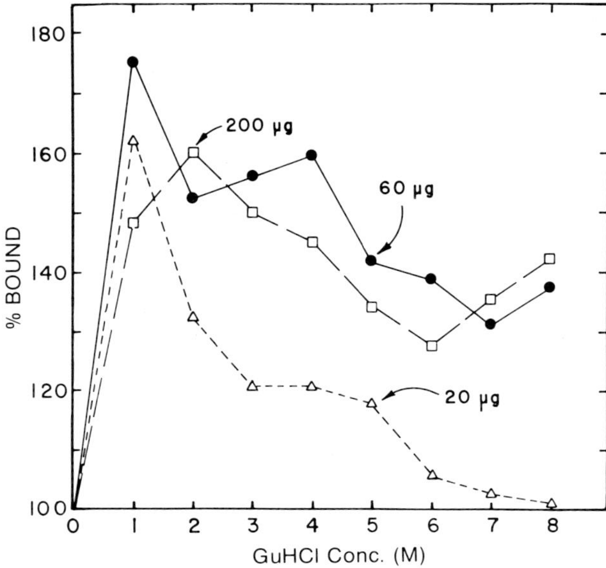

Fig. 4. Effect of varying the protein concentration of the hormone-receptor preparation on binding of [^{3}H]oestradiol-receptor complexes to chromatin-cellulose previously extracted with various concentrations of GuHCl. Protein concentration is expressed as μg per assay tube.

preparations exhibited no proteolytic activity under the above binding conditions. Therefore, it is reasonable to assume that, under the acceptor assay binding conditions, the [^{3}H]E_2-R binding profile to chromatin was not influenced by trypsin-like proteases.

B. Antioestrogen–Receptor Complex Binding to Chromatin-Cellulose

Previous work from our laboratory (Baudendistel and Ruh, 1976; Ruh *et al.*, 1979a) demonstrated that oestrogen-receptor and antioestrogen-receptor complexes bind differently to two or more sites in the uterine nuclei under *in vivo* conditions. In addition, the results from *in vitro* studies presented in this chapter indicate that there are more than one species of high affinity acceptor activity in calf uterine chromatin. In order to elucidate whether the differences in oestrogen versus antioestrogen receptor binding obtained *in vivo* can be demonstrated in the *in vitro* chromatin-cellulose system, we studied antioestrogen–receptor complex binding to deproteinized chromatin-cellulose. When we tested chromatin previously extracted with urea:NaCl for differences in the high affinity binding of oestrogen-receptor and antioestrogen-receptor complexes, we obtained the results shown in Figure 5. Acceptor sites for [^{3}H]tamoxifen-receptor complex ([^{3}H]TAM-R) bound to the same acceptor sites but with a lesser affinity than that found with [^{3}H]E_2-R.

Binding of [^{3}H]TAM-R to GuHCl extracted chromatin (Fig. 6) showed increased acceptor activity in the same two fractions of deproteinized chromatin as [^{3}H]E_2-R, with the additional possibility of a slight increase in binding at 7 M GuHCl. Denatured [^{3}H]E_2-R did not bind to chromatin-cellulose above control levels and showed no peaks of increased binding. However, denatured [^{3}H]TAM-R did display some increased binding to chromatin previously extracted with 2–7 M GuHCl. But, despite the non-specific binding of denatured [^{3}H]TAM-R there did appear to be specific binding of [^{3}H]TAM-R at least to chromatin extracted with1.0 M and 3 M GuHCl.

After obtaining the results in Figures 5 and 6 we purified the oestrogen receptor further in order to decrease non-specific binding. Calf uterine cytosol

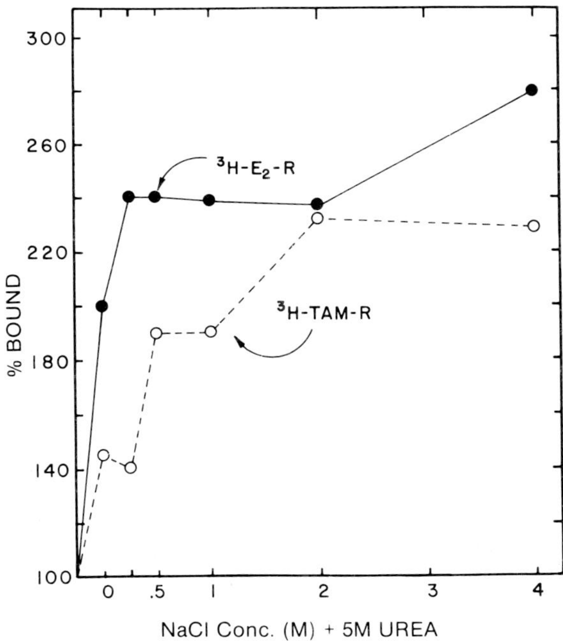

Fig. 5. Comparison of binding of [^{3}H]tamoxifen-receptor complex (○) and [^{3}H]oestradiol-receptor complexes (●) to chromatin-cellulose previously extracted with 5 M urea and increasing concentrations of NaCl.

oestrogen receptors were bound to heparin-Sepharose slurries and eluted with either KCl or NaSCN. As shown in Figure 7 increasing the molarity of KCl was more effective than NaSCN in eluting oestrogen receptor from the bulk of cytosol protein. Since KCl elution gave a receptor preparation of higher purity it was used in subsequent preparations. The further precipitation of the oestrogen receptor by $(NH_4)_2SO_4$ followed by dialysis resulted in a purification of about 200 fold over crude cytosol. The use of this purified receptor preparation revealed the presence of a third region of increased acceptor activity (Fig. 8). Using concentrations of 13–45 μg protein/ml resulted in the detection of three peaks of acceptor activity on chromatin that had been extracted with low (1.0 M) medium (3–5M), and high (7 M) concentrations of GuHCl. These results are in contrast to the chromatin-cellulose data obtained in the progesterone receptor chick oviduct system

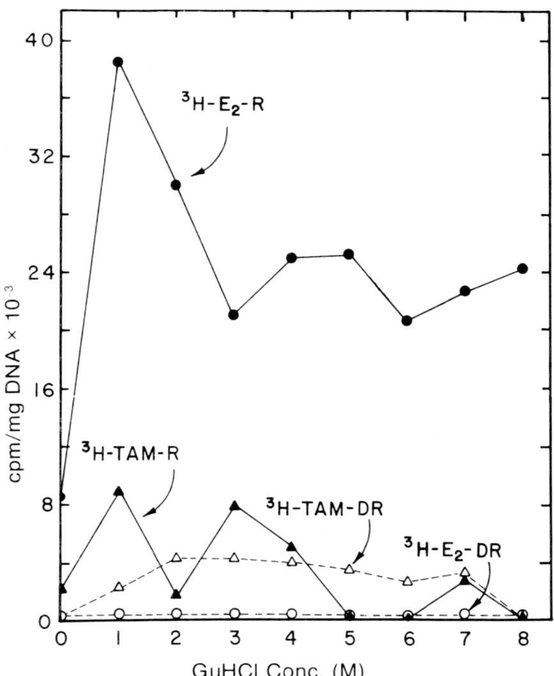

Fig. 6. Comparison of [^{3}H]oestradiol (●) and [^{3}H]tamoxifen (▲) receptor complex binding to GuHCl extracted chromatin-cellulose. As controls, [^{3}H]oestradiol receptor-complex (○) and [^{3}H]tamoxifen receptor-complexes (△) were denatured (40°C for 60 minutes) before incubation with chromatin-cellulose resin.

(Spelsberg *et al.*, 1975), which showed only one area of increased acceptor activity. However, both systems (chick oviduct and calf uterine) share one region of increased acceptor activity, i.e. to chromatin extracted with 4–5 M GuHCl. This would imply that there is at least one group of non-histone proteins with similar functions and affinities for chick oviduct and calf uterine DNA.

The use of antioestrogen-receptor complexes (Fig. 9) further elucidated this general pattern of three areas of increased acceptor activity. Thus both [^{3}H]CI 628 receptor complexes ([^{3}H]CI-R) and [^{3}H]TAM-R showed increased binding at three different chromatin-celluose GuHCl extraction levels. At this point it is difficult to say whether the specific binding peaks of oestrogen-receptor complexes are different from those of antioestrogen-receptor complexes since some shifting in peak binding from experiment to experiment did occur. Neither free [^{3}H]E$_2$ nor [^{3}H]CI 628 can account for the peaks since both were unable to bind above background levels. However, free [^{3}H]tamoxifen did demonstrate some binding and contributed to the 7 M binding peak.

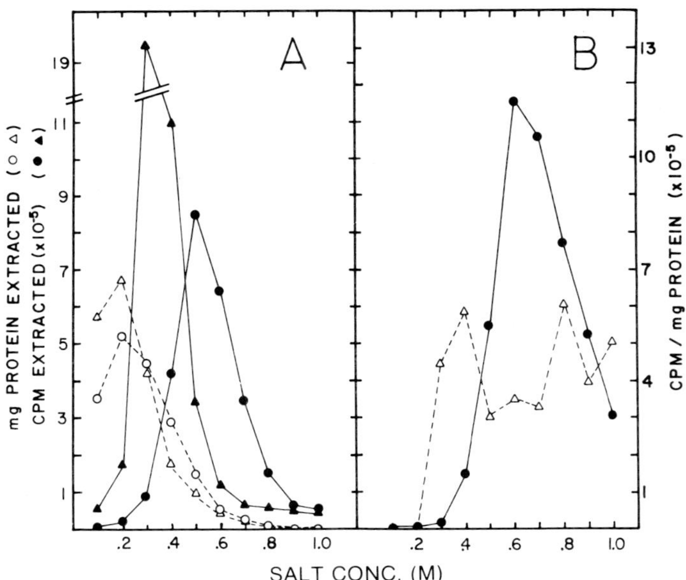

Fig. 7. Purification of oestrogen-receptor complexes using heparin-Sepharose. (A) Elution of proteins bound to heparin-Sepharose with stepwise salt gradient. (B) Specific activity of proteins eluted from heparin-Sepharose. NaSCN elution represented by triangles; KCl elution represented by circles.

It would seem that [^{3}H]tamoxifen, because of both its lower affinity for the oestrogen receptor and its tendency for a higher nonspecific binding to non-receptor components, is not as good a probe for antioestrogen action in this system as [^{3}H]CI 628. However, even [^{3}H]CI 628 is known to display considerable nonspecific binding. Therefore, to further distinguish oestrogen receptor from antioestrogen receptor binding to acceptor sites future studies will use more refined techniques. High affinity antioestrogens such as H 1285 (Collins *et al.*, 1971; Emmens, 1973) will be tritiated and used in conjunction with reconstituted acceptor sites made by acidic protein-DNA reannealing methods.

IV. CONCLUSIONS

We have found evidence for high affinity binding (acceptor sites) of oestrogen-receptor complexes in calf uterine chromatin. It would seem, in

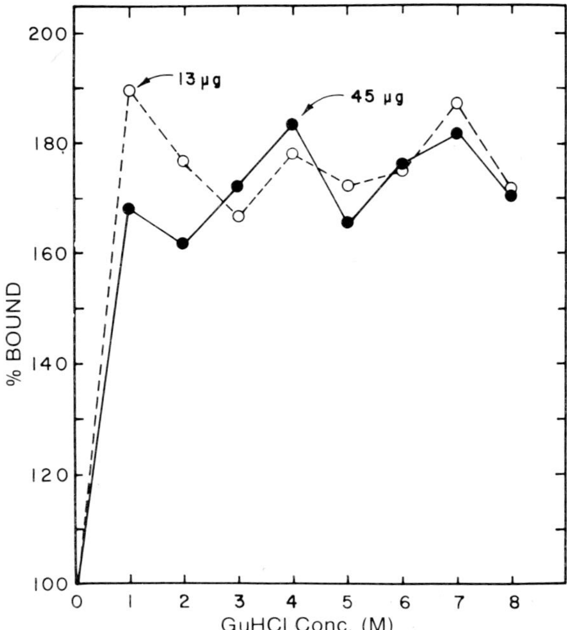

Fig. 8. Effect of varying the protein concentration of the purified receptor solution on binding to chromatin-cellulose previously extracted with various concentrations of GuHCl. Protein concentration is expressed as µg per assay tube.

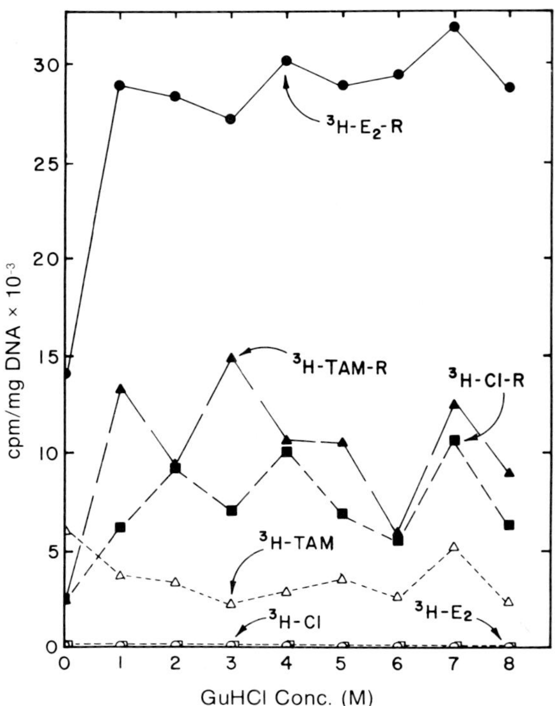

Fig. 9. Comparison of heparin-Sepharose purified oestrogen-receptor and antioestrogen-receptor complex binding to GuHCl extracted chromatin-cellulose. Binding of free oestrogen or antioestrogen was included as controls. Protein concentration of the receptor preparation was 13 μg per assay tube. [^{3}H]oestradiol-receptor complex (●); [^{3}H]tamoxifen-receptor complex (▲); [^{3}H]CI 628-receptor complex (■); [^{3}H]oestradiol (○); [^{3}H]tamoxifen (△); [^{3}H]CI 628 (□).

general, that this increased acceptor activity is similar to that found by Spelsberg *et al.* (1975) in the chick oviduct, by Klyzsejko-Stefanowicz *et al.* (1976) in rat prostrate chromatin, and by Perry and Lopez (1978) in sheep hypothalamic chromatin. In addition we have detected the presence of at least three different species of acceptor activity within the high affinity binding of oestrogen-receptor complexes to calf uterine chromatin. By analogy, these three species of uterine chromatin acceptor activity might be similar to three species of acceptor activity detected by isoelectric focusing of oviduct chromatin acidic proteins in Spelsberg's laboratory (Thrall *et al.*, 1978). Antioestrogen-receptor complexes were also found to bind to three different species of acceptor sites in uterine chromatin. However, more extensive studies are needed before we can determine if the antioestrogen-receptor complexes bind to the same or different acceptor sites as the oestrogen-receptor complexes.

ACKNOWLEDGEMENTS

The authors wish to thank Drs Thomas Spelsberg and Mary Ruh for their many helpful discussions. We would also like to thank Ms Connie Bryant for preparation of the manuscript. This work was supported by NIH HD13425.

REFERENCES

Baudendistel, L. J., and Ruh, T. S. (1976). *Steroids* **28**, 223–237.
Baudendistel, L. J., Ruh, M. F., Nadel, E. M., and Ruh, T. S., (1978). *Acta Endocr.* **89**, 599–611.
Bradford, M. (1976). *Anal. Biochem.* **72**, 248–254.
Burton, K. (1956). *Biochem. J.* **62**, 315–322.
Clark, J. H., Anderson, J. N., and Peck, E. J. Jr., (1973). *Steroids* **22**, 707–718.
Clark, J. H., Eriksson, H. A., and Hardin, J. W. (1976). *J. Steroid Biochem.* **7**, 1039–1043.
Collins, D. J., Hobbs, J. J., and Emmens, C. W. (1971). *J. Med. Chem.* **14**, 952–957.
Cuatrecasas, P. (1970). *J. Biol. Chem.* **245**, 3059–3065.
Emmens, C. W. (1973). *J. Reprod. Fert.* **34**, 23–28.
Gorski, J., and Gannon, F. (1976). *Ann. Rev. Physiol.* **38**, 425–450.
Kallos, J., and Hollander, V. P. (1978). *Nature* **272**, 177–180.
Katzenellenbogen, B. S., and Ferguson, E. R. (1975). *Endocrinology* **97**, 1–12.
Katzenellenbogen, B. S., and Katzenellenbogen, J. A. (1973). *Biochem. Biophys. Res. Commun.* **50**, 1152–1159.
King, R. J. B., and Gordon, J. (1972). *Nature, New Biol.* **240**, 185–187.
Klyzsejko-Stefanowicz, L., Chiu, J., Tsai, Y., and Hnilica, L. S. (1976). *Proc. Natl Acad. Sci. U.S.A.* **73**, 1954–1958.
Korenman, S. G. (1970). *Endocrinology* **87**, 1119–1123.
Liang, T., and Liao, S. (1974). *J. Biol. Chem.* **249**, 4671–4678.
Markaverich, B. M., and Clark, J. H. (1979). *Endocrinology* **105**, 1458–1462.
Molinari, A. M., Medici, N., Moncharmont, B., and Puca, G. A. (1977). *Proc. Natl Acad. Sci. U.S.A.* **74**, 4886–4890.
O'Malley, B. W., and Means, A. R. (1974). *In* "The Cell Nucleus" (H. Busch, ed.), Vol. III, pp. 380–416. Academic Press, New York.
O'Malley, B. W., Spelsberg, T. C., Schrader, W. T., Chytil, F., and Steggles, A. W. (1972). *Nature* **235**, 141–144.
Perry, B. N., and Lopez, A. (1978). *Biochem. J.* **176**, 878–883.
Puca, G. A., Sica, V., and Nola, E. (1974). *Proc. Natl Acad. Sci. U.S.A.* **71**, 979–983.
Rochefort, H., Lignon, F., and Capony, F. (1972). *Biochem. Biophys. Res. Commun.* **47**, 662–670.
Ruh, T. S., and Baudendistel, L. J. (1977). *Endocrinology* **100**, 420–426.
Ruh, T. S., and Ruh, M. F. (1974). *Steroids* **24**, 209–224.
Ruh, T. S., Baudendistel, L. J., Nicholson, W. F., and Ruh, M. F. (1979a). *J. Steroid Biochem.* **11**, 315–322.
Ruh, T. S., Baudendistel, L. J., and Ruh, M. F. (1979b). *In* "Antihormones" (M. K. Agarwal, ed.), pp. 199–217. Elsevier/North Holland, Amsterdam.

Sica, V., and Bresciani, F. (1979). *Biochemistry* **18**, 2369–2378.

Spelsberg, T. C., Webster, R. A., and Pikler, G. M. (1975). *In* "Chromosomal Proteins and Their Role in Regulation of Gene Expression" (G. S. Stein and L. J. Kleinsmith, eds), pp. 153–186. Academic Press, New York.

Spelsberg, T. C., Stake, E., and Witzke, D. (1978). *In* "Methods in Cell Biology", Vol. XVII (G. Stein, J. Stein and L. J. Kleinsmith, eds), pp. 303–324. Academic Press, New York.

Spelsberg, T. C., Thrall, C., Martin-Dani, G., Webster, R. A., and Boyd, P. A. (1979). *In* "Ontogeny of Receptors and Reproductive Hormone Action" (T. H. Hamilton, J. H. Clark, and W. A. Sadler, eds.), pp. 31–63. Raven Press, New York.

Thrall, C. L., Webster, R. A., and Spelsberg, T. C. (1978). *In* "The Cell Nucleus" (H. Busch, ed.), Vol. VI, pp. 461–529. Academic Press, New York.

Webster, R. A., Pikler, G. M., and Spelsberg, T. C. (1976). *Biochem. J.* **156**, 409–418.

15

Oestrogen Receptor Chromatin Interactions: Effect of Antioestrogens

M. C. LEBEAU, N. MASSOL AND E. E. BAULIEU

I. INTRODUCTION

It is generally accepted that hormone-receptor complexes accumulate in the nuclei of target cells exposed to steroids (Maurer and Chalkley, 1967; Gorski *et al.*, 1968; Jensen *et al.*, 1968). However the nature of the nuclear binding sites (usually called "acceptor" sites) for the hormone-receptor complexes is still controversial. It was proposed that these could be DNA (Shyamala Harris, 1971; Musliner and Chader, 1971; King and Gordon, 1972; Toft, 1972; André and Rochefort, 1973; Alberga *et al.*, 1976), although a number of investigators observed that the binding of receptor to isolated nuclei or DNA was non-saturable (Chamness *et al.*, 1974; André and Rochefort, 1975). Yamamoto and Alberts (1975) suggested that the techniques used in these studies mainly measured interactions of the receptor with non-specific sites, while a few high affinity sites to which the receptor binds in order to exert its activity were not detected. In fact, even this concept

NON-STEROIDAL ANTIOESTROGENS
ISBN 0 12 677880 9

of a few specific DNA sites has no experimental basis, and receptor chromatin interactions might involve other chromatin elements than DNA itself.

Other suggestions for "acceptor" sites have included proteins associated with DNA, such as the basic proteins described by Puca *et al.* (1974) for the oestrogen receptor, and the acidic proteins described by Spelsberg *et al.* (1971, 1976) for the progesterone receptor. These sites could also be part of the nuclear matrix proteins (Barrack *et al.*, 1977) or could even be ribonucleoproteins, as reported by Liao *et al.* (1973) for the androgen receptor.

All these studies, however, suffer from a number of technical and theoretical limitations, in particular when they have dealt with salt extracted nuclear material (Bradbury *et al.*, 1973; Christiansen and Griffith, 1977; Spadafora *et al.*, 1979).

In order to solubilize chromatin under mild ionic conditions, without the need of shearing or sonication, specific nucleases were used to partially digest the DNA. One could thus obtain a workable fraction, which, in first approximation, is accepted as still representative of the native state of chromatin (Finch *et al.*, 1975; Noll *et al.*, 1975; Oudet *et al.*, 1975). One could hope that, when using these conditions, protein–DNA interactions would be better preserved than in salt extracts, and that one had a chance of isolating receptors still associated with their physiological acceptor sites, that is at the specific loci where they were placed *in vivo* under the effect of the hormone. A number of investigators have therefore sought to prepare chromatin subfractions, enriched in both receptor and/or oestradiol regulated gene.

Since accumulation and retention of hormone-receptor complexes in the nucleus have been correlated with hormone action (Anderson *et al.*, 1973; Mulvihill and Palmiter, 1977; Sutherland *et al.*, 1977a; Palmiter *et al.*, 1978), it was very interesting to see that accumulation and retention of nuclear receptor complexes were also observed in target cells of animals exposed to antioestrogens. Of course, there was some confusion since, in mammalian systems such as the rat uterus, triphenylethylene antioestrogens such as tamoxifen (ICI 46,474) and nafoxidine (Upjohn 11,100A) display some partial oestrogen-like activity with which the nuclear receptor complexes could be correlated (Clark *et al.*, 1974; Katzenellenbogen and Ferguson, 1975; Jordan *et al.*, 1977b). However, the case was clarified in the chick system, since accumulation and persistency of the receptor in the nucleus was observed, but no oestrogenic effect was recorded (Sutherland *et al.*, 1977b; Sutherland and Foo, 1980). Recently, the same was observed for monohydroxytamoxifen (ICI 79,280) (Binart *et al.*, 1979).

These observations raise questions about the mode of action of these antioestrogens. The answers would bring some insight on the mechanism of action of oestrogens themselves. One of the many questions one can ask is whether the antioestrogen-receptor complexes reach the same acceptor sites as the oestradiol-receptor complexes, but are inactive because of a transconformation of the receptor protein. Perhaps the antioestrogen-receptor complex cannot interact with the oestrogen acceptor sites and attaches elsewhere in the nucleus.

In this report we summarize a number of experiments performed in our laboratory and in others that describe oestrogen receptor in chromatin, and we discuss some recent, as yet unpublished, data which we have obtained using antioestrogens.

II. OESTRADIOL RECEPTOR IN CHROMATIN PREPARED FROM NUCLEASE DIGESTED NUCLEI

To our knowledge, in all the experiments dealing with oestrogen receptors in chromatin, essentially three types of nucleases have been used, DNAase I (3.1.4.5.), DNAase II (3.1.4.6.) and micrococcal nuclease from *Staphylococcus aureus* (3.1.4.7.).

A. DNAase I

Shyamala Harris (1971) first reported the extraction by DNAase I, under certain ionic conditions, of oestradiol receptor from rat uterine nuclei. This receptor, which aggregated in sucrose gradients without KCl, could be stabilized into an 8S sedimenting form in the presence of polyanions. Similar results were reported by Senior and Frankel (1978), who obtained a 6S form of the receptor that which did not aggregate in low salt sucrose gradients when digesting rat uterine nuclei with DNAase I.

We also obtained a non-aggregating 7–8S form of the oestrogen receptor after DNAase I digestion of oviduct nuclei from laying hens or oestradiol stimulated chicks (manuscript in preparation).

DNAase I is, however, better known for its ability to selectively digest active genes characteristically expressed in specialized cells, such as globin in red cells and ovalbumin in oviduct cells (Weintraub and Groudine, 1976; Garel *et al.*, 1977; Palmiter *et al.*, 1978; Bloom and Anderson, 1979). However, this digestion does not depend on the state of active or non-active transcription at the time of exposure to the enzyme. In particular, Palmiter *et al.* (1978) showed that, in chicks previously primed by oestradiol and secondarily treated with oestradiol or tamoxifen, the ovalbumin gene in the oviduct is in both cases digested by DNAase I in a similar way as in the laying hen.

In conclusion these remarkable properties of DNAase I, which result in the destruction of the oestradiol regulated genes and the solubilization of the receptor, are quite opposite to the aim we are pursuing, that is to obtain fractions of chromatin containing both the receptor and the gene(s) controlled by oestradiol.

B. DNAase II

Following a method first described by Gottesfeld *et al.* (1974) to separate actively transcribing from non-transcribing chromatin, Hemminki and Vauhkonen (1976) prepared chromatin subfractions from hen oviduct by digesting the nuclei with DNAase II followed by a fractionation of the solubilized chromatin in the presence of 3 mM $MgCl_2$. They found that the $MgCl_2$-soluble fraction was enriched, compared to the $MgCl_2$-insoluble fraction, in both the concentration of specific oestradiol binding sites per mg DNA and ovalbumin gene copies, as measured by hybridization with ovalbumin cDNA. Therefore, it seems that the combination of DNAase II digestion and $MgCl_2$ fractionation selects a certain fraction of chromatin which contains both actively transcribing genes and oestradiol receptor. Hemminki (1977) also showed that, in primed immature chicks (Oka and Schimke, 1969), after a secondary oestradiol stimulation, the $MgCl_2$-soluble fraction of oviduct chromatin contained 2.7 times more oestradiol receptor per mg DNA than in the unstimulated chicks. He concluded, contrary to the report of Levy and Baxter (1976) for glucocorticoid and thyroid hormone receptor sites in cultured pituitary cells, that hormone stimulation leads to an enrichment in acceptor sites for oestradiol receptors in template-active chromatin fractions.

Using basically the same method, Alberga *et al.* (1979) found similar results in another system. Administration of oestradiol to a male or a female chick results in the increased synthesis by the liver of the yolk protein vitellogenin. This is accompanied by a concomitant increase in hepatic nuclear oestrogen binding sites. Alberga *et al.* (1979) found that, after DNAase II digestion of these nuclei and $MgCl_2$ fractionation, the $MgCl_2$-soluble chromatin fraction was enriched 5-fold, compared to total chromatin, in oestradiol binding sites per mg DNA. Upon further purification of this soluble fraction by ultracentrifugation on metrizamide gradients, they isolated a nucleoprotein peak containing a 2–4 fold receptor enrichment over the Mg-insoluble chromatin fractions and showing a 4-fold enrichment in vitellogenin gene, compared to unfractionated chromatin. It therefore appears, from the results of these two laboratories, that oestrogen receptor is not randomly distributed in chromatin but is associated with a fraction containing actively transcribing genomic sequences in such a tight way that it resists digestion by DNAase II, precipitation by $MgCl_2$ and centrifugation on metrizamide. Whether this observation will remain merely empirical or will bring a mechanistic explanation is not yet known.

C. Micrococcal Nuclease

Micrococcal nuclease from *Staphylococcus aureus* has also been used to prepare solubilized chromatin. Results from our laboratory (Massol *et al.*,

1978) showed that, after a mild digestion of hen oviduct nuclei by this nuclease followed by lysis of the nuclei and ultracentrifugation of the resulting chromatin on 5–20 % sucrose gradients, a typical profile of mono-, di-, and tri-nucleosomes was observed. The oestrogen binding sites sedimented mainly at 13–14S, slightly faster than the 12S mono-nucleosome fraction (Fig. 1).

When one plots the kinetics of appearance of monomers, dimers and trimers, as well as of the 13–14S oestradiol binding peak against enzyme digestion (Fig. 2; Massol *et al.*, 1978), one can see that oestrogen receptor first follows the joint optical density curves and then remains at a plateau value, as do the O.D. values for dimer and trimer appearance. This could be interpreted as an indication that oestrogen receptor is located on the internucleosomal linker, as is also suggested by Rennie (1979) for the androgen receptor in prostate chromatin, and that it is digested away after more extensive enzyme action. Another explanation is that, at very early times of micrococcal

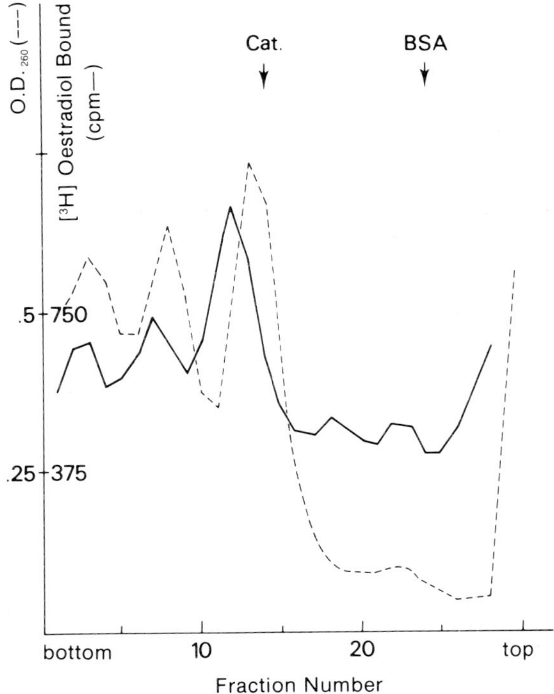

Fig. 1. Typical 5–20 % sucrose density gradient of laying hen chromatin. Oviduct nuclei were digested with 54 U/mg DNA micrococcal nuclease and lysed in 0.2 mM EDTA, pH 7.4. The samples were incubated overnight with 5 nM [^{3}H]oestradiol at 0° and 90 min at 30 °C. The extracts were treated 5 min with charcoal-dextran before layering on the gradient. Run was 4.5 hours at 58,000 rpm in an SW 60 rotor. O.D. $_{260}$ ----; cpm__________;markers were catalase (11.6S) and bovine serum albumin (4.2S).

nuclease digestion, there is a selective excision of receptor bearing nucleosomes. Selective release of mononucleosomes enriched in ovalbumin coding sequences at the onset of micrococcal nuclease digestion has been observed by Bellard *et al.* (1978) and by Bloom and Anderson (1978). This may suggest that we are looking at the same sub-population of mononucleosomes, which contain both receptor binding sites and transcribing ovalbumin genes. This idea is confirmed by the recently published data of Bloom and Anderson (1979). They describe a temporal correlation between the decline observed in the oviduct nuclear oestrogen receptor of oestradiol stimulated chicks acutely withdrawing from the hormone and the concentration of ovalbumin gene in the mononucleosomes generated at early micrococcal nuclease digestion times.

Two other groups have used this nuclease to investigate oestradiol receptor–chromatin relationships in uterine systems. Senior and Frankel (1978), digesting rat uterus nuclei with micrococcal nuclease, found two types of chromatin binding sites for the oestradiol-receptor complex. One type sedimented along with the O.D.$_{260}$ absorbing material, slightly faster than the mono-, di-, and tri-nucleosome fractions on sucrose gradients, with sedimentation coefficients of 12S, 16.5S and slightly more than 20S, the other type sedimented at 7S. The authors present evidence that these two classes of

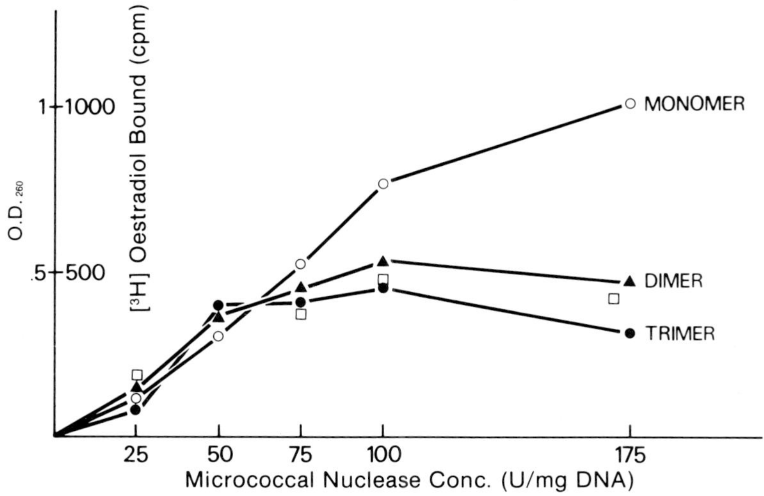

Fig. 2. Equal aliquots of hen oviduct nuclei were digested for 30 seconds at 30 °C with varying concentrations of micrococcal nuclease and centrifuged on a sucrose gradient. O.D.$_{260}$ of the mono- (12–13S) (○), di- (17–18S) (△), and tri-nucleosome (22–23S) (●) fractions, and cpm in the 13–14S peak (□) were plotted against enzyme concentration.

binding sites are not interconvertible and arise independently during enzyme digestion, and show that one could be located on the nucleosome itself, and the other on the inter-nucleosomal linker. André *et al.*, (1978) used extensive micrococcal nuclease digestion of lamb endometrial nuclei in order to generate "free" nuclear oestrogen receptor and compare it to cytosol receptor (8S or Ca^{2+} generated 4S). They concluded that the micrococcal nuclease-extracted nuclear receptor resembles "native" 8S cytosol receptor in its Stokes radius, DNA-binding ability and behaviour in the presence of KCl.

In conclusion, André *et al*'s purpose resembled more that of Shyamala Harris, when she used DNAase I to free the receptor from its chromatin acceptor sites, and they did not study receptor–acceptor interactions. Senior and Frankel's results support our observations and show that a similar picture is obtained in a different system. The reason for quantitative differences between different experiments cannot be explained yet, but since different model systems and different experimental conditions were used, and given the extreme complexity of chromatin, this is not surprising.

III. OESTROGEN RECEPTORS IN CHICK OVIDUCT CHROMATIN AFTER OESTRADIOL BENZOATE, TAMOXIFEN OR MONOHYDROXYTAMOXIFEN ADMINISTRATION

When studying the action of antioestrogens such as tamoxifen and monohydroxytamoxifen researchers have found that the chick oviduct model has the advantage over the mammalian model systems since, in the chick, these compounds are complete antioestrogens (Sutherland *et al.*, 1977b; Binart *et al.*, 1979; Sutherland and Foo, 1980) and have no oestrogen-like activity, according to all the criteria tested (see Chapters 9 and 10). These have included light microscopy (unpublished observations), wet weight and DNA determinations (Sutherland *et al.*, 1977b; Binart *et al.*, 1979; Sutherland and Foo, 1980), measurement of ovalbumin and conalbumin synthesis (Catelli *et al.*, 1980) and of progesterone receptor (Sutherland *et al.*, 1977b; Binart *et al.*, 1979).

Since we wanted to find out if the nucleosome-associated peaks of oestradiol binding sites we observed in our chromatin gradients were related somehow to biological activity, we injected a certain number of hormones and antihormones to primed immature chicks and compared the resulting biological activity with the presence or absence of receptor peaks (Lebeau, Massol and Baulieu, unpublished).

When we injected oestradiol benzoate (1–10 mg/kg) into 4–6 week withdrawn immature chicks, sacrificed the animals 2–12 hours later, digested the nuclei with micrococcal nuclease and analysed the resulting chromatin by ultracentrifugation on sucrose gradients, we found oestrogen receptor sedimenting partly in the 13–14S region of the gradient (as in the laying hen; Fig. 1) and partly at 7S (Fig. 3B). We do not yet know why the 7S form is observed in stimulated chick and not in laying hen chromatin, but this is under investigation. When analysing chromatin from unstimulated control chicks, after incubation with radioactive oestradiol and ultracentrifugation as described in the legend to Figure 3, we observed the same $O.D._{260}$ profiles in the gradients as with chromatin from stimulated animals, but the radioactivity due to bound [^{3}H]oestradiol was extremely low (Fig. 3A). When we administered tamoxifen alone to an identical group of chicks at a dose which is known to translocate the oestrogen receptor to the nucleus (Sutherland *et al.*, 1977b), gradient profiles resembling that of control chicks were obtained (not shown). Although care was taken to prevent ligand dissociation from the receptor and resulting receptor degradation, the oestrogen binding sites missing in the chromatin could not systematically be accounted for in the other sub-nuclear fractions (undigested nuclear pellet, supernatant obtained after enzyme digestion and before nuclear lysis). As it has been shown (Capony and Rochefort, 1978) that tamoxifen dissociates readily from the oestrogen receptor in other systems, we attributed our results to uncontrolled ligand dissociation and receptor degradation, in spite of the precautions used.

When tamoxifen was injected together with oestradiol benzoate, the same chromatin gradient profile was seen as after tamoxifen injection alone. This showed that tamoxifen exerted its antioestrogen action and prevented the appearance of chromatin binding sites. When tamoxifen was given 2–15 hours after oestradiol benzoate, the height of the oestrogen induced 13–14S oestrogen binding peak was reduced proportionally to the length of time tamoxifen was allowed to act as if it progressively chased the oestrogen receptor from its chromatin acceptor sites. These results also show that tamoxifen can reach the nucleus and act at that level at a time when oestradiol receptor is located mainly in the nucleus and cytoplasmic receptor is very low.

Lately, a sufficient quantity of monohydroxytamoxifen became available to us and we were able to use this compound in our experiments. Monohydroxytamoxifen has been shown to be a better antioestrogen than tamoxifen in mammals (Jordan *et al.*, 1977a) and to have an affinity for oestradiol receptor of the same order as oestradiol (Binart *et al.*, 1979; and Chapter 9). For this reason, the tamoxifen-linked disadvantage of ligand dissociation during the experiment was obviated and we hoped to obtain results more clearly interpretable. Two to eleven hours after administration of monohydroxytamoxifen to withdrawn chicks the birds were sacrificed and chromatin prepared and labelled as described for the laying hen (legend to Fig. 3). Some bound [^{3}H]oestradiol was found in the gradient (Fig. 3C), with

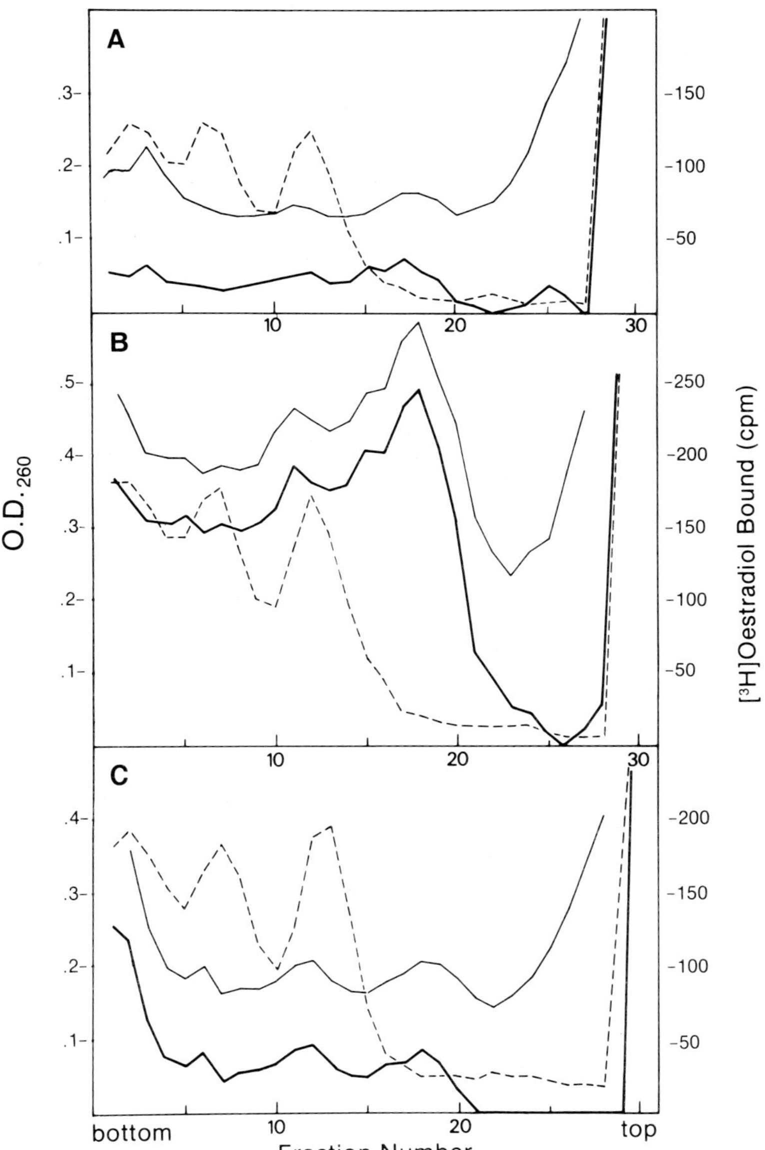

Fig. 3. Oviduct nuclei from withdrawn immature chicks, untreated (A), or 11 hours after injection of oestradiol benzoate (B), or monohydroxytamoxifen (C) were digested with 44, 50 and 51 U/mg DNA micrococcal nuclease and treated as in Figure 1 except that samples were incubated with either 10 nM [^{3}H]oestradiol alone (total cpm, ———) or with 10 nM [^{3}H]oestradiol + 1 μM non-radioactive oestradiol (non-specific cpm). O.D. $_{260}$ (---), specifically bound cpm (———) = total cpm − non-specifically bound cpm.

small peaks sedimenting both in the 13–14S and 7S regions, however these were not much higher than the control values and were nearly all due to non-specific binding.

We find it remarkable that nuclear tamoxifen-receptor and monohydroxytamoxifen-receptor complexes cannot be detected in gradient analyses where we observe receptor–acceptor interactions after oestradiol administration. The correlation between the absence of these nuclear complexes and the lack of biological activity of these two antioestrogens is striking. If nuclear binding of tamoxifen or monohydroxytamoxifen receptor complex does take place, it is quite labile and cannot be of the same type, or to the same acceptor sites, as that of the oestradiol-receptor complex. We are now investigating the nature of this receptor–chromatin interaction and the chromatin elements that are involved.

IV. CONCLUSIONS

In recent years new approaches to the study of chromatin, such as the use of specific nucleases and very precise ionic fractionation techniques, have brought new insights into the complex structure of what, until recently, had remained an intricate entity. It appears that, in a system such as the chick oviduct, where responses to oestrogens and to antioestrogens are clearcut, the antioestrogens are excellent tools to assist our understanding of how oestrogen receptors interact with chromatin. Results from our own and other laboratories suggest that antioestrogens translocate the oestrogen receptor to the nucleus but that these antioestrogen-receptor complexes cannot engage in the same type of interactions with chromatin acceptor sites as oestradiol receptor complexes. The assumption that the antioestrogen-receptor complexes can associate with the "oestrogen" acceptor sites but remain inactive because of a transconformation of the receptor protein might not be correct. We are struck by the fact that we cannot detect these receptor complexes in our chromatin preparations in spite of the fact that we are using monohydroxytamoxifen, which has a sufficiently high affinity for the oestrogen receptor to avoid dissociation resulting in uncontrolled degradation of the receptor.

We therefore hope that, by comparing chromatin subfractions from oestrogen-stimulated chick oviducts and antioestrogen-treated chick oviducts, we can find out what elements are present or absent or what type of modifications the chromatin elements have undergone. In this way one may perhaps understand how hormone carrying receptor molecules can interact with inactive chromatin to promote specific oestrogenic responses.

ACKNOWLEDGEMENTS

The work stemming from Lab. Hormones, Bicêtre was supported by contract INSERM n° 77.5.037.4. and contract Faculty of Medicine Paris-South n° 738. We thank Jean-Claude Lambert for the preparation of the figures.

REFERENCES

Alberga, A., Ferrez, M., and Baulieu, E. E. (1976). *FEBS Letters* **61**, 223–226.
Alberga, A., Tran, A., and Baulieu, E. E. (1979). *Nucl. Acids Res.* **7**, 2031–2044.
Anderson, J. N., Peck, E. J., and Clark, J. H. (1973). *Endocrinology* **92**, 1488–1495.
André, J., and Rochefort, H. (1973). *FEBS Letters* **29**, 135–140.
André, J., and Rochefort, H. (1975). *FEBS Letters* **50**, 319–323.
André, J., Raynaud, A., and Rochefort, H. (1978). *Biochemistry* **17**, 3619–3626.
Barrack, E. R., Hawkins, E. F., Allen, S. L., Hicks, L. L., and Coffey, D. S., (1977). *Biochem. Biophys. Res. Commun.* **79**, 829–836.
Bellard, M., Gannon, F., and Chambon, P. (1978). *Cold Spring Harbor Symp. Quant. Biol.* **42**, 779–791.
Binart, N., Catelli, M. G., Geynet, C., Puri, V., Hähnel, R., Mester, J., and Baulieu, E. E. (1979). *Biochem. Biophys. Res. Commun.* **91**, 812–818.
Bloom, K. S., and Anderson, J. N. (1978). *Cell* **15**, 141–150.
Bloom, K. S., and Anderson, J. N. (1979). *J. Biol. Chem.* **254**, 1532–1539.
Bradbury, E. M., Carpenter, B. G., and Rattle, H. W. E. (1973). *Nature* **241**, 123–126.
Capony, F., and Rochefort, H. (1978). *Mol. Cell. Endocr.* **11**, 181–198.
Catelli, M. G., Binart, N., Elkik, F., and Baulieu, E. E. (1980). *Eur. J. Biochem.* **107**, 165–172.
Chamness, G. C., Jennings, A. W., and McGuire, W. L. (1974). *Biochemistry* **13**, 327–331.
Christiansen, G., and Griffith, J. (1977). *Nucl. Acids Res.* **4**, 1837–1851.
Clark, J. H., Peck, E. J., and Anderson, J. N. (1974). *Nature* **251**, 446–448.
Finch, J. T., Noll, M., and Kornberg, R. D. (1975). *Proc. Natl Acad. Sci. U.S.A.* **72**, 3320–3322.
Garel, A., Zolan, M., and Axel, R. (1977). *Proc. Natl Acad. Sci. U.S.A.* **74**, 4867–4871.
Gorski, J., Toft, D. O., Shyamala, G., Smith, D., and Notides, A. (1968). *Recent Progr. Horm. Res.* **24**, 45–80.
Gottesfeld, J. M., Garrard, W. T., Bagi, G., Wilson, R. F., and Bonner, J. (1974). *Proc. Natl Acad. Sci. U.S.A.* **71**, 2193–2197.
Hemminki, K. (1977). *Acta Endocr.* **84**, 215–224.
Hemminki, K., and Vauhkonen, M. (1976). *J. Steroid Biochem.* **7**, 1087–1090.
Jordan, V. C., Collins, M. M., Rowsby, L., and Prestwich, G. (1977a). *J. Endocr.* **75**, 305–316.
Jordan, V. C., Dix, C. J., Rowsby, L., and Prestwich, G. (1977b). *Mol. Cell. Endocr.* **7**, 177–192.
Jensen, E. V., Suzuki, T., Kawashima, T., Stumpf, W. E., Jungblut, P. W., and DeSombre, E. R. (1968). *Biochemistry* **59**, 632–638.
Katzenellenbogen, B. S., and Ferguson, E. R. (1975). *Endocrinology* **97**, 1–12.
King, R. J. B., and Gordon, J. (1972). *Nature, New Biol.* **240**, 185–187.
Levy, B., and Baxter, J. D. (1976). *Biochim. Biophys. Res. Commun.* **68**, 1045–1051.
Liao, S., Liang, T., and Tymoczko, J. L. (1973). *Nature, New Biol.* **241**, 211–213.
Massol, N., Lebeau, M. C., and Baulieu, E. E. (1978). *Nucl. Acids Res.* **5**, 723–738.

Maurer, J. R., and Chalkley, G. R. (1967). *J. Mol. Biol.* **27**, 431–441.

Mulvihill, E. R., and Palmiter, R. D. (1977). *J. Biol. Chem.* **252**, 2060–2068.

Musliner, T. A., and Chader, G. J. (1971). *Biochem. Biophys. Res. Commun.* **45**, 998–1003.

Noll, M., Thomas, J. O., and Kornberg, R. D. (1975). *Science* **187**, 1203–1206.

Oka, T., and Schimke, R. T. (1969). *J. Cell. Biol.* **43**, 123–137.

Oudet, P., Gross-Bellard, M., and Chambon, P. (1975). *Cell* **4**, 281–300.

Palmiter, R. D., Mulvihill, E. R., McKnight, G. C., and Senear, A. W. (1978). *Cold Spring Harbor Symp. Quant. Biol.* **42**, 639–647.

Puca, G. A., Sica, B., and Nola, E. (1974). *Proc. Natl Acad. Sci. U.S.A.* **71**, 979–983.

Rennie, P. S. (1979). *J. Biol. Chem.* **254**, 3947–3952.

Senior, M. B., and Frankel, F. R. (1978). *Cell* **14**, 857–863.

Shyamala Harris, G. (1971). *Nature, New Biol* **231**, 246–248.

Spadafora, C., Oudet, P., and Chambon, P. (1979). *Eur. J. Biochem.* **100**, 225–235.

Spelsberg, T. C., Steggles, A. W., and O'Malley, B. W. (1971). *J. Biol. Chem.* **246**, 4188–4197.

Spelsberg, T. C., Webster, R. A., and Pikler, G. M. (1976). *Nature* **262**, 65–67.

Sutherland, R. L. and Foo, M. S. (1980). *In* "Steroids and their Mechanism of Action in Non-Mammalian Vertebrates" (G. Del Rio and J. Brachet eds), pp. 221–232. Raven Press, New York.

Sutherland, R. L., Lebeau, M. C., Schmelck, P. H., and Baulieu, E. E. (1977a). *FEBS Letters* **79**, 253–257.

Sutherland, R. L., Mester, J., and Baulieu, E. E. (1977b). *Nature* **267**, 434–435.

Toft, D. (1972). *J. Steroid Biochem.* **3**, 515–522.

Weintraub, H., and Groudine, M. (1976). *Science* **193**, 848–856.

Yamamoto, K. R., and Alberts, B. (1975). *Cell* **4**, 301–310.

16

Effects of Antioestrogens in Carcinogen-Induced Rat Mammary Cancer

V. CRAIG JORDAN, C. J. DIX AND KAREN E. ALLEN

I. INTRODUCTION

In the search for effective therapeutic agents it is essential to develop reliable and meaningful laboratory models. The model must be completely investigated and its limitations, advantages and disadvantages adequately defined. Models of human breast cancer which occur with a high incidence and are hormone-dependent were first described by Huggins *et al.* (1959) who reviewed the known information on carcinogen-induced rat mammary tumours and demonstrated the induction of hormone-dependent tumours by

NON-STEROIDAL ANTIOESTROGENS
ISBN 0 12 677880 9

dimethylbenzanthracene (DMBA). Subsequent studies (Huggins *et al.*, 1961; Huggins and Yang, 1962) refined the methodology and established a valuable model for the investigation of hormone-dependent cancer.

During the past 20 years the biology of the tumours has been extensively studied, but many problems concerning the precise control mechanisms for tumour growth remain unresolved. It has also become clear that the animal model is more dependent upon prolactin than its human counterpart and the carcinogen-induced tumours rarely metastasize. The aim of this chapter is to consider the control mechanisms of tumour homeostasis and how pharmacological agents can interfere with tumour growth by direct and indirect means.

A. The Dimethylbenzanthracene (DMBA)-Induced Rat Mammary Carcinoma Model

Carcinogen-induced mammary cancer production is a dose-related phenomenon; however the age at which the carcinogen is administered is critical (Huggins *et al.*, 1961). It has been suggested that this is related to the sensitivity of mammary tissue to stimulate DNA synthesis in response to prolactin secretion (Nagasawa *et al.*, 1976). The hormonal environment is certainly critical for mammary carcinogenesis since long term ovariectomized rats are resistant to carcinogen administration (Dao, 1962). In general, a single intragastric administration of DMBA (20 mg in 2 ml peanut oil) to female Sprague Dawley rats (50–60 days of age) results in tumour appearance 30–150 days later.

The early definition of hormone dependency was based upon the regression of carcinogen-induced tumours after ovariectomy and hypophysectomy (Huggins *et al.*, 1959). Administration of oestrogen causes tumours to regrow in ovariectomized rats; however, the tumours do not regrow in ovariectomized and hypophysectomized rats (Sterental *et al.*, 1963). The pituitary clearly has a role in the growth and homeostasis of DMBA-induced tumours, and the finding that oestrogen stimulated the release of prolactin (Chen and Meites, 1970) suggested a primary role for this hormone. It has been claimed, however, that oestrogen is also a prerequisite for tumour growth. This conclusion is based on the observation that rats with a median eminence lesion of the hypothalamus, having, as a result, high circulating levels of prolactin, had tumour regression after ovariectomy and regrowth only after the grafting of ovarian tissue (Sinha *et al.*, 1973).

It can also be argued that oestrogen has a role within the tumour cells because of the identification (King *et al.*, 1969; McGuire and Julian, 1971; Leclercq and Heuson, 1973) of an oestrogen receptor protein similar to that described in the rat uterus (Gorski *et al.*, 1968; Jensen and DeSombre, 1973).

Certainly some positive functions have been ascribed to the oestrogen receptor system since hormone-dependent tumours contain higher receptor concentrations than hormone-independent tumours (Mobbs, 1966; McGuire and Julian, 1971; Nomura *et al.*, 1974). However, several studies have shown that the hormonal responses of many tumours do not correlate with their oestrogen receptor status (Mobbs and Johnson, 1974; Boylan and Wittliff, 1975; DeSombre *et al.*, 1976). This situation has focused attention upon other hormone receptor systems to determine their interrelationship with oestrogen receptor concentrations.

A direct role for prolactin action was suggested by the identification of prolactin receptors (Turkington, 1974; Kelly *et al.*, 1974; Costlow *et al.*, 1976). It is of interest that prolactin administration, as well as stimulating tumour growth (Leung *et al.*, 1975), increases tumour concentrations of oestrogen receptors both *in vivo* (Vignon and Rochefort, 1976) and *in vitro* (Sasaki and Leung, 1975). It was also found that insulin had a synergistic effect on the prolactin-stimulated rise in oestrogen receptors (Sasaki and Leung, 1975) which may be related to the observation that insulin is required for tumour growth (Heuson and Legros, 1972; Heuson *et al.*, 1972). Insulin receptors have been identified in the plasma membranes of DMBA-induced tumours (Holdaway and Friesen, 1976). The role of insulin is further implicated in receptor modulation and tumour growth, by the reports that chemically-induced diabetes decreases oestrogen receptors in the tumours (Gibson and Hilf, 1976). However, there is no consistent decrease in tumour prolactin binding during regression induced by diabetes (Smith *et al.*, 1977).

Finally, progesterone has been implicated in the growth of DMBA-induced tumours (Jabara, 1967; Jabara and Harcourt, 1970; Jabara and Harcourt, 1971) although combination with oestrogen results in tumour regression (Huggins *et al.*, 1959; Huggins *et al.*, 1961). A progesterone receptor has been identified in the tumour (Terenius, 1973; Asselin *et al.*, 1976; Goral and Wittliff, 1976) which can be induced by oestrogen administration (Asselin *et al.*, 1977; Horwitz and McGuire, 1977).

As yet the physiological and biochemical roles of these hormone receptor systems *in vivo* are unresolved. Ideally endocrine regulations should be studied *in vitro*. There have only been a few reports of the direct effects of hormones but these are consistent with the findings *in vivo*. Oestrogen stimulates RNA polymerase (Arbogast and DeSombre, 1975) and protein synthesis (Lee and Oyasu, 1974). In contrast oestrogen has little effect on DNA synthesis, whilst combinations of insulin, prolactin and progesterone are stimulatory (Pasteels *et al.*, 1976).

It is clear from all the pharmacological and biochemical studies that have been undertaken that prolactin is the dominant endocrine factor in tumour growth, but the precise subcellular mechanisms remain unclear. The complex hormone interrelationships serve to highlight the difficulties that must be considered when evaluating the mode of action of pharmacological agents for future human use.

B. The DMBA-Induced Mammary Tumour Model as a Drug Evaluation System

Early studies using established hormonal (Griswold *et al.*, 1966; Teller *et al.*, 1966a) and chemotherapeutic (Teller *et al.*, 1966b) modalities showed that the DMBA-induced mammary carcinoma model was useful for the evaluation of new drugs. However, it is important to realize that hormonal sensitivity in this model is related to time after DMBA administration: young tumours are more sensitive to hormonal manipulation than older, established tumours (Griswold and Green, 1970).

The potential multiple hormone dependency of the mammary tumours, and the requirement for a balanced hormonal milieu, provide many sites for attack by pharmacological agents. Inhibitors of pituitary function cause tumour regression. 2 Br α Ergocryptine (Heuson *et al.*, 1970) and ergocornine (Nagasawa and Meites, 1970; Cassell *et al.*, 1971), both inhibitors of prolactin release and inhibitors of gonadotrophin release like GP 48,989 (Schmidt-Ruppin *et al.*, 1973; Jordan *et al.*, 1979b) cause tumour regression. It is perhaps interesting to note that synthetic gonadotrophin-releasing hormone analogues are also effective in this respect (DeSombre *et al.*, 1976; Danguy *et al.*, 1977; Nicholson and Maynard, 1979). For one such compound, A-43,818, it has been suggested that its primary function is to disrupt the release of prolactin (Danguy *et al.*, 1977), but whether this is a direct mechanism or an effect via the ovary is unknown.

As another point of attack, compounds that inhibit steroidogenesis predictably cause DMBA-induced tumours to regress (Levin *et al.*, 1976; Brodie *et al.*, 1979).

Finally, compounds have been studied which are believed to have direct antitumour activity. Pharmacological doses of androgens (Griswold and Green, 1970; Horn *et al.*, 1976) and oestrogens (Meites *et al.*, 1971; Kledzik *et al.*, 1976) will cause tumour regression as will the administration of the antioestrogens nafoxidine (Terenius, 1971), enclomiphene (Schulz *et al.*, 1971), CI 628 (DeSombre and Arbogast, 1974), tamoxifen (Jordan, 1974; Nicholson and Golder, 1975) and U 23,469 (Tsai and Katzenellenbogen, 1977). However, it should be borne in mind that tumour regression by these agents can be reversed by prolactin (Meites *et al.*, 1971) or perphenazine administration (Manni *et al.*, 1977). This chapter will focus attention on the non-steroidal antioestrogen tamoxifen and consider various potential mechanisms for its antitumour actions in this model.

II. POTENTIAL MODES OF ACTION FOR TAMOXIFEN

Tamoxifen (*trans* 1-(p-β-dimethylaminoethoxyphenyl)-1,2 diphenyl but-1-ene) inhibits the initiation (Jordan, 1974, 1976a) and growth (Nicholson and Golder, 1975; Jordan and Koerner, 1976) of DMBA-induced mammary tumours. The effect of different daily doses of tamoxifen on the growth of young DMBA-induced tumours is illustrated in Figure 1. In general the tumours regress in response to therapy, but it should be noted that some tumours are refractory to treatment. The age of the tumour is also important since older tumours are less sensitive to tamoxifen (Jordan *et al.*, 1980). This is consistent with the general refractoriness of older tumours to endocrine manipulation (Griswold and Green, 1970).

There are several mechanisms by which tamoxifen could provoke tumour regression. These are illustrated in Figure 2. In general, tamoxifen could either affect the direct action of oestrogen and prolactin or modify the hormonal environment in which the tumour cells are growing.

The major sites that may be involved in the mode of action of tamoxifen are (a) inhibition of oestrogen binding in the tumour; (b) inhibition of ovarian oestrogen synthesis; (c) inhibition of gonadotrophin release; and (d) inhibition of prolactin secretion.

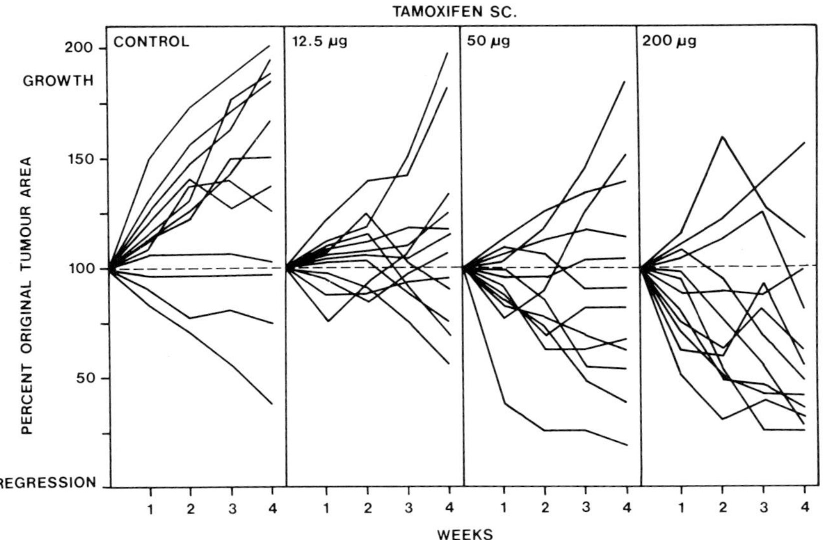

Fig. 1. The effect of different daily doses of tamoxifen (s.c. in 0.1 ml peanut oil) on the percentage growth or regression of DMBA-induced mammary tumours (100–150 days after DMBA). Controls received vehicle alone.

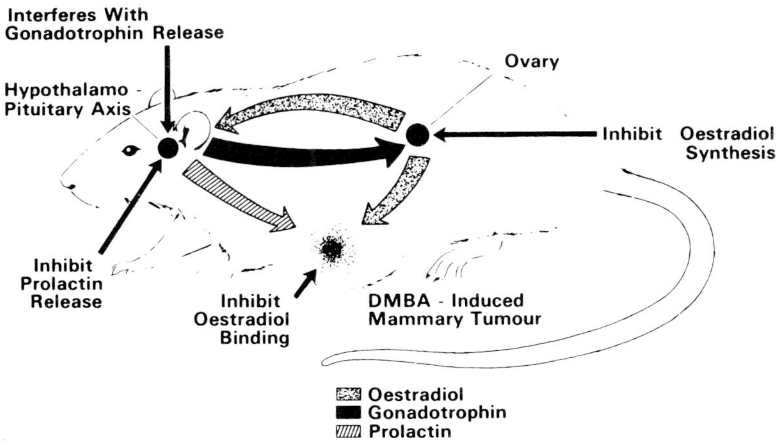

Fig. 2. Potential sites of action of antioestrogens that could result in DMBA-induced tumour regression.

A. Inhibition of Oestrogen Binding in the Tumour

Tamoxifen inhibits the binding of [^{3}H]oestradiol in DMBA-induced tumour tissue whether determined *in vivo* (Jordan, 1976a; Jordan and Dowse, 1976) or *in vitro* (Nicholson and Golder, 1975; Jordan and Jaspan, 1976). At the subcellular level tamoxifen inhibits the binding of [^{3}H]oestradiol to the 8S oestrogen receptor protein derived from DMBA-induced tumours (Powell-Jones *et al.*, 1975; Jordan and Dowse, 1976), and recently it has been shown that [^{3}H]tamoxifen can bind directly to the oestrogen receptor from human mammary tumours (Nicholson *et al.*, 1979).

The oestrogen receptor system in DMBA-induced tumours has been studied extensively (Nicholson *et al.*, 1976; 1977a). Tamoxifen, like oestradiol, will translocate cytoplasmic oestrogen receptors to the nuclear compartment, but, unlike oestradiol, tamoxifen cannot maintain rises in tumour RNA polymerase (Nicholson *et al.*, 1977b). If tamoxifen has an antitumour action via this sequence of events, then a decrease in the protein synthetic capacity of the cells may be an important first step in tumour regression.

The significance of oestrogen receptors in the tumours is poorly understood but it is possible that they are indicators of hormone dependency. Low levels of oestrogen receptor indicate that the tumours will not respond to tamoxifen therapy (Jordan and Jaspan, 1976). Similarly, transplantable rat mammary tumours with low levels of oestrogen receptors do not respond to either tamoxifen therapy or ovariectomy (Jordan *et al.*, 1979b). However, the tumours may not be dependent on oestrogens alone.

B. Inhibition of Ovarian Oestrogen Synthesis

An inhibition of oestrogen synthesis and the resulting reduction in circulating levels of oestradiol-17β would facilitate the competitive blockade of oestrogen receptors by tamoxifen within the tumour cells. Tamoxifen reduces the levels of circulating oestradiol in the rat (Watson *et al.*, 1975) by inhibiting synthesis of oestradiol in the ovary (Watson and Alam, 1976; Watson and Howson, 1977). There is very little information about the long term effects of tamoxifen on ovarian function in rats with DMBA-induced tumours. The few published reports suggest that antioestrogens can lower circulating oestrogen concentrations (Nicholson and Golder, 1975; Jordan and Koerner, 1976). It is clear though, that any fluctuations in the cyclical synthesis of oestrogen will have a profound effect on the regulation of both gonadotrophin and prolactin secretion.

C. Inhibition of Gonadotrophin Release

Evidence from studies in rats and hamsters suggest that antioestrogens can inhibit the positive feedback effects of oestrogens for the ovulatory release of LH (Labhsetwar, 1970a, 1970b, 1972; Yokoyama *et al.*, 1973). In ovariectomized rats, tamoxifen (Döhler *et al.*, 1977) and CI 628 (Callantine *et al.*, 1966) are apparently unable to lower circulating LH levels. In contrast with earlier findings we have observed a partial decrease in LH levels after 1 month of tamoxifen therapy (Table I) and Nicholson (1979) has reported dramatic decreases in LH levels within a few days of initiating therapy. This confusing situation suggested that the effect of tamoxifen and monohydroxytamoxifen should be investigated in some detail, and experiments were performed in collaboration with Dr Barry Furr at ICI Ltd., Pharmaceutical Division.

The daily administration of 200 μg tamoxifen to ovariectomized rats over a 4 week period slowly, but effectively, reduced the concentrations of serum LH (Fig. 3). Fifty μg tamoxifen is equally effective but 12.5 μg appears to be ineffective. It is perhaps relevant to note that the latter dose regimen only produces tumour stasis rather than regression (Fig. 1). With regard to monohydroxytamoxifen the slight effect produced when the drug (50 μg) is given intraperitoneally for 5 days per week (Table I) is not seen when the drug is given daily subcutaneously. The difference probably reflects the rapid clearance of monohydroxytamoxifen when given by the intraperitoneal route. The greater effect of tamoxifen (Table I) emphasizes its longer biological half-life.

Unfortunately there is no information about the effects of antioestrogens on FSH levels in the ovariectomized rat. Nevertheless, the oestrogenic action

TABLE I
Effect of Four Weeks of Therapy on Ovariectomized Rat Serum Luteinizing Hormone (LH) and Prolactin[a]

Treatment	LH (ng/ml)	Prolactin (ng/ml)
Control	51.44 ± 5.66	1.75 ± 0.07
Oestradiol[b]	6.04 ± 1.58[d]	57.7 ± 10.5[d]
Tamoxifen[c]	34.60 ± 4.63[e]	1.88 ± 0.22
Monohydroxytamoxifen[c]	42.18 ± 2.78	2.2 ± 0.31

[a] 8 rats per group.
[b] 50 μg s.c. daily (in 0.1 ml peanut oil) 5 times per week.
[c] 50 μg i.p. daily (in 0.1 ml peanut oil) 5 times per week.
[d] $p < 0.001$ comparison of group mean with control by Student's *t*-test.
[e] $p < 0.05$ comparison of group mean with control by Student's *t*-test.
Other values $p > 0.05$.

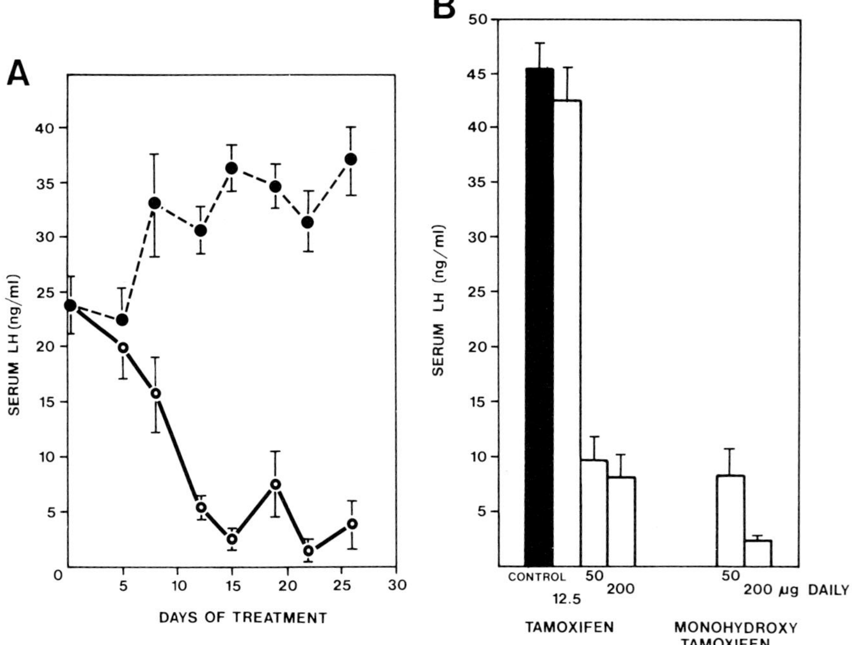

Fig. 3. (A) Effect of daily injections of tamoxifen (200 μg s.c., ○) on ovariectomized rat serum LH levels. Controls (●) received peanut oil vehicle alone. (B) Dose-response effects of tamoxifen and monohydroxytamoxifen upon ovariectomized rat LH after 4 weeks of treatment. Six rats per group.

of tamoxifen and monohydroxytamoxifen at the hypothalamo-pituitary axis indicates that the normal ovarian-pituitary feedback systems will be interrupted.

D. Inhibition of Prolactin Secretion

Non-steroidal antioestrogens inhibit oestrogen-stimulated increases in plasma prolactin (Heuson *et al.*, 1971; Jordan *et al.*, 1975), however this inhibition is incomplete (Jordan and Koerner, 1976). Unlike oestrogen, tamoxifen and monohydroxytamoxifen do not stimulate large rises in circulating prolactin in ovariectomized rats (Table I), which indicates that different oestrogen mediated regulatory systems are operating at the hypothalamo-pituitary axis to control LH and prolactin release.

Results in the intact rat have been confusing. Antioestrogens inhibit (or delay) the surge of prolactin at pro-oestrus (Yokoyama *et al.*, 1973; Jordan *et al.*, 1975), but studies in rats with DMBA-induced tumours have failed to show a uniform decrease in the concentrations of circulating prolactin (Nicholson and Golder, 1975; Jordan and Koerner, 1976). It is interesting to note, however, that tamoxifen-induced regression of tumours can be reversed by perphenazine, a stimulant of prolactin release (Manni *et al.*, 1977).

We believed it was important to re-examine the effects of tamoxifen in DMBA-treated rats. Before the start of the experiment all animals had determinations of serum prolactin at various stages of the oestrous cycle. This defined the known rise in prolactin levels at pro-oestrus (Table II). Daily treatment of the animals with tamoxifen (50 μg i.p. 5 days per week) for 2 and 4 weeks resulted in a uniform decrease in plasma prolactin (Table II). Levels were comparable to those observed in ovariectomized rats (Table I). The result strongly suggests that tamoxifen can reduce the circulating concentrations of prolactin.

TABLE II
Effect of Tamoxifen Therapy (50 μg i.p. 5 times per week) on Serum Prolactin Levels

Cycle time or treatment	N[a]	Serum prolactin (ng/ml)
Control: Dioestrus	6	5.4 ± 2.83
Pro-oestrus	10	56.46 ± 15.19
Oestrus	8	31.94 ± 10.59
Metoestrus	3	10.09 ± 6.15
Tamoxifen: 2 weeks	12	6.43 ± 1.93
4 weeks	11	3.31 ± 0.62

[a] Number of rats per group.

E. Conclusions

The view that non-steroidal antioestrogens produce their antitumour actions exclusively by blocking oestrogen receptors in DMBA-induced tumours (Terenius, 1971; Jordan, 1976b) must be modified in the light of the foregoing discussion. The general endocrine effects of tamoxifen are summarized in Figure 4; all of these probably contribute to tumour regression. It is now perhaps relevant to compare these findings with observations in the treatment of clinical disease to focus upon similarities and differences.

Tamoxifen inhibits oestrogen binding to the oestrogen receptor derived from rat and human mammary tumours (Jordan and Koerner, 1975; Powell-Jones *et al.*, 1975). However, unlike the rat, the greater dependency of human tumours on oestrogen is confirmed by studies on the direct effects of antioestrogens on human cancer cells in culture (Lippman and Bolan, 1975). Again, unlike the rat, tamoxifen, increases plasma oestradiol in women (Groom and Griffiths, 1976), but in both systems tamoxifen can reduce oestrogen-stimulated rises in plasma prolactin. It is also interesting to note that tamoxifen has been found to completely suppress prolactin release by the use of a breast pump (Masala *et al.*, 1978). Tamoxifen lowers plasma LH in postmenopausal women (Golder *et al.*, 1976; Willis *et al.*, 1977) and ovariectomized rats (Fig. 3).

Although there are many similarities and differences between the clinical and laboratory studies it must be stressed that, unlike the rat model, no positive role, as yet, has been ascribed for prolactin in the clinical disease. As

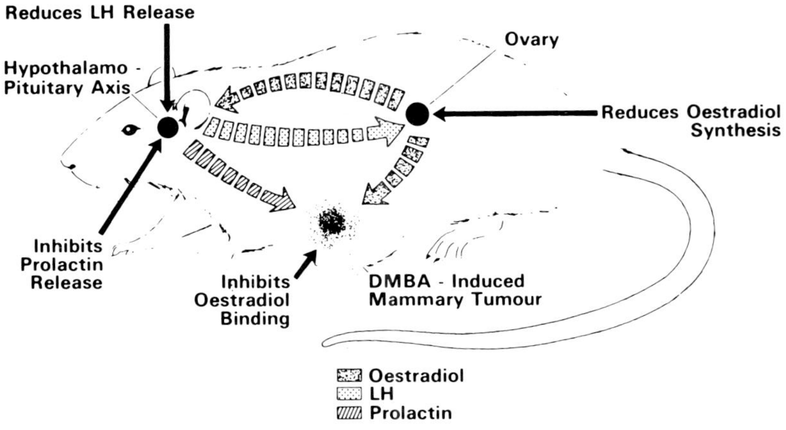

Fig. 4. Summary of the endocrine effects of tamoxifen.

long as the mode of action of a pharmacological agent is appreciated, the DMBA-induced rat mammary carcinoma model remains a useful system for testing therapeutic regimens that might have application in the clinic.

III. A MODEL FOR ADJUVANT THERAPY

Although the simultaneous administration of tamoxifen and DMBA inhibits the initiation of mammary cancer (Jordan, 1974, 1976a), this is a poor model for evaluating the likelihood that antioestrogens will destroy micrometastases during the postmastectomy period. Since prolactin-stimulated DNA synthesis may be important for DMBA-induced carcinogenesis (Nagasawa *et al.*, 1976) and tamoxifen can inhibit oestrogen-stimulated prolactin release (Jordan *et al.*, 1975) and oestrogen-stimulated cell division (Jordan and Dix, 1979), then it is possible that tamoxifen can inhibit the fundamental process of carcinogenesis. In a revised model for adjuvant therapy, at least 28 days are allowed for DMBA to produce the carcinogenic insult before the drug regimen is administered to eradicate the microfoci of deranged cells.

A. Comparison of Tamoxifen and Monohydroxytamoxifen

To compare the antitumour properties of tamoxifen and monohydroxytamoxifen, we used smaller doses of monohydroxytamoxifen because of its greater antioestrogenic potency (Jordan *et al.*, 1977). Compounds were administered 5 days each week for 4 weeks between 30 and 60 days after DMBA administration. In contrast to its apparent weaker antioestrogenic potency, tamoxifen was a much more potent antitumour agent when considering both the numbers of animals remaining tumour-free (Fig. 5) and numbers of tumours formed (Fig. 6). However, the antitumour effect of both agents was only transient and by 200 days nearly all animals had tumours.

Two conclusions can be made from this result: antioestrogenic potency is not related to antitumour activity in this model and short courses of therapy are unable to destroy microfoci of deranged cells by direct action. The tumours that do appear after antioestrogen therapy are sensitive to ovariectomy (Jordan and Allen, 1980).

With regard to the inability of short-term antioestrogen therapy to eradicate tumour foci, it is possible that the one month allowed for DMBA to produce the cellular insult is too long and the cells are biologically too well established. However, earlier therapy with tamoxifen (as early as 5 days after DMBA) using the same treatment regimen has proved to be ineffective (Jordan *et al.*, 1979a).

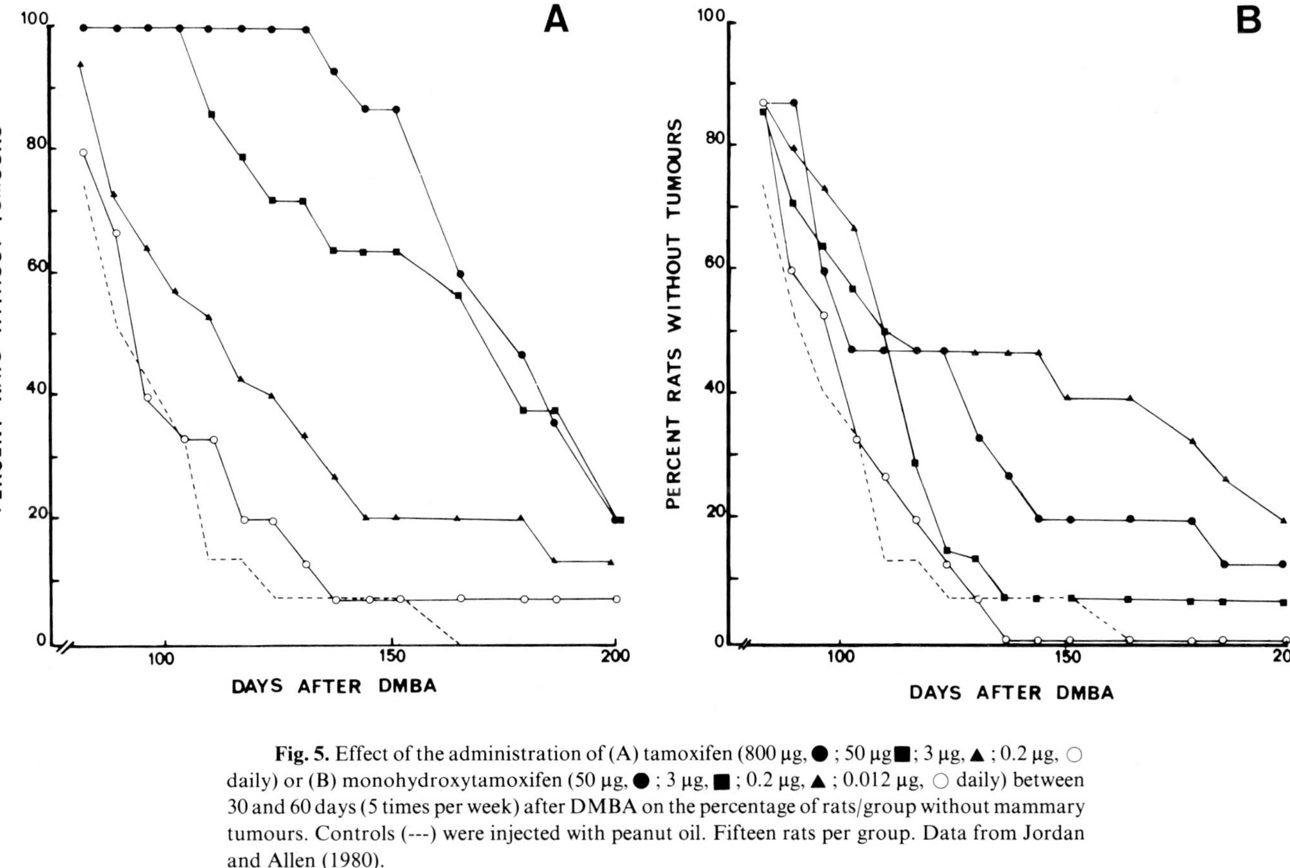

Fig. 5. Effect of the administration of (A) tamoxifen (800 µg, ●; 50 µg ■; 3 µg, ▲; 0.2 µg, ○ daily) or (B) monohydroxytamoxifen (50 µg, ●; 3 µg, ■; 0.2 µg, ▲; 0.012 µg, ○ daily) between 30 and 60 days (5 times per week) after DMBA on the percentage of rats/group without mammary tumours. Controls (---) were injected with peanut oil. Fifteen rats per group. Data from Jordan and Allen (1980).

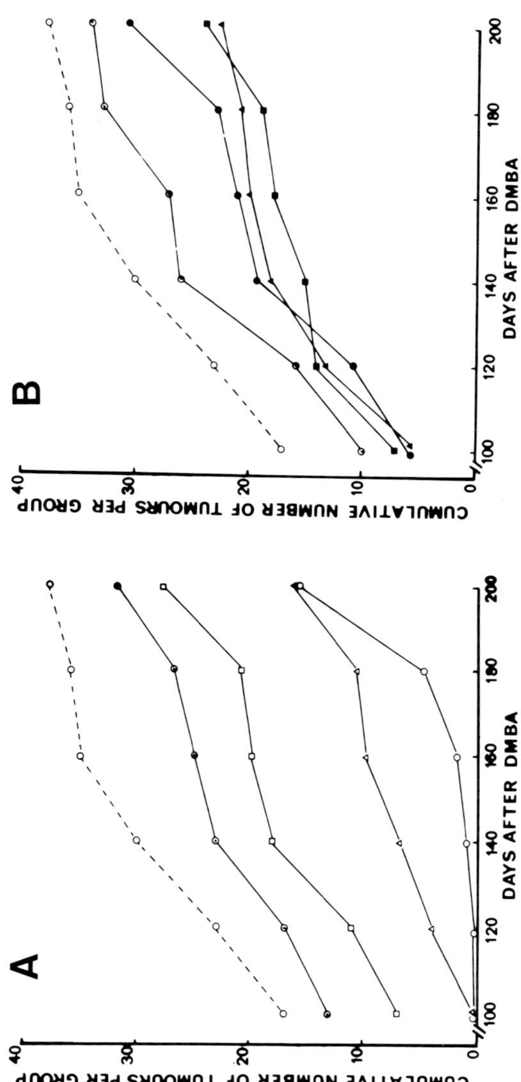

Fig. 6. Cumulative number of mammary tumours after the administration of (A) tamoxifen (800 µg, ○; 50 µg, △; 3 µg, □; 0.2 µg, ⊙ daily) or (B) monohydroxytamoxifen (50 µg, ▲; 3 µg, ●; 0.2 µg, ■; 0.12 µg ⊙ daily) between 30 and 60 days after DMBA. Controls (○ -- ○) received injections of peanut oil alone. Fifteen rats per group. Data from Jordan and Allen (1980).

B. Continuous Antioestrogen Therapy and Ovariectomy

The inability of short courses of tamoxifen and monohydroxytamoxifen to cure animals completely by destroying the microfoci of deranged cells is in complete contrast to the effects of antioestrogens on the survival of human breast cancer cells maintained in long term tissue culture (Lippman and Bolan, 1975). Unlike the situation *in vitro* with a possibly unrepresentative breast cancer cell line, the cancer cells in the rat model seem to be protected from complete destruction. This may be related to observations on the rat uterus, where tamoxifen and monohydroxytamoxifen inhibit cell division rather than elicit a specific cytotoxic action (Jordan and Dix, 1979). It appears, therefore, that the effects of antioestrogens are readily reversible and tumour development is only inhibited in the presence of the drug.

To test this theory, continuous tamoxifen therapy was started 30 days after DMBA and compared with ovariectomy 30 days after DMBA. As previously found (Dao, 1962) ovariectomy retarded tumour appearance (Fig. 7a) but approximately 50% of animals had tumours by 200 days. By comparison, tamoxifen therapy maintained 90% of animals tumour-free throughout the experiment. However, the reduction in the number of tumours when tamoxifen was combined with ovariectomy (Fig. 7b) suggests that the tumours that appear in the ovariectomized group are hormone-dependent. Since it is known that adrenal glands produce steroids (Shaikh and Shaikh, 1975) which can be converted in peripheral tissues to oestrogen (Naftolin *et al.*, 1972; Schindler *et al.*, 1972) it may be these steroids which support the development of tumours in ovariectomized rats. The effectiveness of tamoxifen in the ovariectomized rat could therefore be explained by its ability to inhibit the action of peripherally synthesized oestrogens.

The suggestion that tumour development is suppressed in the continued presence of antioestrogens is supported by the finding that daily administration of monohydroxytamoxifen inhibited tumour development (Fig. 8). It was interesting to find that one hormone-dependent tumour continued to grow during antioestrogen therapy; however, this may be due to inadequate dosage.

In general it is apparent that continued antioestrogen therapy is essential to the suppression of tumour development, and a combination of ovariectomy and antioestrogen therapy is the most effective method of controlling the appearance of overt tumours.

C. Clinical Implications

It has been found that the oestrogen receptor status of the primary tumour is a useful prognostic factor for predicting whether a breast tumour

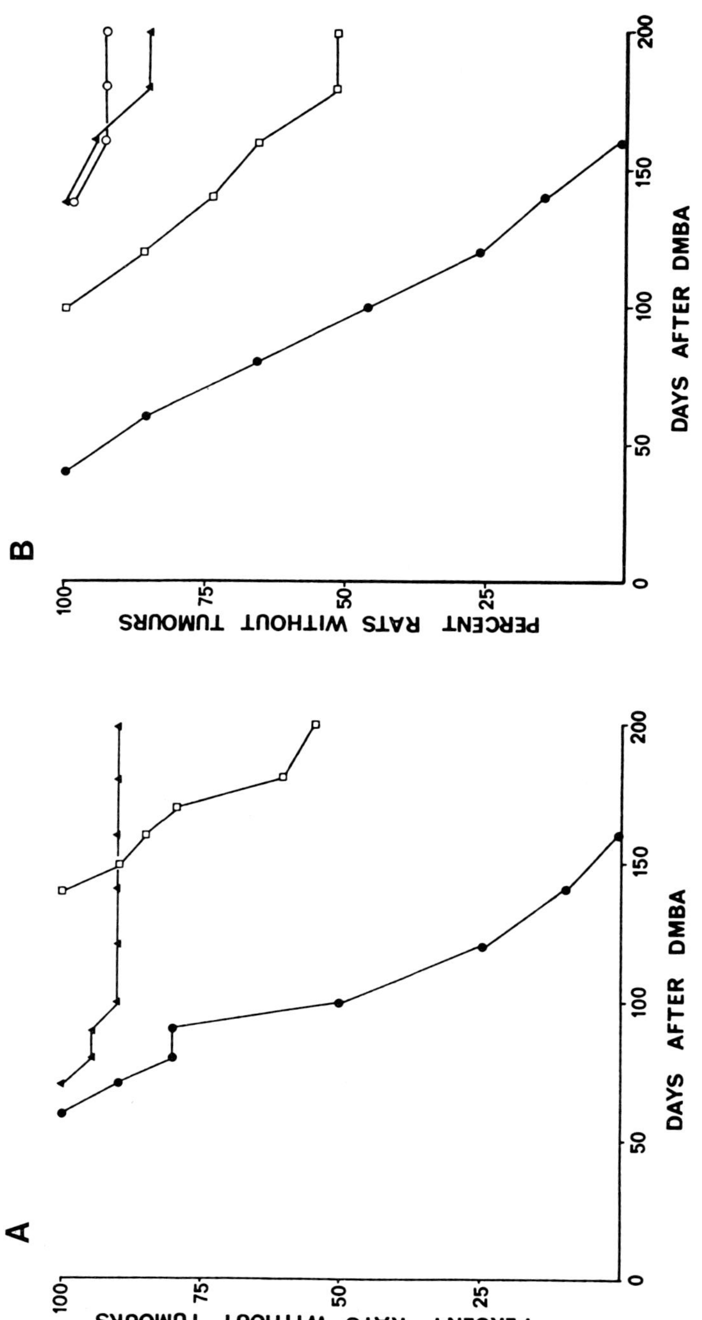

Fig. 7. Effect of (A) tamoxifen (▲, 50 µg daily 5 times per week starting 30 days after DMBA) and ovariectomy (□) 30 days after DMBA and (B) tamoxifen (▲, 50 µg daily 5 times per week starting 30 days after DMBA), ovariectomy (□) 30 days after DMBA and tamoxifen and ovariectomy (○), on the percentage of rats without tumours. Controls (●) were treated daily with peanut oil. Twenty rats per group.

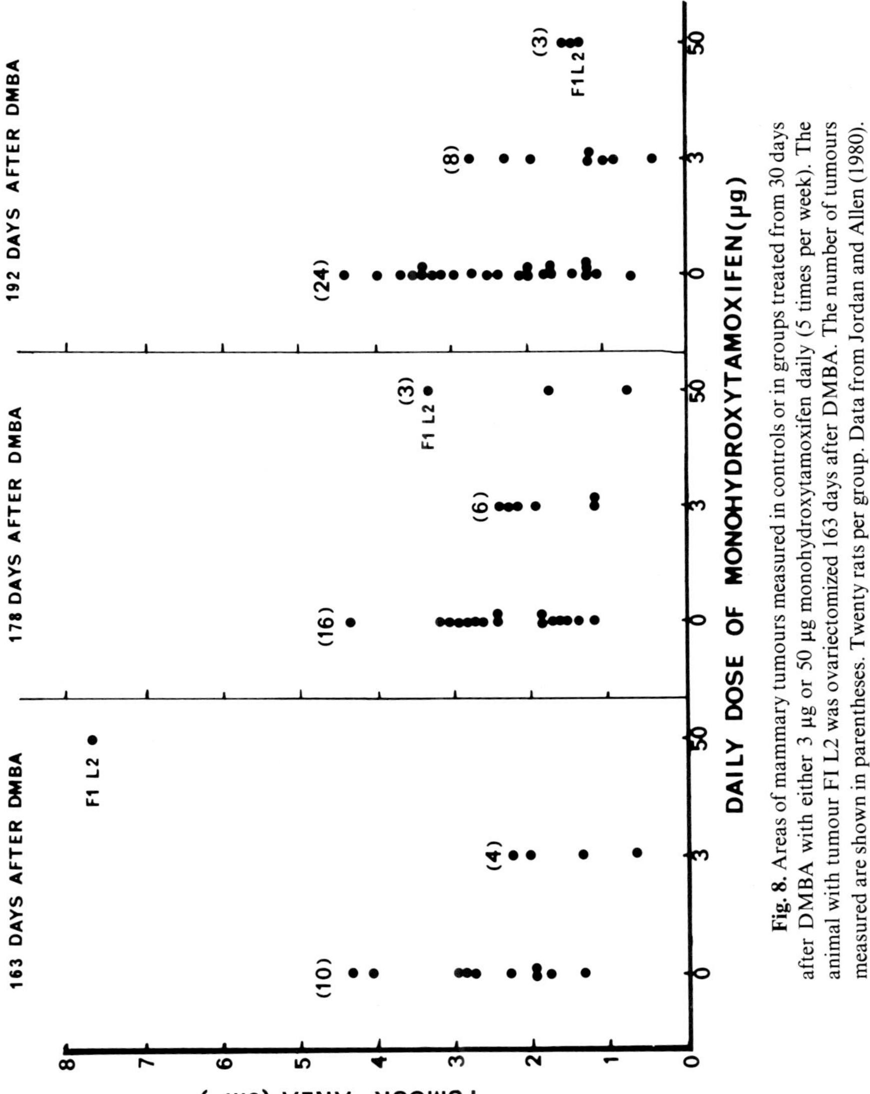

Fig. 8. Areas of mammary tumours measured in controls or in groups treated from 30 days after DMBA with either 3 μg or 50 μg monohydroxytamoxifen daily (5 times per week). The animal with tumour FI L2 was ovariectomized 163 days after DMBA. The number of tumours measured are shown in parentheses. Twenty rats per group. Data from Jordan and Allen (1980).

will recur early or late (Knight *et al.*, 1977; Maynard *et al.*, 1978). Primary tumours that are oestrogen receptor poor recur earlier than oestrogen receptor rich tumours. Many large national and international clinical trials are using tamoxifen, alone or in combination with other cytotoxic agents, as an adjuvant to surgery in breast cancer. However, whether oestrogen receptor rich tumours will be controlled more effectively than oestrogen receptor poor tumours has not been established. If oestrogen receptor rich tumours respond to tamoxifen, then it might be possible to control tumour recurrence in a highly selected sub-population of patients.

How long therapy should be continued, however, is the question that now arises. Although there are many fundamental biological differences between the DMBA-induced rat mammary carcinoma model and human breast cancer, the principles for the control of hormone-dependent growth may be similar. As suggested by the present experiments, a short course of tamoxifen therapy (1 month in a rat with a 3 year life span) does not destroy all the hormone-dependent tumour cells, and only longer treatment regimens are effective. Whether human breast cancer cells are protected from antioestrogen action *in vivo* must await the completion of the clinical trials using the present one or two year treatment regimens, but clearly longer treatment regimens may be necessary if the disease-free interval is to be markedly lengthened.

REFERENCES

Arbogast, L. Y., and DeSombre, E. R. (1975). *J. Natl Cancer Inst.* **54**, 483–485.

Asselin, J., Labrie, F., Kelly, P. A., Philibert, D., and Raynaud, J. P. (1976). *Steroids* **27**, 395–404.

Asselin, J., Kelly, P. A., Caron, M. G., and Labrie, F. (1977). *Endocrinology* **101**, 666–671.

Boylan, E. S., and Wittliff, J. L. (1975). *Cancer Res.* **35**, 506–511.

Brodie, A. M. H., Marsh, D., and Brodie, H. T. (1979). *J. Steroid Biochem.* **10**, 423–429.

Callantine, M. R., Humphrey, R. R., Lee, S. L., Windsor, B. L., Schottin, N. H., and O'Brien, O. P. (1966). *Endocrinology* **79**, 153–169.

Cassell, E. E., Meites, J., and Welsch, C. W. (1971). *Cancer Res.* **31**, 1051–1053.

Chen, C. L., and Meites, J. (1970). *Endocrinology* **86**, 503–505.

Costlow, M. E., Buschow, R. A., and McGuire, W. L. (1976). *Cancer Res.* **36**, 3324–3329.

Danguy, A., Legros, N., Heuson-Stiennon, J. A., Pasteels, J. L., Atassi, G., and Heuson, J. C. (1977). *Eur. J. Cancer* **13**, 1089–1094.

Dao, T. L. (1962). *Cancer Res.* **22**, 973–981.

DeSombre, E. R., and Arbogast, L. Y. (1974). *Cancer Res.* **34**, 1971–1976.

DeSombre, E. R., Kledzik, G., Marshall, S., and Meites, J. (1976). *Cancer Res.* **36**, 354–358.

Döhler, K. D., von zur Mühlen, A., and Döhler, U. (1977). *IRCS Med. Sci.* **5**, 185.

Gibson, S. L., and Hilf, R. (1976). *Cancer Res.* **36**, 3736–3741.

Golder, M. P., Phillips, M. E. A., Fahmy, D. R., Preece, P. E., Jones, V., Henk, J. M., and Griffiths, K. (1976). *Eur. J. Cancer* **12**, 719–723.

Goral, J. E., and Wittliff, J. L. (1976). *Cancer Res.* **36**, 1886–1893.

Gorski, J., Toft, D. O., Shyamala, G., Smith, D., and Notides, A. (1968). *Recent Progr. Horm. Res.* **24**, 45–80.
Griswold, D. P., and Green, C. H. (1970). *Cancer Res.* **30**, 819–826.
Griswold, D. P., Skipper, H. E., Laster, W. R., Wilcox, W. E., and Schabel, F. M. (1966). *Cancer Res.* **26**, 2169–2180.
Groom, G. V., and Griffiths, K. (1976). *J. Endocr.* **70**, 421–428.
Heuson, J. C., and Legros, N. (1972). *Cancer Res.* **32**, 226–232.
Heuson, J. C., Waelbroeck von Gaver, C., and Legros, N. (1970). *Eur. J. Cancer* **6**, 353–356.
Heuson, J. C., Waelbroeck, C., Legros, N., Gallez, G., Robyn, C., and L'Hermite, M. (1971). *Gynec. Invest.* **2**, 130–137.
Heuson, J. C., Legros, N., and Heinmann, R. (1972). *Cancer Res.* **32**, 233–238.
Holdaway, I. M., and Friesen, H. G. (1976). *Cancer Res.* **36**, 1562–1567.
Horn, H., Erlichman, I., and Levij, I. S. (1976). *Br. J. Cancer* **33**, 336–341.
Horwitz, K. B., and McGuire, W. L. (1977). *Cancer Res.* **37**, 1733–1738.
Huggins, C., and Yang, N. C. (1962). *Science* **137**, 257–262.
Huggins, C., Briziarelli, G., and Sutton, H. (1959). *J. Exp. Med.* **109**, 25–41.
Huggins, C., Grand, L. C., and Brillantes, F. P. (1961). *Nature* **189**, 204–207.
Jabara, A. G. (1967). *Br. J. Cancer* **21**, 418–429.
Jabara, A. G., and Harcourt, A. G. (1970). *Pathology* **2**, 115–123.
Jabara, A. G., and Harcourt, A. G. (1971). *Pathology* **3**, 209–214.
Jensen, E. V., and DeSombre, E. R. (1973). *Science* **182**, 126–134.
Jordan, V. C. (1974). *J. Steroid. Biochem.* **5**, 354.
Jordan, V. C. (1976a). *Eur. J. Cancer* **12**, 419–424.
Jordan, V. C. (1976b). *Cancer Treat. Rep.* **60**, 1409–1419.
Jordan, V. C., and Allen, K. E. (1980). *Eur. J. Cancer* **16**, 239–252.
Jordan, V. C., and Dix, C. J. (1979). *J. Steroid Biochem.* **11**, 285–291.
Jordan, V. C., and Dowse, L. J. (1976). *J. Endocr.* **68**, 297–303.
Jordan, V. C., and Jaspan, T. (1976). *J. Endocr.* **68**, 453–460.
Jordan, V. C., and Koerner, S. (1975). *Eur. J. Cancer* **11**, 205–206.
Jordan, V. C., and Koerner, S. (1976). *J. Endocr.* **68**, 305–311.
Jordan, V. C., Koerner, S., and Robinson, C. (1975). *J. Endocr.* **65**, 151–152.
Jordan, V. C., Collins, M. M., Rowsby, L., and Prestwich, G. (1977). *J. Endocr.* **75**, 305–316.
Jordan, V. C., Dix, C. J., and Allen, K. E. (1979a). *In* "Adjuvant Therapy of Cancer II" (S. E. Jones and S. E. Salmon, eds), pp. 19–26. Grune and Stratton. New York.
Jordan, V. C., Dixon, B., Prestwich, G., and Furr, B. J. A. (1979b). *Eur. J. Cancer* **15**, 755–761.
Jordan, V. C., Naylor, K. E., Dix, C. J., and Prestwich, G. (1980). *In* "Recent Results in Cancer Research" (B. Henningsen, F. Linder, and C. Steichele, eds), Vol. 71, pp. 30–44. Springer-Verlag, Berlin.
Kelly, P. A., Bradley, C., Shiu, R. P. C., Meites, J., and Friesen, H. G. (1974). *Proc. Soc. Exptl. Biol. Med.* **146**, 816–819.
King, R. J. B., Gordon, J., and Steggles, A. W. (1969). *Biochem. J.* **114**, 649–657.
Kledzik, G. S., Bradley, C. J., Marshall, S., Campbell, G. A., and Meites, J. (1976). *Cancer Res.* **36**, 3265–3268.
Knight, W. A., Livingston, R. B., Gregory, E. J., and McGuire, W. L. (1977). *Cancer Res.* **37**, 4669–4671.
Labhsetwar, A. P. (1970a). *Endocrinology* **87**, 542–551.
Labhsetwar, A. P. (1970b). *J. Endocr.* **47**, 481–493.
Labhsetwar, A. P. (1972). *Endocrinology* **90**, 941–946.
Leclercq, G., and Heuson, J. C. (1973). *Eur. J. Cancer* **9**, 675–680.
Lee, C., and Oyasu, R. (1974). *J. Natl Cancer Inst.* **52**, 283–284.

Leung, B. S., Sasaki, G. H., and Leung, J. S. (1975). *Cancer Res.* **35**, 621–627.
Levin, J. M., Goldman, A. S., Rosato, F. E., and Rosato, E. E. (1976). *Cancer* **38**, 56–61.
Lippman, M. E., and Bolan, G. (1975). *Nature* **256**, 592–593.
Manni, A., Trujillo, J. E., and Pearson, O. H. (1977). *Cancer Res.* **37**, 1216–1219.
Masala, A., Delitala, G., LoDico, G., Stopelli, I., Alagra, S., and Devilla, L. (1978). *Br. J. Obstet. Gynaecol.* **85**, 134–137.
Maynard, P. V., Blamey, R. W., Elston, C. W., and Griffiths, K. (1978). *Cancer Res.* **38**, 4292–4295.
McGuire, W. L., and Julian, J. A. (1971). *Cancer Res.* **31**, 1440–1445.
Meites, J., Cassell, E., and Clark, J. (1971). *Proc. Soc. Exptl. Biol. Med.* **137**, 1225–1227.
Mobbs, B. G. (1966). *J. Endocr.* **36**, 409–414.
Mobbs, B. G., and Johnson, I. E. (1974). *Eur. J. Cancer* **10**, 757–763.
Naftolin, F., Ryan, K. J., and Petro, Z. (1972). *Endocrinology* **90**, 295–298.
Nagasawa, H., and Meites, J. (1970). *Proc. Soc. Exptl. Biol. Med.* **135**, 469–472.
Nagasawa, H., Yanai, R., and Taniguchi, H. (1976). *Cancer Res.* **36**, 2223–2226.
Nicholson, R. I. (1979). *Reviews on Endocrine-Related Cancer* **3**, 31–39.
Nicholson, R. I., and Golder, M. P. (1975). *Eur. J. Cancer* **11**, 571–579.
Nicholson, R. I., and Maynard, P. V. (1979). *Br. J. Cancer* **39**, 268–273.
Nicholson, R. I., Golder, M. P., Davis, P., and Griffiths, K. (1976). *Eur. J. Cancer* **12**, 711–717.
Nicholson, R. I., Davis, P., and Griffiths, K. (1977a). *Eur. J. Cancer* **13**, 201–208.
Nicholson, R. I., Davis, P., and Griffiths, K. (1977b). *J. Endocr.* **73**, 135–142.
Nicholson, R. I., Syne, J. S., Daniel, C. P., and Griffiths, K. (1979). *Eur. J. Cancer* **15**, 317–329.
Nomura, Y., Abe, Y., and Inokuchi, K. (1974). *Gann* **65**, 523–528.
Pasteels, J. L., Heuson, J. C., Heuson-Stiennon, J., and Legros, N. (1976). *Cancer Res.* **36**, 2162–2170.
Powell-Jones, W., Jenner, D. A., Blamey, R. W., Davis, P., and Griffiths, K. (1975). *Biochem. J.* **150**, 71–75.
Sasaki, G. H., and Leung, B. S. (1975). *Cancer* **35**, 645–651.
Schindler, A. E., Ebert, A., and Friedrich, E. (1972). *J. Clin. Endocr. Metab.* **35**, 627–630.
Schmidt-Ruppin, K. H., Meisels, A., Schott, E., Storni, A., and Schieweck, K. (1973). *Experientia* **29**, 823–825.
Schulz, K. D., Haselmayer, B., and Hölzel, F. (1971). *In* "Basic Actions of Sex Steroids on Target Organs" (P. O. Hubinont, F. Leroy and P. Galand, eds), pp. 274–299. Karger, Basle.
Shaikh, A. A., and Shaikh, S. A. (1975). *Endocrinology* **96**, 37–44.
Sinha, S., Cooper, D., and Dao, T. L. (1973). *Cancer Res.* **33**, 411–414.
Smith, R. D., Hilf, R., and Senior, A. E. (1977). *Cancer Res.* **37**, 4070–4074.
Sterental, A., Dominguez, J. M., Weissman, C., and Pearson, O. H. (1963). *Cancer Res.* **23**, 481–484.
Teller, M. N., Stock, C. C., and Bowie, M. (1966a). *Cancer Res.* **26**, 2329–2333.
Teller, M. N., Stock, C. C., Stohr, G., Merker, P. C., Kaufman, R. J., Escher, G. C. and Bowie, M. (1966b). *Cancer Res.* **26**, 245–252.
Terenius, L. (1971). *Eur. J. Cancer* **7**, 57–64.
Terenius, L. (1973). *Eur. J. Cancer* **9**, 291–294.
Tsai, T. L. S., and Katzenellenbogen, B. S. (1977). *Cancer Res.* **37**, 1537–1543.
Turkington, R. W. (1974). *Cancer Res.* **34**, 658–763.
Vignon, F., and Rochefort, H. (1976). *Endocrinology* **98**, 722–729.
Watson, J., and Alam, M. (1976). *Contraception* **13**, 101–107.
Watson, J., and Howson, J. W. H. (1977). *J. Reprod. Fert.* **49**, 375–380.
Watson, J., Anderson, F. B., Alam, M., O'Grady, J. E., and Heald, P. J. (1975). *J. Endocr.* **65**, 7–17.

Willis, K. J., London, D. R., Ward, H. W. C., Butt, W. R., Lynch, S. S., and Rudd, B. T. (1977). *Br. Med. J.* **1**, 425–428.

Yokoyama, A., Tomogane, H., and Ota, K. (1973). *Acta Endocr.* **74**, 769–774.

17

Biochemical Basis of Tamoxifen Action in Hormone-Dependent Breast Cancer

R. I. NICHOLSON, N. M. BORTHWICK, C. P. DANIEL, J. S. SYNE AND P. DAVIES

I. INTRODUCTION

The low incidence of side effects associated with the long-term use of the non-steroidal antioestrogen tamoxifen (trans-1-(4-β-dimethylamino-ethoxyphenyl)1,2-diphenylbut-1-ene; "Nolvadex") has led to its increased employment in the therapy of advanced breast cancer where, like other forms of endocrine therapy, it produces objective clinical responses in approximately 20–40 % of patients (Mouridsen *et al.*, 1978) with an average remission interval of about twelve months (Ward, 1973). Regressions occur primarily in those patients whose secondary tumours contain oestrogen receptor proteins; tumours lacking oestrogen receptors have a much lower response rate to the drug (Mouridsen *et al.*, 1978). In addition, the lack of toxicity of tamoxifen has more recently led to its use in the adjuvant treatment of breast cancer after mastectomy. Preliminary results indicate that postmenopausal patients with oestrogen receptor positive tumours may derive some benefit from this treatment regime (Palshof *et al.*, 1980).

NON-STEROIDAL ANTIOESTROGENS
ISBN 0 12 677880 9

The clinical efficacy of tamoxifen and its widespread use in the management of breast cancer has inspired a marked interest in its mode of action and necessitated a wider understanding of its biochemistry and pharmacokinetics. Some novel data concerning these aspects are presented in this chapter.

II. PHARMACOLOGY OF TAMOXIFEN

As an antioestrogen, tamoxifen must at least in part directly oppose the trophic actions of oestrogens. This aspect of its mode of action is illustrated in Figure 1 by the effect of the drug alone and in combination with oestradiol on the weight of the uterus in ovariectomized rats. It is quite clear that the daily administration of high doses of tamoxifen for 4 days decreased the tissue response to oestradiol and eventually reduced uterine weights to those observed in animals treated with tamoxifen alone. Tamoxifen also possesses weak oestrogenic activity. At 300 μg/rat/day it was approximately 30% as effective as oestradiol (0.5 μg/rat/day) in producing a uterotrophic response. Larger doses of tamoxifen (900 μg or 9 mg/rat/day) did not induce any appreciable further increase in uterine weights. These observations regarding the long-term action of tamoxifen are also evident with respect to the release of luteinizing hormone from the pituitary gland of ovariectomized animals (Nicholson, 1979a) and also on a number of biochemical end-points of oestrogen action measured in DMBA-induced mammary tumours prior to regression (Nicholson *et al.*, 1978; Nicholson, 1979b; Nicholson and Griffiths, 1980). Similarly, in women, experimental data are consistent with tamoxifen antagonizing the actions of oestrogens, although showing a degree of oestrogen-like activity in some tissues (Furr *et al.*, 1979).

It is also of interest that within 24 hours of administration tamoxifen promotes a whole series of biological responses which are indistinguishable from those produced after a single injection of oestradiol. These include increased uterine weights and macromolecular synthesis, including that of the production of the cytoplasmic progesterone receptor (Fig. 2). Furthermore, unlike the effects of the drug which occur after multiple injections (Fig. 1), no antagonism between tamoxifen and oestradiol was evident at this early time point (Fig. 2). Other authors have made similar observations about tamoxifen (Cowan and Leake, 1979) and other non-steroidal antioestrogens (Clark *et al.*, 1974).

These studies suggest that the antagonistic properties of tamoxifen in certain oestrogen-responsive tissues of the rat, and possibly human beings, are due to the inability of the drug to promote a full, long-term oestrogenic response. In tissues which require a full oestrogenic stimulus for their continued growth and function, an interference with this stimulus by the antioestrogen would cause regression in oestrogen-primed tissue. Moreover, in the case of breast cancer, where a degree of oestrogen-dependence has been implicated in the growth of both human (Stoll, 1969) and rat (Dao and Sinha, 1972) mammary tumours, the substitution of a partial oestrogenic stimulus by

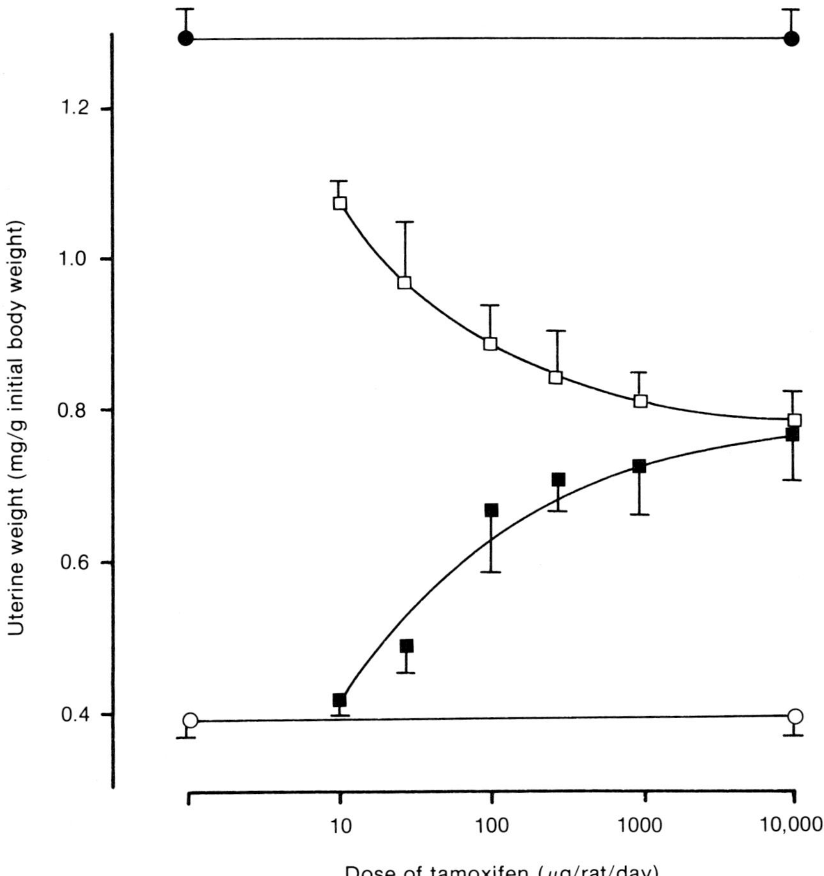

Fig. 1. Effect of tamoxifen and oestradiol on uterine weights in ovariectomized rats. Three-week ovariectomized animals were injected daily (subcutaneously, s.c.) with various doses of tamoxifen (10 μg to 9 mg/day) alone and in combination with oestradiol benzoate (0.5 μg/day) for 4 days. Uterine wet weight is expressed in relation to total body weight and each point represents the mean ± S.D. of six uteri. Control, sesame oil injected animals (○), oestradiol (●), tamoxifen (■), tamoxifen plus oestradiol (□).

the antioestrogen might be conducive to tumour remission. However, the early oestrogen-like properties of tamoxifen, equivalent to those produced by oestradiol (Fig. 2), do not support a model for the mode of action of the drug in which its antioestrogenic and antitumour properties reside solely in a weak oestrogenic activity. Further information regarding this phenomenon was sought originally in an examination of the interaction of the drug with oestrogen receptor proteins.

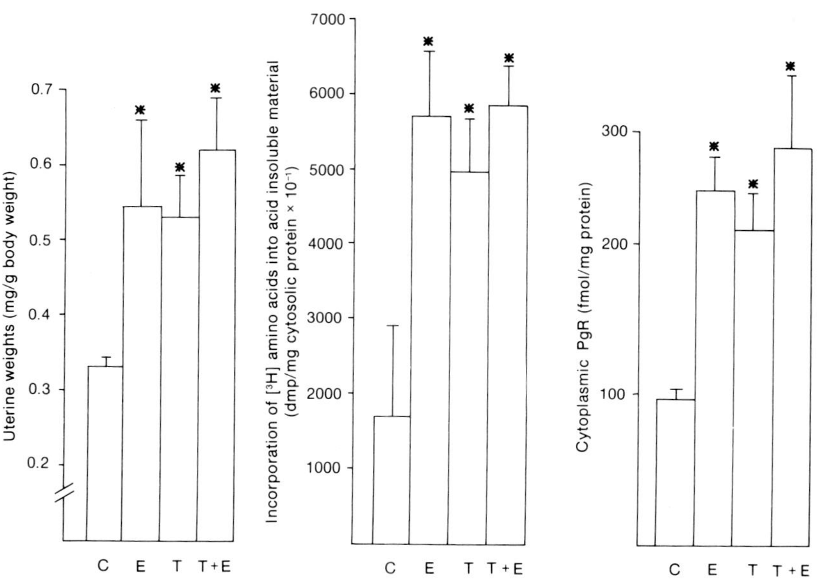

Fig. 2. Response of the rat uterus to tamoxifen and oestradiol. Three-week ovariectomized animals were given a single (s.c.) injection of either vehicle (C, sesame oil, 100 μl,) oestradiol (E, 0.5 μg), tamoxifen (T, 300 μg) or tamoxifen plus oestradiol (T + E). After 24 hours the uterus was ligated under sagatal anaesthesia and 5 μCi of [^{3}H]amino acids in 50 μl saline (0.16 M) introduced directly into the lumen at each uterine horn 30 minutes prior to sacrifice. On removal, uteri were blotted dry, weighed and washed thoroughly in saline. The uteri from 5 animals from each experimental group were homogenized separately in 1 ml 0.05 mM EDTA solution, pH 8.0 and centrifuged at 105,000 g for one hour. Aliquots of the supernatant fraction (cytosol) were added to two volumes 10% (w/v) TCA at 4°C and allowed to flocculate for 15 minutes at this temperature. Precipitates were washed twice with 5% (w/v) TCA, the final pellets redissolved in 0.5 M NaOH and radioactivity counted. Proteins were determined by the method of Lowry *et al.* (1951). Cytoplasmic progesterone receptor (PgR) levels were measured in uteri from age and treatment matched animals as described by Davies *et al.* (1979). Values are the mean ± S.D. of 5 uteri per group. *$p < 0.05$.

III. INTERACTION OF TAMOXIFEN WITH THE OESTROGEN RECEPTOR

There is now convincing evidence to suggest that, at the molecular level, the phenotypic response of breast tumour cells to oestrogens may be related to the presence of cytoplasmic receptor proteins which bind oestradiol with selective high affinity (Jensen *et al.*, 1974). The binding of the hormone is thought to aid the transfer of the receptor to, or its retention within, the nucleus, enhancing the transcription of the DNA template by RNA and DNA polymerases and thereby resulting in the production of components essential for continued cell growth and function. Based on this model system for the action of oestradiol in breast tumour tissue, any drug which interferes with the ability of the tissue, or more specifically the receptor protein, to bind the oestrogen or process its message is theoretically capable of causing tumour regression and ultimately cell death.

Sucrose density gradient analysis has shown that tamoxifen can compete with oestradiol for its specific 4 or 8S binding protein (Jordan, 1975; Jordan and Koerner, 1975; Powell-Jones *et al.*, 1975; Nicholson *et al.*, 1978). In rodents the drug associated with approximately the same number of binding sites as oestradiol does, but with only 5–10% of its affinity (Capony and Rochefort, 1978; Nicholson *et al.*, 1978, 1979a). Since the receptor proteins for tamoxifen and oestradiol are commonly precipitated by protamine sulphate (Capony and Rochefort, 1978; Nicholson *et al.*, 1979a) and ammonium sulphate (Capony and Rochefort, 1978) and show a similar specificity of binding (Capony and Rochefort, 1978; Nicholson *et al.*, 1978; 1979a), the experimental data provide good evidence of a common binding protein, and possibly of a common binding site for both oestradiol and tamoxifen on the oestrogen receptor protein.

Tamoxifen, like oestradiol, is also capable of translocating the receptor to nuclei of both rat mammary tumours (Nicholson *et al.*, 1976; 1977a) and rat uteri (Jordan *et al.*, 1977a; Koseki *et al.*, 1977; Davies *et al.*, 1979). Moreover, tamoxifen as monitored by gas-chromatography-high resolution mass spectrometry, is present in human and rat plasma (Gaskell *et al.*, 1978; Daniel *et al.*, 1979; Nicholson, 1979a, 1979b) and also in rat mammary tumour tissue (Fig. 11, Section IV) during tamoxifen therapy, in approximately a 1000-fold molar excess over oestradiol, a situation that strongly favours the formation of the antioestrogen receptor complex as opposed to the oestrogen receptor complex (Nicholson, 1979b; 1981). Furthermore, there is now substantial evidence that the antagonistic properties of tamoxifen towards oestradiol reside in a competition between oestrogen and antioestrogen receptor complexes for a limited number of specific acceptor sites on chromatin (Jordan *et al.*, 1977a; Koseki *et al.*, 1977; Nicholson, 1979b; Nicholson and

Griffiths, 1980) and that the antioestrogenic and antitumour properties of the drug are manifest, at least in part, through the antioestrogen receptor complex (Nicholson and Griffiths, 1980). Unfortunately, no physical or chemical properties which characterize the overall activity of the tamoxifen receptor-complex or its binding to chromatin have, as yet, been identified (see Nicholson and Griffiths, 1980). However, useful information has been gained from studies into the effect of tamoxifen on RNA synthesis.

IV. COMPARATIVE EFFECTS OF TAMOXIFEN AND OESTRADIOL ON RNA SYNTHESIS

As stated earlier, it is now accepted that one of the first responses of oestrogen-dependent tissues to oestradiol is a rapid stimulation of RNA synthesis, resulting from transcription of the DNA template by RNA polymerases (Gorski, 1964; Hamilton, 1968). These enzymes catalyse the initiation, elongation and termination of polyribonucleotide chains employing ribonucleoside triphosphates as substrates. Eukaryotic cells contain several distinct classes of RNA polymerases: RNA polymerase I or A is normally found in nucleoli and is deemed responsible for ribosomal RNA (rRNA) synthesis; RNA polymerase II or B, and III or C are nucleoplasmic enzymes which are thought to synthesize heterogeneous nuclear RNA (HnRNA; precursor for messenger RNA) and 5S rRNA plus transfer RNA (tRNA), respectively (Chambon, 1975; Roeder, 1976). Increases in RNA synthesis in response to oestradiol are manifested by a transient rise in RNA polymerase II activity, which occurs within the first hour and is obligatory for the subsequent elevation of RNA polymerase I and a major prolonged enhancement of RNA polymerase II (Glasser *et al.*, 1972; Borthwick and Smellie, 1975). The stimulation of a second rise in RNA polymerase II and an elevated and sustained activity of RNA polymerase I appear essential for true oestrogen-dependent tissue growth (Hardin *et al.*, 1976). Increases in RNA polymerase III activity have recently been shown to parallel those for RNA polymerase I (Weil *et al.*, 1977).

Investigations using DMBA-induced rat mammary tumours, have shown that increases in RNA polymerase II activity resulting from the administration of tamoxifen, at a dose (100 μg/day) known to cause tumour regression (Nicholson and Golder, 1975), are qualitatively similar to those produced by oestradiol during the first peak of activity (0–60 min), and also during the early phase of the second peak (1–4 hours), although tamoxifen appears unable to maintain the secondary stimulation of the activity of this enzyme (Figs 3 and 4; Nicholson *et al.*, 1977b). The effects of tamoxifen on RNA polymerase I are, however, quantitatively inferior to those initiated by oestradiol. Identical findings have also been observed in uteri from ovariectomized rats, where tamoxifen induced early alterations in RNA polymerase II activity (2–4 hours), but without substantial effect on RNA polymerase I (Fig. 5; Davies *et al.*, 1979). Similarly, Kurl and Borthwick (1980) have demonstrated that tamoxifen, in comparison with oestradiol, is a poor inducer of immature rat uterine nuclear RNA polymerase I activity, although they reported substantial and maintained elevations in RNA polymerase II. The comparative effects of tamoxifen and oestradiol on RNA polymerase III are less easy to define due to appreciable variations in enzyme activity following the administration of oestradiol (Fig. 5). Nevertheless, it is clear that tamoxifen is unable to promote large alterations in the activity of this enzyme. Simultaneous administration of tamoxifen with oestradiol antagonizes the

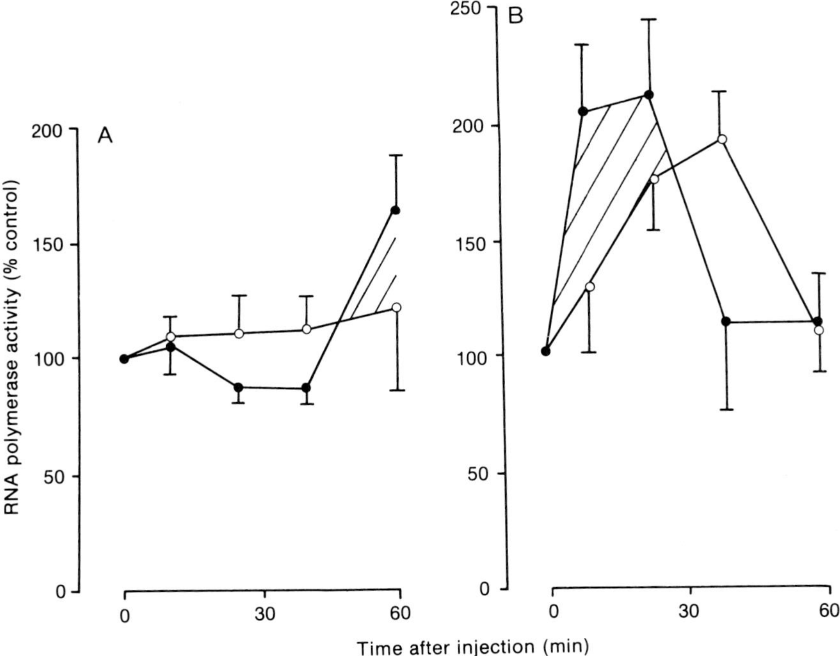

Fig. 3. Alterations in activity of nuclear RNA polymerases I (A) and II (B) in DMBA-induced mammary tumours resulting from administration of oestradiol or tamoxifen. Mammary tumour bearing rats were given a single dose of 5 μg oestradiol (●), 100 μg tamoxifen (○) or vehicle alone by intravenous injections, and biopsy samples were removed at various times up to 60 minutes after treatment. RNA polymerase I and II activity was determined as described by Nicholson *et al.* (1977b). Values are expressed as percentages of control activity (zero time) and are the mean ± S.E.M. of four or five animals.

action of oestradiol on RNA polymerases I and III, but is without considerable effect on the oestradiol-induced increase in RNA polymerase II (Fig. 6).

As stated earlier, tamoxifen possesses some uterotrophic activity in the ovariectomized rat, which is dose related after either 24 hours (Fig. 7A) or 96 hours (Fig. 1). It was of some interest therefore, to determine if any such relationship existed between this parameter and alterations in RNA polymerase activities. The data presented in Figures 7 and 8B indicate that tamoxifen, at dose levels (300 µg and 9 mg) which, at 24 hours, produced increases in uterine weights equivalent to those stimulated by oestradiol, also stimulated RNA polymerase II activity at 4 hours to a value which was indistinguishable from that brought about by oestradiol. Indeed, in addition

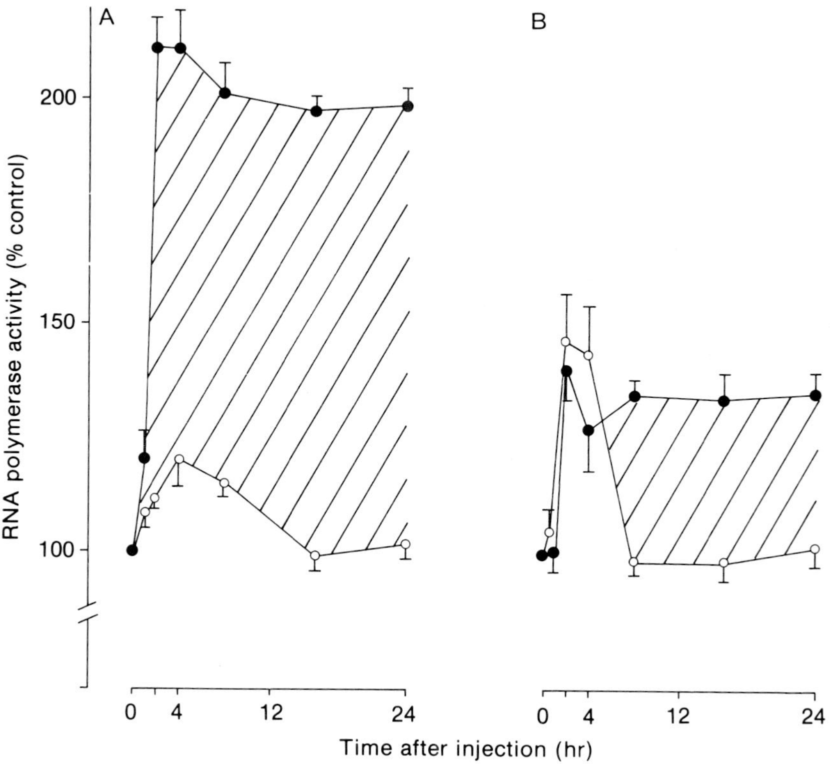

Fig. 4. Effect of oestradiol and tamoxifen on activities of nuclear RNA polymerases I (A) and II (B) in DMBA-induced mammary tumours of the rat. The experimental procedure was as described in the legend to Figure 3, except that biopsies were removed at times up to 24 hours.

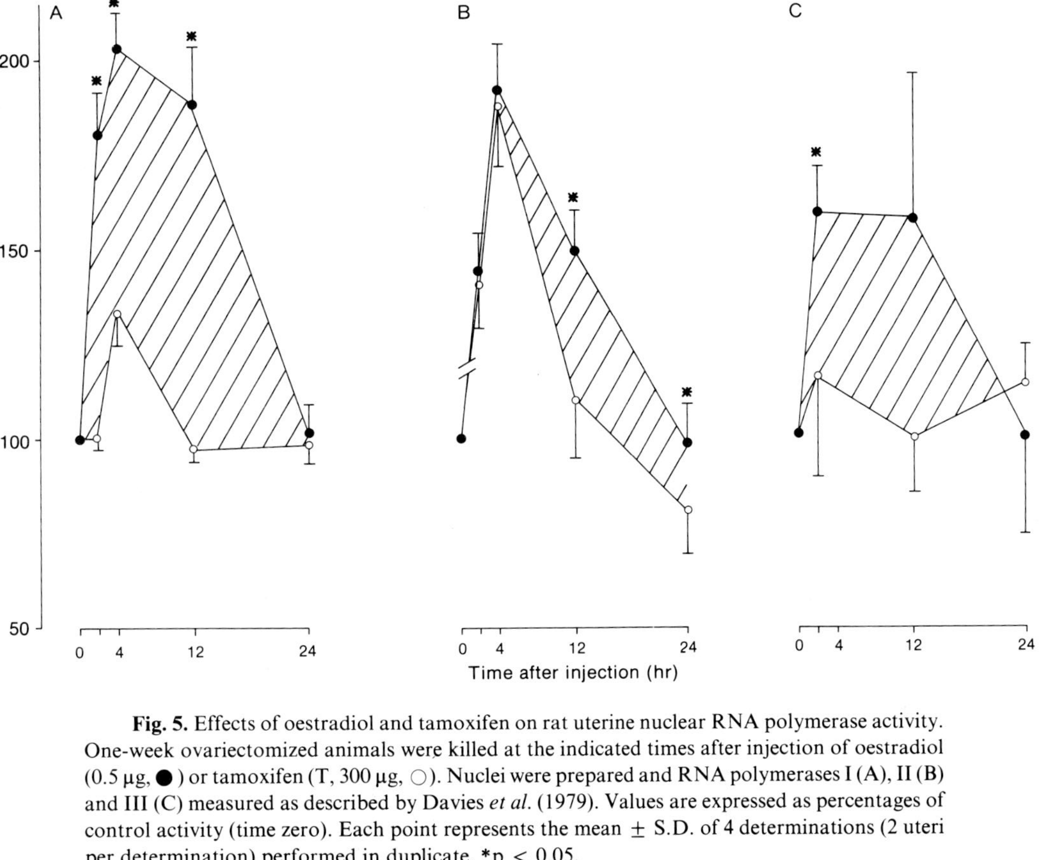

Fig. 5. Effects of oestradiol and tamoxifen on rat uterine nuclear RNA polymerase activity. One-week ovariectomized animals were killed at the indicated times after injection of oestradiol (0.5 μg, ●) or tamoxifen (T, 300 μg, ○). Nuclei were prepared and RNA polymerases I (A), II (B) and III (C) measured as described by Davies *et al.* (1979). Values are expressed as percentages of control activity (time zero). Each point represents the mean ± S.D. of 4 determinations (2 uteri per determination) performed in duplicate. *$p < 0.05$.

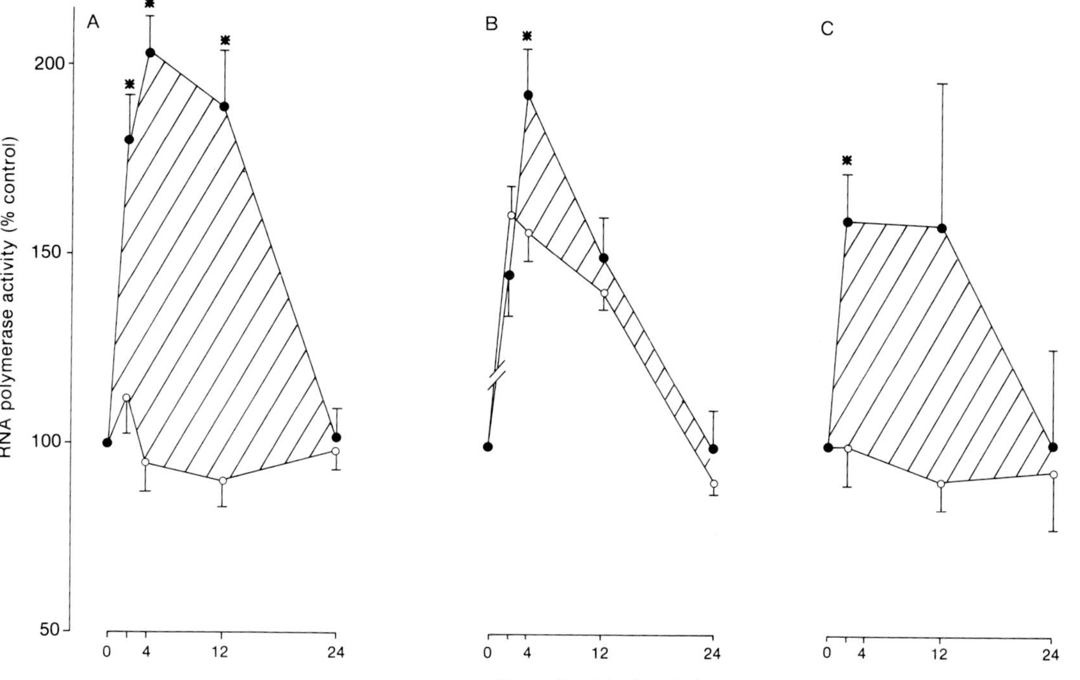

Fig. 6. Effect of oestradiol and oestradiol in combination with tamoxifen on rat uterine nuclear RNA polymerase I (A), II (B) and III (C) activity. Details are essentially as described for Figure 5. 0.5 μg oestradiol (●), 0.5 μg oestradiol plus tamoxifen 300μg (○).

to its stimulatory effect on RNA polymerase II at 4 hours, a single injection of 9 mg of tamoxifen produced an equivalent response to oestradiol at 12 hours. Furthermore, the stimulation of RNA polymerase II by tamoxifen also appears to produce functional mRNA, since a dose-related increase in the level of cytoplasmic progesterone receptor was observed at 12 hours (Fig. 7B). The administration of 30 μg tamoxifen was without substantial effect on either RNA polymerase II activity (at 4 or 12 hours), uterine weights (24 hours) or cytoplasmic progesterone receptor levels (12 hours).

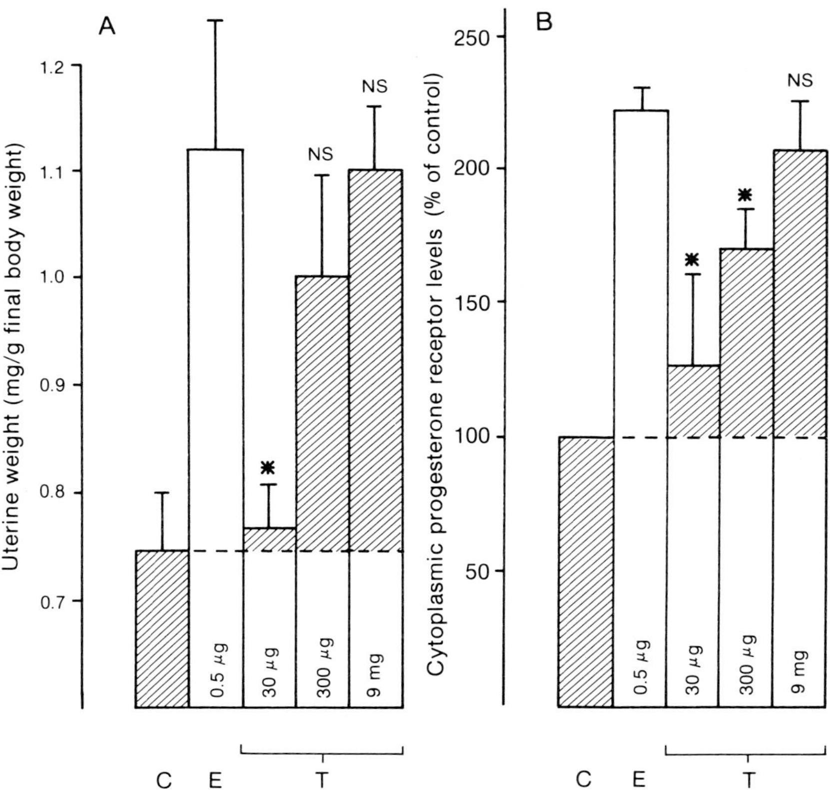

Fig. 7. Dose effect of tamoxifen on uterine weights and cytoplasmic progesterone receptor levels in ovariectomized rats. One-week ovariectomized animals were given a single injection of either vehicle (sesame oil, 100 μl), oestradiol (E, 0.5 μg), or tamoxifen (30 μg, 300 μg or 9 mg) Uterine wet weights (A) were measured 24 hours after injection and cytoplasmic progesterone receptor concentrations (B) were determined 12 hours after injection using the method described by Davies *et al.* (1979). Each value represents the mean ± S.D. of six determinations. $*p < 0.05$.

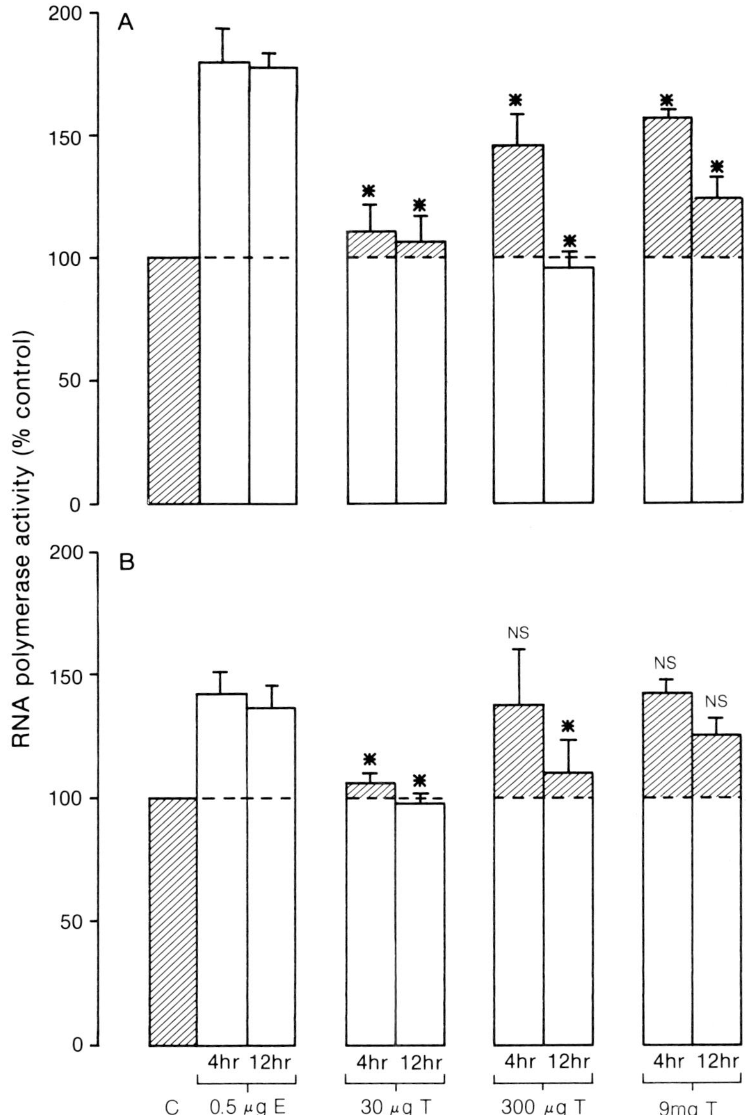

Fig. 8. Dose effect of tamoxifen on uterine nuclear RNA polymerases I and II in ovariectomized rats. One-week ovariectomized animals were given a single injection of either vehicle (sesame oil, 100 μl), oestradiol (E, 0.5 μg) or tamoxifen (30 μg, 300 μg or 9 mg) 4 hours or 12 hours prior to sacrifice. Nuclear RNA polymerases I (A) and II (B) were assayed as described by Davies *et al.* (1979). Each value represents the mean ± S.D. of 5 determinations (2 uteri per determination). *$p < 0.05$.

The effects of tamoxifen on RNA polymerase I were less striking than those achieved by oestradiol (Fig. 8A). Nevertheless, a correlation was observed between the increasing dose level of the drug and the degree of stimulation of RNA polymerase I activity at 4 hours. Interestingly, the pattern of response of this enzyme to tamoxifen and oestradiol was similar to the increased uterine weights observed after 4 daily injections of the compounds (Fig. 1), i.e. the cumulative response to tamoxifen, at doses of either 300 μg or 9 mg, was approximately one-third of the response shown to oestradiol.

In the rat uterus, both tamoxifen and oestradiol apparently increase RNA polymerase II activity by making more initiation sites available (Fig. 9), rather than affecting the size of the RNA product (Davies *et al.*, 1979). Furthermore, using chick oviduct it has been shown that the number of initiation sites is dependent upon the concentration of the nuclear oestrogen receptor complexes (Tsai *et al.*, 1975). This also appears to be the case in the rat uterus for oestradiol but not for tamoxifen, since the nuclear presence of the tamoxifen receptor complex is maintained after the number of initiation sites returns to pre-stimulation levels (Fig. 7; Davies *et al.*, 1979). The initiation site assay has limitations, e.g. using exogenous RNA polymerase II, the enzyme may overcome normal physiological regulatory systems and measure all potentially available sites, and may not yield information regarding the amount and similarities between transcripts initiating at these sites. However it does reflect overall structural changes in uterine chromatin caused by the oestrogen-receptor and antioestrogen-receptor complexes and as such is qualitatively relevant. These data (Fig. 7; Davies *et al.*, 1979) could, therefore, point to a basic inefficacy of the tamoxifen-receptor complex in its association with chromatin, which ultimately is manifested by a failure to promote a full oestrogenic response with respect to RNA polymerase activity and hence may mediate the antioestrogenic and antitumour properties of the drug. It is also possible that the early similarities observed between tamoxifen and oestradiol on RNA polymerase II activity during the first 4 hours of treatment (Figs 4 and 5) may relate to their early equipotent biological effects on the rat uterus (Fig. 2) and DMBA-induced mammary tumours (Nicholson *et al.*, 1979b; Nicholson and Griffiths, 1980). The inability of tamoxifen to antagonize the effects of oestradiol on RNA polymerase II at this time (Fig. 6) would add weight to this hypothesis. In this light, it is also of interest that tamoxifen brings about almost identical increases in the activity of RNA polymerases I and II to oestradiol in mouse uteri (Fig. 10), a tissue where it elicits a full uterotrophic effect (Terenius, 1970; 1971).

As the effects on extranucleolar chromatin, as manifested by increases in RNA polymerase II, may be effected directly (Fig. 7A), the tamoxifen-receptor complex may initially accomplish these. However, in the rat, the continued presence of the tamoxifen-receptor complex in the nucleus may not

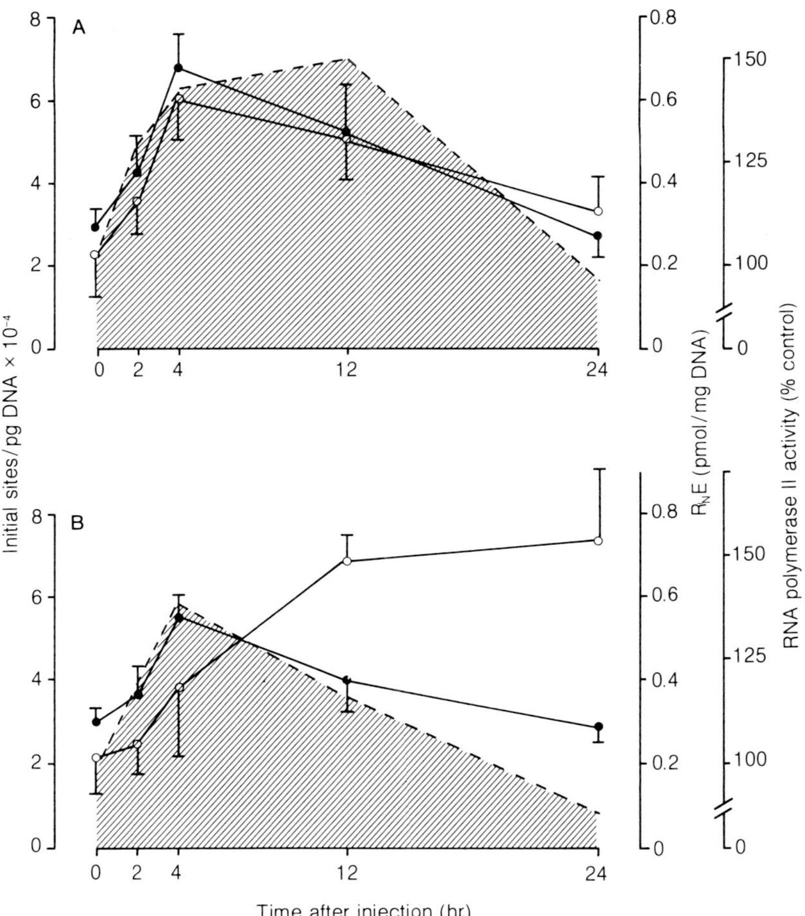

Fig. 9. Effect of oestradiol and tamoxifen on nuclear oestrogen receptor levels and numbers of initiation sites on rat uterine chromatin for RNA polymerase II. One-week ovariectomized animals were killed at the indicated times after injection of (A) oestradiol (0.5 μg) or (B) tamoxifen (300 μg). Nuclei were prepared and the nuclear oestrogen receptor levels (○), together with number of initiation sites (●) available for exogenous RNA polymerase II were measured as described by Anderson *et al.* (1972) and Davies *et al.* (1979), respectively. Values are the mean ± S.D. of 4 determinations (2 uteri per determination). The hatched area represents the activity of RNA polymerase II (see Figure 5).

result in the correct or sufficient cellular products necessary for the promotion of an efficient response at either the nucleolar or nucleoplasmic level and hence the maintenance of the species of RNA necessary to sustain oestrogen-dependent tissue growth. As stated earlier, a controlling mechanism for this could lie with an inherent defect in the antioestrogen-receptor complex and its binding to specific sites on chromatin, thereby influencing the variety and quantity of transcripts produced by RNA polymerase II. Alternatively, its antioestrogenic properties might reside in a direct interaction and inhibitory effect of tamoxifen with some other cellular component(s) normally associated with the propagation of the secondary events. Certainly, after 14 days of tamoxifen treatment (300 μg/day) tamoxifen is present in both the cytoplasmic and also the nuclear fraction of rat mammary tumour tissue in a massive excess over both oestradiol (Fig. 11) and the oestrogen receptor (not illustrated). It is feasible that the high levels of the drug may interfere with

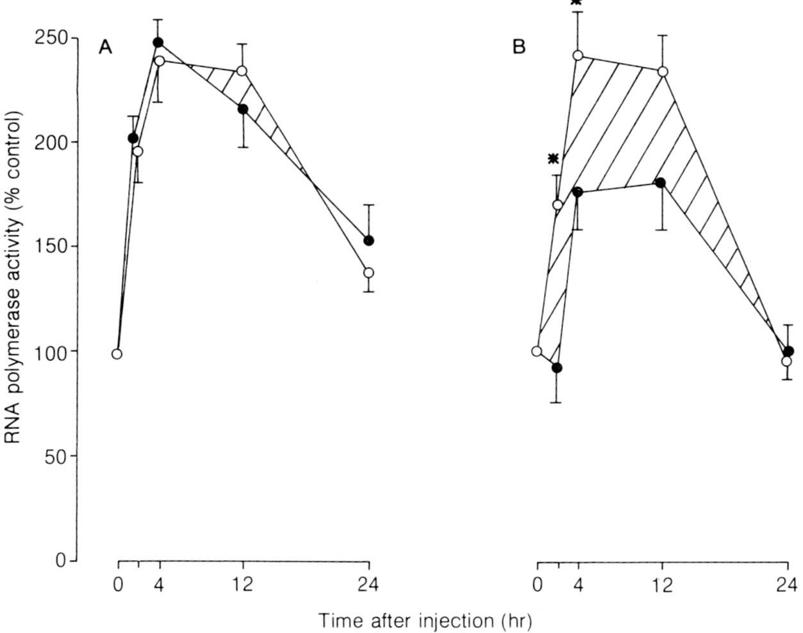

Fig. 10. Effect of oestradiol and tamoxifen on nuclear RNA polymerase activities in uteri from ovariectomized mice. One-week ovariectomized mice were killed at the indicated times after injection of oestradiol (E, ○, 0.1 μg) or tamoxifen (●, 50 μg). Nuclei were prepared and RNA polymerases I (A) and II (B) measured as described by Davies *et al.* (1979). Values are expressed as percentages of control activity (time zero). Each point represents the mean ± S.D. of 4 determinations in duplicate. *$p < 0.05$.

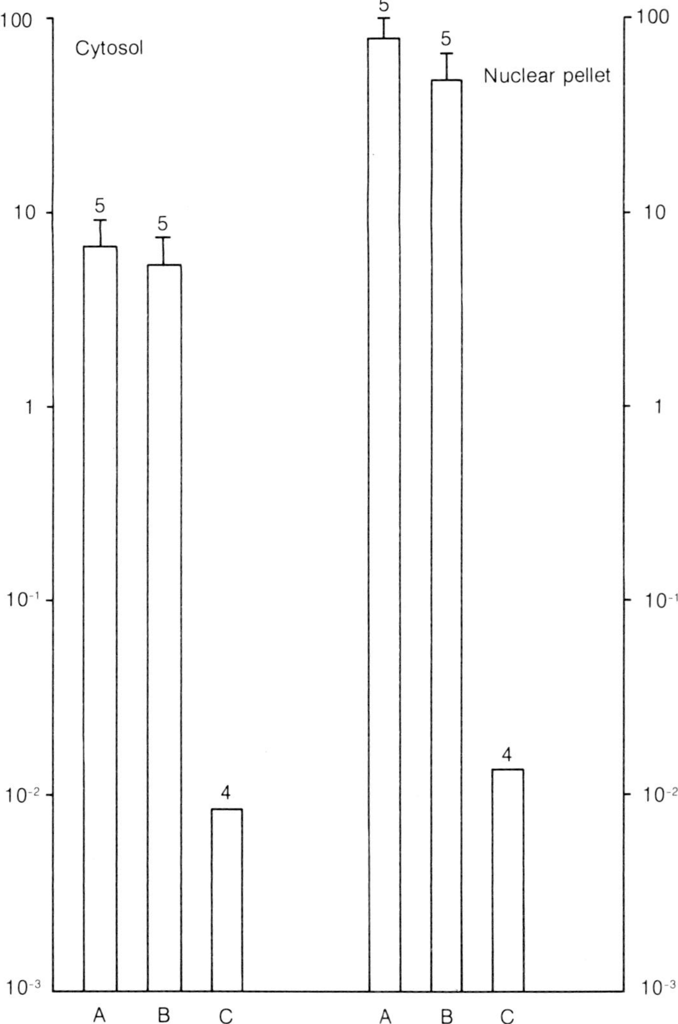

Fig. 11. Concentration of tamoxifen, metabolite X and oestradiol in DMBA-induced mammary tumours. Five tumour-bearing rats were administered tamoxifen (300 μg/day) for 14 days and sacrificed 18 hours after the last injection. Cytosol and nuclear fractions were prepared as described in Nicholson *et al.* (1977a) and tamoxifen (A), and metabolite X (B) were determined in each fraction by gas chromatography-high resolution mass spectrometry (Daniel *et al.*, 1979). Oestradiol (C) was assayed by radioimmunoassay in 4 tumours from similarly treated animals. The results are expressed as mean ± S.D.

some post-receptor, yet receptor linked, event. The early activity of tamoxifen might therefore be seen as tamoxifen acting directly through the oestrogen receptor and promoting a response identical to that of oestradiol, while its later properties could parallel a toxic accumulation of the drug within the tissue. It is an interesting prospect that varying species and tissue responses to tamoxifen (Furr *et al.*, 1979; Martin, 1980) might reflect their ability to accumulate the drug, rather than process its message through the oestrogen receptor system.

It is also noteworthy that, while considerable amounts of unchanged drug are present in rat plasma 24 hours after the administration of 300 μg of tamoxifen (approx. 10 ng/ml; Nicholson *et al.*, 1979b), a second injection of the drug at this time is able to promote a further stimulation of nuclear RNA polymerases I and II in rat uteri (Fig. 12). However, after 4 daily injections of tamoxifen, no stimulation of the RNA polymerases was observed. Obviously a critical evaluation of the plasma and tissue levels of tamoxifen and its metabolites in relation to the various tissue responses is crucial to our understanding of antioestrogen action.

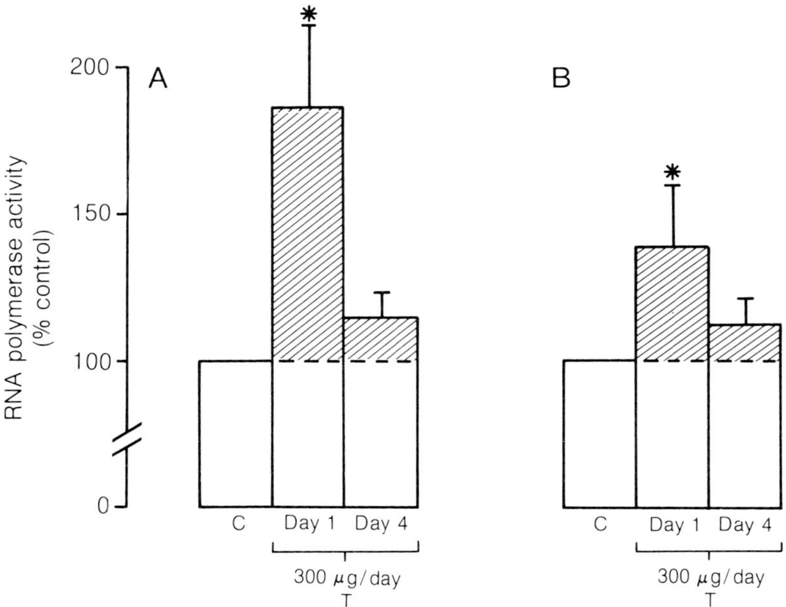

Fig. 12. Effect of multiple injections of tamoxifen on nuclear RNA polymerases in rat uteri from ovariectomized animals. Groups of 1 week ovariectomized animals were administered (s.c.) tamoxifen (300 μg/day) daily for periods up to 4 days. Uteri were removed 4 hours after the last injection of tamoxifen and their nuclei assayed for RNA polymerase I (A) or II (B) activity. The data are presented as a percentage of control activity (non-treated animals) and are the mean ± S.D. of 4 determinations (2 uteri per determination). $^*p < 0.05$.

V. SIGNIFICANCE OF METABOLITES TO THE ACTION OF THE DRUG

The studies previously described in this chapter have illustrated a series of events which have been attributed to the direct action of the parent drug tamoxifen. Indeed, such a concept is reinforced by experiments using the MCF 7 human mammary tumour cell line, where the characteristic properties of the molecule are recorded in the apparent absence of drug metabolism (Horwitz *et al.*, 1978). However, in the intact animal and patient, a number of metabolites have been identified following the *in vivo* administration of [^{14}C]tamoxifen (Fromson *et al.*, 1973a, 1973b), and it is feasible that they may influence the action of the parent drug.

The principal metabolite described by Fromson *et al.* (1973a, 1973b) was a monohydroxylated derivative, metabolite B (1-(4-β-dimethylamino-ethoxyphenyl)1-4-hydroxyphenyl,2-phenylbut-1-ene). This compound is thought to be formed from tamoxifen by aromatic hydroxylation in the liver and then to undergo enterohepatic recirculation. It is present in the plasma of postmenopausal patients undergoing tamoxifen therapy (10 or 20 mg b.d.) for advanced breast cancer, reaching some 5–10 ng/ml by day 20 and plateauing thereafter (Daniel *et al.*, 1979). This concentration of metabolite B is approximately 100 times higher than that of oestradiol, but only 2% that of tamoxifen. More recently, a *des*-methyl derivative of tamoxifen, metabolite X (1-(4-β-methylaminoethoxyphenyl)1,2-diphenylbut-1-ene) has also been identified and is present in plasma of women on tamoxifen therapy in amounts equivalent to or higher than tamoxifen itself (Adam *et al.*, 1979). The tissue distribution of these compounds in rat mammary tumours after 14 days of tamoxifen treatment (300 μg/rat/day) is shown in Figure 11. Ratios of approximately 800:1 were recorded for both tamoxifen and metabolite X to oestradiol in the cytoplasmic fraction and 5,000:1 in the nuclear fraction respectively. Metabolite B was also detected at about 1 ng/mg cytosolic protein and 5 ng/mg DNA (100–500 times higher than the corresponding concentration of oestradiol), although the relatively low concentration of this metabolite in mammary tumours makes its precise quantification by gas chromatography-high resolution mass spectrometry difficult.

Competitive binding studies from this laboratory have indicated that metabolite B and metabolite X, like tamoxifen, bind to cytoplasmic oestrogen receptor preparations and displace radioactive oestradiol from its specific 4S and 8S binding protein (Nicholson and Griffiths, 1980). Approximately 50% inhibition of [^{3}H]oestradiol binding (5 nM) may be achieved by 50 nM metabolite B, 150 nM metabolite X and 500 nM tamoxifen. Similar data have been recorded for tamoxifen and metabolite B using human mammary tumour (Nicholson *et al.*, 1979a) and rat uterus (Jordan *et al.*, 1977b; Nicholson *et al.*, 1979a). Moreover, metabolite B, like tamoxifen, is capable of eliciting the translocation of the oestrogen receptor to the rat uterine nucleus, although its nuclear retention profile is closer to that of oestradiol than to that of tamoxifen (Jordan *et al.*, 1978). Furthermore, administration *in vivo* of either metabolite B or metabolite X reduced uterine weights and caused the regression of oestrogen-receptor positive mammary tumours (Nicholson, 1981). In each case, however, tumour regressions were less marked than with tamoxifen. Jordan and Naylor (1978) have presented similar data for metabolite B, administered at a lower dose level.

The possibility therefore exists that metabolite B and metabolite X may effectively sequester available oestrogen receptor and play a supportive, or possibly primary, role in determining the receptor-mediated properties of the drug. Their influence, however, on other, as yet theoretical receptor-linked events remains unknown.

VI. CONCLUSIONS

The data of RNA polymerase activity in the nuclei of rat mammary tumours and rat uteri appear consistent with the properties of tamoxifen outlined earlier (Section I) where it was observed that, during the early phase of the action of the drug, it promotes similar tissue effects to oestradiol, but subsequently fails to maintain its initial oestrogenic potential in terms of growth. However it is evident that there are still fundamental questions which remain unanswered. In particular, the plasma and tissue concentrations of the drug and its metabolites in relation to transcriptional and post-transcriptional events will be invaluable to our understanding of the action of the drug and in the development of a more effective treatment regime. Studies to this end are currently in progress.

ACKNOWLEDGEMENTS

The authors wish to thank the Tenovus Organization and ICI (UK) for their generous and continued financial support and Professor K. Griffiths for his helpful criticism and advice. C.P.D. and J.S.S. are recipients of Tenovus and ICI Scholarships respectively.

REFERENCES

Adam, H. K., Douglas, E. J., and Kemp, J. V. (1979). *Biochem. Pharmacol.* **28**, 145–147.
Anderson, J., Clark, J. H., and Peck, E. J. (1972). *Biochem. J.* **126**, 561–567.
Borthwick, N. M., and Smellie, R. M. S. (1975). *Biochem. J.* **147**, 91–101.
Capony, F., and Rochefort, H. (1978). *Mol. Cell. Endocr.* **11**, 181–198.

Chambon, P. (1975). *Ann. Rev. Biochem.* **44**, 613–638.

Clark, J. H., Peck, E. J., and Anderson, J. N. (1974). *Nature* **251**, 446–448.

Cowan, S., and Leake, R. E. (1979). *In* "Antihormones" (M. K. Agarwal, ed.), pp. 283–292. Elsevier/North Holland, Amsterdam.

Daniel, C. P., Gaskell, S. J., Bishop, H., and Nicholson, R. I. (1979). *J. Endocr.* **83**, 401–408.

Dao, T. L., and Sinha, D. (1972). *In* "Prolactin and Carcinogenesis" (A. R. Boyns and K. Griffiths, eds), pp. 189–194. Alpha Omega Alpha Publishing, U.K.

Davies, P., Syne, J. S., and Nicholson, R. I. (1979). *Endocrinology* **105**, 1336–1342.

Fromson, J. M., Pearson, S., and Bramah, S. (1973a). *Xenobiotica* **3**, 693–709.

Fromson, J. M., Pearson, S., and Bramah, S. (1973b). *Xenobiotica* **3**, 711–714.

Furr, B. J. A., Patterson, J. S., Richardson, D. H., Slater, S. R., and Wakeling, A. E. (1979). *In* "Pharmacological and Biochemical Properties of Drug Substances" (M. E. Goldberg, ed.), Vol. II, pp. 355–399. American Pharmacological Association, Washington, U.S.A.

Gaskell, S. J., Daniel, C. P., and Nicholson, R. I. (1978). *J. Endocr.* **78**, 293–394.

Glasser, S. R., Chytil, F., and Spelsberg, T. C. (1972). *Biochem. J.* **130**, 947–957.

Gorski, J. (1964). *J. Biol. Chem.* **239**, 889–892.

Hamilton, T. H. (1968). *Science* **161**, 649–661.

Hardin, J. W., Clark, J. H., Glasser, S. R., and Peck, E. J. (1976). *Biochemistry* **7**, 1370–1374.

Horwitz, K. B., Koseki, Y., and McGuire, W. L. (1978). *Endocrinology* **103**, 1742–1751.

Jensen, E. V., Mohla, S., Gorell, T. A., and DeSombre, E. R. (1974). *Vitamins and Hormones* **32**, 89–127.

Jordan, V. C. (1975). *In* "The Hormonal Control of Breast Cancer" Alderley Park, 24th Sept. pp. 11–17. I. C. I. Publications, U.K.

Jordan, V. C., and Koerner, S. (1975). *Eur. J. Cancer* **2**, 205–206.

Jordan, V. C., and Naylor, K. E. (1978). *Brit. J. Pharmacol.* **64**, 37P.

Jordan, V. C., Collins, M. M., Rowsby, L., and Prestwich, G. (1977a). *J. Endocr.* **75**, 305–316.

Jordan, V. C., Dix, C. J., Rowsby, L., and Prestwich, G. (1977b). *Mol. Cell. Endocr.* **7**, 177–192.

Jordan, V. C., Dix, C. J., Naylor, K. E., Prestwich, G. and Rowsby, L. (1978). *J. Toxicol. Environ. Health* **4**, 363–390.

Koseki, Y., Zava, D. T., Chamness, G. C., and McGuire, W. L. (1977). *Endocrinology* **101**, 1104–1110.

Kurl, R. L., and Borthwick, N. M. (1980). *J. Endocr.* **85**, 519–524.

Lowry, O. H., Rosebrough, N. J., Farr, A. L., and Randell, R. J. (1951). *J. Biol. Chem.* **193**, 265–272.

Martin, L. (1980). *In* "Oestrogens in the Environment" (J. McLachlan, ed.), Elsevier/North Holland, Amsterdam (In Press).

Mouridsen, H., Palshof, T., Patterson, J., and Battersby, L. (1978). *Cancer Treat. Reviews* **5**, 131–141.

Nicholson, R. I. (1979a). *Reviews in Endocrine-Related* **3,** 31–39.

Nicholson, R. I. (1979b). *Biochem. Soc. Transactions,* 577th Meeting, pp. 569–572.

Nicholson, R. I. (1981). *J. Reprod. Fert.* (In Press).

Nicholson, R. I., and Golder, M. P. (1975). *Eur. J. Cancer* **12**, 571–579.

Nicholson, R. I., and Griffiths, K. (1980). *In* "Advances in Steroid Hormone Research" (E. Thomas, ed.), Vol. IV, pp. 119–152. Urban and Schwartzenberg, Baltimore-Munich.

Nicholson, R. I., Golder, M. P., Davies, P., and Griffiths, K. (1976). *Eur. J. Cancer* **12**, 711–717.

Nicholson, R. I., Davies, P., and Griffiths, K. (1977a). *Eur. J. Cancer* **13**, 201–218.

Nicholson, R. I., Davies, P., and Griffiths, K. (1977b). *J. Endocr.* **73**, 135–142.

Nicholson, R. I., Davies, P., and Griffiths, K. (1978). *Reviews in Endocrine-Related Cancer* April Supplement, pp. 306–318.

Nicholson, R. I., Daniel, C. P., Gaskell, S. J., Syne, J. S., Davies, P., and Griffiths, K. (1979a). *In* "Antihormones" (M. K. Agarwal, ed.), pp. 253–267. Elsevier/North Holland, Amsterdam.

Nicholson, R. I., Syne, J. S., Daniel, C. P., and Griffiths, K. (1979b). *Eur. J. Cancer* **15**, 317–239.

Palshof, T., Mouridsen, H. T., and Daehnfeldt, J. L. (1980). *In* "Breast Cancer: Experimental and Clinical Aspects" (H. T. Mouridsen and T. Palshof, eds.), pp. 183–188. Pergamon Press, Oxford.

Powell-Jones, W., Jenner, D. A., Blamey, R. W., Davies, P., and Griffiths, K. (1975). *Biochem. J.* **150**, 71–75.

Roeder, R. G. (1976). *Cold Spring Harbor Symp. Quant. Biol.* **40**, 285–329.

Stoll, B. A. (1969). "Hormonal Management of Breast Cancer". Pitman Medical, London.

Terenius, L. (1970). *Acta Endocr.* **64**, 47–58.

Terenius, L. (1971). *Acta Endocr.* **66**, 431–447.

Tsai, S. Y., Tsai, M. J., Schwartz, R., Kalimi, M., Clark, J. H., and O'Malley, B. W. (1975). *Proc. Natl Acad. Sci. U.S.A.* **72**, 4228–4232.

Ward, H. W. C. (1973). *Brit. Med. J.* **1**, 13–14.

Weil, P. A., Sidikaro, J., Stancel, G. M., and Blatti, S. P. (1977). *J. Biol. Chem.* **252**, 1092–1098.

18

Antioestrogen Action in Ovarian-Dependent and Ovarian-Autonomous Experimental Mammary Tumours

BENITA S. KATZENELLENBOGEN, TEN-LIN S. TSAI AND ELLEN A. RORKE

I. INTRODUCTION: ANTITUMOUR ACTION OF ANTIOESTROGENS

Antioestrogens are compounds that block, at least in part, the action of oestrogens in target tissues. While the pursuit of compounds with such activity was initially prompted by the search for effective contraceptive agents for the human female, interest has refocused on these compounds because of their potential for controlling the growth of hormone-dependent neoplasms, particularly tumours of the breast (Horwitz and McGuire, 1978). Since antioestrogens are able to antagonize the actions of oestrogens, these compounds hold the potential of being noninvasive, nonsurgical agents capable of controlling the growth of hormone-dependent tumours. Hence, we have analysed the effectiveness of several antioestrogens, previously shown to be potent in antagonizing oestrogen-induced uterine growth (Ferguson

NON-STEROIDAL ANTIOESTROGENS
ISBN 0 12 677880 9

and Katzenellenbogen, 1977), in preventing the development of 7,12-dimethylbenzanthracene (DMBA)-induced rat mammary tumours and in eliciting the regression of established tumours, and have attempted to elucidate the mechanisms of their tumour antagonism. An additional aim has been to assess the possible effects of antioestrogens on the growth of mammary tumours that are recalcitrant to endocrine ablation. For these studies we have compared the effects of antioestrogens on the growth and properties of ovarian-dependent, DMBA-induced mammary tumours and the ovarian-autonomous, but oestrogen-sensitive R3230AC rat mammary adenocarcinoma. Inasmuch as one of the problems frequently associated with antioestrogen therapy has been the development of photosensitivity in patients (Bloom and Boesen, 1974; Heuson *et al*; 1975), we were particularly interested in using the antioestrogen U 23,469 which is structurally related to the antioestrogen nafoxidine (see Fig. 1), but which is nonphototoxic and hence may prove to be more suitable for human use.

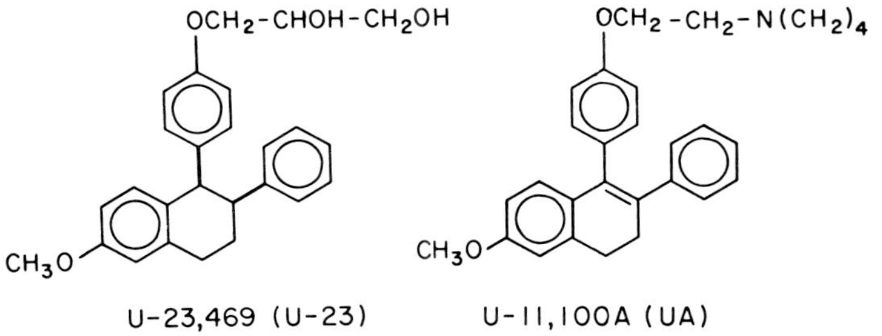

Fig. 1. Structure of the nonsteroidal antioestrogen U 23,469, and the structure of a related antioestrogen U 11,100A.

II. INFLUENCE OF ANTIHORMONAL AND HORMONAL TREATMENTS ON DMBA-INDUCED MAMMARY TUMOUR DEVELOPMENT AND RECEPTOR LEVELS

Virgin female Sprague-Dawley rats that receive DMBA at 47–50 days of age and then receive U 23,469 (U-23; 250 μg s.c. in 0.15 M NaCl daily) have a greatly reduced number of mammary tumours and a markedly decreased tumour area. Treatment with U-23 for increasing time periods (3, 6 or 12 weeks) beginning 2 weeks after DMBA results in a progressive decrease in tumour size and number and a progressive delay in onset of tumour appearance; U-23 treatment beginning 1 week after DMBA or given prior to DMBA is even more effective (Fig. 2).

The time course of tumour regression (3 months after DMBA) by U-23 or ovariectomy is similar with 50% regression in about 2 weeks, and both elicit regression of almost all tumours (> 90%) (Fig. 3). Treatments with the antioestrogens U 11,100A and CI 628, or with high doses of oestradiol-17β or oestradiol benzoate, also elicited the regression or disappearance of many of the tumours within two weeks (Tsai *et al.*, 1979). As seen in Figure 4, oestradiol (5 μg/rat/day) is able to reactivate these regressed tumours; tumours which had regressed following ovariectomy or antioestrogen treatment began to regrow soon after the administration of oestradiol.

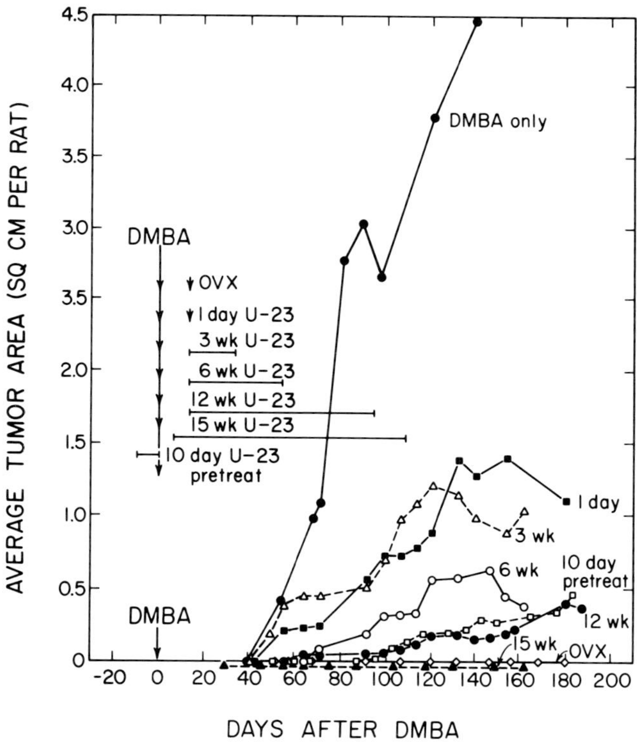

Fig. 2. The influence of treatments on the development and growth of DMBA-induced rat mammary tumours. Female Sprague-Dawley rats received DMBA at 47–50 days of age then, following a 2 week period, groups of rats were ovariectomized (OVX) or they received U 23,469 (U-23) injections of 250 μg/day either for 1 day or for 3, 6 or 12 weeks. Another group was pretreated with U 23,469 for 10 days before DMBA administration and another group received 15 weeks of U 23,469 exposure starting at only 1 week after DMBA. There were 8–13 rats per treatment group and 58 rats in the control group. Values represent the average tumour area per rat in these different groups. From Tsai and Katzenellenbogen (1977).

In an attempt to understand the mechanism by which this antioestrogen might be eliciting tumour regression, we examined its effects on tumour oestrogen, progesterone and prolactin receptors. Table I summarizes the effects of these different treatments on receptor levels in mammary tumours. We have determined here the levels of nuclear oestrogen receptor, cytosol oestrogen receptor and cytosol progesterone receptor, and the ratio of nuclear to total oestrogen receptor. In tumours induced by DMBA, we find approximately 0.2 pmole of cytoplasmic oestrogen receptor per 100 mg tissue (59 ± 9 [n = 30] fmoles/mg cytosol protein) and approximately one-half of the receptor is in the nucleus. Likewise, high levels of progesterone cytosol receptor are found. This appears to be the case whether tumours are assayed from cycling animals at random stages during the oestrous cycle (Table I, Group 1a) or whether tumours are assayed from animals at 19 hours after ovariectomy (Table I, Group 1b). Hence, these data have been pooled (Group

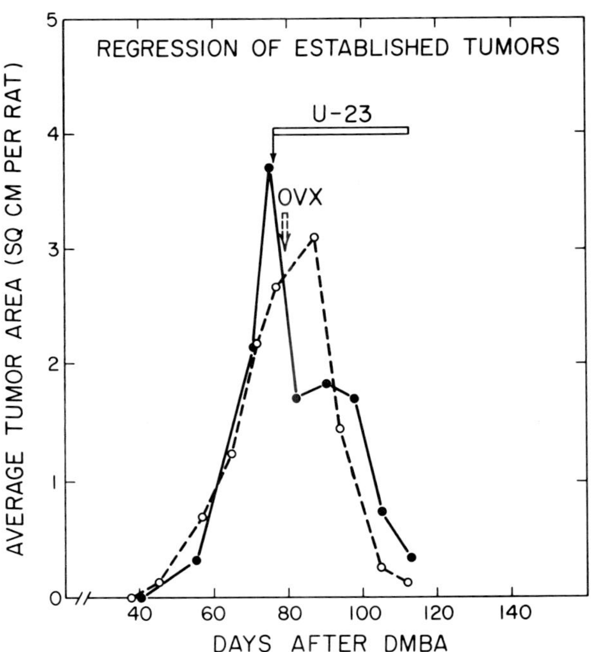

Fig. 3. The effect of U 23,469 (U-23) treatment for ovariectomy (OVX) on the regression of established tumours. At the time indicated (arrow) after DMBA treatment, animals (15/group) received U 23,469 injections (250 μg s.c. in 0.5 ml of 0.15 M NaCl/day, 6 days/week) for 36 days or were ovariectomized and followed for 34 days. Values represent the average tumour area per rat for each group of 15 rats. From Tsai and Katzenellenbogen (1977).

1c) and are used for statistical comparison with the other experimental treatment groups (Table I, Groups 2–5).

The statistically significant changes induced by the treatments are as follows. After U-23 treatment (Table I, Group 4), as tumours regress, approximately 90 % of the receptor is found in the nucleus. After ovariectomy (Table I, Group 2), little (30 %) of the total receptor is in the nucleus and cytoplasmic receptor levels are high; as expected in the absence of ovarian oestrogen, the progesterone cytosol receptor level is very low. In tumours regressing under U-23 treatment (Table I, Group 4), the progesterone receptor level is similar to that of controls and is considerably higher than that seen in mammary tumours regressing due to ovariectomy. This may reflect some oestrogen-like action of this compound U 23,469. Receptor levels were also studied during tumour reactivation by oestradiol. In both cases (Table I,

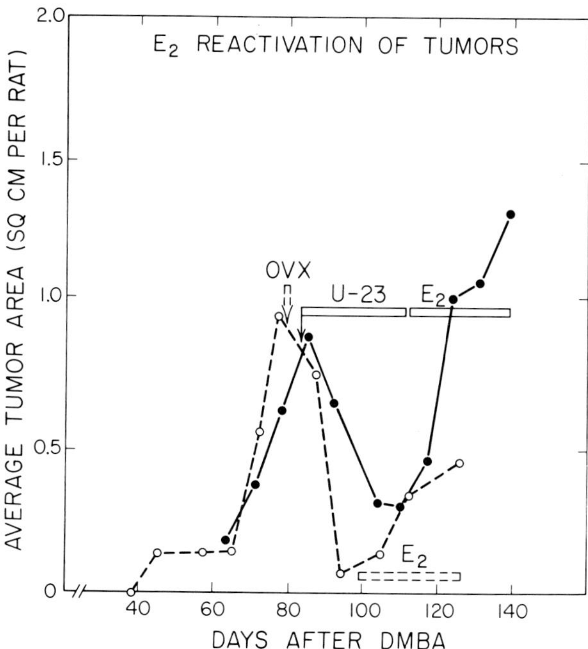

Fig. 4. The ability of oestradiol (E_2) to elicit regrowth of tumours caused to regress by U 23,469 (U-23) treatment or ovariectomy (OVX). Animals received DMBA at 47 days of age and at the times indicated (arrows), rats (6/group) were ovariectomized or received U 23,469 injections (250 μg s.c. in 0.15 M NaCl/day) for 28 days prior to administration of oestradiol (5 μg s.c. in 0.15 M NaCl/day) for 27 days. Values represent the average tumour area per rat for the six rats in each group. From Tsai and Katzenellenbogen (1977).

TABLE I
Oestrogen and Progesterone Receptor Levels in DMBA-Induced Mammary Tumours[a]

Treatment	$\frac{ER_n}{ER_n + ER_c}$[b] (%)	pmoles/100 mg tissue		
		ER_n	ER_c	PR_c
1a. DMBA only (no 19 h OVX)	60	0.28 ± 0.09[c] (20)[d]	0.19 ± 0.03 (19)	1.33 ± 0.18 (10)
1b. DMBA only[e] (19 h OVX)	43	0.19 ± 0.03 (22)	0.25 ± 0.06 (11)	1.48 ± 0.15 (20)
1c. DMBA only (pooled)	52	0.23 ± 0.04 (42)	0.21 ± 0.03 (30)	1.43 ± 0.12 (30)
2. OVX-regressing[f]	30	0.33 ± 0.07 (8)	0.79 ± 0.31[g] (6)	0.14 ± 0.07[g] (6)
3. OVX → E_2[h]	62	0.26 ± 0.06 (5)	0.16 ± 0.04 (5)	0.42 ± 0.16[g] (5)
4. U 23,469-regressing[i]	90	0.54 ± 0.06[g] (18)	0.06 ± 0.02[j] (18)	1.14 ± 0.23 (17)
5. U 23,469 → E_2[k]	58	0.21 ± 0.03 (10)	0.15 ± 0.05 (7)	1.05 ± 0.06 (11)

[a] From Tsai and Katzenellenbogen (1977).
[b] ER_n, nuclear oestrogen receptor; ER_c, cytosol oestrogen receptor; PR_c, cytosol progesterone receptor; OVX, ovariectomy; E_2, 17β-oestradiol.
[c] Mean ± S.E.M.
[d] Numbers in parentheses = number of tumours assayed.
[e] Tumours were assayed 19 hours after bilateral OVX.
[f] Regressing tumours were assayed 3 to 5 weeks after OVX.
[g] $p < 0.01$ versus DMBA-only pooled value.
[h] At 3 weeks after OVX, each rat received s.c. injections of 5 μg E_2 in 0.5 ml 0.15 M NaCl daily 6 days/week for 3 weeks. The tumours were assayed 24 hours after the last E_2 injection.
[i] Each rat received s.c. injections of 250 μg U 23,469 in 0.5 ml 0.15 M NaCl daily 6 days/week for approximately 4 weeks. The tumours were assayed 24 hours after the last U 23,469 injection and 19 hours after bilateral OVX.
[j] $p < 0.05$ versus DMBA-only pooled value.
[k] After 4 weeks of U 23,469 injections, each rat received E_2 injections for 4 weeks. Tumours were assayed 24 hours after the last E_2 injection.

Groups 3 and 5), receptor assays were done 24 hours after the last injection of oestradiol. Oestradiol treatment shifted the oestrogen receptor distribution towards that seen in the DMBA-only control group (Table I, Group 1c).

A similar picture is seen when uteri are also studied (Tsai and Katzenellenbogen, 1977). After ovariectomy, cytosol progesterone receptor levels are greatly diminished in uteri, as in tumours, while cytosol oestrogen receptor levels are high, and in both tissues, little (approximately one-third) oestrogen receptor is in the nucleus. During U-23 treatment, cytosol oestrogen receptor content is very low in the uterus, as in the regressing tumour, with over 90% of the receptor in the nucleus.

Antioestrogens also influence the level of prolactin binding in DMBA-induced mammary tumours (Table II). Tumour prolactin receptor content is greatly reduced in tumours regressing during treatment with a variety of antioestrogens, or with high doses of oestrogen. Ovariectomy results in an even more marked reduction in tumour prolactin receptor.

TABLE II
Prolactin Receptor in DMBA-Induced Mammary Tumours[a]

Group[b]	% Specific binding[c]
1. Control	8.0 ± 0.8[d] (31)[e]
2. U 23,469 (250 μg/day)	4.5 ± 0.8[f] (16)
3. U 11,100A (250 μg/day)	4.9 ± 0.6[f] (7)
4. CI 628 (200 μg/day)	5.4 ± 0.9[f] (18)
5. Oestradiol-17β (50 μg/day)	3.7 ± 0.9[f] (19)
6. Oestradiol benzoate (50 μg/day)	2.8 ± 0.3[f] (11)
7. Ovariectomy	1.3 ± 0.4[f] (8)

[a] From Tsai *et al.* (1979).

[b] Each rat bearing tumours (approx. 60–80 days after DMBA) received s.c. injections of antioestrogen or oestrogen in 0.5 ml 0.15 M NaCl daily for 2–4 weeks. Controls received 0.15 M NaCl alone and rats that were ovariectomized received no injections. The tumours were assayed 19–23 hours after the last injection, or approximately 2 weeks after ovariectomy.

[c] The difference in bound [^{125}I]prolactin with or without excess cold prolactin expressed as the percentage of total radioactivity added in each tube.

[d] Mean ± S.E.M.

[e] Numbers in parentheses = number of tumours assayed.

[f] $p < 0.05$ versus control value.

Hence, as was seen in the uterus, high doses of antioestrogen perturb the normal distribution of oestrogen receptor so that much of the receptor is found in the nucleus with low levels of cytoplasmic receptor. This situation may render the mammary tumour incapable of responding to the animal's own endogenous oestrogens and hence it will be unable to grow. In addition, antioestrogens may also influence mammary tumour growth in this system by reducing the tumour content of prolactin receptors (Table II; and Kelly *et al.* 1977).

III. INFLUENCE OF ANTIHORMONAL AND HORMONAL TREATMENTS ON R3230AC MAMMARY TUMOUR DEVELOPMENT AND RECEPTOR LEVELS

Antioestrogen treatment was also found to markedly depress the growth of the ovarian autonomous but oestrogen-sensitive R3230AC rat mammary tumour (Katzenellenbogen *et al.*, 1979; Tsai *et al.*, 1979). Administration of the antioestrogen U 23,469 and two related antioestrogens, U 11,100A and CI 628, beginning at the time of tumour transplantation into Fischer 344 host rats results in a 2–4 fold depression in tumour growth rate; the degree of growth reduction is related to the dose of antioestrogen (Fig. 5). Oestradiol-17β (15 μg) also depresses R3230AC tumour growth, while growth is at or slightly above the control rate in ovariectomized host (OVX group), as has been previously reported (Hilf *et al.*, 1965). These findings suggest that antioestrogens may provide palliative benefit in the case of some ovarian-unresponsive but oestrogen-sensitive breast cancers, in addition to being highly beneficial in the treatment of ovarian-dependent breast cancers.

In the hope of determining the possible bases for the depressive effect of antioestrogen and high dose oestradiol on tumour growth, oestrogen receptor levels were determined in some tumours harvested at 25 days after transplantation. As seen in Table III, antioestrogen treatments resulted in some changes in oestrogen receptor distribution similar to those seen in the DMBA mammary tumour system. For example, treatment with U 23,469 or U 11,100A resulted in a significant reduction of cytoplasmic oestrogen receptors and an increase in nuclear oestrogen receptor sites so that over 60 % of total receptors were in the nucleus 19–24 hours after the last injection of these antioestrogens. (Note that the control receptor level in R3230AC tumours is about 20 % that of control DMBA tumours). Oestradiol treatment likewise reduced the level of cytoplasmic receptor very markedly, without a corresponding increase in the nuclear receptor content, so that total tissue oestrogen receptor content was only approximately half of the control level. A similar effect of oestradiol treatment was seen in DBMA tumours (Tsai *et al.*,

1979). In contrast to the situation seen in DMBA tumours (Tsai *et al.*, 1979), however, the antioestrogen CI 628 did not affect the oestrogen receptor distribution pattern in the R3230AC tumours, although it did significantly depress tumour growth rate. Ovariectomy (Table III, Group 6) had no effect on oestrogen receptor levels, in agreement with the report of Wittliff *et al.* (1972).

There was also no significant difference in plasma prolactin and oestradiol levels between any of the R3230AC treatment groups and the controls (Tsai *et al.*, 1979). Since we found the level of prolactin receptor in control R3230AC mammary tumours to be quite low (approximately 12% that of DMBA tumours as reported also by Smith *et al.*, 1976 and 1977), we were not able to measure reliably any possible changes in tumour prolactin receptors in the different treatment groups.

Interestingly, although antioestrogens or high doses of oestradiol both depressed the growth of R3230AC mammary tumours, their effects on tumour enzyme activities differed (Katzenellenbogen *et al.*, 1979; Rorke and Katzenellenbogen, 1980). While oestradiol increased the activity of glucose-6-phosphate dehydrogenase and malic enzyme 2-fold and decreased the activity

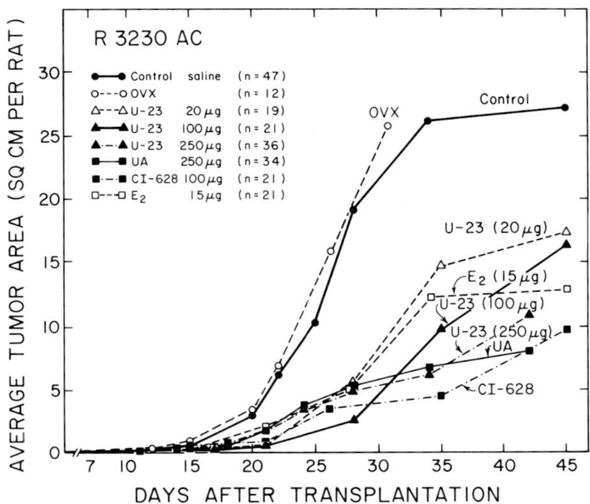

Fig. 5. The influence of treatment with antioestrogens or oestrogen on the growth of R3230AC mammary tumours. Tumours were transplanted into intact female Fischer 344 host rats, and beginning on the day after tumour transplantation, rats received the indicated daily doses of antioestrogen or oestradiol (E_2). In one group, tumours were transplanted into host rats that had been ovariectomized 4 days prior to the time of tumour transplantation (OVX). The antioestrogens utilized were U 23,469, U 11,100A and CI 628. From Tsai *et al.* (1979).

TABLE III
R3230AC Mammary Tumour Oestrogen Receptor Levels[a]

Treatment group	fmoles/100 mg tissue			$\frac{ER_n}{ER_n + ER_c}$ (%)
	ER_n[b]	ER_c[b]	$ER_n + ER_c$	
1. Control	21 ± 5[c] (12)[d]	46 ± 7 (12)[d]	67 ± 9 (12)[d]	31
2. U 23,469[e] (250 μg/day)	39 ± 5[g] (16)	14 ± 3[g] (16)	53 ± 6 (16)	74
3. U 11,100A[e] (250 μg/day)	39 ± 5[g] (9)	25 ± 5[g] (9)	64 ± 7 (9)	61
4. CI 628[e] (100 μg/day)	25 ± 8 (9)	48 ± 8 (10)	73 ± 11 (9)	34
5. E_2-17β[e] (15 μg/day)	19 ± 8 (6)	9 ± 6[g] (6)	28 ± 10[g] (6)	68
6. OVX[f]	23 ± 5 (14)	60 ± 9 (13)	83 ± 9 (13)	28

[a] From Tsai *et al.* (1979).
[b] ER_n, nuclear oestrogen receptor; ER_c, cytosol oestrogen receptor; OVX, ovariectomy.
[c] Mean ± S.E.M.
[d] Numbers in parentheses = number of tumours assayed.
[e] Each rat received s.c. injections of antioestrogens or oestradiol-17β in 0.5 ml 0.15 M NaCl daily for approximately 25 days post-R3230AC tumour transplant. The tumours were assayed 19–23 hours after the last injection.
[f] Rats were ovariectomized 5 days before receiving R3230AC tumour transplants.
[g] $p < 0.05$ versus Control value.

of α-glycerolphosphate dehydrogenase 2-fold, in keeping with previous reports (Hilf *et al.*, 1965), ovariectomy and antioestrogen treatments did not alter the activity from that of control tumours, and administration of antioestrogen along with oestradiol blocked the oestradiol stimulation almost completely.

IV. HORMONAL DEPENDENCE AND HORMONAL SENSITIVITIES OF BREAST CANCERS

The studies reported here with DMBA and R3230AC mammary tumours indicate significant differences in their spectrum and degree of responsiveness to additive (hormonal and antihormonal) therapy and endocrine ablative therapy. Likewise, human breast cancer probably consists of a spectrum of diseases in terms of its hormonal dependence, as evidenced by the responses of patients to endocrine therapy. Antioestrogens depress growth of the R3230AC mammary tumour, although the growth of this tumour is not affected by ovariectomy. Likewise, we find that high levels of oestrogen also depress growth, as reported previously by Hilf *et al.* (1965). This tumour is also sensitive to other hormones, with high levels of androgen (Hilf *et al.*, 1965), insulin (Cohen and Hilf, 1975), and prolactin (Smith *et al.*, 1977) also reducing growth. However, although antioestrogens markedly reduce the growth of R3230AC tumours, these agents do not elicit tumour regression or the complete suppression of tumour development, as is seen in the DMBA tumour system.

In contrast to the R3230AC mammary tumours, the large majority (approximately 85%) of DMBA-induced mammary tumours are ovarian-dependent for their growth and many are effectively suppressed by antioestrogen treatment or by large doses of oestrogen (DeSombre and Arbogast, 1974; Heuson *et al.*, 1971; Jordan, 1976; Kelly *et al.*, 1977; Tsai and Katzenellenbogen, 1977). However, it is well known that DMBA tumours show considerable variability in terms of their hormonal dependence or responsiveness (DeSombre *et al.*, 1976; Leung *et al.*, 1975; Mobbs, 1966). Of the small proportion of DMBA tumours that are ovarian unresponsive, our data, with a small number of these tumours, indicate that they usually do not respond to subsequent antioestrogen, and likewise, antioestrogen-insensitive tumours rarely are arrested by subsequent ovariectomy. In addition, some tumours that are growth arrested or stabilized by ovariectomy or antioestrogen treatment may be further inhibited by subsequent anti-oestrogen or endocrine ablative treatment (Tsai *et al.*, 1979). The extent to which antioestrogens are capable of inducing decreases in tumour size beyond that achieved by ovariectomy may be a reflection of their ability to antagonize the low levels of endogenous oestrogens (e.g. adrenal oestrogens) that still may be present after ovariectomy.

During DMBA tumour regression by the 3 antioestrogens we have studied (U 23,469, U 11,100A, and CI 628), prolactin receptor was reduced in all cases (as also reported by Kelly *et al.*, 1977, for the steroidal antioestrogen RU 16117). Likewise, oestrogen receptor distribution is perturbed by antioestrogens in a manner that causes much of the receptor to be found in the nucleus with low levels of cytoplasmic receptor. Hence, changes in both oestrogen receptors and prolactin receptors may account for growth inhibition in this tumour system. Kledzik *et al.* (1976) and Smith *et al.* (1976) have also reported that high levels of oestrogen depress prolactin receptors in this tumour.

In R3230AC tumours, however, growth is markedly depressed but not completely eliminated by antioestrogens or oestrogen. With 2 of the antioestrogens (U 23,469 and U 11,100A), there is the suggestion that oestrogen receptor distribution changes (Table III) parallel those seen in the DMBA tumour system. However, this was not always the case as CI 628, which effectively reduced tumour growth (Fig. 5), did not alter the subcellular distribution of oestrogen receptor (Table III). There was also no effect of any of these antihormonal treatments on the blood level of oestradiol, and little, if any, decrease in the blood level of prolactin.

Smith *et al.* (1977) have reported that very high doses of oestradiol valerate (7.5 mg/kg/week in oil) slightly decrease (by 20–25%) prolactin receptor levels in R3230AC tumours. However, lower doses of oestradiol valerate (0.5 mg/kg/week) which do not reduce prolactin receptor levels are effective in converting the tumour to a lactation-like morphology (Klein and Loizzi, 1977). Hence, the data suggest that the basis of the ovarian-autonomy yet oestrogen-responsiveness and antioestrogen-sensitivity of the R3230AC mammary tumour is likely complex with possibly subtle interrelationships between levels of oestrogen and prolactin receptors and blood levels of these hormones. It is also possible that other hormones, such as insulin (Cohen and Hilf, 1975), which may be involved in growth regulation of breast cancer, may influence the effects of antioestrogens in this tumour.

One hypothesis that has been raised to account for the differences in hormonal dependence of mammary tumours suggests that hormonal dependence is related to the level of hormone receptors in the tumour. Earlier studies have suggested that the markedly lower levels of oestrogen receptor (found by us and McGuire *et al.*, 1971 to be about 20% that of DMBA tumours) and prolactin receptor (found by us and Smith *et al.*, 1976, 1977, to be about 12% that of DMBA tumours) in R3230AC tumours, as compared with the DMBA-induced mammary tumour, may account for the ovarian-autonomy yet oestrogen-responsiveness of this tumour. This concept is also supported by the report of reduced prolactin receptor and oestrogen receptor levels in a hormone-independent transplantable mammary tumour (MTW9) compared with its hormone-dependent counterpart (Costlow *et al.*, 1975). However, even in the DMBA mammary tumour system where prolactin and oestrogen receptor levels are, as a rule, considerably higher than in R3230AC tumours, and where there is generally a good correlation between receptor levels and hormonal responsiveness, absolute correlations between levels of oestrogen and prolactin receptors and hormonal dependence frequently do not occur (DeSombre *et al.*, 1976). In addition, our observations that antioestrogens and oestrogen interact with oestrogen receptors and modulate the subcellular distribution and level of oestrogen receptors in R3230AC tumours, while ovariectomy does not appear to influence these parameters, may explain the oestrogen and antioestrogen sensitivity but ovarian autonomy of this tumour.

Since human breast cancers cover a broad spectrum in terms of their hormonal dependence, the DMBA and R3230AC mammary tumour systems appear to represent at least 3 portions of the spectrum: (1) ovarian-dependent tumours which are effectively regressed by antioestrogens; (2) ovarian-independent tumours (such as some DMBA tumours, Tsai *et al.*, 1979) which are largely unresponsive to antioestrogens; and (3) ovarian-independent tumours (such as the R3230AC tumour) whose growth is depressed by antioestrogens. It is possible that tumours of class 3, represented by the R3230AC tumour model, may derive some palliative benefit from anti-oestrogen treatment despite a lack of responsiveness to endocrine ablative therapy.

ACKNOWLEDGEMENTS

We are grateful to Dr Bogden of the Mason Research Institute for supplying us with donor rats bearing R3230AC tumours, to Drs Janice Bahr and Victor Ramirez for assistance with oestradiol and prolactin radio-immunoassays, to the Parke-Davis and Upjohn Companies for providing us with antioestrogens, and to the Upjohn Company for the supply of DMBA emulsions. We also thank the NIAMDD Hormone Distribution program for providing us with ovine prolactin.

The studies reported in this chapter were supported in part by NIH grants USPHS CA18119 (to B.S.K.) and HD07028 (postdoctoral traineeship, E.A.R.).

REFERENCES

Bloom, H. J. G., and Boesen, E. (1974). *British Med. J.* **2**, 7–10.

Cohen, N. D., and Hilf, R. (1975). *Cancer Res.* **35**, 560–567.

Costlow, M. E., Buschow, R. A., Richert, N. J., and McGuire, W. L. (1975). *Cancer Res.* **35**, 970–974.

DeSombre, E. R., and Arbogast, L. Y. (1974). *Cancer Res.* **34**, 1971–1976.

DeSombre, E. R., Kledzik, G., Marshall, S., and Meites, J. (1976). *Cancer Res.* **36**, 354–358.

Ferguson, E. R., and Katzenellenbogen, B. S. (1977). *Endocrinology* **100**, 1242–1251.

Heuson, J. C., Waelbroeck, C., Legros, N., Gallez, G., Robyn, C., and L'Hermite, M. (1971). *Gynecol. Invest.* **2**, 130–137.

Heuson, J. C., Engelsman, E., Blonk-Vander Wijst, J., Maass, H., Drochmans, A., Michel, J., Nowakowski, H., and Gorins, A. (1975). *British Med. J.* **2**, 711–713.

Hilf, R., Michel, I., Bell, J. J., and Borman, A. (1965). *Cancer Res.* **25**, 286–299.

Horwitz, K. B., and McGuire, W. L. (1978). *In* "Breast Cancer 2 — Advances in Research and Treatment" (W. L. McGuire, ed.), pp. 155–204. Plenum Press, New York.

Jordan, V. C. (1976). *Eur. J. Cancer* **11**, 419–424.

Katzenellenbogen, B. S., Tsai, T. L., Rorke, E., and Rutledge, S. (1979). *Proceedings 61st Annual Endocrine Society Meeting,* Abstract 296, p. 146.

Kelly, P. A., Asselin, J., Caron, M. G., Raynaud, J. P., and Labrie, F. (1977). *Cancer Res.* **37**, 76–81.

Kledzik, G. S., Bradley, C. J., Marshall, S., Campbell, G. A., and Meites, J. (1976). *Cancer Res.* **36**, 3265–3268.

Klein, D. M., and Loizzi, R. F. (1977). *J. Natl Cancer Inst.* **48**, 813–818.

Leung, B. S., Sasaki, G. H., and Leung, J. S. (1975). *Cancer Res.* **35**, 621–627.

McGuire, W. L., Julian, J. A., and Chamness, G. C. (1971). *Endocrinology* **89**, 969–973.

Mobbs, B. G. (1966). *J. Endocr.* **36**, 409–414.

Rorke, E. A., and Katzenellenbogen, B. S. (1980). *Cancer Res.* **40**, 3158–3162.

Smith, R. D., Hilf, R., and Senior, A. E. (1976). *Cancer Res.* **36**, 3726–3731.

Smith, R. D., Hilf, R., and Senior, A. E. (1977). *Cancer Res.* **37**, 595–598.

Tsai, T. L. S., and Katzenellenbogen, B. S. (1977). *Cancer Res.* **37**, 1537–1543.

Tsai, T. L. S., Rutledge, S., and Katzenellenbogen, B. S. (1979). *Cancer Res.* **39**, 5043–5050.

Wittliff, J. L., Gardner, D. G., Battema, W. L., and Gilbert, P. J. (1972). *Biochem. Biophys. Res. Commun.* **48**, 119–125.

19

Binding of Non-Steroidal Antioestrogens to Saturable Binding Sites Distinct from the Oestrogen Receptor in Normal and Neoplastic Tissues

L. C. MURPHY, M. S. FOO, M. D. GREEN, B. K. MILTHORPE, A. M. WHYBOURNE, Z. S. KROZOWSKI AND R. L. SUTHERLAND

I. INTRODUCTION

The molecular mechanisms by which synthetic non-steroidal antioestrogens antagonize the effects of oestrogens at the target tissue level have yet to be fully elucidated. There are, however, many studies which indicate that these drugs mediate their effects, at least in part, through the specific oestrogen receptor protein of oestrogen target tissues. This hypothesis was derived to some extent from experiments which demonstrated that unlabelled antioestrogens could inhibit the binding of tritiated oestradiol to its saturable

NON-STEROIDAL ANTIOESTROGENS
ISBN 0 12 677880 9

binding sites in the cytosol of several oestrogen target tissues, supplying strong circumstantial evidence that these compounds bind to the oestrogen binding site of the oestrogen receptor protein (Korenman, 1970; Skidmore *et al.*, 1972; Lippman *et al.*, 1976; Horwitz and McGuire, 1978; Jordan *et al.*, 1978; Sutherland and Foo, 1979). More direct evidence to support this concept has come from binding studies with tritiated CI 628 and tamoxifen. These recent studies illustrated that, in the rat uterus and DMBA-induced rat mammary carcinoma, oestradiol and antioestrogens were bound to approximately the same number of saturable binding sites. Moreover, both groups of compounds could completely inhibit the binding of oestrogens and antioestrogens to their saturable binding sites (Katzenellenbogen *et al.*, 1978; Capony and Rochefort, 1978; Nicholson *et al.*, 1979), suggesting that oestrogens and antioestrogens were mutually competitive for the same binding sites.

In a recent publication from this laboratory (Sutherland and Foo, 1979), it was confirmed that tamoxifen, CI 628 and oestradiol were bound to a similar number of saturable binding sites in immature rat uterine cytosol and that oestradiol could completely inhibit the binding of tritiated antioestrogens to their saturable binding sites. Data from similar experiments using chick oviduct cytosol were substantially different. In this tissue cytosol the concentration of saturable binding sites for tamoxifen and CI 628 was three fold greater than that for oestradiol, and high concentrations of oestradiol could only partially inhibit the binding of tritiated antioestrogens to their saturable binding sites (Sutherland and Foo, 1979). Together these data illustrated the presence, in chick oviduct cytosol, of a hitherto undescribed, high affinity, saturable antioestrogen binding site distinct from the oestrogen binding site of the classical oestrogen receptor.

In this chapter we report our successful search for a similar specific antioestrogen binding site in several normal and neoplastic tissues and further documentation of its binding characteristics.

II. ANTIOESTROGEN BINDING TO NORMAL OESTROGEN TARGET TISSUE CYTOSOL

The experimental data which illustrate the existence of the novel antioestrogen binding site have been derived from two types of experiments, viz. direct saturation analysis using tritiated antioestrogens (CI 628 and tamoxifen) and increasing concentrations of the same ligand, and competition experiments in which series of steroidal and non-steroidal compounds were tested for their ability to compete with tritiated antioestrogen for its saturable binding sites.

A. Direct Binding Studies

In these studies, designed to compare the number of saturable binding sites for oestrogens and antioestrogens in a series of oestrogen target tissues, aliquots of cytosol were incubated at 4°C with a fixed concentration of tritiated tamoxifen or CI 628 (1.25 nM) and increasing concentrations of unlabelled ligand in the range 1.25 nM to 2 μM. After 16 hours incubation protein-bound and unbound ligand were separated by charcoal adsorption (0.5% charcoal for 30 minutes at 4°C) and the bound and unbound ligand concentrations calculated. The apparent equilibrium dissociation constants (K_d) and binding site concentrations (C) of the saturable antioestrogen binding sites were calculated from measured bound and unbound ligand concentrations by a previously described non-linear regression analysis technique (Sutherland and Simpson-Morgan, 1975).

Typical data from these direct binding studies are illustrated in Figure 1 where they are presented as Scatchard plots. Binding curves for three oestrogen target tissues (human endometrium, rat liver and mature rat uterus) and one non-target tissue (chicken skeletal muscle) are shown. The Scatchard plots for the three oestrogen target tissues were curvilinear (Fig. 1) but could be readily resolved into a high affinity saturable binding component and non-specific binding using either the computer assisted non-linear regression technique of Sutherland and Simpson-Morgan (1975) or a graphical analysis as described by Chamness and McGuire (1976). Results using this latter technique are presented in Chapter 12 for CI 628 binding to chick oviduct cytosol. There was no saturable antioestrogen binding site in the skeletal muscle cytosol.

Table I summarizes the apparent affinities and concentrations of saturable binding sites for oestradiol and tamoxifen in eight different oestrogen target tissue cytosols. With the exception of the immature rat uterus all target tissues contained a significantly greater number of saturable antioestrogen binding sites than could be accounted for by the binding of antioestrogens to the oestrogen receptor alone. It should be remembered that the values for the antioestrogen binding parameters include the binding of antioestrogen to the oestrogen receptor as well as the specific antioestrogen binding site. For this reason only first approximations of the true K_d values for tamoxifen binding to the specific antioestrogen binding site can be obtained from the apparent K_d values reported in Table I.

B. Competition Studies

In these experiments, designed to test the ability of oestradiol to inhibit the binding of tritiated antioestrogen to its saturable binding sites, aliquots of

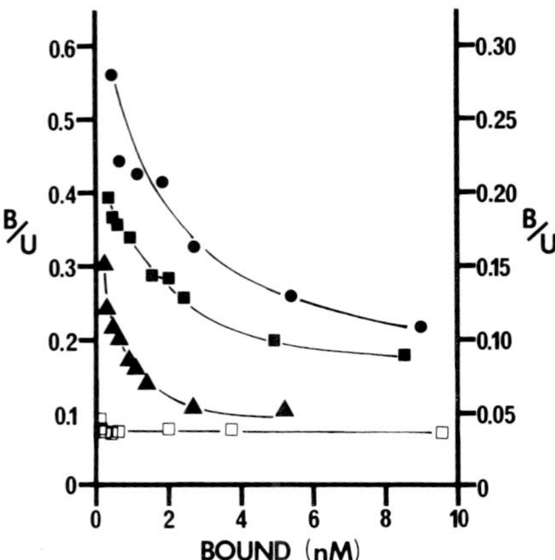

Fig. 1. Scatchard plots of antioestrogen binding to human endometrium, rat liver, mature rat uterus and chick muscle cytosol. All tissues were homogenized with a Polytron and/or teflon-glass tissue grinder, in 10–25 volumes (w/v) of 10 mM Tris-HCl buffer, pH 7.4, containing 1.5 mM EDTA and 0.5 mM dithiothreitol. A high speed cytosol was prepared. Saturation analysis was performed as described in the text. CI 628 binding to human endometrium cytosol (●); CI 628 binding to rat liver cytosol (■); tamoxifen binding to mature rat uterine cytosol (▲); tamoxifen binding to chick skeletal muscle cytosol (□). The scale of the left hand ordinate applies to human endometrium only. From Sutherland *et al.* (1980).

cytosol were incubated for 16 hours at 4°C with 1.25 nM tritiated antioestrogen (CI 628 or tamoxifen) and increasing concentrations of unlabelled oestradiol or antioestrogen. Protein-bound radioactivity was assessed at various ligand concentrations by charcoal adsorption. Data from four different tissues, human endometrium, chick oviduct, mature rat uterus and chick skeletal muscle, are illustrated in Figure 2 where it can be seen that the degree of inhibition of tritiated antioestrogen binding induced by oestradiol varies appreciably with the tissue under study. In the immature rat uterus, oestradiol can completely inhibit saturable antioestrogen binding (Capony and Rochefort, 1978; Katzenellenbogen *et al.*, 1978; Sutherland and Foo, 1979), while in the mature rat uterus and chicken oviduct partial inhibition by oestrogen occurs (Fig. 2). Interestingly, in human endometrial cytosol, oestradiol was unable to cause any inhibition of antioestrogen binding. These results can probably be explained by the relative affinities and concentrations of oestrogen and antioestrogen binding sites in individual cytosols. These binding parameters will govern the amount of tritiated antioestrogen bound to the oestrogen receptor and thus the proportion of the label that can be displaced by oestradiol.

TABLE I

Binding Parameters for the Interactions between Oestradiol, Tamoxifen and Cytosol from Eight Oestrogen Target Tissues[a]

Tissue	Oestradiol		Tamoxifen		Tamoxifen/Oestradiol	
	K_d (nM)	C (nM)	K_d (nM)	C (nM)	K_d (nM)	C (nM)
Rat uterus (immature)	0.17	0.99	2.54	1.08	14.9	1.09
Rat uterus (mature)	0.24	0.13	4.11	0.56	17.1	4.30
Rat liver	0.46	0.28	4.06	1.74	8.8	6.15
Rat kidney	0.14	0.12	3.25	1.76	23.2	6.20
Chick oviduct	0.07	0.19	9.82	0.66	140.3	3.47
Chick liver	0.93	0.11	3.62	0.50	3.9	4.55
Human endometrium	0.52	0.21	3.43	0.74	6.7	3.45
Human mammary carcinoma (ER+)	0.18	0.17	6.04	1.47	33.6	8.65

[a] The experimental procedures are described in the text. The binding site concentration (C) is expressed as nmoles of oestradiol or tamoxifen specifically bound per litre of the reaction mixture which is a 2 fold dilution of the cytosol. The data represent the means of estimates on 2–10 different cytosol preparations. From Sutherland *et al.* (1980).

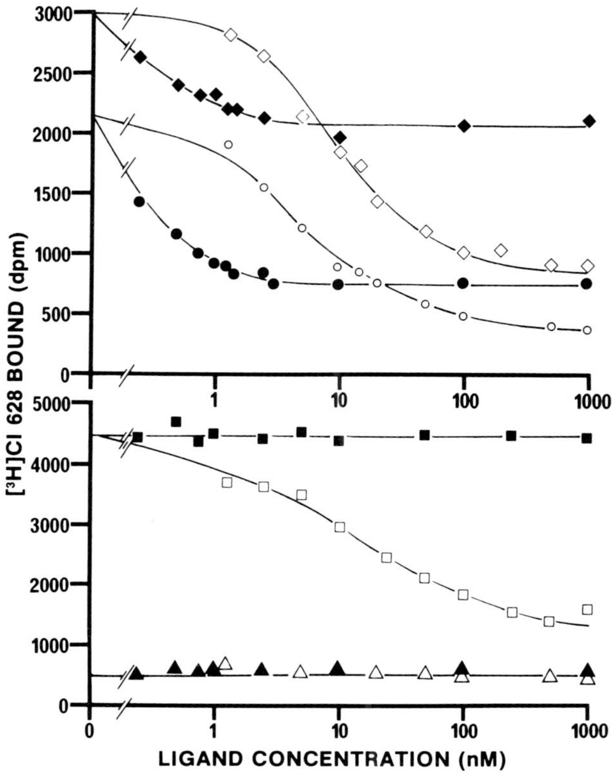

Fig. 2. Competition of oestradiol and CI 628 for antioestrogen binding sites in chick oviduct, mature rat uterus, human endometrium and chick muscle cytosol. Aliquots of cytosol were incubated for 16 hours at 4°C with 1.25 nM tritiated CI 628 and increasing concentrations of unlabelled oestradiol or CI 628. Protein-bound radioactivity was separated by charcoal adsorption and the data plotted as dpm tritiated CI 628 bound versus log of the added ligand concentration. Results for chick oviduct (diamonds), rat uterus (circles), human endometrium (squares) and chick skeletal muscle cytosols (triangles) are illustrated. Tritiated CI 628 binding in the presence of oestradiol and CI 628 are represented by solid and open symbols respectively. From Sutherland *et al.* (1980).

III. ANTIOESTROGEN BINDING TO IMMATURE RAT UTERINE CYTOSOL FOLLOWING RECEPTOR TRANSLOCATION

Since the immature rat uterus was the only oestrogen target tissue studied which did not appear to possess an antioestrogen binding site distinct from the oestrogen receptor (Table I; Sutherland and Foo, 1979) further experiments were conducted in an attempt to locate such a site in this tissue. It appeared likely that, if a specific antioestrogen site was present, it would be masked by the significantly higher oestradiol binding capacity of immature rat uterine cytosol, seen under the present experimental conditions (Table I). To overcome this problem cytoplasmic oestrogen receptor levels were depleted by administering 1.0 μg oestradiol to immature Hooded rats (21–23 days) one hour before sacrifice (Mester and Baulieu, 1975). As can be seen in Table II treatment with this dose of oestradiol resulted in a depletion of cytoplasmic oestrogen receptor concentration to about 10% of pre-injection levels. In addition the antioestrogen was now bound to a significantly greater number of saturable binding sites than could be accounted for by the residual oestrogen receptor (Table II). When this residual oestrogen receptor binding was completely obliterated by saturating the cytosol with 6 μM oestradiol *in vitro*, the antioestrogen was still able to bind to a high affinity, saturable binding site (Fig. 3, Table II). The presence of the specific antioestrogen binding site was confirmed in competition studies which illustrated that, while oestradiol could completely inhibit antioestrogen binding in normal rat uterine cytosol, it could only partially inhibit this binding in the oestrogen receptor depleted cytosol (Fig. 4).

TABLE II
Binding Parameters for the Interactions between Oestradiol, CI 628 and Immature Rat Uterine Cytosol before and after Oestrogen Receptor Translocation to the Nucleus[a]

Experimental conditions	Oestradiol		CI 628	
	K_d (nM)	C (nM)	K_d (nM)	C (nM)
Control	0.40 ± 0.08	1.11 ± 0.11	3.96 ± 0.41	1.40 ± 0.38
Translocated	0.74 ± 0.18	0.14 ± 0.01	2.79 ± 0.62	0.37 ± 0.03
Translocated + 6 μm E_2 *in vitro*	—	—	2.52 ± 0.52	0.26 ± 0.04

[a] The experimental procedures are described in the test. Uteri were homogenized in 15 volumes of buffer, cf. 25 volumes for the uteri in Table I. Binding site concentrations are as in Table I. The data represent the mean ± S.E.M. of 3 experiments per group.

IV. ANTIOESTROGEN BINDING TO HUMAN MAMMARY CARCINOMA CYTOSOL

Although tamoxifen is used clinically in the treatment of human breast cancer, there is little published data on the interactions between tamoxifen and its binding components in cellular extracts of human mammary tumours. In view of the previous finding of a specific, high affinity antioestrogen binding site in normal oestrogen target tissues, we investigated the binding of tritiated tamoxifen to cytosol from oestrogen receptor positive (ER+) and oestrogen receptor negative (ER−) human mammary carcinoma biopsies.

The experimental design was identical to that described in Section II, i.e. saturation analysis and competition studies. The data from these experiments have been described in detail elsewhere (Sutherland and Murphy, 1980). Saturation analysis studies using oestradiol and tamoxifen revealed that both ligands were bound to high affinity, saturable binding sites in ER+ but not ER− tumour cytosols. Replicate estimates of the binding parameters illustrated that the saturable tamoxifen binding sites were present at 8.6 times the concentration of saturable oestradiol binding sites (the cytoplasmic oestrogen receptor) and that the affinity of tamoxifen for its saturable binding site was about 34 fold less than the affinity of oestradiol for the oestrogen receptor (Table III). Non-specific binding of tamoxifen was 2.3 times that of oestradiol measured in the same samples (Table III).

Competition studies employing a fixed amount of tracer oestradiol and increasing concentrations of unlabelled oestradiol or tamoxifen demonstrated that tamoxifen could completely inhibit the binding of [^{3}H]oestradiol to the cytoplasmic oestrogen receptor in ER+ tumours with a mean (± S.E.M.) relative binding affinity 0.87 ± 0.35% that of oestradiol (Fig. 5). Neither

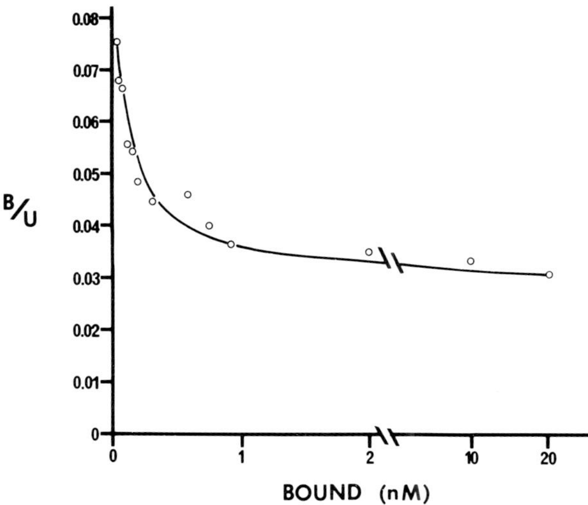

Fig. 3. Scatchard plot of tamoxifen binding to oestrogen receptor depleted immature rat uterine cytosol in the presence of a saturating concentration of oestradiol. Immature Hooded rats (21–23 days) received a single s.c. injection of 1 μg oestradiol in saline, and were sacrificed 1 hour later. Uteri were removed, a cytosol prepared, preincubated with 6 μM oestradiol for 30 minutes at 4°C and binding assays conducted as described in Figure 1.

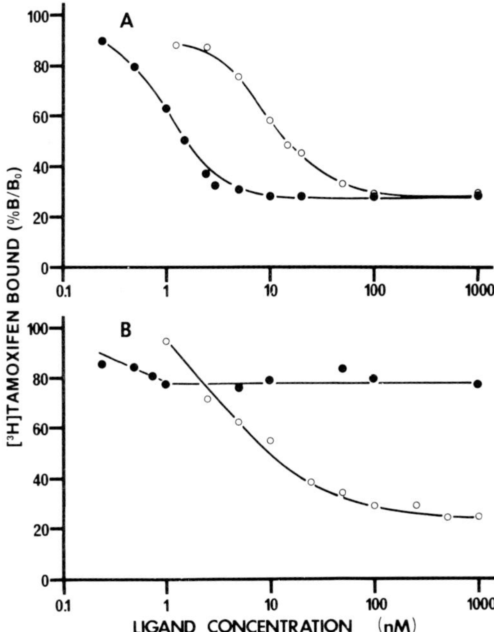

Fig. 4. Competition of oestradiol and tamoxifen for antioestrogen binding sites in immature rat uterine cytosol before and after receptor depletion by a single injection of oestradiol. Rats were treated with oestradiol or saline as described in Figure 3; uterine cytosols were prepared and competition experiments performed as described in Figure 2. Data are presented as percent B/B_O versus log of the added ligand concentration, where B = dpm bound at each level of unlabelled ligand and B_O = dpm bound in the absence of unlabelled ligand. (A) Control cytosol — oestradiol (●), tamoxifen (○). (B) Treated cytosol — oestradiol (●), tamoxifen (○). From Murphy and Sutherland (1981).

TABLE III
Binding Parameters for the Interactions between Oestradiol, Tamoxifen and Human Mammary Carcinoma Cytosols[a]

Ligand	Tissue	K_d (nM)	C (nM)	K_{ns}
Oestradiol	ER+	0.18 ± 0.07	0.17 ± 0.05	0.05 ± 0.01
	ER−	—	—	0.06 ± 0.02
Tamoxifen	ER+	6.0 ± 1.6	1.5 ± 0.5	0.12 ± 0.02
	ER−	—	—	0.14 ± 0.03

[a] The experimental procedures and methods of analysis are described in the text. The binding site concentration (C) is expressed as nmoles of oestradiol or tamoxifen bound per litre of the reaction mixture which is a 2 fold dilution of the cytosol. Non-specific binding, K_{ns}, is a unitless parameter. Data are presented as mean ± S.E.M. of 5 replicates/group. From Sutherland and Murphy (1980).

oestradiol nor tamoxifen could inhibit the binding of [^{3}H]oestradiol to ER – tumour cytosols, confirming the non-specific nature of such binding.

When attempts were then made to inhibit the binding of [^{3}H]tamoxifen to its saturable binding sites with increasing concentrations of oestradiol, no inhibition was observed even when unlabelled oestradiol was present at a 10,000 fold excess over tracer tamoxifen (Fig. 5). This result illustrates that under these *in vitro* assay conditions little or no tracer tamoxifen was bound to the oestrogen receptor and that the saturable antioestrogen binding site does not bind oestradiol.

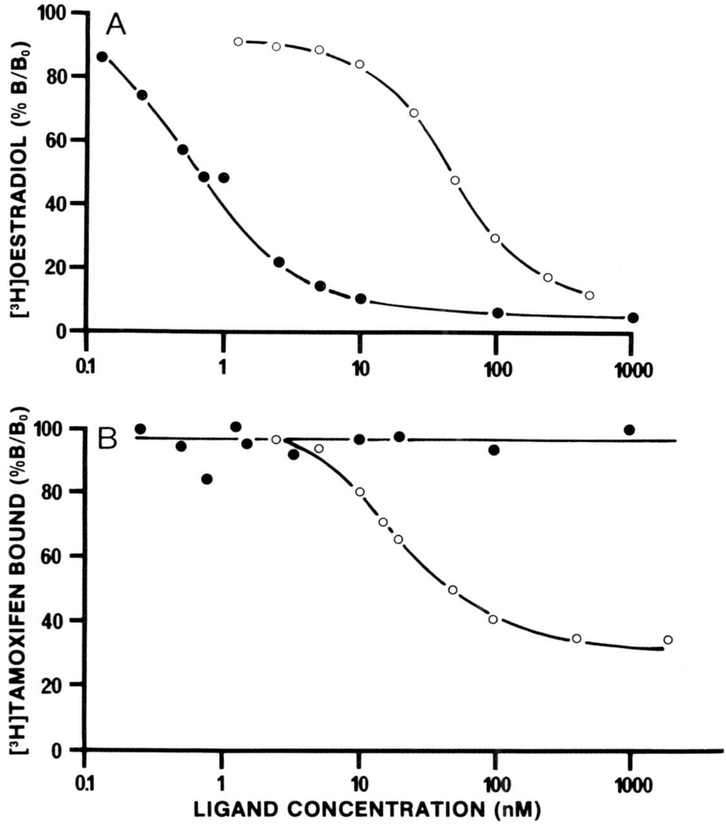

Fig. 5. Competition of oestradiol and tamoxifen for saturable oestrogen and antioestrogen binding sites in human mammary carcinoma cytosol. The experimental procedures were similar to those described in Figure 2 and data presentation as in Figure 4. (A) Oestradiol (●) and tamoxifen (○) inhibition of tritiated oestradiol binding. (B) Oestradiol (●) and tamoxifen (○) inhibition of tritiated tamoxifen binding. From Sutherland and Murphy (1980).

Although these binding data are not incompatible with tamoxifen binding to the oestrogen receptor in human mammary carcinoma *in vivo*, they are at a variance with the recently published data of Nicholson *et al.* (1979). These workers were able to demonstrate that oestradiol and tamoxifen were bound to a similar number of high affinity, saturable binding sites in ER+ human mammary carcinoma cytosol. However, their experiments employed much lower concentrations (0.4–30 nM) of tamoxifen and 5–10 fold higher protein concentrations than we report here. The overall effect of Nicholson's experimental design would be to facilitate estimates of bound and unbound ligand concentrations at much lower degrees of saturation than the experiments described in Table III and Figure 5.

In an attempt to further explain the differences between the results of Nicholson *et al.* (1979) and Sutherland and Murphy (1980) the binding of lower concentrations of [^{3}H]tamoxifen (0.10–1.25 nM) to a tumour cytosol with high concentration of oestrogen receptor (i.e. > 300 fmol/mg protein) was studied. Under these experimental conditions an additional high affinity (K_d = 0.5 nM) antioestrogen binding site was revealed (Fig. 6). This site was present at the same concentration as the oestrogen receptor site, indicating that it probably represented binding of tamoxifen to the classical oestrogen receptor site (Table IV). When the *in vitro* binding assay was conducted on the same material, under the experimental conditions described by Sutherland and Murphy (1980), i.e. 1.25 nM [^{3}H]tamoxifen plus increasing concentrations of unlabelled tamoxifen, similar results to those described in Table III were obtained. Under these conditions a high affinity (K_d = 8 nM) antioestrogen binding site was present in 5 fold excess over the oestrogen receptor (Table IV, Fig. 6).

The binding of tamoxifen to the oestrogen receptor in cytosol from this tumour, containing high concentrations of oestrogen receptor, was further supported by data which illustrated that in this material unlabelled oestradiol could partially inhibit the binding of [^{3}H]tamoxifen to its saturable binding sites in cytosol (Fig. 7).

These data indicate that tamoxifen is bound to three distinct binding components in the cytosol of ER+ human mammary tumours. These binding components are the cytoplasmic oestrogen receptor, the antioestrogen binding site and non-specific binding. Although the affinity is highest for the oestrogen receptor (K_d=0.5 nM), significant amounts of tamoxifen are also bound to the antioestrogen binding site due to its relatively high affinity (K_d =6–8 nM) and the fact that it is present in approximately 8 fold excess over the oestrogen receptor.

The relative distribution of tamoxifen between these three binding components *in vitro* was further studied using a computer simulation technique. In these studies the total concentration of protein-bound

TABLE IV
Binding Parameters for the Interactions between Oestradiol, Tamoxifen and a Human Mammary Carcinoma Cytosol at Low (0.10 nM) and High (1.25 nM) Initial Tamoxifen Concentrations[a]

Ligand	Ligand range (nM)	K_d (nM)	C (nM)
Oestradiol	0.28– 100	0.08	0.21
Tamoxifen	0.10–1,000	0.45	0.19
Tamoxifen	1.25–1,000	7.97	0.99

[a] The experimental conditions are described in the legend to Figure 6.

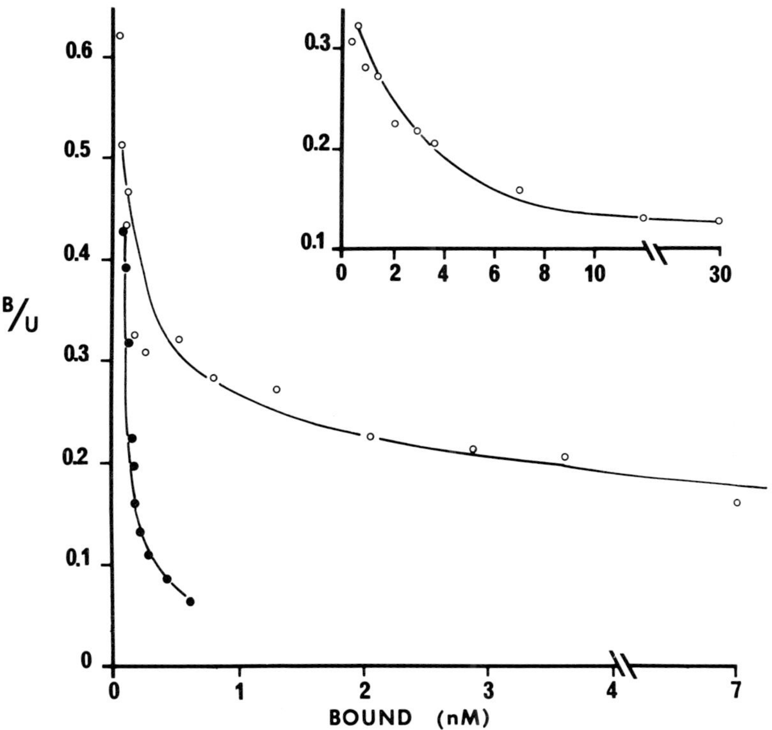

Fig. 6. Scatchard plots of oestradiol and tamoxifen binding to cytosol from a human mammary carcinoma with a high oestrogen receptor concentration, i.e. > 300 fmol/mg protein. Saturation analysis was performed at 4°C by incubating 100 μl of cytosol (protein concentration = 1.95 mg/ml) with increasing concentrations of oestradiol or tamoxifen. Both labelled and unlabelled ligand were used to cover the appropriate concentration ranges which were 0.28–100 nM for oestradiol and 0.10 nM–1 μM for tamoxifen. After 16 hours incubation protein-bound and unbound ligand were separated by charcoal adsorption (0.5 % charcoal for 30 minutes at 4°C)

tamoxifen, [B], was calculated from nominated unbound tamoxifen concentrations, [U], according to the formula:

$$[B] = \frac{C_1 [U]}{(K_1 + [U])} + \frac{C_2 [U]}{(K_2 + [U])} + K_{ns} [U] \quad (1)$$

where K_1 and K_2 are the apparent equilibrium dissociation constants for the oestrogen receptor and antioestrogen binding site, respectively, and C_1 and C_2 are the concentrations of these two sites. K_{ns} is the non-specific binding parameter. The contribution of each binding component to the total amount of tamoxifen bound was calculated according to the following equations:

$$[B_1] = \frac{C_1 [U]}{(K_1 + [U])} \quad (2)$$

$$[B_2] = \frac{C_2 [U]}{(K_2 + [U])} \quad (3)$$

$$[B_3] = K_{ns} [U] \quad (4)$$

where B_1, B_2 and B_3 are the oestrogen receptor (Binding Site 1), the antioestrogen binding site (Binding Site 2) and non-specific binding components (Non-specific), respectively.

Two separate simulation studies are illustrated in Figure 8. The values for the binding parameters used to obtain the curves presented in Figure 8A are taken from the data presented in Table IV, and those for Figure 8B are taken from Table III. Since the data in Table III did not include an estimate of the affinity of tamoxifen for the oestrogen receptor, this parameter ($K_1 = 3.7$ nM) was taken from the data of Nicholson *et al.* (1979). The distribution of tamoxifen between the various binding components was markedly different in the two studies presented with the major difference being that, at low total tamoxifen concentrations, significantly more tamoxifen was bound to the oestrogen receptor in Figure 8A. When the proportion of tamoxifen bound to the oestrogen receptor was calculated at a total tamoxifen concentration of 1.25 nM (i.e. the concentration of tracer tamoxifen used in our competition studies), it was found that approximately 30% of the tamoxifen was bound to the oestrogen receptor in Figure 8A and approximately 7% in Figure 8B. This probably explains why we were able to detect significant displacement of [^{3}H]tamoxifen with oestradiol in Figure 7, where a cytosol preparation with

---

and the bound and unbound ligand concentrations calculated. The tamoxifen binding curve derived from the same cytosol but using the experimental conditions described by Sutherland and Murphy (1980), i.e. 1.25 nM [^{3}H]tamoxifen plus increasing concentrations of unlabelled tamoxifen is shown in the inset. The apparent equilibrium dissociation constants and binding site concentrations were calculated for each binding curve as described in the text and are summarized in Table IV.

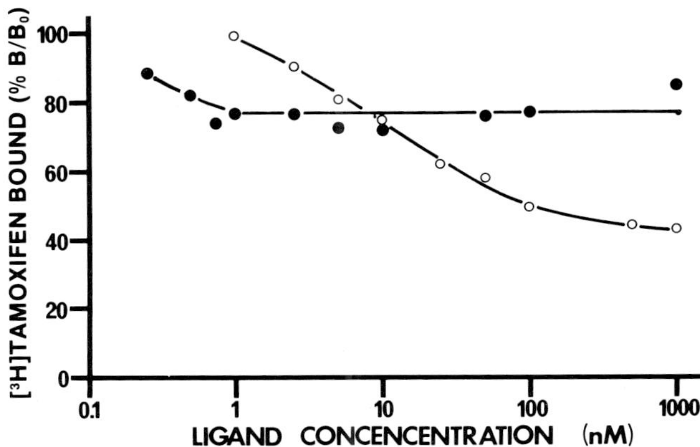

Fig. 7. Competition of oestradiol and tamoxifen for antioestrogen binding sites in the same human mammary carcinoma cytosol depicted in Figure 6. Experimental conditions were as described in Figure 2 while data are plotted as in Figure 4. Oestradiol (●), tamoxifen (○).

the binding properties recorded in Table IV and simulated in Figure 8A was used, but not in Figure 5, where a cytosol with the binding properties reported in Table III and Figure 8B was employed. It is worth noting that in the competition experiments illustrated in Figures 5 and 7 the degree of inhibition of [^{3}H]tamoxifen binding by oestradiol was somewhat less than predicted by the simulation studies (i.e. less than 5% in Fig. 5 and approximately 20% in Fig. 7). This may be due to an underestimation of the apparent equilibrium dissociation constant for the antioestrogen binding site in these studies.

V. LIGAND SPECIFICITY OF THE HIGH AFFINITY ANTIOESTROGEN BINDING SITE

Further experiments were conducted to assess the ligand specificity of the antioestrogen binding site. In these experiments cytosols from the MCF 7 and T 47D human mammary carcinoma cell lines were used. These cells were cultured in the presence of oestrogen (i.e. 10% foetal calf serum) which depleted cytoplasmic oestrogen receptor levels and thus elevated the concentration of antioestrogen binding sites relative to oestrogen receptor sites. As a result an insignificant amount of the 1.25 nM tritiated CI 628 was bound to the oestrogen receptor under the experimental conditions described in Figures 9–11 and therefore the competition curves represent the inhibition of tritiated CI 628 binding to the antioestrogen binding site alone. A series of structurally related synthetic non-steroidal antioestrogens (tamoxifen, CI

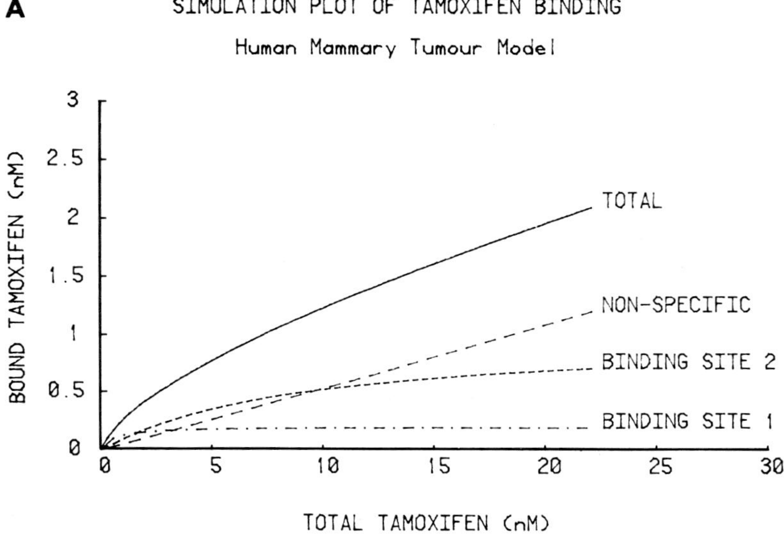

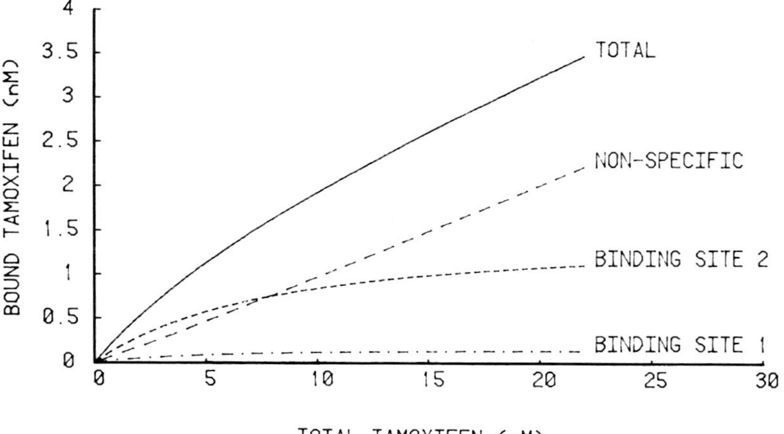

Fig. 8. Computer simulation studies of the distribution of tamoxifen between the oestrogen receptor (Binding Site 1), the antioestrogen binding site (Binding Site 2) and non-specific binding components in human mammary carcinoma cytosol at varying tamoxifen concentrations. The simulation studies were conducted as described in the text using the following binding parameters:

(A) $K_1 = 0.45$ nM, $C_1 = 0.19$ nM, $K_2 = 7.97$ nM, $C_2 = 0.99$ nM and $K_{ns} = 0.06$.

(B) $K_1 = 3.70$ nM, $C_1 = 0.17$ nM, $K_2 = 6.04$ nM, $C_2 = 1.47$ nM and $K_{ns} = 0.12$.

628, CI 680, nafoxidine and clomiphene) was capable of inhibiting the binding of tritiated CI 628 to its saturable binding sites (Figs 9 and 10). By contrast, a series of natural and synthetic oestrogens (oestrone, oestradiol, oestriol, diethystilboestrol), androgens (testosterone, 5α-dihydrotestosterone, R 1881) and progestins (progesterone, R5020) was incapable of inducing inhibition (Fig. 9), indicating that the high affinity antioestrogen binding site was not a sex steroid hormone receptor.

The effect of geometric isomerism was next investigated. We have previously demonstrated that the *cis*-isomers of tamoxifen (ICI 47,699) and clomiphene (zuclomiphene) have an affinity for the oestrogen receptor which is 5–10 % that of the corresponding *trans*-isomers (Sutherland and Foo, 1981). The binding of the same four compounds, tamoxifen, ICI 47,699, enclomiphene and zuclomiphene, to the antioestrogen binding site is presented in Figure 10. These data illustrate that the structural requirements for binding to the antioestrogen binding site are markedly different from those required for binding to the oestrogen receptor. Although the *cis*-isomers were again bound with lower affinity than the corresponding *trans*-isomers, their relative potencies were significantly greater, i.e. zuclomiphene had 75 % of the activity of enclomiphene while ICI 47,699 had 40 % of the potency of tamoxifen.

The major metabolites of tamoxifen in the human are 4-hydroxytamoxifen and N-desmethyltamoxifen (Fromson *et al.*, 1973; Adam *et al.*,

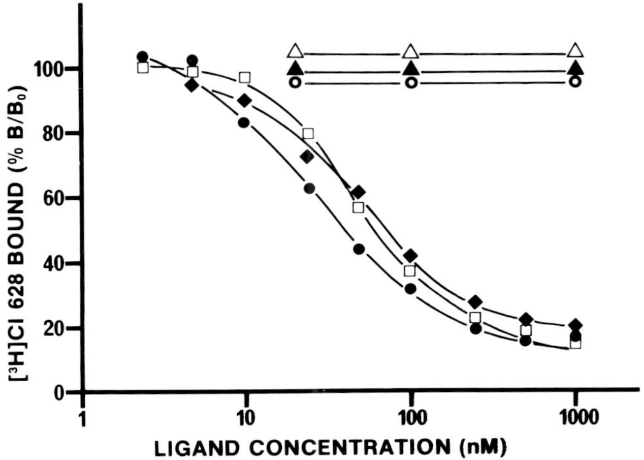

Fig. 9. Specificity of the saturable antioestrogen binding site in MCF 7 human mammary carcinoma cell cytosol. The experiments were performed as described in Figure 2 and the data presented as in Figure 4. Inhibition of [^{3}H]CI 628 binding by tamoxifen (●), CI 628 (□), and nafoxidine (◆); and a series of natural and synthetic oestrogens (▲), androgens (○), and progestins (△) described in the text. From Sutherland *et al.* (1980).

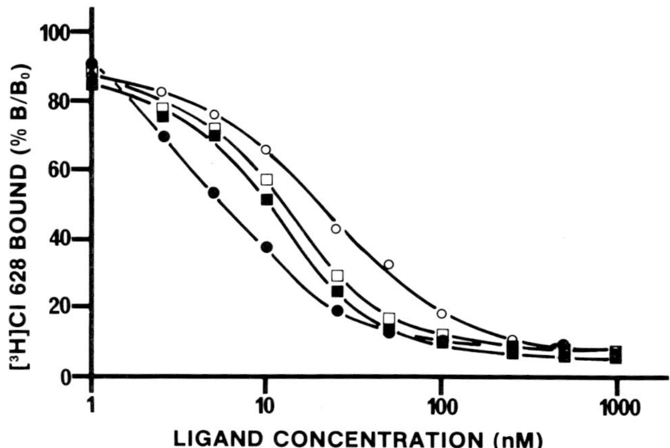

Fig. 10. Influence of the *cis*- and *trans*- configuration on the affinity of two triphenylethylene derivatives for the saturable antioestrogen binding site in MCF 7 cell cytosol. The experiments were performed as described in Figure 2 and the data presented as in Figure 4. Inhibition of [^{3}H]Cl 628 binding by enclomiphene (■), zuclomiphene (□), tamoxifen (●) and ICI 47,699 (○).

1979; Daniel et al., 1979). Studies on the binding of these metabolites to oestrogen receptor sites have demonstrated that the 4-hydroxylation markedly increased the affinity of the compound for the oestrogen receptor, while demethylation in the alkylaminoethoxy side chain had little effect on the binding to receptor (Jordan *et al.*, 1977; Binart *et al.*, 1979; Wakeling and Slater, 1980; Sutherland and Whybourne, 1981). The situation was markedly different when the binding of these three compounds to the antioestrogen binding site was investigated. Monohydroxytamoxifen and tamoxifen had similar affinities for this site, while the desmethyl derivative had only about 30% of the potency of these two compounds (Fig. 11). This adds further support to the idea that the structural requirements for binding to the oestrogen receptor and antioestrogen binding site are markedly different.

VI. DISCUSSION

The data presented herein, which demonstrate an excess of high affinity, saturable antioestrogen binding sites over oestrogen receptor sites in a number of oestrogen target tissues (Table I and II), and the inability of oestradiol to compete for all these sites (Figs 2, 4, 5, 7 and 9), supply strong evidence for the existence of a high affinity antioestrogen binding site in oestrogen target tissues. The site has a high affinity ($K_d \simeq$ 2–10 nM) for CI 628

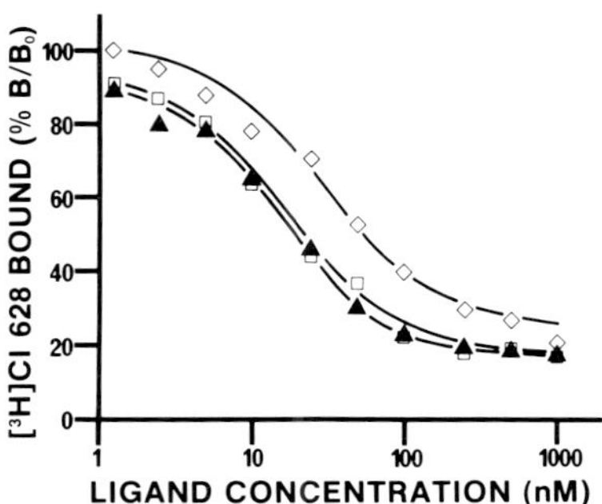

Fig. 11. Binding of tamoxifen and its metabolites 4-hydroxytamoxifen and N-desmethyltamoxifen to the antioestrogen binding site. The experiments were performed as described in Figure 2 using cytosol from the T 47D human mammary carcinoma cell line. Inhibition of [^{3}H]Cl 628 binding by tamoxifen (▲), 4-hydroxytamoxifen (□) and N-desmethyltamoxifen (◇).

and tamoxifen and is saturable at nanomolar concentrations of the drugs. Such concentrations are readily attained in the plasma, and presumably the cellular and extracellular fluid, of humans receiving tamoxifen chronically (Daniel *et al.*, 1979; Adam *et al.*, 1980). This intracellular binding site shows a surprising degree of ligand specificity since it binds a series of structurally related synthetic non-steroidal antioestrogens but does not bind a number of natural and synthetic oestrogens, androgens and progestins (Fig. 9) indicating that it is not one of the common steroid hormone receptor sites. In addition, the structural requirements for the binding of non-steroidal antioestrogens to this site are markedly different from those for binding to the oestrogen receptor (Figs 10 and 11). There is also an indication of tissue specificity for this site as it was present in all oestrogen target tissues studied but was absent from oestrogen receptor negative human mammary carcinoma biopsies, rat plasma and chick skeletal muscle (Figs 1 and 2, Table III). However, at this stage insufficient non-target tissues for oestrogen have been studied in detail to confirm that the antioestrogen binding site is confined to oestrogen target tissues.

It is important to give some consideration to why previous experimentation did not reveal this specific antioestrogen binding site and why the early data from this laboratory (Sutherland and Murphy, 1980) appears to be at variance with other published data (Nicholson *et al.*, 1979; Rochefort *et al.*, 1981). Most of the anomalies that have occurred can be attributed entirely to experimental design. In the first instance the early direct binding studies using tritiated antioestrogens employed rat uterine cytosol as the source of binding sites (Katzenellenbogen *et al.*, 1978; Capony and Rochefort, 1978). This tissue is rich in oestrogen receptor and for this reason almost all the tritiated antioestrogen is bound to the oestrogen receptor at the expense of other sites. Interestingly, had the same experimental design been applied to other oestrogen target tissues with relatively less receptor and a higher anti-oestrogen binding site to oestrogen receptor concentration ratio the results would have been different and the antioestrogen binding site revealed. When the oestrogen receptor content of rat uterine cytosol was selectively depleted by translocation of the cytoplasmic receptor to the nucleus, and a concommitant decrease in the oestrogen receptor to antioestrogen binding site concentration ratio, results similar to those seen with other oestrogen target tissue cytosols became apparent (Fig. 3, Table II). Similar arguments apply to the data of Rochefort *et al.* (1981) where MCF 7 cell cytosol was used. Again this tissue cytosol is rich in oestrogen receptor when the cells are grown in charcoal stripped foetal calf serum, and if the cytosol protein concentration is high, the majority of antioestrogen will be bound to the oestrogen receptor thus reducing the likelihood of revealing the antioestrogen binding site. When these cells are grown in the continuous presence of oestrogen (i.e. 10% foetal calf serum), the cytoplasmic oestrogen receptor level is depleted, the oestrogen receptor to antioestrogen binding site concentration ratio is decreased, and results similar to those seen with ER+ human mammary tumour biopsies are observed (Murphy and Sutherland, unpublished observation).

We have gone to some length to explain the differences between our data and those of Nicholson *et al.* (1979) and these experiments have been summarized in Figures 5–8 and Tables III and IV. Clearly, these data illustrate that antioestrogens bind to three cellular components *in vitro*, i.e. the oestrogen receptor, the antioestrogen binding site and non-specific binding components. The relative contribution of each of these binding components to the overall binding of antioestrogens *in vitro* will depend on their concentration ratios in the materials under study and the *in vitro* conditions under which the binding assays are performed.

Although the presence of a specific antioestrogen binding site distinct from the oestrogen receptor has only been revealed by the use of tritiated antioestrogens, earlier experimental data may support the existence of such a site. In these earlier relative binding studies tamoxifen was shown to inhibit the binding of tritiated oestradiol to the oestrogen receptor of human mammary carcinoma cytosol in a dose-dependent manner but with an affinity considerably lower than that of oestradiol, i.e. in the range 0.4–1.0% that of oestradiol (Hahnel *et al.*, 1973; Powell-Jones *et al.*, 1978; Lippman *et al.*, 1976; Tanaka *et al.*, 1978). Such estimates of the relative binding affinity of tamoxifen for the oestrogen receptor are significantly lower than those found in some other oestrogen target tissues. For example, studies carried out under identical assay conditions in this laboratory have yielded estimates for the relative binding affinities of tamoxifen in rat uterus, chick oviduct, and human mammary carcinoma cytosols of 13, 5, and 0.9%, respectively (Sutherland and Foo, 1981). These differences could be due to a number of factors including tissue and species differences in the structure and specificity of the oestrogen binding site, different degrees of tamoxifen degradation and metabolism *in vitro* in different tissue cytosols, different ratios of receptor binding to non-specific binding in different tissues, and the presence of additional tamoxifen binding components which reduce the availability of tamoxifen for binding to the classical oestrogen receptor site. It is the latter possibility which we favour since the relative binding affinities of tamoxifen for the oestrogen receptor in these three tissue cytosols is highly correlated with the concentration ratios of the oestrogen receptor and antioestrogen binding site, i.e. a low relative binding affinity is accompanied by a high antioestrogen binding site to oestrogen receptor concentration ratio (Table I).

In conclusion, we have described the binding properties of a specific, high affinity, saturable cytoplasmic binding site for the synthetic non-steroidal antioestrogens. To date we have no data that indicate a specific role for this site in mediating the effects of antioestrogen at the target tissue level. The possibility that the antioestrogen binding site has a natural ligand and may be involved in mediating the antagonistic effects of the drugs while agonist effects are mediated through the oestrogen receptor are interesting suggestions which warrant further investigation. Even if this site has no direct role in mediating the effect of antioestrogens, its affinity and concentrations are such that it will be responsible for binding a significant proportion of the drug *in vivo* and as a result may regulate the tissue concentrations of the drugs and their metabolites and the amounts of antioestrogen available for binding to the oestrogen receptor.

ACKNOWLEDGEMENTS

We thank ICI, Parke-Davis, Upjohn and Merrell for their kind donations of the antioestrogens used in this study.

REFERENCES

Adam, H. K., Douglas, E. J., and Kemp, J. V. (1979). *Biochem. Pharmacol.* **27**, 145–147.

Adam, H. K., Gay, M. A., and Moore, R. H. (1980). *J. Endocr.* **84**, 35–42.

Binart, N., Catelli, M. G., Geynet, C., Puri, B., Hahnel, R., Mester, J., and Baulieu, E. E. (1979). *Biochem. Biophys. Res. Commun.* **91**, 812–818.

Capony, F., and Rochefort, J. (1978). *Mol. Cell. Endocr.* **11**, 181–198.

Chamness, G. C., and McGuire, W. L. (1976). *Steroids* **26**, 538–542.

Daniel, C. P., Gaskell, S. J., Bishop, H., and Nicholson, R. I. (1979). *J. Endocr.* **83**, 401–408.

Fromson, J. M., Pearson, S., and Bramah, S. (1973). *Xenobiotica* **3**, 711–714.

Hahnel, R., Twaddle, E., and Ratajczah, T. (1973). *J. Steroid Biochem.* **4**, 687–695.

Horwitz, K. B., and McGuire, W. L. (1978). *J. Biol. Chem.* **253**, 8185–8191.

Jordan, V. C., Collins, M. M., Rowsby, L., and Prestwich, G. (1977). *J. Endocr.* **75**, 305–316.

Jordan, V. C., Dix, C. J., Naylor, K. E., Prestwich, F., and Rowsby, L. (1978). *J. Toxicol. Environ. Health* **4**, 363–390.

Katzenellenbogen, B. S., Katzenellenbogen, J. A., Ferguson, E. R., and Krauthammer, N. (1978). *J. Biol. Chem.* **253**, 697–707.

Korenman, S. G. (1970). *Endocrinology* **87**, 1119–1123.

Lippman, M., Bolan, G., Monaco, M., Pinkus, L., and Engel, L. (1976). *J. Steroid Biochem.* **7**, 1045–1051.

Mester, J., and Baulieu, E. E. (1975). *Biochem. J.* **146**, 617–623.

Murphy, L. C., and Sutherland, R. L. (1981). *J. Endocr.* (In Press).

Nicholson, R. I., Syne, J. S., Daniel, C. P., and Griffiths, K. (1979). *Eur. J. Cancer* **15**, 317–329.

Powell-Jones, W., Jenner, D. A., Blumey, R. W., Davies, P., and Griffiths, K. (1975). *Biochem. J.* **150**, 71–75.

Rochefort, J., Borgna, J. L., Coezy, E., Vignon, F., and Westley, B. (1981). This volume. pp. 355–364.

Skidmore, J., Walpole, A. L., and Woodburn, J. (1972). *J. Endocr.* **52**, 289–298.

Sutherland, R. L., and Foo, M. S. (1979). *Biochem. Biophys. Res. Commun.* **91**, 183–191.

Sutherland, R. L., and Foo, M. S. (1981). This volume, pp. 195–214.

Sutherland, R. L., and Murphy, L. C. (1980). *Eur. J. Cancer* **16**, 1141–1148.

Sutherland, R. L., and Simpson-Morgan, M. W. (1975). *J. Endocr.* **65**, 319–332.

Sutherland, R. L., and Whybourne, A. M. (1981). This volume. pp. 75–84

Sutherland, R. L., Murphy, L. C., Foo, M. S., Green, M. D., Whybourne, A. M., and Krozowski, Z. S. (1980). *Nature* **288**, 273–275.

Tanaka, M., Abe, K., Ohnami, S., Adachi, I., Yamaguchi, K., and Miyakawa, S. (1978). *Jap. J. Clin. Oncol.* **8**, 141–148.

Wakeling, A. E., and Slater, S. R. (1980). *Cancer Treat. Rep.* **64**, 741–744.

20

Antioestrogen and Oestrogen Action in Breast Cancer Cells

W. L. McGUIRE, D. P. EDWARDS, D. J. ADAMS AND N. SAVAGE

I. INTRODUCTION

Since the original identification of cytoplasmic oestrogen receptors (ER) in human breast cancer (Jensen *et al.*, 1971; Jensen and DeSombre, 1972), rapid progress has been made towards linking presence of the receptor with endocrine responsiveness of the tumour. It is now known that the likelihood of a successful response to endocrine therapy is increased at least 10-fold in

NON-STEROIDAL ANTIOESTROGENS
ISBN 0 12 677880 9

patients whose tumours are positive for ER (McGuire *et al.*, 1975). However, not all ER-containing tumours respond, and this has led to the concept that ER are necessary but not sufficient markers of hormone dependence.

We have demonstrated progesterone receptors (PgR) in human breast tumours (Horwitz *et al.*, 1975a) and have proposed that this receptor, whose synthesis is known to be controlled by oestrogen in the uterus, might serve as a marker of oestrogen action in breast cancer (Horwitz *et al.*, 1975b). Thus, the presence of PgR in a tumour would indicate that the entire sequence involving oestrogen binding to cytoplasmic receptor, movement of the receptor complex into the nucleus and stimulation of a specific end product can be achieved in the tumour cell, and would rule out the existence of a defect beyond the binding step.

Though this proposal assumes that PgR are under control of oestrogen acting through ER, this priming effect has not been demonstrated in human breast cancer. We have used the MCF 7 human breast cancer cell line to study the response of PgR to oestrogens and antioestrogens. The MCF 7 cell line, derived from a patient with metastatic breast cancer (Soule *et al.*, 1973), is ideally suited to study the mechanism of PgR induction. These cells are in permanent tissue culture, contain oestrogen receptors (Brooks *et al.*, 1973, Horwitz *et al.*, 1975a) and are oestrogen responsive (Lippman *et al.*, 1976). Cells grown without oestradiol have low PgR levels (Horwitz *et al.*, 1975a). This chapter summarizes our recent work in this model system which shows that PgR are under oestrogen control and that PgR synthesis involves the oestrogen receptor. We have also studied the effects of antioestrogens and find that tamoxifen is a potent inducer of progesterone receptor in these cells. This oestrogenic property (Leavitt *et al.*, 1977) of tamoxifen is masked at very high doses (1 μM) which also inhibit cell growth. Another antioestrogen, nafoxidine, has by contrast, little if any effect on PgR when tested over a wide dose range. The fact that growth inhibitory effects of both antioestrogens can be reversed by oestradiol (Lippman *et al.*, 1976) suggests that the effects of these compounds are mediated through the oestrogen receptor system.

Furthermore, we describe (Horwitz and McGuire, 1978a) a complex response system in these cells in which oestrogen receptor binding, translocation and turnover of nuclear receptors or their "processing" mediate induction of PgR by oestradiol. Though antioestrogens can bind and translocate receptor, the subsequent nuclear receptor processing step is partially (tamoxifen) or completely (nafoxidine) impaired. This may explain the differential effect of these two antioestrogens on PgR induction.

Finally, we demonstrate oestrogen stimulation of specific protein synthesis in antioestrogen blocked cells.

II. OESTRADIOL: EFFECTS ON PROGESTERONE RECEPTOR MEDIATED THROUGH THE OESTROGEN RECEPTOR

A. Binding, Translocation and Processing of Oestrogen Receptor

Oestradiol enters the cell and binds to unfilled receptor sites that are found mostly in cytosol (Rc) or that are loosely associated with nuclear components (Rn). The newly formed hormone-receptor complex (RnE) is rapidly translocated to sites in the nucleus from which it can only be extracted with buffers of high ionic strength. Bound nuclear receptors then undergo rapid turnover or "processing"; within 3 to 5 hours, 70% or more of RnE sites are lost from the cells without reappearance of unfilled sites in any compartment. Much later (a period of several days for progesterone receptor induction) we see formation of specific products or effects on growth or DNA synthesis.

The data from an experiment in which we follow these movements and changes in oestrogen receptor levels are shown in Figure 1. The untreated cells (C) have unfilled sites associated with the nucleus (Rn) and the cytoplasm (Rc). There are no filled nuclear sites (RnE). Within 5 minutes of 10^{-8}M oestradiol addition, Rc and Rn are no longer measurable and all cellular receptors appear in the nucleus bound to oestradiol. Starting at about 30 minutes and continuing for 3 to 5 hours we see a progressive loss of RnE. Processing is essentially complete after 5 hours; thereafter RnE levels stabilize at the new steady state level as long as the cells are kept on oestradiol. If the hormone is removed (Horwitz and McGuire, 1978a) there are several effects. The binding of oestradiol as RnE is remarkably prolonged. At least some oestrogen always remains bound to nuclear receptors even 8 days after the hormone has been removed. However, in addition, unfilled cytoplasmic and nuclear sites are restored. Restoration of cellular ER cannot be explained by loss of E from the nuclear receptor followed by redistribution of the newly emptied sites. Instead, both cytoplasmic receptors (Rc) and nuclear receptors (Rn) are clearly being synthesized *de novo*, and this synthesis is reflected in the restoration of total cellular ER.

B. Oestrogen Receptor Processing and Progesterone Receptor Induction

Figure 2 compares the amount of PgR induced. The extent of free receptor binding and processing parallels PgR induction. Induction is incomplete at low doses if receptor binding and processing is incomplete, reaches a maximum at 0.1 nM when RnE processing is maximal, and is not increased further by accumulation of unprocessed RnE. This suggests that processing may be an essential step in induction of a specific protein by

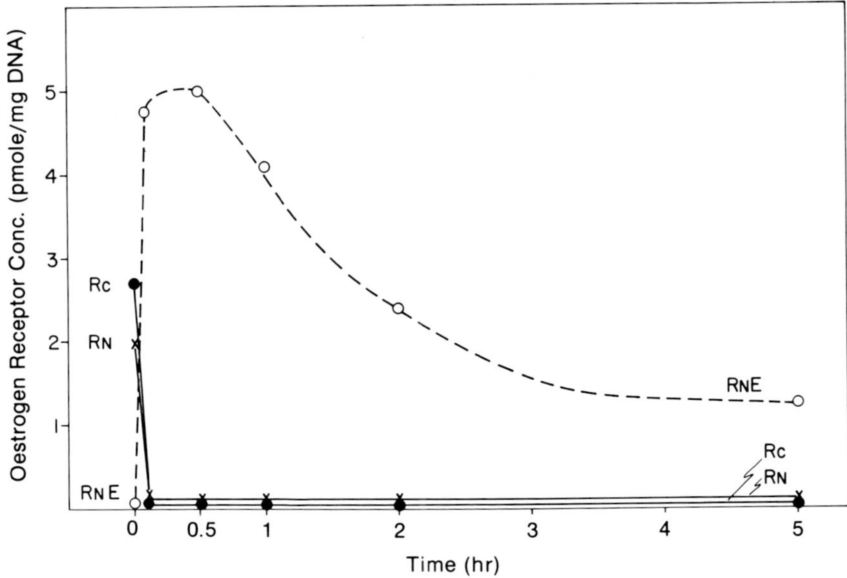

Fig. 1. Effect of oestradiol on oestrogen receptor distribution in MCF 7 cells. Cells were treated for the times indicated with 10 nM oestradiol added to MEM containing stripped calf serum, insulin, hydrocortisone and prolactin. Control flasks received the same medium without oestradiol. Cytoplasmic and nuclear oestrogen receptors were measured by the single saturating dose protamine assay. Values have been corrected for nonspecific binding. Unoccupied cytoplasmic receptors (●, Rc, 4°C incubation), unoccupied nuclear receptors (x, Rn, 4°C incubation), occupied nuclear receptors (○, RnE, 30°C-4°C incubations). Adapted from Horwitz and McGuire (1978c).

oestradiol. However, the nature of processing is unclear. It may be an active state in which a new equilibrium between receptor degradation and synthesis is achieved (Sarff and Gorski, 1971, Williams and Gorski, 1972), or a redistribution of receptor within nuclear binding sites of differing affinities (De Hertogh *et al.*, 1973) or specificities (Schrader *et al.*, 1972), or sequestration of receptor to sites inaccessible to salt extraction (Clark and Peck, 1976, Ruh and Baudendistel, 1977). We will return to these questions later. Regardless, our data would suggest that the processing step is saturable, and that peak activation occurs when RnE processing is maximal.

These studies with cells of human breast cancer origin show that one response to oestradiol treatment is an increase in levels of PgR, as would be predicted from studies of chick oviduct (Sherman *et al.*, 1970), rat uterine PgR priming (Faber *et al.*, 1972), and cyclic changes in PgR levels observed in the

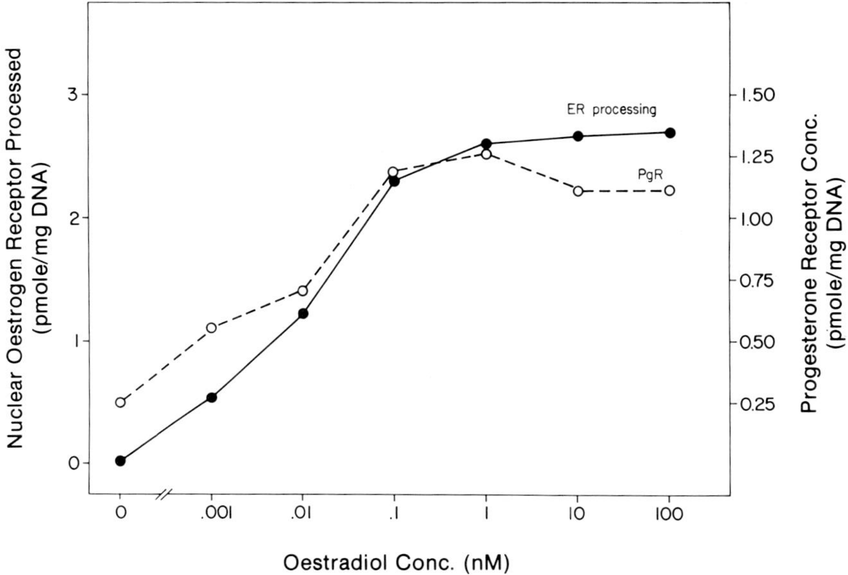

Fig. 2. Comparison of oestrogen receptor processing and progesterone receptor induction. Oestrogen receptor was measured and the amount of oestrogen receptor lost at each dose (control–total) is plotted. Progesterone receptor measured by single saturating dose assay: 200 μl cytosol incubated 4 hours at 4°C, in triplicate, with 20 nM [^{3}H]R 5020 alone or with 100-fold excess R 5020. After 15 minutes incubation with dextran-coated charcoal suspension, cytosols were centrifuged, and aliquots of the supernatant counted to determine bound radioactivity. Data shown are corrected for nonspecific binding. Adapted from Horwitz and McGuire (1978c).

human endometrium (Bayard *et al.*, 1975). Our results clearly show that human breast cells that have undergone malignant transformation can continue to synthesize a specific protein under hormone control. Furthermore, these results lend credence to our hypothesis (Horwitz *et al.*, 1975b) that presence of PgR in biopsies of human breast tumours indicates that *in situ* the tumour was exposed to, and was capable of responding to, circulating oestrogens. Since the tumour, in one instance, has remained hormone responsive, one might suspect that other oestrogen-sensitive effects have also been retained.

Our studies suggest that oestrogen stimulation of PgR involves ER. First, the extent of PgR induction parallels closely both the binding and translocation of Rc and the binding of Rn. Second, PgR induction is correlated with ER processing during oestradiol stimulation.

III. ANTIOESTROGENS: EFFECTS ON PROGESTERONE RECEPTOR AND OESTROGEN RECEPTOR PROCESSING

A. Oestrogen Receptor Compartmentalization and Processing

Tamoxifen (Tam) and nafoxidine (Naf), two non-steroidal anti-oestrogens, are potent growth inhibitors of MCF 7 cells when present in high doses (Lippman *et al.*, 1976, Horwitz *et al.*, 1978). Doses above 50 nM are inhibitory for nafoxidine, above 100 nM are inhibitory for tamoxifen. These effects are probably mediated through the ER system and are not simply toxic effects of the compounds, since they can be reversed by addition of oestradiol at concentrations 100 to 1000-fold lower than the antioestrogen.

With increasing doses of tamoxifen, Rc are progressively depleted. At 100 nM more than 95 % of Rc are translocated. However, total receptor levels fall to only 70 % of control values even at the highest doses. No processing at all is seen with nafoxidine despite complete Rc depletion.

Again, with antioestrogens, as with oestradiol, processing of nuclear receptor parallels PgR induction. Tamoxifen is a potent inducer of PgR. While low doses have only minimal effects at intermediate doses, PgR induction equals or exceeds that obtained with oestradiol. When doses are raised further, PgR levels are suppressed even below control levels. This high tamoxifen dose (1 μM) is markedly antioestrogenic: at this dose, but not at lower doses, we see inhibition of cell growth and eventual cell death. Nafoxidine, in contrast to tamoxifen, has little or no effect on PgR at any dose studied.

These results suggest that in breast cancer cells of human origin, the ER system mediates antioestrogen action. Antioestrogens bind and translocate cytoplasmic ER. In these respects oestrogen antagonists resemble oestradiol. However, the subsequent nuclear processing reactions of oestrogen-bound and antioestrogen-bound receptors are dissimilar. After oestradiol, nuclear hormone-receptor complexes fall rapidly to less than one third of control values. This pathway of receptor processing is either impaired (tamoxifen) or fails entirely (nafoxidine) for the antioestrogen-receptor complex. Our data with antioestrogens would further suggest that processing is an active step in ER function at least in the special case of PgR induction and does not simply serve to return receptor to the cytoplasm.

With oestradiol and tamoxifen, processing of receptor occurs in MCF 7 cells despite the continuous presence of the hormones. This differs from the loss of nuclear ER described in the rat uterus by Giannopoulos and Gorski (1971) and Anderson *et al.*, (1975) following a single pulse of oestradiol. The latter have shown that if oestradiol is administered to the rat so as to maintain elevated blood levels of the hormone, nuclear receptors rise to very high levels.

Thus, significant differences are found in the early nuclear reactions of the oestrogen receptor-hormone complex of human tumour cells compared to the rat uterus, the usual model of oestrogen action. Other tissue differences in mechanisms of ER action have also been reported (Lazier and Alford, 1977, Cidlowski and Muldoon, 1976), suggesting perhaps that studies of oestrogen action in uteri may not be extrapolated to other tissues.

Oestrogenic and antioestrogenic responses in the rat uterus are characterized as early (< 6 hours) or late (24 hours) and different control mechanisms may be required for each (Hardin *et al.*, 1976, Lan and Katzenellenbogen, 1976, Stormshak *et al.*, 1976). Upon initial injection both responses are evoked by antioestrogens (Clark *et al.*, 1974, Katzenellenbogen and Ferguson, 1975, Capony and Rochefort, 1975); however, late responses cannot be elicited either by oestradiol or by antioestrogens if preceded 24 hours by a primary antioestrogen injection (Katzenellenbogen *et al.*, 1977, Ferguson and Katzenellenbogen, 1977). This has led to models of oestrogen action having at least 2 nuclear binding sites for the ER-complex, one of which is accessible to antioestrogen-receptor complexes. These models are further supported by evidence of differential salt extractability of oestrogen-bound and antioestrogen-bound nuclear receptors (Clark and Peck, 1976, Mester and Baulieu, 1975, Juliano and Stancel, 1976, Ruh and Buadendistel, 1977) and by their differential nuclear retention time (Clark *et al.*, 1973). Our data lend support to the concept of dual nuclear sites of action of ER complexes; they suggest, moreover, that processing of ER occurs at only one of these. These sites may be temporally as well as structurally distinct, since, as we show below, binding to the processing site can be prevented without affecting initial nuclear binding.

IV. ACTINOMYCIN D: EFFECTS ON OESTROGEN RECEPTOR COMPARTMENTALIZATION AND PROCESSING

A. Inhibition of Oestrogen Receptor Processing

Actinomycin D (AcD) has been a powerful tool in investigations into the biochemistry of nucleic acids and their involvement in replication and transcription (Goldberg and Friedman, 1971). The antibiotic intercalates into double-stranded DNA with its chromophore between successive G-C base pairs; two pentapeptides lie in the minor groove of the double helix (Sobel and Jain, 1972). Two binding sites distinguished by different affinities for DNA have been described; both are partially blocked by the presence of chromosomal proteins (Kleiman and Huang, 1971).

The nature of the inhibitory action of AcD is complex and partially concentration dependent. High dose AcD suppresses the synthesis of all cellular RNA fractions by preferentially blocking chain elongation catalysed by DNA-directed RNA polymerase. However, at low concentrations there is differential inhibition of various RNA classes with ribosomal RNA being most sensitive (Goldberg and Friedman, 1971). DNA synthesis in intact cells or by isolated DNA polymerases is also sensitive to AcD but requires the presence of much higher inhibitor concentrations (Hyman and Davidson, 1970).

More recently it has been further suggested that AcD may inhibit protein synthesis through direct effects on mRNA movement or translation (Leinwand and Ruddle, 1977, Bastos and Aviv, 1977).

Figure 3 shows the effect of addition of AcD (2 μM) to oestradiol-treated cells. In this study cells were treated simultaneously with the hormone, and inhibitor and receptor levels were measured at the indicated times. AcD completely inhibits the normal processing of oestrogen-charged nuclear receptor. The result is analogous to the effects of nafoxidine. Interestingly,

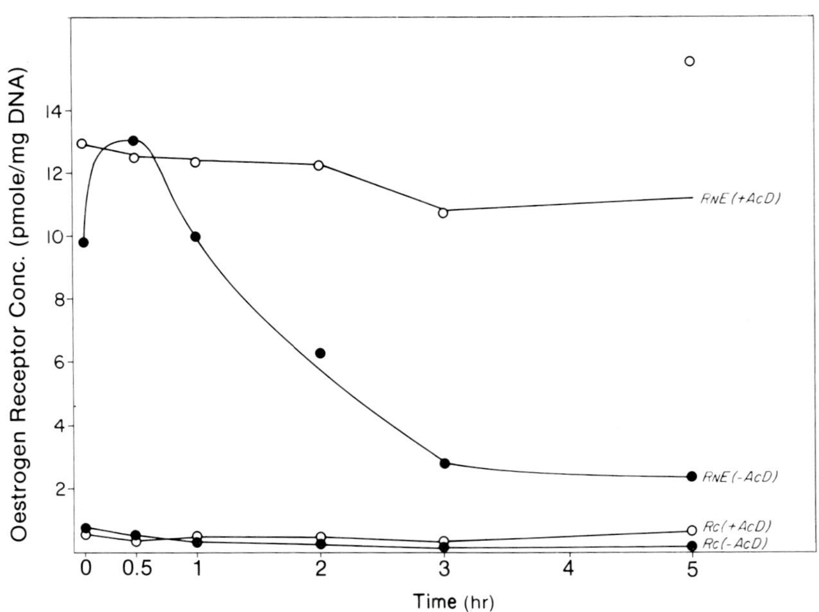

Fig. 3. Effect of continuous actinomycin D treatment on processing of MCF 7 oestrogen receptor. Cells were treated at time 0 with 10 nM oestradiol alone (●) or together with 2 μM actinomycin D (○). At the indicated times cells were harvested and assayed for oestrogen receptor by protamine sulphate precipitation. Adapted from Horwitz and McGuire, (1978b).

neither the initial binding of oestradiol to unfilled sites, nor the translocation of the hormone-receptor complex to the nucleus is affected by actinomycin.

These measurements were made with an exchange assay on protamine precipitated receptor extracted from nuclei with high salt. However, actinomycin is not simply enhancing salt extractability of RnE since a similar loss of ER, and its inhibition by AcD, can be demonstrated when nuclear receptors are labelled directly with [^{3}H]oestradiol, thereby obviating the need to extract receptors (not shown) (Horwitz and McGuire, 1978b).

Actinomycin could be working in at least two ways. Its effect could be direct, physically blocking ER access to a specific DNA binding site. Alternatively, its effect may be indirect, inhibiting RNA and protein synthesis. We have several indirect lines of evidence based on the rate of inhibition and the effects of other inhibitors which suggest that AcD acts directly to block processing.

B. Rate of Actinomycin D Block and Effect of Other Inhibitors

First, the inhibitory effect of AcD is rapid (Fig. 4). In this study cells were treated with oestradiol, while addition of AcD was delayed from 5 minutes to 2 hours. The effect of AcD is to immediately fix ER at the levels they had reached before addition of the inhibitor. If oestradiol and AcD are added together at the start of treatment (Fig. 3), oestrogen binding to unfilled receptors and initial accumulation of receptor in the nucleus are not impaired. However, all subsequent processing stops. The slight downward slopes of the dotted lines show that the effect on ER processing occurs within 15 minutes of AcD addition, so that entry of AcD into nuclei must be quite rapid, and an intermediate effect of AcD on protein synthesis is unlikely.

We have also tested several other inhibitors of cell function for their effect on ER binding, translocation and processing during oestradiol treatment. At 1 μM all other intercalators and inhibitors tested were ineffective; the list includes other inhibitors of transcription (daunomycin, adriamycin, distamycin A, α-amanatin), inhibitors of replication (chloroquine, nalidixic acid, mytomycin C, novobiocin, ethidium bromide), a translation inhibitor (cycloheximide) and inhibitors of other cell processes (colchicine, cytochalasin B). The sole exception was chromomycin A_3. This compound behaves identically to AcD, and like AcD is the only inhibitor which shows specificity for G-C base pairs (Goldberg and Friedman, 1971).

The failure of other intercalators and translation inhibitors to prevent ER processing suggests that the AcD effect is not indirect, resulting from its property of inhibiting RNA and protein synthesis. Instead, AcD (and chromomycin) may directly block ER insertion into specific sites on DNA. AcD may distinguish between two RnE binding sites in nuclei. Newly translocated receptor binds to a site on chromatin or DNA insensitive to

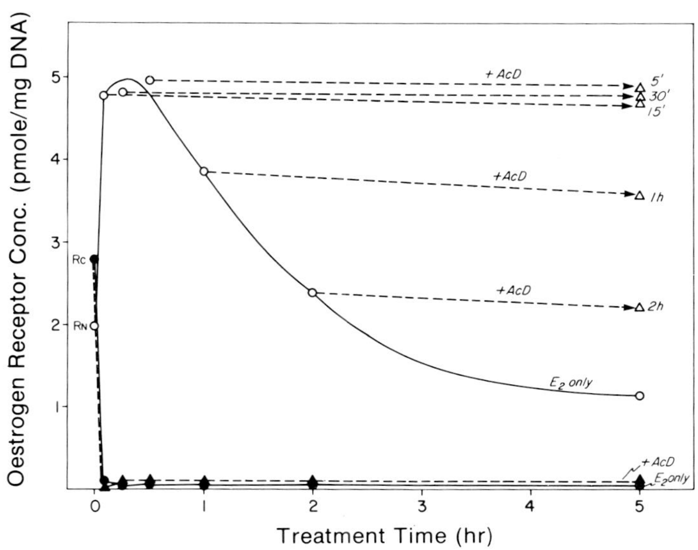

Fig. 4. Effect of delayed actinomycin D treatment on oestrogen receptor levels. MCF 7 cells were treated with 10 nM oestradiol alone (○) or with oestradiol, followed by actinomycin D given 5 minutes to 2 hours later (△). Cells were harvested at the end of 5 hours of oestradiol treatment and assayed for oestrogen receptor. Dashed lines represent the changes in oestrogen receptor levels from the time of antinomycin D addition to the end of the experiment. From Horwitz and McGuire (1978b).

inhibition. AcD or chromomycin A_3 stop subsequent processing by preventing RnE insertion at a second base specific region on DNA or by preventing its release from those sites. The existence of two receptor binding sites in nuclei, one for chromatin, another for DNA, have been postulated in the chick oviduct for PgR (Schrader *et al.*, 1972). Palmiter *et al.* (1976) have also proposed a two-step nuclear receptor translocation mechanism involving a rate-limited movement of steroid receptors from initial nonproductive chromatin binding sites to productive sites.

As described above, the actions of AcD are complex and there are several models which can explain our data. A model involving only one binding site requires that nuclear ER binding is immediately to DNA; AcD may then mechanically prevent ER release from this site. It is also possible that actinomycin is somehow preventing ER egress from the nucleus (Bastos and Aviv, 1977) or altering its turnover at some extra-nuclear site.

In summary, we have provocative data which suggest that the nuclear oestrogen-receptor complex interacts with DNA, that this interaction is required for appropriate receptor turnover or processing, and that processing may be essential for induction of a specific protein by oestrogen. If the receptor is improperly inserted into DNA, for instance when it is bound by nafoxidine, processing fails and the biological effect is blunted.

V. OESTROGEN STIMULATION OF SPECIFIC PROTEINS IN ANTIOESTROGEN BLOCKED BREAST CANCER CELLS

Proliferation of our MCF 7 cells is not reproducibly enhanced by addition of oestradiol to the growth medium. However, incubation with antioestrogens such as tamoxifen or nafoxidine inhibits cellular proliferation and this inhibition can be rapidly reversed by oestradiol. We have analysed protein synthesis in MCF 7 cells during this period of oestrogen reversal of growth inhibition. Growth conditions under which we examined protein synthesis are shown in Figure 5. Cells were grown for 6 days in the continuous presence of 1 μM nafoxidine and then switched to either control medium or medium containing 10 nM oestradiol. By day 6, nafoxidine has arrested cellular proliferation, and changing at this time to control medium is without effect on growth. Growth inhibition, however, is rapidly overcome by incubating with oestradiol. Radio-labelled proteins were analysed by SDS-gel electrophoresis after 4 days of treatment of nafoxidine inhibited cells with oestradiol. Proteins extracted from oestrogen-treated cells were labelled with [^{3}H]leucine while proteins from nafoxidine-pretreated cells served as controls and were labelled

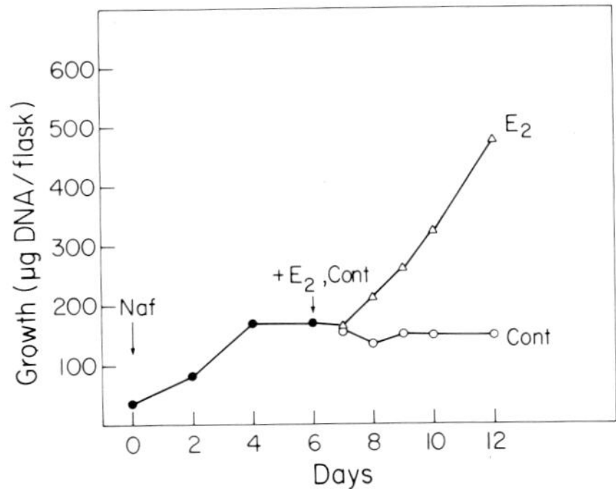

Fig. 5. Antioestrogen effect on cell growth and reversal with oestradiol. Two days after plating, cells were maintained on 1.0 μM nafoxidine (●) in experimental medium for 6 days, then changed to medium containing either 0.01 % ethanol vehicle (control) (○), or 10 nM oestradiol (△) and grown for an additional 6 days. Total DNA per flask was determined at the times indicated. Values represent the mean determinations from duplicate T-75 flasks. Adapted from Edwards *et al.* (1980).

with [^{14}C]leucine. The results of a representative experiment showing the [^{3}H] and [^{14}C] dpm in each gel slice is illustrated in Figure 6. A pronounced increase in the ^{3}H/^{14}C ratio over baseline was detected at a molecular weight of about 24,000 daltons. A distinct but smaller increase was detected at a molecular weight of 36,000 daltons. Data from several independent experiments showed a mean value of 24,183 (range, 23,202-26,467) and 35,510 (range 34,455-37,638) daltons respectively for these oestrogen-induced ratio peaks. No substantial or consistent increase over the basal values were observed in the rest of the gel.

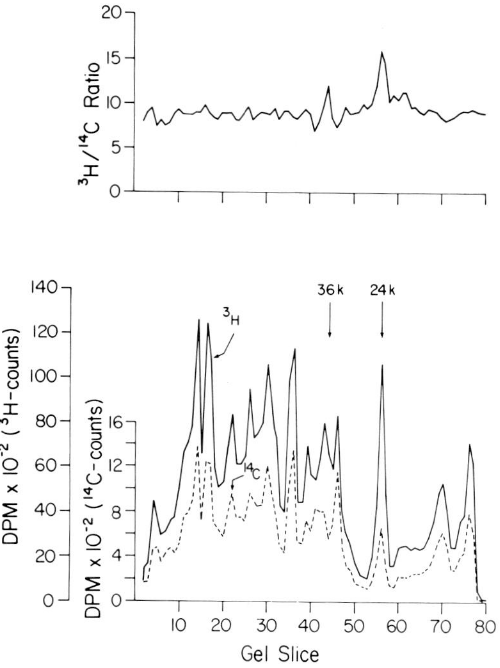

Fig. 6. SDS gel electrophoresis of proteins synthesized by nafoxidine treated cells [^{14}C] and cells rescued from nafoxidine inhibition by oestradiol [^{3}H]. Two days after plating, cells were incubated continuously for 6 days with growth medium containing 1.0 μM nafoxidine. At the end of 6 days pretreatment with nafoxidine, two T-75 flasks were continued on nafoxidine for another 4 days and two flasks were changed to medium with 10 nM oestradiol for 4 days. Nafoxidine treated cells served as controls and were labelled for 2 hours with [^{14}C]leucine, while oestrogen treated cells were labelled for 2 hours with [^{3}H]leucine. Equal numbers of control and oestrogen treated cells were mixed together, homogenized and run on SDS-gels. The arrows indicate the positions and molecular weight estimates of the induced [^{3}H]/[^{14}C] ratio peaks. The upper panel shows the ratio [^{3}H]/[^{14}C] dpm in each gel slice. The bottom panel shows the total dpm in each gel slice for both [^{3}H] and [^{14}C]. Adapted from Edwards *et al.* (1980).

The relative prominence of the two induced peaks seemed to vary with each experiment. By way of example, the $^3H/^{14}C$ ratios measured in a separate but identical experiment at 4 days of oestrogen treatment are shown in Figure 7 (upper panel). Here the major induced peak is 36,000 daltons, which shows about a 2 fold increase over baseline, compared with the induced peak at 24,000 daltons, which shows an increase of about 1.5 fold over baseline. We have estimated these relative increases in seven independent experiments and find that considerable variation occurs not only in the magnitude of the induction, but also in the protein band that is induced to the greater extent. This is apparently due to variable effects either in the cell's response to oestrogen or in extraction of these proteins and is not due to inconsistencies in gel electrophoresis, since frozen aliquots of the same labelled cytosol proteins re-run on SDS-gel give very consistent $^3H/^{14}C$ ratio patterns. The mean increase from separate experiments (n = 7) was 1.54 fold at 24,000 daltons and 1.6 fold at 36,000 daltons.

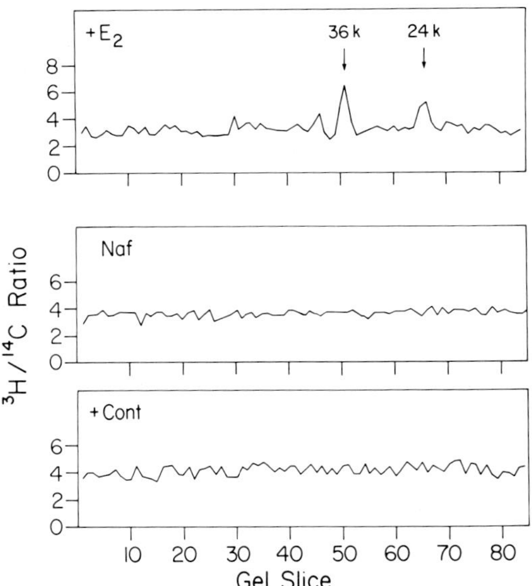

Fig. 7. SDS-gel electrophoresis of labelled MCF 7 cytosol proteins. Upper panel (+ E_2): the experimental protocol was the same as described in Figure 6. This is an identical but independent experiment. Middle panel (Naf): cells were grown for 6 days on 1.0 μM nafoxidine and then two flasks were labelled with [^{3}H]leucine and two with [^{14}C]leucine. Proteins from both groups of nafoxidine treated cells were run simultaneously on one gel. Lower panel (+ Cont): at the end of 6 days incubation with 1.0 μM nafoxidine, cells were either continued for 4 days on nafoxidine and then labelled with [^{14}C]leucine or changed to control media for 4 days and then labelled with [^{3}H]leucine. Proteins from both labelling groups were run simultaneously on the same gel. Adapted from Edwards *et al.* (1980).

In control experiments, proteins were extracted and co-electrophoresed on SDS-gels from cells incubated only with nafoxidine and labelled with both isotopes. Proteins were also extracted and co-electrophoresed from nafoxidine-treated cells (pulsed with [^{14}C] leucine) and from nafoxidine-pretreated cells changed to control medium for 4 days (pulsed with [^{3}H]leucine). These control experiments (Fig. 7, middle and lower panel) show no induced ratio peaks, indicating that the increased ratio observed at 24,000 and 36,000 daltons in the previous experiment is the result of oestradiol stimulation.

We have observed that oestradiol in MCF 7 human breast cancer cells directly stimulates synthesis of specific proteins which migrate on SDS-gel electrophoresis at molecular weights of 24,000 and 36,000 daltons. Induction of these proteins does not occur following nafoxidine treatment or in cells maintained on control growth medium for the same length of time as on oestradiol. We have consistently detected induction of these proteins by the double label ratio method in several independent experiments.

Induction of specific proteins is observed only during the period of oestrogen stimulation of cells whose growth has been arrested by the antioestrogen nafoxidine. We do not detect an induction of these proteins when cells grown on control medium are treated with oestradiol alone (data not shown). Growth of MCF 7 cells in our laboratory also does not appear to be reproducibly influenced by oestrogen alone, and we believe that cells maintained on control growth medium (medium freed of endogenous steroids) may be proliferating at maximal rates in the absence of oestrogens. The oestrogen-induced proteins therefore may be related to oestrogen effects on cell growth, since oestrogen rescue after antioestrogen growth inhibition is the only condition under which we observe either the specific protein induction or growth stimulation. To further test this hypothesis we are currently investigating whether oestrogens induce these same proteins in other human breast cancer cell lines, some of which show different levels of sensitivity in their growth to antioestrogens and oestrogens.

Westley and Rochefort (1979) recently demonstrated that oestrogens induce an MCF 7 cell secretory protein, found only in the medium, which constitutes a major fraction of all secretory proteins. By two-dimensional electrophoresis they were also able to show that oestrogen regulates several intracellular proteins. However, the molecular weights of the oestrogen-induced proteins described by Westley and Rochefort are higher than those of the proteins detected in our studies.

These oestrogen-induced proteins in MCF 7 cells may be excellent markers of oestrogen action in human breast cancer. If they are present in abundance, these induced proteins may be the specific probes needed to permit isolation of hormone regulated messages and to further study oestrogen regulation of gene expression in breast tumours.

ACKNOWLEDGEMENTS

This work was supported in part by the National Cancer Institute CA11378, CA09042, HD07139, and the American Cancer Society.

REFERENCES

Anderson, J. N., Peck, E. J. Jr., and Clark, J. H. (1975). *Endocrinology* **96**, 160–167.
Bastos, R. N., and Aviv, H. (1977). *Cell* **11**, 641–650.
Bayard, R., Damilano, S., Robel, P., and Baulieu, E. E. (1975). *C. R. Acad. Sci.* **281**, 1341–1344.
Brooks, S. C., Locke, E. R., and Soule, H. D. (1973). *J. Biol. Chem.* **248**, 6251–6253.
Capony, F., and Rochefort, H. (1975). *Mol. Cell. Endocr.* **3**, 233–251.
Cidlowski, J. A., and Muldoon, T. G. (1976). *Biol. Reprod.* **15**, 381–398.
Clark, J. H., and Peck, E. J. Jr. (1976). *Nature* **260**, 635–637.
Clark. J. H., Anderson, J. N., and Peck, E. J. Jr. (1973). *Steroids* **22**, 707–718.
Clark, J. H., Peck, E. J. Jr., and Anderson, J. N. (1974). *Nature* **251**, 446–448.
De Hertogh, R., Ekka, E., Vanderheyden, I., and Hoet, J. J. (1973). *J. Steroid Biochem.* **4**, 313–320.
Edwards, D. P., Adams, D. J., Savage, N., and McGuire, W. L. (1980). *Biochem. Biophys. Res. Commun.* **93**, 804–812.
Faber, L. E., Sandman, M. L., and Stavely, H. E. (1972). *J. Biol. Chem.* **247**, 5648–5649.
Ferguson, E. R., and Katzenellenbogen, B. S. (1977). *Endocrinology* **100**, 1242–1251.
Giannopoulos, G., and Gorski, J. (1971). *J. Biol. Chem.* **246**, 2524–2529.
Goldberg, I. H., and Friedman, P. A. (1971). *Ann. Rev. Biochem.* **40**, 775–810.
Hardin, J. W., Clark, J. H., Glasser, S. R., and Peck, E. J. Jr. (1976). *Biochemistry*. **15**, 1370–1374.
Horwitz, K. B., and McGuire, W. L. (1978a). *J. Biol. Chem.* **253**, 2223–2228.
Horwitz, K. B., and McGuire, W. L. (1978b). *J. Biol. Chem.* **253**, 6319–6322.
Horwitz, K. B., and McGuire, W. L. (1978c). *J. Biol. Chem.* **253**, 8185–8191.
Horwitz, K. B., Costlow, M. E., and McGuire, W. L. (1975a). *Steroids* **26**, 785–795.
Horwitz, K. B., McGuire, W. L., Pearson, O. H., and Segaloff, A. (1975b). *Science* **189**, 726–727.
Horwitz, K. B., Koseki, Y., and McGuire, W. L. (1978). *Endocrinology* **103**, 1742–1751.
Hyman, R. W., and Davidson, N. (1970). *J. Mol. Biol* **50**, 421–438.
Jensen, E. V., and DeSombre, E. R. (1972). *Ann. Rev. Biochem.* **41**, 203–230.
Jensen, E. V., Block, G. E., Smith, S., Kyser, K., and DeSombre, E. R. (1971). *Natl Cancer Inst. Monographs* **34**, 55–79.
Juliano, J. V., and Stancel, G. H. (1976). *Biochemistry* **15**, 916–920.
Katzenellenbogen, B. S., and Ferguson, E. R. (1975). *Endocrinology* **97**, 1–12.
Katzenellenbogen, B. S., Ferguson, E. R., and Lan, N. C. (1977). *Endocrinology* **100**, 1252–1259.
Kleiman, L., and Huang, R. C. C. (1971). *J. Mol. Biol.* **55**, 503–521.
Lan, N. C., and Katzenellenbogen, B. S. (1976). *Endocrinology* **98**, 220–227.
Lazier, C. B., and Alford, W. S. (1977). *Biochem. J.* **164**, 659–667.
Leavitt, W. W., Chen, T. J., and Allen, T. C. (1977). *Ann. N.Y. Acad. Sci.* **286**, 210–225.
Leinwand, L., and Ruddle, F. H. (1977). *Science* **197**, 381–383.
Lippman, M., Bolan, G., and Huff, K. (1976). *Cancer Res.* **36**, 4610–4618.
McGuire, W. L., Carbone, P. O., Sears, M. E., and Escher, G. C. (1975). *In* "Oestrogen Receptors in Human Breast Cancer" (W. L. McGuire, P. P. Carbone and E. P. Vollmer, eds), pp.1–7. Raven Press, New York.
Mester, J., and Baulieu, E. E. (1975). *Biochem. J.* **146**, 617–623.

Palmiter, R. D., Moore, P. B., Mulvihill, E. R., and Emtage, S. (1976). *Cell* **8**, 557–572.
Ruh, T. S., and Baudendistel, L. J. (1977). *Endocrinology* **100**, 420–426.
Sarff, M., and Gorski, J. (1971). *Biochemistry* **10**, 2557–2563.
Schrader, W. T., Toft, D. O., and O'Malley, B. W. (1972). *J. Biol. Chem.* **247**, 2401–2407.
Sherman, M. R., Corval, P. I., and O'Malley, B. W. (1970). *J. Biol. Chem.* **245**, 6085–6096.
Sobel, H. M., and Jain, S. C. (1972). *J. Mol. Biol.* **68**, 21–24.
Sonnenschein, C., Soto, A. M., Colofiore, J., and Farookhi, R. (1976). *Expl Cell Res.* **101**, 15–22.
Soule, H. D., Vazquez, J., Long, A., Albert, S., and Brennan, M. H. (1973). *J. Natl Cancer Inst.* **51**, 1409–1416.
Stormshak, F., Leake, R., Wertz, N., and Gorski, J. (1976). *Endocrinology* **99**, 1501–1511.
Westley, B., and Rochefort, H. (1979). *Biochem. Biophys. Res. Commun.* **90**, 410–416.
Williams, D., and Gorski, J. (1972). *Proc. Natl Acad. Sci. U.S.A.* **69**, 3464–3468.

21

Mechanism of Action of Tamoxifen and Metabolites in MCF 7 Human Breast Cancer Cells

H. ROCHEFORT, J. L. BORGNA, E. COEZY, F. VIGNON AND B. WESTLEY

I. INTRODUCTION

It is difficult to approach the mechanism of action of antioestrogens *in vivo* in the whole animal since some of the effects can be indirect and the drug can be metabolized before being able to act. Conversely, the *in vitro* cell culture approach has the advantage of being simple and of avoiding metabolism problems. Oestrogen responsive human breast cancer cell lines such as the MCF 7 (Lippman *et al.*, 1976a) and the ZR 75-1 (Engel *et al.*, 1978) cell lines are now available. They represent excellent *in vitro* systems for studying the mechanism of action of antioestrogens and for screening

NON-STEROIDAL ANTIOESTROGENS
ISBN 0 12 677880 9

potential antioestrogens for use in the treatment of breast cancer. In fact, their growth is prevented by antioestrogens like that of the oestrogen receptor positive human breast cancers (Lippman *et al.*, 1976b, Horwitz *et al.*, 1978). We have therefore chosen the MCF 7 cell line to answer several questions concerning the action of tamoxifen: 1. Does tamoxifen bind directly to the oestrogen receptor and/or to another receptor specific for antioestrogens? 2. Is tamoxifen metabolized in the MCF 7 cells? 3. Are tamoxifen and 4-hydroxytamoxifen (one of the metabolites of tamoxifen formed *in vivo*) full oestrogen antagonists or partial agonists for all the responses studied? 4. What is the mechanism of cell growth blockade?

II. BINDING OF [^{3}H]TAMOXIFEN TO MCF 7 CELLS EXTRACTS *IN VITRO*

The availability of [^{3}H]tamoxifen of high specific activity (SA 15.8 Ci/mmole) from ICI Laboratories (England) allowed us to specify the binding characteristics of this antioestrogen in extracts prepared from different oestrogen target tissues (Capony and Rochefort, 1978; Jordan and Prestwich, 1977; Nicholson *et al.*, 1979). The conclusion that [^{3}H]tamoxifen was binding directly to the 8S oestrogen receptor was based on the following observations: binding specificity, number of saturable binding sites and physicochemical properties of the binding proteins. It has been postulated that, in breast cancer, tamoxifen can bind to sites specific for antioestrogens but not for oestrogens (Sutherland and Murphy, 1980). We therefore looked at the binding of [^{3}H]tamoxifen to the cytosol and KCl nuclear extract prepared from MCF 7 cells cultured for 4 days in Dulbecco's modified Eagle's medium containing 5% charcoal treated foetal calf serum, in order to remove, at least partly, plasma oestrogens (see Section V). This binding was evaluated, after 3–4 hours incubation at 0–2°C, with dextran-coated charcoal suspension as previously described (Capony and Rochefort, 1975). Scatchard plot analysis indicated a single class of binding sites of high affinity, and the comparison of the number of sites indicated similar values for oestradiol (E_2) and tamoxifen (Table I). The higher values obtained for oestrogen receptors in the nuclear extract (cf. the cytosol) are consistent with previous results of Zava and McGuire (1977) on free nuclear receptor sites. However, according to the same laboratory, these sites are in fact due to cytoplasmic contamination of the nuclear preparation (Edwards *et al.*, 1980). The binding specificity was studied by competition of [^{3}H]tamoxifen with several non-radioactive oestrogens and antioestrogens. It showed that the efficiency for competition was related to the affinity of each ligand for the oestrogen receptor. Diethylstilboestrol and oestradiol were more active than the antioestrogens tamoxifen or nafoxidine and we could not find any [^{3}H]tamoxifen saturable

TABLE I
[^{3}H]Oestradiol and [^{3}H]Tamoxifen Binding Sites in MCF 7 Cells[a]

	Binding site concentration (fmol/mg protein)		
	R_c	R_n	Total
E_2	171 ± 69 (9)	251 ± 81 (9)	422 ± 150
Tam	135 ± 91 (6)	331 ± 73 (6)	466 ± 164

[a] The [^{3}H]oestradiol (E_2) and [^{3}H]tamoxifen (Tam) binding sites were determined by Scatchard Plots on cytosol (R_c) and KCl-nuclear extract (R_n) prepared from MCF 7 cells. The bound [^{3}H]oestradiol and [^{3}H]tamoxifen were determined by charcoal assay as described in Capony and Rochefort (1978). Results are the means ± S.D. of n different experiments.

binding sites which were resistant to oestrogen competition. As for the uterine cytosol, we conclude that [^{3}H]tamoxifen binds directly to the oestrogen receptor, the only saturable binding protein that we could demonstrate. The non-specific, non-saturable binding of [^{3}H]tamoxifen was, however, higher than that of [^{3}H]oestradiol in the MCF 7 cells as in the uterine extracts.

III. METABOLISM OF [^{3}H]TAMOXIFEN BY MCF 7 CELLS

Since hydroxylated metabolites with higher affinity for the oestrogen receptor than tamoxifen itself (Jordan *et al.*, 1977) have been described after injection of tamoxifen *in vivo* (Fromson *et al.*, 1973), we looked to see whether tamoxifen was acting by itself or through its transformation into more active metabolites. We incubated MCF 7 cells for 3–72 hours with 50 nM [^{3}H]tamoxifen. Then the cytosol, the KCl-nuclear fraction and the medium were extracted by ethyl acetate and the extract analysed by thin layer chromatography as described by Borgna and Rochefort (1979). The migrating conditions allowed us to separate monohydroxytamoxifen, N-desmethyltamoxifen and tamoxifen. We found less than 0.5 % metabolism of tamoxifen, and we did not find any monohydroxytamoxifen or N-desmethyltamoxifen under these conditions. We concluded, in agreement with the finding of Horwitz *et al.* (1978), that tamoxifen is most likely acting directly in these cells and not via higher affinity metabolites.

IV. EFFECT OF TAMOXIFEN AND MONOHYDROXYTAMOXIFEN ON SPECIFIC OESTROGEN-INDUCED PROTEINS

The progesterone receptor is the only oestrogen induced protein currently known in MCF 7 cells (Horwitz *et al.*, 1978). Antioestrogens increased the concentration of progesterone receptor thus behaving as partial oestrogen agonists. This contrasted with their full antagonist effect on cell growth. We then looked for other oestrogen induced proteins that might be more closely related to tumour growth using [^{35}S]methionine labelled proteins analysed by SDS polyacrylamide gel electrophoresis (Bonner and Laskey, 1974). The MCF 7 cells were first withdrawn from oestrogen in a medium containing 10% charcoal-treated serum; they were then cultured in the same medium containing different hormones or antihormones and then finally labelled with [^{35}S] methionine. The labelled proteins of a cell lysate and of the medium were analysed by SDS polyacrylamide gel electrophoresis. The fluorograms of these gels revealed different bands of which the intensity could be quantified in a gel scanner. We found no clear effect of oestradiol on the labelling of intracellular proteins by this technique. Using the two-dimensional technique of O'Farrell (1975), we found 3 spots constantly stimulated by oestradiol (Westley and Rochefort, 1979). However, the most dramatic effect of oestradiol was seen with the secreted proteins. We found that starting from 12 hours after treatment, a protein of 46,000 daltons molecular weight (46 K) was induced by oestradiol. Near optimal induction was obtained with 0.1 nM oestradiol. In addition to this 46 K protein, some other proteins were also stimulated. The induction was found to be specific for oestrogen receptor ligands since oestrone and oestriol were 10-fold less efficient than oestradiol while progesterone and dexamethasone were inactive. Dihydrotestosterone (DHT) was only active at a concentration of 5 nM (Rochefort *et al.*, 1979a) which is consistent with an effect of DHT mediated by the oestrogen receptor (Garcia and Rochefort, 1977; Rochefort *et al.*, 1979b, 1979c). Tamoxifen and monohydroxytamoxifen were then tested under the same conditions. When added separately to MCF 7 cells, they did not induce any secretory proteins. When added with oestradiol they fully prevented the induction of the 46 K protein by oestradiol (Fig. 1) and also by DHT (Rochefort *et al.*, 1979a). Monohydroxytamoxifen was 10 fold more potent than tamoxifen in blocking the induction of the secreted protein by oestradiol. We also found that these two antioestrogens inhibited the induction of the 46 K protein by DHT in a ratio corresponding roughly to the relative affinities of these 3 ligands for the oestrogen receptor. The efficient molar ratio of tamoxifen/oestradiol needed to inhibit the oestradiol induction of the 46 K protein by 50% varied from 10^4 to 10^2 depending on whether tamoxifen was added together with or before the addition of oestradiol. This was consistent with a slower rate of entry of tamoxifen into the cells as compared with oestradiol.

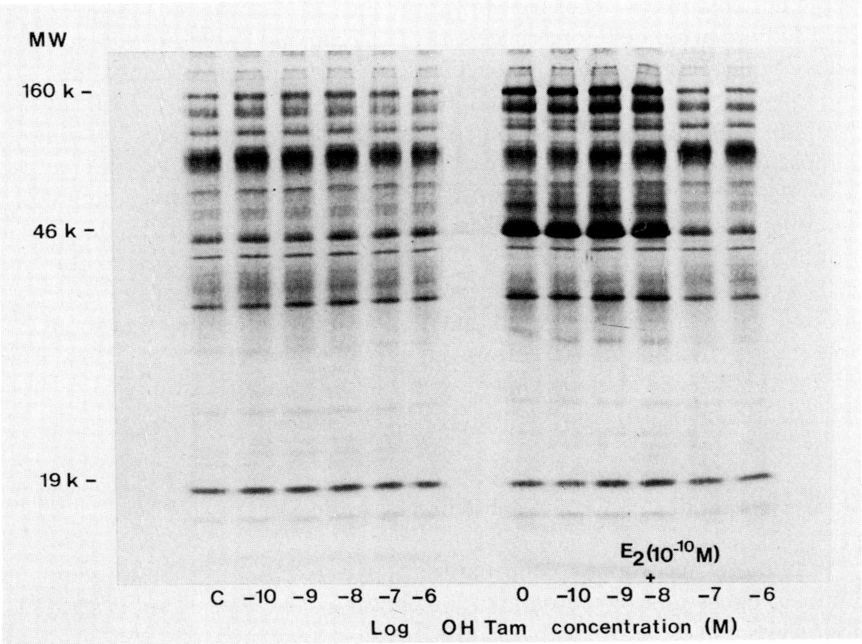

Fig. 1. Effect of 4-hydroxytamoxifen on secretory proteins in MCF 7 cells. Increasing concentrations of 4-hydroxytamoxifen (OH Tam) were incubated with MCF 7 cells for 2 days either without or with oestradiol (0.1 nM). The secreted proteins, labelled by [^{35}S]methionine, were then analysed by SDS polyacrylamide gel electrophoresis. The major oestrogen induced proteins are seen at molecular weights of 46 K and 160 K daltons.

V. EFFECT OF TAMOXIFEN AND MONOHYDROXYTAMOXIFEN ON CELL GROWTH

It is well documented that tamoxifen and other non-steroidal anti-oestrogens prevent cell growth (Lippman *et al.*, 1976a; Horwitz *et al.*, 1978). This inhibition appears to be oestrogen receptor specific since it is not found in oestrogen receptor negative cells and is totally overcome in the presence of an excess of oestradiol.

A. Relative Efficiency of Tamoxifen and Monohydroxytamoxifen on the Growth of MCF 7 Cells

Two 5 x 10 cells were plated in Dulbecco's modified Eagle's medium containing 1% dextran coated charcoal treated serum for 13 days with or without antioestrogens. Cell growth was evaluated both by counting the cells in a Coulter Counter, after trypsinization, and by assaying the total DNA by an ethidium bromide fluorescence assay (Le Pecq and Paoletti, 1966; Karsten and Wollenberger, 1977). Concentrations of 0.1 μM tamoxifen and monohydroxytamoxifen inhibited the cell growth from day 7 of culture. Monohydroxytamoxifen was much more efficient than tamoxifen since it almost totally prevented cell growth. Moreover, oestradiol (10 nM) added secondarily at day 9 was effective in rescuing the cells from tamoxifen treatment but not from monohydroxytamoxifen treatment. In the control, the doubling time was approximately 3 days. A dose response experiment where cells were incubated 8 days with increasing concentrations of tamoxifen or monohydroxytamoxifen showed that monohydroxytamoxifen was about 100 fold more efficient in preventing cell growth than tamoxifen itself. This different efficiency is in agreement with the difference of affinity of the two ligands for the oestrogen receptor (Rochefort *et al.*, 1979c).

B. Mechanism of Cell Growth Inhibition by Antioestrogens

A priori, according to the nature of the receptor for oestrogens and antioestrogens and of the pathways mediating the effect of antioestrogens, four series of mechanisms can be considered to explain how antioestrogens are working to prevent cell growth (Fig. 2). We believe that the action of antioestrogens is mediated by the oestrogen receptor rather than by different receptors specific for antioestrogens, since we have shown (Section II) that the antioestrogen binds specifically to the oestrogen receptor and not to other saturable proteins. This is also consistent with the fact that no growth inhibition could be seen in the presence of oestrogens. Subsequent to binding to receptors, antioestrogens would either stimulate a pathway inhibiting cell growth or inhibit a pathway stimulating cell growth. The stimulation of an inhibitory pathway can be proposed since antioestrogens decreased the growth of cells cultured in "steroid free" medium. However, we have not seen any proteins induced specifically by antioestrogens in looking at secretory and intracellular proteins by the two-dimensional gel electrophoresis technique (O'Farrell, 1975). Another possibility is that antioestrogens block a stimulatory pathway which would be stimulated by the oestrogen receptor either free or occupied by oestrogens. It is unlikely that the unoccupied oestrogen receptors in MCF 7 cells are biologically active, since they are not located in purified nuclei (Edwards *et al.*, 1980). One has therefore to postulate that the stimulation of cell growth is due to oestrogen receptor occupied by the oestrogens remaining in the cell and eventually in the culture medium. We have considered this last possibility since the cells are currently plated and grown in a medium containing up to 10% foetal calf serum. We confirmed that the treatment of serum by charcoal was totally efficient in removing the

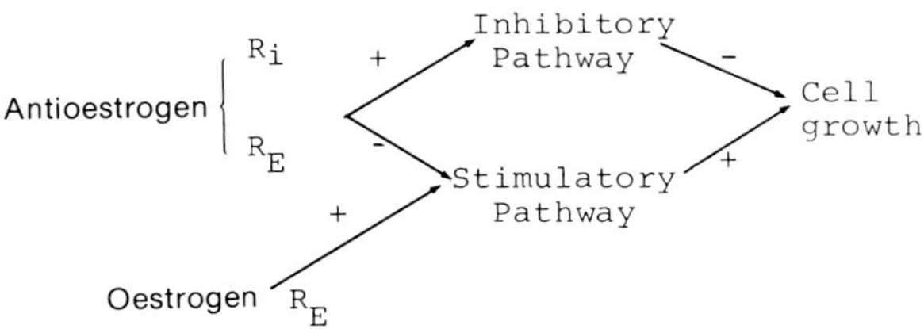

Fig. 2. Possible mechanisms to explain the blockade of MCF 7 cell growth by antioestrogens. Four possibilities can be schematically considered. Antioestrogens might act via their binding to the oestrogen receptor (R_E) and/or to another receptor specific for antioestrogens (R_i). We are in favour of a binding to the oestrogen receptor. Thereafter the antioestrogen-receptor complexes might stimulate either a growth inhibitory pathway (inhibitor growth factor) or they might inhibit a stimulatory pathway (such as the induction of oestrogen induced growth factors). We favour this second possibility.

free oestrogens as shown by others (Armelin *et al.*, 1974). However, we found that the same treatment was inefficient in removing the oestrogen sulphates which are present in high concentrations in plasma. We found up to 30 nM oestrogen conjugates remaining after our charcoal treatment (Vignon *et al.*, 1980). We then demonstrated that the MCF 7 cells were able to hydrolyse the sulphate ester bond of [^{3}H]oestrone sulphate, thus liberating [^{3}H]oestrogens which were recovered bound to the nuclear oestrogen receptor. This showed that the cells contained an aryl sulphatase activity. Finally, oestrone and oestradiol-3-sulphate, but not the oestradiol-17-sulphate, induced the 46 K protein in MCF 7 cells. These results led us to propose that the culture medium contains oestrogen sulphate which can be used by the cells as biologically active oestrogens. Even though this does not demonstrate that cell growth is really oestrogen-dependent in this system, it nevertheless remains a good possibility.

We conclude that the most likely hypothesis is that antioestrogens block the growth of human breast cancer by antagonizing the stimulation of growth by oestrogens. To demonstrate this, cell growth studies in chemically defined media (Bottenstein *et al.*, 1979) are in progress.

VI. CONCLUSIONS

We propose that tamoxifen and monohydroxytamoxifen are full oestrogen antagonists in the MCF 7 human breast cancer cells at least for one parameter, the induction of a 46 K secretory glycoprotein. They are, however, partial agonists for the progesterone receptor (Fig. 3). According to metabolism studies, tamoxifen appears to be active by itself without needing any activation into hydroxylated metabolites such as monohydroxytamoxifen which have high affinity for the oestrogen receptor. However, *in vivo*, monohydroxytamoxifen is formed by human liver, and according to the relative plasma concentrations of monohydroxytamoxifen, tamoxifen and oestradiol (Daniel *et al.*, 1979) it is most likely that monohydroxytamoxifen will be the active metabolite at the target cell level (Borgna and Rochefort, 1981). The mechanism of action of tamoxifen or monohydroxytamoxifen in the MCF 7 breast cancer cells is still unknown. It is striking that no difference could be detected between the interaction of the oestrogen receptor with oestradiol or monohydroxytamoxifen (Chapter 5). Thus, it appears particularly interesting to analyse carefully the interaction with chromatin of the oestrogen receptor bound to oestradiol or to monohydroxytamoxifen in order to detect any difference which might explain the partial inefficiency of the oestrogen receptor when occupied by antioestrogen.

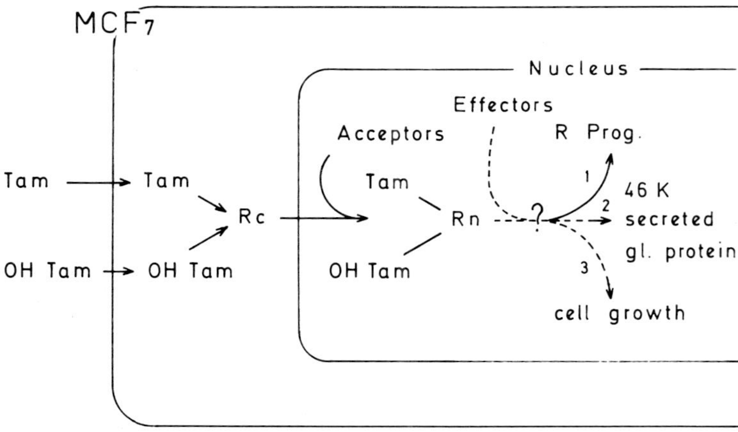

Fig. 3. Interaction and mechanism of action of tamoxifen (Tam) and monohydroxytamoxifen (OH Tam) in MCF 7 cells. Both antioestrogens are acting by themselves in MCF 7 cells. They induce the nuclear translocation of oestrogen receptor and provoke three types of responses (1, 2, 3) which are differently altered by antioestrogens. Tamoxifen is a partial agonist in pathway 1, is a full antagonist in pathway 2, and might be a full antagonist on cell growth in pathway 3, though this has not yet been proved.

ACKNOWLEDGEMENTS

We are grateful to D. Derocq and J. Vanbiervliet for their excellent technical help and to E. Barrié and H. Spoward for preparing the manuscript. We thank ICI Laboratories (England, Dr Patterson) for kindly providing us with [^{3}H]tamoxifen and monohydroxytamoxifen. This work was supported by the Institut National de la Santé et de la Recherche Médicale, the Centre National de la Recherche Scientifique and the Medical Research Council (Great Britain).

REFERENCES

Armelin, H. A., Wishikawa, K., and Sato, G. H. (1974). *In* "Control of Proliferation in Animal Cells" (B. Clarkson and R. Baserga, eds), pp. 97–104. Cold Spring Harbor, New York.

Bonner, W. M., and Laskey, R. A. (1974). *Eur. J. Biochem.* **46**, 83–88.

Borgna, J. L., and Rochefort, H. (1979). *C. R. Acad. Sci.* **289**, 1141–1144.

Borgna, J. L., and Rochefort, H. (1981). *J. Biol. Chem.* **256,** 859-868.

Bottenstein, J., Hayashi, I., Hutchings, S., Masui, H., Mather, J., McClure, D. B., Ohasa, S., Rizzino, A., Sato, G., Serrero, G., Wolfe, R., and Wu, R. (1979). *In* "Methods in Enzymology" Vol. LVII (W. B. Jacoby and I. H. Pastan, eds), pp. 94–109. Academic Press, New York.

Capony, F., and Rochefort, H. (1975). *Mol. Cell. Endocr.* **3**, 233–251.

Capony, F., and Rochefort, H. (1978). *Mol. Cell. Endocr.* **11**, 181–198.

Daniel, C. P., Gaskell, S. J., and Nicholson, R. I. (1979). *J. Endocr.* **81**, 148P–149P.

Edwards, D. P., Martin, P. M., Horwitz, K. B., Chamness, G. C., and McGuire, W. L. (1980). *Expl Cell Res.* **127**, 197–214.

Engel, L. W., Young, N. A., Tralka, T. S., Lippman, M. E., O'Brien, S. J., and Joyce, M. J. (1978). *Cancer Res.* **38**, 3352–3364.

Fromson, J. M., Pearson, S., and Brahman, S. (1973). *Xenobiotica* **3**, 693–709.

Garcia, M., and Rochefort, H. (1977). *Steroids* **29**, 11–26.

Horwitz, K. B., Koseki, Y., and McGuire, W. L. (1978). *Endocrinology* **105**, 1742–1758.

Jordan, V. C., and Prestwich, G. (1977). *Mol. Cell. Endocr.* **8**, 179–188.

Jordan, V. C., Collins, M. M., Rowsby, L., and Prestwich, G. (1977). *J. Endocr.* **75**, 305–316.

Karsten, U., and Wollenberger, A. (1977). *Anal. Biochem.* **77**, 464–470.

Le Pecq, J. B., and Paoletti, C. (1966). *Anal. Biochem.* **17**, 100–107.

Lippman, M., Bolan, G., and Huff, K. (1976a). *Cancer Res.* **36**, 4595–4601.

Lippman, M., Bolan, G., and Huff, K. (1976b). *Cancer Treat. Rep.* **60**, 1421–1429.

Nicholson, R. I., Syne, J. S., Daniel, C. P., and Griffiths, K. (1979). *Eur. J. Cancer.* **15**, 317–329.

O'Farrell, P. H. (1975). *J. Biol. Chem.* **250**, 4007–4021.

Rochefort, H., Garcia, M., Vignon, F., and Westley, B. (1979a). *In* "Steroid Induced Uterine Proteins" (M. Beato, ed.), Raven Press, New York.

Rochefort, J., Capony, F., and Garcia, M. (1979b). *J. Steroid. Biochem.* **11**, 1635–1638.

Rochefort, H., Garcia, M., and Borgna, J. L. (1979c). *Biochem. Biophys. Res. Commun.* **88**, 351–357.

Sutherland, R. L., and Murphy, L. C. (1980). *Eur. J. Cancer* **16**, 1141–1148.

Vignon, F., Terqui, M., Westley, B., Derocq, D., and Rochefort, H. (1980). *Endocrinology* **106**, 1079–1086.

Westley, B., and Rochefort, H. (1979). *Biochem. Biophys. Res. Commun.* **90**, 410–416.

Zava, D. T., and McGuire, W. L. (1977). *J. Biol. Chem.* **252**, 3703–3708.

22

Regulation of Growth and DNA Synthesis by Oestrogens and Antioestrogens in Human Breast Cancer Cell Lines

MARC E. LIPPMAN, SUSAN C. AITKEN AND JOSEPH C. ALLEGRA

I. INTRODUCTION

Oestrogens and antioestrogens have profound effects on the growth of human breast cancer. Since the work of Beatson nearly a century ago, investigators have been attempting to understand the basis for endocrine regulation of cell proliferation. Studies in the intact animal are difficult. It is impossible to administer a hormone without altering the activities or levels of a host of other factors. Similarly, it is impossible to assume that the effects observed can be attributed to a direct action of the hormone on the target tissue. Effects on vasculature, the immune system or supporting stroma are all possible. Finally, "growth" itself is a very difficult parameter to dissect and measure on a cellular basis. For these reasons, we have attempted over the

NON-STEROIDAL ANTIOESTROGENS
ISBN 0 12 677880 9

past few years to develop cell systems in which oestrogenic effects on growth could be elicited. In this review, we will summarize some of our work in which we have been able to demonstrate specific effects of oestrogens and antioestrogens on human breast cancer cell lines. We have developed a defined medium which permits further amplification of these oestrogenic effects. In addition, we have recently begun to study the mechanisms of hormonal stimulation of growth by a detailed analysis of the regulation of DNA synthesis. These experiments will be discussed in detail below.

Previously published data from our laboratory have provided support for the notion that human breast cancer cells in long-term tissue culture might retain hormone responsiveness (Lippman *et al.*, 1976a, 1976b, 1976c, 1977; Osborne *et al.*, 1976; Allegra and Lippman, 1978; Strobl and Lippman, 1979). Physiological concentrations of oestradiol stimulate incorporation of precursors into macromolecules. Antioestrogens such as tamoxifen, nafoxidine and clomiphene strongly inhibit macromolecular synthesis and are eventually lethal to cells. These inhibitory effects are specific in that they are only seen in breast cancer cell lines which are oestrogen receptor positive, prevented by similtaneous addition of oestradiol and reversed by subsequent addition of oestradiol for up to 48 hours following the addition of antioestrogen. In this chapter we will review more recent experimental work which both clarifies the degree of this stimulation and probes its mechanism.

II. EFFECT OF OESTROGENS AND ANTIOESTROGENS ON CELL GROWTH

All the work summarized in this review was performed on two cell lines: MCF 7 (generously provided by Marvin Rich of the Michigan Cancer Foundation) and ZR 75-1. The human and mammary nature of these cell lines have been summarized in detail elsewhere (Soule *et al.*, 1973; Engel *et al.*, 1978; Engel and Young, 1978).

While a degree of oestrogenic and antioestrogenic effects on breast cancer cell lines had been reported previously (Lippman *et al.*, 1976a; 1977) we found that the degree of stimulation was variable. A variety of explanations presented themselves. First, in standard tissue culture media without serum supplementation MCF 7 and ZR 75-1 cells cease growth and die after a variable period. Thus, experiments in which a single trophic factor was added to medium were often ambiguous in interpretation. Second, the effect on cells of endogenous hormones contained in serum was an unknown factor. Prior work had shown that at least two weeks might be required for removal of oestradiol from intracellular sites (Strobl and Lippman, 1979).

One approach to some of these difficulties which we have employed is the development of defined, serum free conditions which support the indefinite exponential growth of human breast cancer cells at a rate equivalent to optimal concentrations of serum supplements. We have succeeded for the ZR 75-1 cell line in developing such a medium (Allegra and Lippman, 1978; Lippman *et al.*, 1979). Based in part upon some suggestions of Sato and his colleagues (Hayashi and Sato, 1976; Hayashi *et al.*, 1978), we empirically developed a hormone supplemented medium. The basic nutrient system was Improved Minimal Essential Medium (Richter *et al.*, 1972) which we had previously employed for serum free growth of hepatoma tissue culture cells (Thompson *et al.*, 1975). This medium was supplemented with 17β oestradiol (10^{-9} M), insulin (10^{-7} M), triiodothyronine (10^{-8}M), transferrin (5 μg/ml) and dexamethasone (10^{-8}M), and termed "IMEM-HS". ZR 75-1 cells grow in this medium at a rate equivalent to optimal supplementation with foetal calf serum (Fig. 1). Cells can be passaged either by scraping with a rubber policeman or using EDTA. Plating efficiency is approximately 1.2% in IMEM-HS but can be increased to 3.4% by additional supplementation with cytidine, uridine, thymidine and adenosine (all at 10^{-8} M), nonessential amino acids and fibroblast growth factor (0.025 μg/ml). Conditioned medium derived from ZR 75-1 cells, human placental lactogen, epidermal growth factor, androgens, vasopressin, or oxytocin had no further effect on either

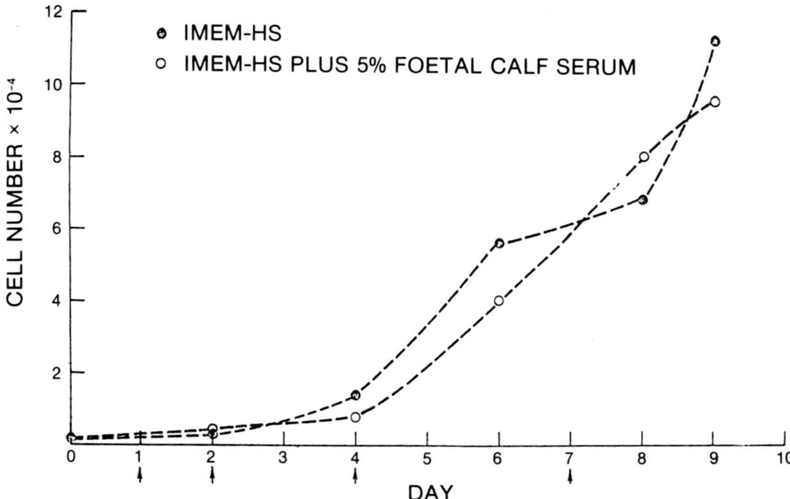

Fig. 1. Comparison of ZR 75-1 cell accumulation in IMEM-HS defined medium with cell growth in that same medium plus optimal concentration of foetal calf serum. Detailed methods can be found in Allegra and Lippman (1978).

growth or plating efficiency at any concentrations we employed. Cells have been maintained under these conditions for at least 6 months through 13 passages without obvious morphologic change or alterations in hormonal responsiveness.

The effects of omission of any of the growth factors on cell number are shown in Figure 2. As shown, cells in IMEM-HS grow rapidly throughout the experimental period. Control cells in IMEM alone remain viable for a variable period of time (about 7 days in the experiment shown). Conditions prior to the initiation of the experiment (density, charcoal treated calf serum *vs* foetal calf serum, etc.) strongly influence this period of preserved viability. Omission of transferrin from the medium results in cell death after about 4–5 days in culture; as little as 0.25 μg/ml can stimulate cell number over control cells. About 2.5 μg/ml is optimal. If either triiodothyronine (T_3), oestradiol, or insulin is omitted from the medium the cells grow slowly for 4–7 days and then enter a prolonged period (lasting up to at least 23 weeks) during which time there is no net increase in cell number. T_3 stimulates growth at 10^{-10} M but

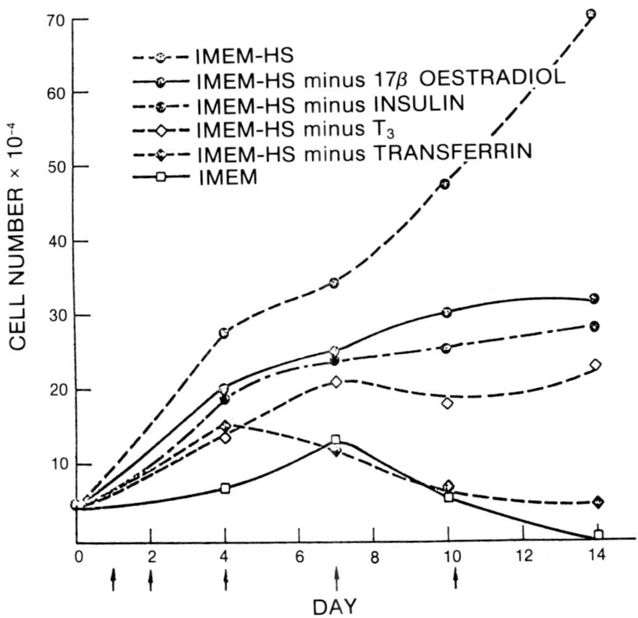

Fig. 2. Detailed effects of omission of various components of IMEM-HS on net cell accumulation of ZR 75-1 human breast cancer. Detailed methods can be found in Allegra and Lippman (1978) and Strobl and Lippman (1979).

10^{-8} provides greatest stimulation. Insulin is active at 10^{-11} M and maximal at 10^{-10} M. We use 10^{-7} M insulin since these higher concentrations are no less stimulatory and the ZR 75-1 cells can metabolize insulin very rapidly (Osborne *et al.*, 1978).

It is important to note that, while there is no net change in cell number in cells deprived of oestradiol, for the following reasons this does not appear to be due simply to a cessation of growth. First, oestradiol free cells continue to incorporate thymidine though at a lower rate than hormone treated cells; second, if the cells are prelabelled with thymidine there is a loss of radioactivity into the medium in oestrogen deprived cells but not in oestrogen treated cells (oestrogen treated cells, 1% loss; oestrogen deprived cells, 60% loss); third, there is an obvious decrease in cell adhesiveness in oestrogen deprived cells and detached cells are easily seen in the medium. Thus, it is likely that the ZR 75-1 cells are capable of low growth in oestrogen free medium, an effect masked by continued cell loss from the dish.

A detailed example of the effects of oestradiol on growth of ZR 75-1 cells in defined medium is shown in Figure 3. If oestradiol is removed from cells in IMEM-HS, they double about once and then enter the prolonged phase of no net growth previously described. As shown, the continued presence of oestradiol in IMEM-HS induces exponential growth of ZR 75-1 cells until density induced inhibition of cell proliferation is achieved.

This experiment strongly suggests that oestradiol is an immediate mitogen of at least some oestrogen-dependent human breast cancer cells. Of course, it is possible that oestrogen induces increases in the activity of a diffusable mitogen for breast cancer cells, but this appears unlikely on two bases. First, conditioned medium obtained from ZR 75-1 cells grown in IMEM-HS will not stimulate MCF 7 human breast cancer cells nor support their serum free growth. Second, conditioned medium plus IMEM-HS without oestradiol will not replace oestradiol as a stimulator of ZR 75-1 cells.

More quantitative information on oestrogen stimulation of ZR 75-1 cells may be found in Figure 4. In this experiment, a prolonged period (11 days) of daily media changes employing oestrogen free medium was employed prior to the start of the experiment to rid the cells of oestradiol. Thus, at the initiation of the experiment little further growth is seen in ZR 75-1 cells without further addition of oestradiol. Addition of 10^{-12} M oestradiol fails to stimulate the cells, whereas 10^{-11} M stimulates cell division about half as well as 10^{-10} M and 10^{-9} M which are optimally active. Oestradiol at 10^{-8} M is about equal to 10^{-11} M, and 10^{-7} M is substantially less stimulatory. Whether or not these suboptimal effects of higher concentrations of oestradiol are simply nonspecifically toxic or specific regulatory mechanisms analogous to the inhibitory effect of high concentrations of oestrogen on human breast cancer growth will require further work.

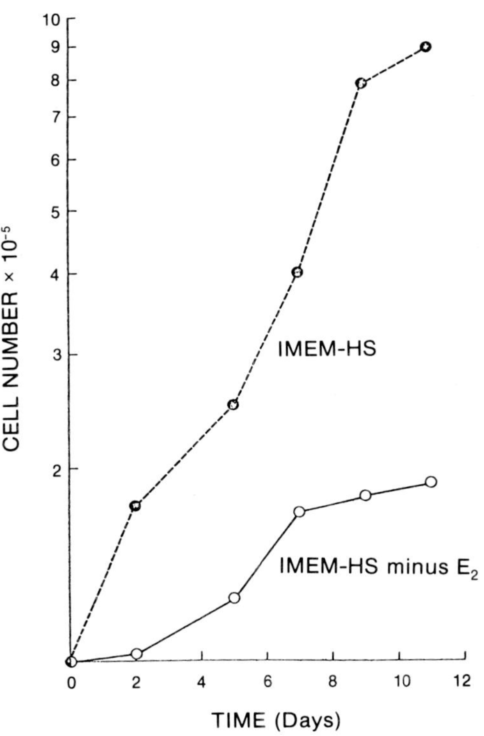

Fig. 3. Effects of omission of oestradiol from IMEM-HS on cell growth in ZR 75-1 cells. Methods are detailed in Allegra and Lippman (1978) and Strobl and Lippman (1979).

Also, as shown in Figure 4, addition of tamoxifen (10^{-6} M) to cells results in cell death. It is important to understand why tamoxifen is more inhibitory than simple oestrogen lack. As previously shown, tamoxifen effects are specific. Also from previous work (Strobl and Lippman, 1979), it appears extremely unlikely that this lethal effect of tamoxifen can be attributed to competition with oestradiol remaining within cells for binding to specific receptor sites. Another conceivable explanation is that the cells are able to synthesize biologically active oestrogens from small molecules. This seems unlikely for several reasons. While all cells capable of growth in defined media must be able to synthesize cholesterol, at least six separate enzymatic biotransformations would have to occur to reach oestradiol and most of these enzymes have not been found outside the gonads and adrenals. Second, if oestradiol was synthesized slowly by these cells in culture, one would expect that after a few days in IMEM-HS without exogenous oestradiol,

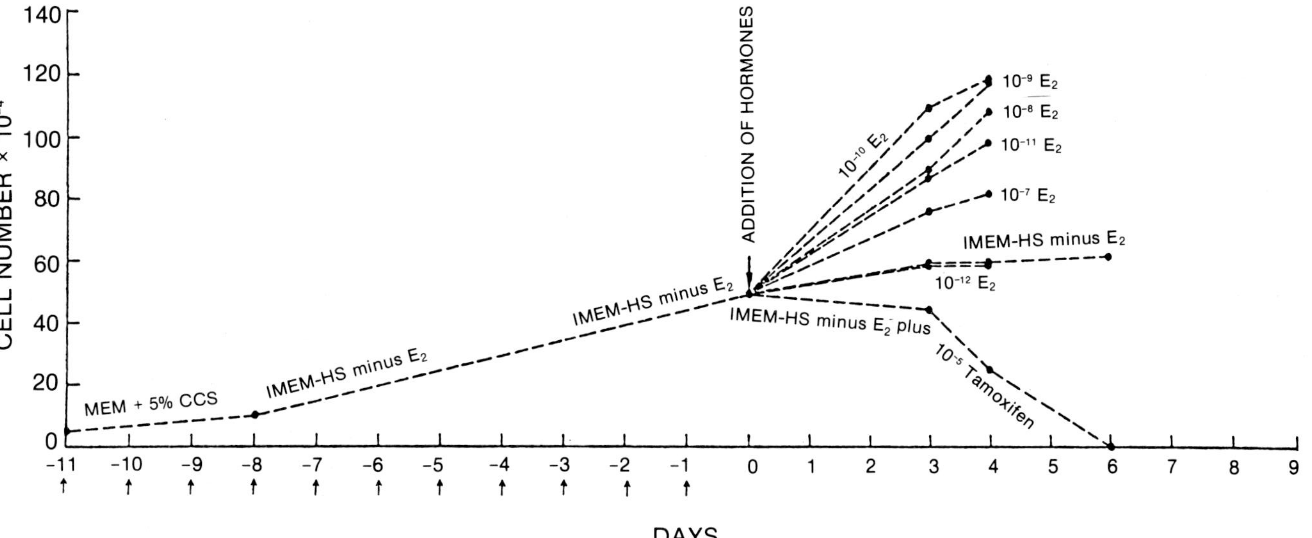

Fig. 4. Dose-response curve of ZR 75-1 human breast cancer cells to oestradiol. Cells were depleted of oestradiol for the 11 days prior to the initiation of the experiment. CCS is charcoal treated foetal calf serum. E_2 stands for 17β oestradiol. Methods are described in Strobl and Lippman (1979).

concentrations would approach those required for growth stimulation. We have never observed this. Third, radioimmunoassay of supernatant medium following prolonged maintenance in IMEM-HS without exogenous oestradiol fails to reveal significant concentrations of oestradiol.

On the other hand, the effects of tamoxifen are not explicable on the basis of nonspecific toxicity. As we have previously shown (Lippman *et al*., 1976a; 1977), antioestrogen effects are seen only in oestrogen receptor containing cells, are prevented by simultaneous addition of oestradiol and, finally, once initiated are reversible for up to 60 hours by addition of oestradiol. This latter point is dealt with in greater detail below.

There are at least two viable explanations for this inhibitory effect of tamoxifen in the absence of oestradiol. First, one may imagine some intrinsic activity of the oestrogen receptor in the absence of hormone. This activity is stimulated by hormone and inhibited by antihormone. Alternatively, it is possible that human breast cancer cells produce some gene product(s) required for growth. In the absence of hormone receptor complexes, these DNA segments are transcribed at some constitutive rate consistent with cell survival and perhaps minimal growth. The addition of hormone results in substantial gene activation by hormone receptor complexes leading to enhanced cell growth. Antioestrogen receptor complexes are known to translocate to the nucleus. Conceivably, these antioestrogen receptor complexes further suppress transcription of these segments of the genome leading to eventual cell death.

A more detailed examination of the interaction of tamoxifen and oestrogen is shown in Figure 5. In this experiment, ZR 75-1 cells which had been maintained for 11 days in IMEM-HS without oestradiol were treated beginning at time 0 with 10^{-6} M tamoxifen. At the times indicated by the arrows, 10^{-9} M oestradiol was added to the medium without removing the tamoxifen, and thymidine incorporation was assessed at the times indicated. As shown, oestradiol treatment strikingly reverses tamoxifen inhibition for the first 12 hours. For the next 24 hours, oestradiol prevents further tamoxifen inhibition, but stimulation of DNA synthesis above levels seen at the times of the oestradiol addition does not occur. In data not shown, cells at these time points would eventually show complete reversal of antioestrogen effects. At later time points, 60 hours and later, addition of oestradiol to antioestrogen treated cells has no ability to alter the irreversible and lethal inhibition of antioestrogen treated cells.

The effects on cell number are mirrored by effects on mitotic index. As shown in Table I, oestradiol treatment induces a substantial increase in mitotic index in MCF 7 human breast cancer cells deprived of both insulin and oestradiol. It is of interest that insulin is largely able to replace oestradiol as a mitogen in MCF 7 cells (though not in ZR 75-1 cells). However, insulin

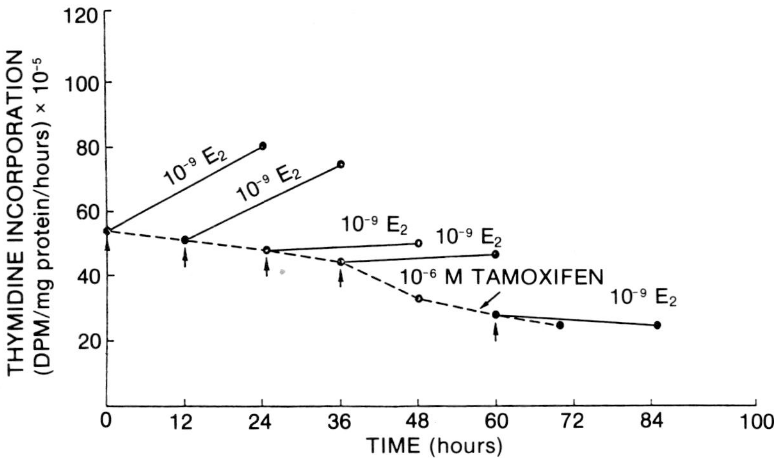

Fig. 5. Effect of 17β oestradiol addition on tamoxifen induced inhibition of thymidine incorporation of ZR 75-1 human breast cancer cells. At time 0, oestrogen depleted cells were treated with 10^{-6} M tamoxifen. At the arrows, either vehicle or 10^{-9} M oestradiol was added to the cells and thymidine incorporation assessed for the hour prior to harvest. Detailed methods can be found in Allegra and Lippman (1978) and Strobl and Lippman (1979).

TABLE I
Effect of Oestradiol on the Mitotic Index of MCF 7 Cells

Experiment number	Control cells			Oestradiol-treated cells		
	M.I.[a] (%)	Number of cells counted	Number of fields counted	M.I. (%)	Number of cells counted	Number of fields counted
1[b]	1.28	2195	8	1.94	2988	8
2[c]						
24 hrs	3.43	611	4	4.74	674	8
48 hrs	4.89	429	11	8.45	331	10
72 hrs	4.48	735	10	15.34	1199	7
96 hrs	8.96	736	18	5.07	1044	7

[a] M.I. = Mitotic Index = $\dfrac{\text{Number of Cells in Mitosis}}{\text{Total number of cells}}$

[b] In experiment 1, control cells were grown in serum free medium and oestradiol treated cells in serum free medium + 2 nM oestradiol for 72 hours. Colchicine was added 4 hours before harvesting the cells.

[c] In experiment 2, control cells were grown in medium supplemented with 1 % charcoal-treated calf serum and oestradiol treated cells in medium supplemented with 1 % charcoal-treated calf serum + 2 nM oestradiol. Different flasks of cells were harvested at 24, 48, 72 and 96 hours after colchicine addition at 20, 44, 68 and 92 hours.

growth effects are unaccompanied by progesterone receptor induction and insulin cannot reverse antioestrogen effects.

In work which will be discussed shortly, we have shown that oestrogen stimulation leads to a parasynchronous recruitment of cells from a nondividing state (Lippman and Aitken, 1980a, 1980b). Such recruitment is accompanied by inductions of several enzymes involved in DNA synthesis including thymidine kinase (Lippman *et al.*, 1976d) and DNA polymerase (Edwards *et al.*, 1980).

Thus, hormones can exert profound regulatory effects on growth of human mammary cancer cells. The use of completely defined serum free medium and cloned lines of human breast cancer cells of unequivocal pedigree will likely permit further insights into mechanisms of hormonal regulation of neoplastic cell growth.

III. EFFECT OF OESTROGENS AND ANTIOESTROGENS ON DNA SYNTHESIS

While such oestrogenic effects on growth appear incontrovertible, a true understanding of the exact mechanism by which oestrogens regulate DNA synthesis and a convenient short-term method of quantification of this stimulation requires alternative approaches.

The experiments discussed below are directed toward establishing a set of techniques which will permit an accurate determination of the net rate of DNA synthesis in tissue culture systems. We will review such a set of methods and discuss their technical application to oestrogenic and antioestrogenic effects on DNA synthesis in MCF 7 cells. $[^{32}P]P_i$ is employed to monitor net DNA synthesis. A number of problems are associated with the use of this tracer in estimating rates of net DNA synthesis:

1. Equilibrium conditions must exist with respect to precursor pools of deoxynucleotides.
2. The effective specific activity of $[^{32}P]P_i$ in the tissue culture system must be known.
3. A differentiation between repair and replicative DNA synthesis must be made. It is possible that a part of the incorporation of labelled precursors into DNA represents repair activity rather than net DNA synthesis.
4. Biochemical techniques employed must accurately reflect what is intended to be measured, i.e. material represented as DNA must be verified as indeed being DNA.

Each of the above areas will be investigated and a number of closely related issues in the analysis of oestrogen mediated effects on DNA synthesis will be addressed. 1. Does the effect of oestrogen represent a synchronization of responsive cells with respect to cell cycle kinetics and can the effect be localized to a particular phase such as a shortening of S or release of cells from G_1 arrest? 2. How does oestrogen administration affect labelling kinetics and to what extent are transport processes and pool sizes influencing the appearance of label in DNA and intracellular precursor pools for DNA synthesis? 3. The response of MCF 7 cells to tamoxifen is also reviewed.

In order to interpret data derived from the incorporation of labelled precursors appropriately, information on transport and pool size is critical. Consequently, the kinetics of phosphate transport and utilization in MCF 7 cells under relevant experimental conditions were investigated prior to consideration of hormonal regulation of phosphate incorporation into DNA.

A. Kinetics of Phosphate Transport and Utilization in MCF 7 Cells

[^{32}P]P_i has frequently been employed as a precursor in measurements of DNA synthesis. In order to generate measurable incorporation into DNA in our tissue culture system it was necessary to reduce the ambient phosphate concentration in the culture medium to 10^{-5} M. Figure 6 demonstrates the continued growth of MCF 7 cells in low phosphate medium, indicating that lowering ambient phosphate concentration would not perturb cell viability. DNA and protein content per dish increased steadily for 60 hours after transfer of cells to 10^{-5} M phosphate medium. In addition, the rate of incorporation of a variety of labelled precursors into acid-precipitable material was examined at three different times after cells were placed in serum free conditions. The ratios of incorporation of [^{3}H]dThd (DNA), [^{3}H]Urd (RNA), [^{14}C]Leu (protein), and [^{14}C]acetate (a variety of macromolecular cell components) in low phosphate medium to the incorporation observed in standard medium are presented in Table II. Little or no effect on rates of macromolecular synthesis was apparent. At the time periods examined, it was also evident that intracellular acid-soluble phosphate (column 3) and cell protein (column 2) were similarly unaffected by reduction in extracellular phosphate to 10^{-5} M. It is probable, therefore, that data derived under these circumstances can be validly compared with previous information on MCF 7 cells obtained in standard medium.

Analysis of the kinetics of phosphate incorporation into the acid-soluble pool of MCF 7 cells is critical to validate the experimental circumstances of labelling. The period chosen to measure incorporation must be one in which labelled precursor has equilibrated with competing intracellular pools. This period could well be subject to considerable experimental variation. It can be seen (Fig. 7) that approximately 6 hours were the minimum required in this tissue culture system. Hormonal treatment (control, tamoxifen, oestradiol)

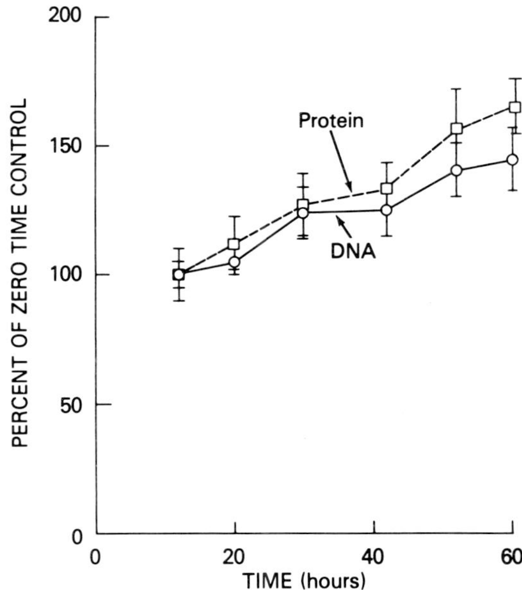

Fig. 6. Growth of MCF 7 cells in 10^{-5} M phosphate medium. Cells were placed in 10^{-5} M phosphate medium at time 0 and harvested at the times indicated. Protein (□) and DNA (○) content were determined as previously described (Lippman and Aitken, 1980a, 1980b). Values reported represent the average of 3 determinations ± 1 S.D.

TABLE II
Effect of Lowered Phosphate Concentration on Incorporation of Label into Acid-Precipitable Material in MCF 7 Cells[a]

Time (hours)	Protein	P_i	[^{3}H]dThd	[^{14}C]Acetate	[^{3}H]Urd	[^{14}C]Leu
12	0.97 ± 0.05	0.93 ± 0.12	1.10 ± 0.05	1.10 ± 0.22 (0.79 ± 0.24)	1.04	1.37
30	0.97 ± 0.07	1.18 ± 0.27	0.97 ± 0.01	0.95 ± 0.16 (0.77 ± 0.05)	0.99	1.18
48	1.04 ± 0.03	1.24 ± 0.18	1.27 ± 0.12	1.03 ± 0.22 (1.40 ± 0.03)	1.45	0.91

[a] Cells were labelled with [^{14}C]acetate (5 μCi/ml, 8 hours), [^{3}H]dThd (1 μCi/ml, 2 hours) or [^{3}H]Urd (1 μCi/ml, 2 hours) plus [^{14}C] Leu (1 μCi/ml, 2 hours) and harvested at the times indicated after transfer to either 10^{-5} M phosphate IMEM or standard IMEM (10^{-3} M phosphate). Incorporation of label was normalized per unit protein. The incorporation of [^{14}C]acetate into DNA was also determined (values in parentheses). Numbers are presented as the ratio of values observed in 10^{-5} M phosphate IMEM to values obtained in standard IMEM (10^{-3} M phosphate). Determination of protein and P_i was based on 5 independent samples, determination of [^{3}H]dThd and [^{14}C]acetate incorporation on 2 independent samples, and determination of [^{3}H]Urd + [^{14}C]Leu incorporation on a single sample. Values reported are the mean ± 1 S.D.

did not appreciably alter the time required for equilibration of [^{32}]P]P_i with intracellular acid-soluble phosphate pools. However, the amount of label accumulating in oestrogen-treated cells was significantly greater than that in controls ($p < 0.005$). The particular experiment illustrated represents a time between 20 and 32 hours following hormone treatment. A similar experiment conducted between 48 and 60 hours after hormone addition yielded similar results (data not presented). [^{32}P]P_i equilibrated approximately 6 hours after administration of label.

Unfortunately, though the deoxynucleotide pool, in which we are specifically interested, is the immediate precursor pool for DNA synthesis, it may represent less than 1% of the total acid-soluble pool. It is possible that equilibration of the larger acid-soluble pool may not reflect equilibrium in the deoxynucleotide pool serving DNA synthesis. Examination of the time course of [^{32}P]P_i incorporation into DNA demonstrates that linearity was achieved in all experimental circumstances within 4–6 hours of exposure to radioactive

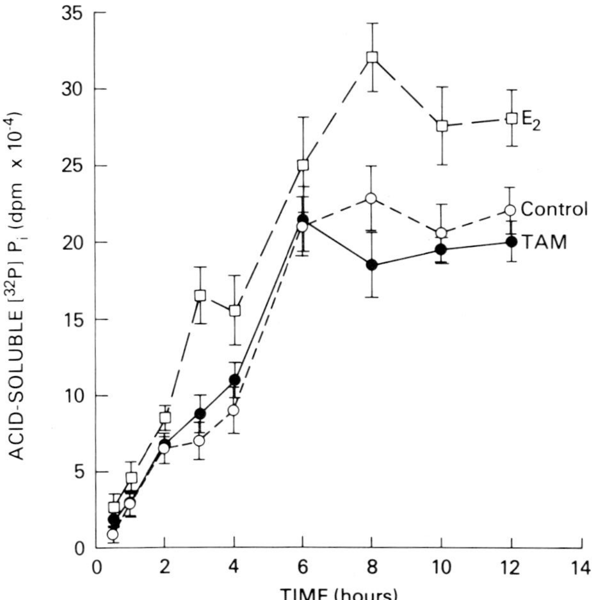

Fig. 7. Incorporation of [^{32}P]P_i into the acid-soluble pool of MCF 7 cells. Cells were transferred to 10^{-5} M phosphate medium 32 hours before time 0. Twenty-four hours before time 0 cells were again transferred to fresh low phosphate medium + oestradiol (5×10^{-9} M) or tamoxifen (2×10^{-6} M). [^{32}P]P_i was added at time 0 and cells were harvested at the times indicated. The acid-soluble fraction was obtained as previously described and analysed for radioactivity (Lippman and Aitken, 1980a, 1980b). Values were normalized per unit protein and represent the average of 3 determinations ± S.D. Control (○); tamoxifen (●); oestradiol (□).

trace (Fig. 8). The experiment illustrated also refers to the period between 20 and 32 hours after hormonal administration. In a second experiment involving a time period of between 48 and 60 hours, it was observed that control and tamoxifen-treated cells required 6 hours for ^{32}P incorporation into DNA to become linear (data not presented). This is strong evidence that the deoxynucleotide pool has also come to equilibrium with $[^{32}P]P_i$.

In spite of the similar equilibration time requirements of the total acid-soluble pool and linear DNA synthesis versus time, there remains some question about whether the specific activity of the acid-soluble pool is truly an accurate reflection of the specific activity of the deoxynucleotide pool. The former can be directly determined as previously described (Lippman and Aitken, 1980a, 1980b). The deoxynucleotide pool, on the other hand, is relatively small and routine determination of specific activity of $[^{32}P]P_i$ isolated in deoxynucleotides would be impossible when dealing with small numbers of cells. Regardless of whether one is to extrapolate from units of incorporation (dpm) to units of mass in DNA, an accurate determination of phosphate specific activity is essential. The acid-soluble pool of approximately

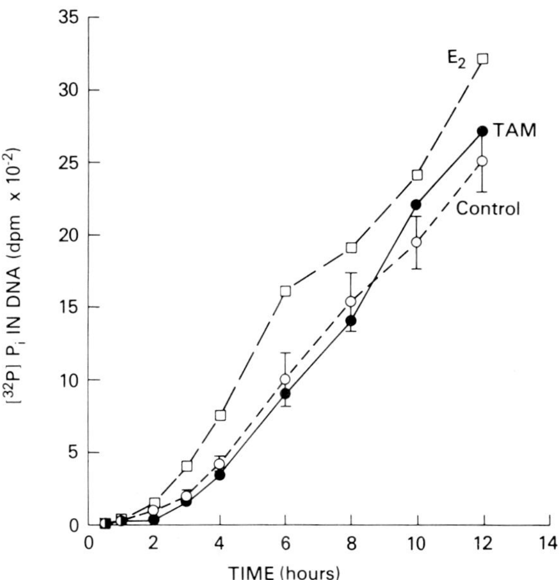

Fig. 8. Incorporation of $[^{32}P]P_i$ into DNA of MCF 7 cells. Cells were treated as previously described (Fig. 7). DNA was isolated by treatment of sonicates with RNAase + pronase and hydroxylapatite chromatography as previously described (Lippman and Aitken, 1980a, 1980b). For reasons of clarity, standard deviations are depicted only for control samples although variation among all experimental groups was similar and in no case exceeded 15% of the reported value. Control (○); tamoxifen (●); oestradiol (□).

10^9 MCF 7 cells pulsed with [^{32}P]P_i and [^{3}H]dThd was subjected to sequential fractionation as shown in Table III. It can be seen from column 2 (in which [^{3}H]dThd is utilized as a trace for the distribution and recovery of nucleotides) that charcoal treatment of the acid-soluble fraction resulted in adsorption of virtually all nucleotides to the charcoal pellet. The supernatant remaining after charcoal treatment is considered to represent true inorganic phosphate (row 2). Extraction of nucleotides from the charcoal pellet with ammoniacal ethanol is represented in row 3. This extraction procedure is relatively specific for nucleotides. Isolation of the dTMP component employing thin-layer chromatography was also performed. The results of three separate experiments (A, B, C) are present in column 3. It can be seen from examination of these data that the specific activity of [^{32}P]P_i in all components of the acid-soluble pool is identical.

TABLE III
Distribution of [^{32}P]P_i amongst Components of the Acid-Soluble Pool in MCF 7 Cells[a]

Fraction	% Recovery ([^{3}H]dThd)	Specific activity (dpm[^{32}P]/pmol P_i)
Acid-soluble	100 ± 10	A. 12.8
		B. 4.67 ± 1.80
		C. 10.51 ± 2.37
Charcoal-treated supernatant	8.7 ± 2.8	A. 11.0
		B. 4.54 ± 0.23
		C. 9.48 ± 2.47
Charcoal pellet	63.6 ± 16.8	A. 11.05
		B. 4.54 ± 0.37
		C. 11.30 ± 0.95
Thymidine	27.8 ± 8.6	A. N.D.
		B. N.D.
		C. 10.07 ± 0.66

[a] Approximately 10^9 cells were pulsed with [^{32}P]P_i (1 μCi/ml, 8 hours) and with [^{3}H]dThd (1 μCi/ml, 2 hours). Cells were transferred to 10^{-5} M phosphate medium 24 hours prior to addition of [^{32}P]P_i. The acid-soluble fraction (row 1) was obtained as previously described (Lippman and Aitken, 1980a, 1980b). Aliquots were taken for determination of radioactivity and P_i. A third aliquot was treated with dextran-coated charcoal (2.5 mg Norit A + 0.25 mg dextran) and centrifuged (10 minutes, 1500 g). The resultant supernatant (row 2) was similarly analysed for radioactivity and P_i. The charcoal precipitate was then extracted with ammoniacal ethanol. A portion of this extract (row 3) was analysed for radioactivity and P_i. A second portion was lyophilized and chromatographed as previously described. The fraction corresponding to a dTMP standard run in parallel was eluted with 0.01N HCl (row 4). Aliquots were again taken for counting and determination of P_i. Column 1 presents these fractions. Column 2 (recovery of [^{3}H]dThd) provides a marker for the distribution of nucleotides among soluble pool components. Radioactivity in the acid-soluble pool is taken as 100%. Column 3 (^{32}P specific activity) is obtained by dividing the observed ^{32}P dpm in the sample by the mass of phosphate detected. In column 3, A, B, and C represent different experiments. N.D. = not determined.

The above experiments strongly suggest that estimates of the specific activity of the DNA precursor pool based on data derived from the acid-soluble pool are accurate, provided equilibrium conditions are established. True estimates of the rate of net DNA synthesis then become possible under a variety of experimental conditions provided that equilibrium conditions are met for each type of experimental manipulation performed.

1. *Effect of Oestradiol and Tamoxifen*

It is important to investigate the time course and dose response to hormonal treatment of phosphate pools in MCF 7 cells since preliminary analyses at 24 and 48 hours indicated pool kinetics could be profoundly altered by administration of oestrogen or tamoxifen. MCF 7 cells were

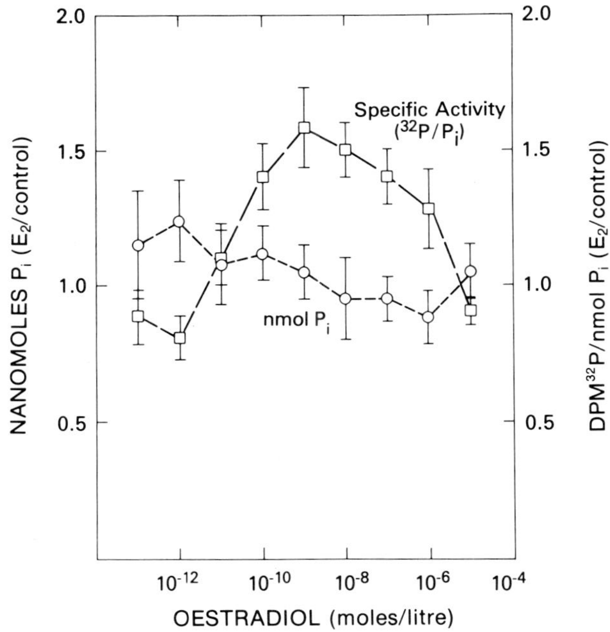

Fig. 9. Effect of varying concentrations of oestradiol on phosphate pools in MCF 7 cells. Eight hours before time 0, cells were transferred to low phosphate medium ± varying concentrations of oestradiol as indicated. After 24 hours, [^{32}P]P$_i$ (1 μCi/ml) was added to wells. Cells were harvested 32 hours after exposure to hormone. The radioactivity and phosphate content of acid-soluble pools were determined as previously described (Lippman and Aitken, 1980a, 1980b). The protein content of sonicates was also determined. Values were normalized per unit protein and are presented as the average of at least 2 independent determinations ± S.D. (□) = specific activity (dpm/nmol); (○) = mass (nmol).

exposed to varying concentrations of 17β oestradiol between 10^{-13} and 10^{-5} M for a period of 32 hours. The effect of hormone treatment on acid-soluble pool size and specific activity is shown in Figure 9. Values are expressed as the ratio to values seen in control MCF 7 cells. Oestrogen treatment did not significantly alter phosphate pool size (nmol P_i) at any concentration tested at this 32 hour time point. In contrast, the specific activity of phosphate pools (dpm ^{32}P/nmol P_i) rose significantly in a dose-dependent fashion and was maximal at 10^{-9} M.

Figure 10 demonstrates the change in the size of acid-soluble phosphate pools as a function of hormone treatment (control, tamoxifen, oestradiol + tamoxifen) and time. Phosphate pools in MCF 7 cells appear to be extremely stable over prolonged incubations in low phosphate medium although pool sizes may decrease slightly after 48 hours.

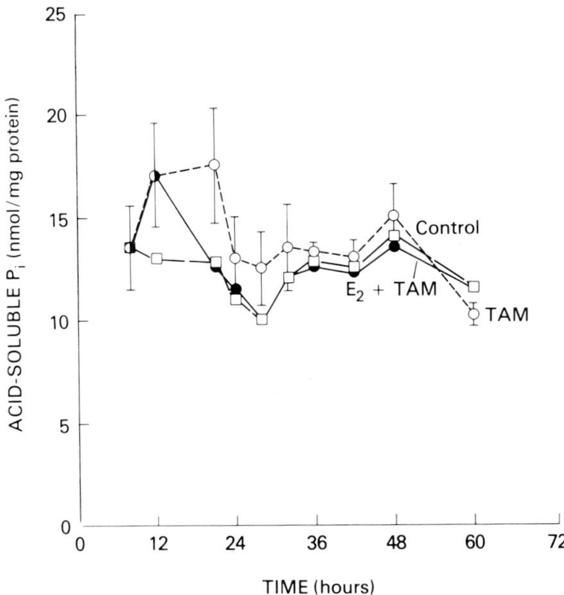

Fig. 10. Hormonal regulation of the size of acid-soluble phosphate pools in MCF 7 cells. Cells were transferred to 10^{-5} M phosphate medium 8 hours before a second medium change and hormone addition at time 0. Samples were harvested at the times indicated and the acid-soluble fraction analysed for phosphate content and ^{32}P as previously described. Values were normalized per unit protein in the sonicate and are presented as the average of at least 2 determinations ± S.D. For reasons of clarity, only the standard deviations of control samples are presented although standard deviations did not exceed 10% in any group. Control (○); tamoxifen (□); oestradiol + tamoxifen (●).

On the other hand, both time and experimental treatment significantly affect specific activity of acid-soluble phosphate pools (Fig. 11). The effective specific activity of acid-soluble phosphate rose steadily over time in all experimental conditions (control, tamoxifen, oestradiol + tamoxifen). All points represent values at equilibrium (8 hours after addition of $[^{32}P]P_i$) but varying times after transfer to 10^{-5} M phosphate medium ± hormones. Oestradiol increased the specific activity of acid-soluble phosphate over controls at all times greater than 16 hours and differences were especially marked at later time periods. Tamoxifen treatment resulted in increased specific activities relative to controls between 20 and 40 hours after administration. This general pattern would be predicted if extracellular phosphate (which has been substantially reduced to 10^{-5} M) were being progressively depleted by MCF 7 cells at rates which are additionally influenced by hormonal treatment. The specific activity of label in the medium would therefore vary depending on the incubation time at which trace was added. Intracellular specific activities would then tend to reflect extracellular

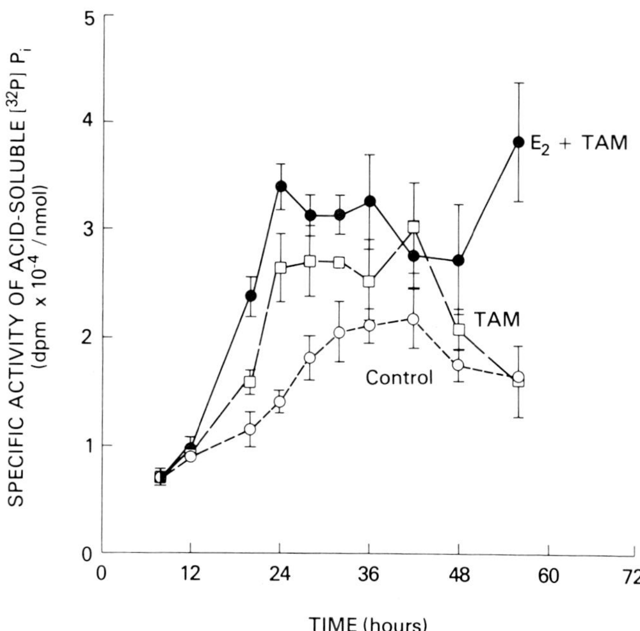

Fig. 11. Hormonal regulation of specific activity of acid-soluble phosphate pools. Cells were treated as previously described (Fig. 10). Represented values are the average of at least 2 determinations ± S.D. Control (○); tamoxifen (□); oestradiol + tamoxifen (●).

values. In data not shown, this hypothesis was confirmed by direct analysis of the phosphate content and radioactivity in medium at varying times after transfer of cells to low phosphate medium. A progressive depletion in mass of phosphate with time (0–60 hours) was seen, and increased specific activity of phosphate as a consequence of this decrease in pool size was also observed.

Thus, the status of intracellular phosphate pools in MCF 7 cells is affected by hormone treatment. Independent determination of the specific activity of phosphate pools is mandatory if extrapolation to determination of DNA synthetic rates is to be valid. Our data also suggest that the measurement of DNA synthesis should be based on a brief period of labelling time after equilibrium conditions have been established in DNA precursor pools. The time period of between 6 and 8 hours exposure to label was chosen as being convenient and as fulfilling equilibration requirements and will be used in subsequent experimental data summarized below.

Since we are concerned with the incorporation of $[^{32}P]P_i$ into DNA, and in view of the fact that ^{32}P is an effective precursor for a variety of other cellular materials, it is critical to deal with preparations which are unequivocally DNA if incorporation of label is to be validly interpreted.

Table IV shows the recovery profile from MCF 7 cells pulsed with either $[^3H]$dThd, $[^3H]$Urd or $[^3H]$Leu, effective precursors for DNA, RNA and protein, respectively. Column 1 describes the steps in a typical fractionation process. The remainder of the table presents the percentage of radioactivity recovered following acid-precipitation on millipore filters. Total acid-precipitable counts are taken as 100%. At this time only the top 4 rows of the table are of interest. It is clear that hydroxylapatite (HAP) chromatography, RNAase + pronase incubation, or HAP chromatography subsequent to RNAase + pronase incubation all yield excellent recovery of DNA ($[^3H]$dThd incorporation, column 2). However, considerable amounts of uridine and leucine label remain following RNAase + pronase treatment alone, and uridine is a substantial contaminant when samples are directly applied to HAP columns without prior enzymatic hydrolysis. HAP chromatography and enzymatic hydrolysis together, however, reduce uridine and leucine label to background levels, yielding high recovery of DNA free from contamination with protein or RNA. This procedure was followed in all subsequent experiments.

To confirm that all ^{32}P eluted from HAP columns represents only label in DNA, an MCF 7 cell extract from samples labelled with $[^{32}P]P_i$ and $[^3H]$dThd was processed for isolation of a variety of cell fractions (Table V). The eluate from HAP chromatography + enzymatic hydrolysis was divided into 2 aliquots, one for acid-precipitation and a second for acid-precipitation and hydrolysis to constituent nucleotides. A $[^{14}C]$dTMP standard was added to the acid-precipitate from unlabelled MCF 7 cells in order to estimate recovery

TABLE IV
Recovery of Radioactivity during Purification of DNA and dTMP[a]

Fraction	[^{3}H]dThd	[^{3}H]Urd	[^{3}H]Leu
1. Total acid-precipitable	100 ± 18	100 ± 9	100 ± 22
2. RNAase + pronase incubation	82 ± 17	15 ± 4	42 ± 11
3. Hydroxylapatite chromatography	96 ± 16	11 ± 6	2 ± 0.7
4. RNAase + pronase + hydroxylapatite chromatography	94 ± 11	1 ± 0.5	1 ± 0.2
5. Acid-hydrolyzed precipitate	61 ± 1	10 ± 4	12 ± 2
6. TLC eluate, (dThd, dTMP)	42 ± 6	0.5 ± 0.1	0.5 ± 0.1

[a] Approximately 10^6 cells were pulsed with either [^{3}H]dThd (1 μCi/ml, 1 hour), [^{3}H]Urd (1 μCi/ml, 1 hour), or [^{3}H]Leu (1 μCi/ml, 1 hour). At steps 1–4 of purification, acid-precipitable material was collected by the millipore filter technique for determination of radioactivity. Aliquots were taken directly for counting at steps 5 (differential acid hydrolysis of total acid-precipitable material) and 6 (eluate from thin layer chromatography of fraction 5). All values are reported as the mean of 3 independent determinations divided by the value obtained for total acid-precipitable material (row 1) ± 1 S.D. and were normalized per unit protein in the sonicate.

during the course of further fractionation. Following lyophilization of solubilized material samples were chromatographed (Lippman and Aitken, 1980b). The fractions corresponding to appropriate markers (dTMP, dCMP) were identified, cut from the plate and counted directly. Values are presented as a percentage of recovery (sonicate = 100%) and where of special interest they are presented as dpm. In column 2 [^{3}H]dThd provides an index of the efficiency of DNA recovery through the hydrolysis step. It can be seen that virtually all acid-precipitable thymidine label was recovered in the HAP eluate following acid-hydrolysis. Much of the label was subsequently lost during lyophilization and chromatography, probably due to exchange of tritium label with water, and subsequent values relating to [^{3}H]dThd are not reliable indices of the actual recovery of thymidine. The use of [^{14}C]dTMP markers permitted accurate assessment of recovery during these later steps. The pattern of recovery of ^{32}P label is presented in column 3. Approximately 2% of total ^{32}P is recovered in DNA. On further chromatography approximately 25% of ^{32}P seen in the HAP eluate could be identified in dTMP, the value which would be anticipated if the HAP eluate is indeed highly purified DNA, and if thymidine represents approximately 25% of the total nucleotide bases in DNA.

The above results strongly suggest that label eluted from hydroxylapatite following enzymatic hydrolysis is indeed a valid index of net DNA synthesis. Obviously, the conversion from dpm to mass units of incorporation is contingent upon the accurate determination of the specific activity of [^{32}P]P_i in acid-soluble pools as described previously.

TABLE V
Recovery of [^{32}P]P_i from Hydroxylapatite and Thin Layer Chromatography[a]

Fraction	[^{3}H]dThd %	[^{3}H]dThd dpm	[^{32}P]P_i %	[^{32}P]P_i dpm
Sonicate	100 ± 10	213,745	100 ± 13	1.71×10^7
Acid-precipitable	81 ± 11	171,587	28 ± 1	4.80×10^6
Acid-soluble	19 ± 1		71 ± 2	
charcoal-treated supernatant	1 ± 0.2		33 ± 5	
charcoal pellet extract	11 ± 2.5		12 ± 2	
HAP eluate (DNA)	80 ± 8	170,996	2 ± 0.1	167,220 ± 8,763
acid-hydrolysis	83 ± 4		2 ± 0.1	
lyophilization			2 ± 0.1	
Chromatography			0.5 ± 0.05	35,510 ± 3,473
recovery standard [^{14}C]dTMP				0.81
dpm corrected for recovery				43,840 ± 4,339
% of dpm recovered from HAP				0.26

[a] MCF 7 cells were transferred to 10^{-5} M phosphate medium 24 hours prior to labelling with [^{3}H]dThd (1 μCi/ml, 2 hours) and [^{32}P]P_i (1 μCi/ml, 8 hours). Dpm in the sonicate were taken as 100%. Cell sonicates were processed as previously described (Lippman and Aitken, 1980a, 1980b). Known amounts of [^{14}C]dTMP (0.1 μCi) were added to the acid-precipitable pellet from unlabelled MCF 7 cells just prior to acid-hydrolysis as an index of recovery for chromatography. All values are the mean of three determinations ± 1 S.D. and were normalized per unit protein in the sonicate.

B. Differentiation between Repair and Replicative DNA Synthesis

Given the availability of two independent methods for determining mass of DNA synthesized ([^{32}P]P_i incorporation and ethidium bromide fluorometry) it was considered possible to investigate the issue of the possible contribution of unscheduled DNA synthesis or repair to DNA synthesis in MCF 7 cells. Measurements based on ^{32}P incorporation could overestimate the amount of net DNA synthesized under conditions in which repair constitutes a significant contribution to incorporated label. Therefore, a comparison was made between the mass of DNA synthesized (based on incorporation of ^{32}P of known specific activity into DNA over a 72 hour period) with measurements of mass (based on ethidium bromide fluorometry) at the start and at various points during that 72 hour period. These data are presented in Table VI. It can be seen that even under circumstances in which prolonged administration of ^{32}P may induce cell and DNA damage, the amount of repair is in fact not measurable against a background of replicative DNA synthesis. It is, however, possible that under other circumstances in which replicative DNA synthesis is blocked (i.e. drug administration) a small background of repair synthesis could be demonstrated.

TABLE VI
Contribution of Repair DNA Synthesis to Measurements of Net DNA based on ^{32}P Incorporation[a]

Time (hours)	nmol DNA (P_i)	nmol DNA (EtBr)	Specific activity (dpm/nmol P_i)	ratio (^{32}P/EtBr)
0	0	31.33 ± 4.4	0	0
24	18.2 ± 3.6	53.6 ± 7.8	10.7 ± 1.26	0.186
48	29.6 ± 3.7	60.7 ± 12.6	15.9 ± 3.7	1.006
72	34.0 ± 6.2	65.4 ± 7.0	11.4 ± 2.4	0.997

[a] Cells were replicately plated in IMEM + 2.5% charcoal treated foetal calf serum + 10^{-7} M insulin. When cells were subconfluent medium was replaced with IMEM containing 10^{-5} M phosphate. At time 0 medium was again replaced with IMEM + 10^{-5} M phosphate, 5×10^{-9} M 17β oestradiol, and approximately 1 μCi/ml [^{32}P]P_i. One group of samples was immediately harvested (time 0) and other groups were harvested at successive 24 hour intervals. DNA synthesis was measured by ethidium bromide fluorometry (column 3) and by conversion of ^{32}P incorporation to mass units based on the specific activity of ^{32}P in the acid soluble pool (column 4). Isolation of DNA was performed as previously described (Lippman and Aitken, 1980a, 1980b). The ratio of DNA synthesized (^{32}P) to the difference in mass between 0 time and the indicated time points (EtBr) is shown in column 5.

C. Experimental Protocol for Assessment of Net DNA Synthesis

Given the ability to validly isolate DNA and determine specific activity of acid-soluble phosphate pools, it is possible to develop an experimental protocol to produce and to reduce data. In any given experiment each experimental group is divided into three: one subset is labelled for 6 hours with [^{32}P]P_i; a second is similarly labelled for 8 hours; and a third is labelled for 8 hours and in addition is pulsed for the 2 hours prior to harvest with [^{3}H]dThd. This protocol is necessitated by the extended period required for equilibration of [^{32}P]P_i with intracellular phosphate pools and by the fact that dThd administration, as will be demonstrated later, affects the pattern of net DNA synthesis in MCF 7 cells and thus constitutes an independent variable in experimental design. A typical experiment in which the major variable is oestrogen administration is seen in Table VII. These data can be transformed to mass of phosphate incorporated based on the experimentally determined specific activity of acid-soluble phosphate. Such data reduction is illustrated in Table VIII. Data can be still further reduced (Table IX) on the basis of observed differences in values between 6 and 8 hours of labelling and then, if desired, shown as a set of ratios between groups. Thus, final analysis involves three sets of values: the effect of thymidine on the system (dThd/control); the effect of the experimental manipulation (oestrogen/control); and the effect of thymidine coupled with the effect of oestrogen (oestrogen + dThd/control).

TABLE VII
Effect of Oestradiol and Thymidine on DNA Synthesis[a]

Group	Protein (mg)	DNA (μg)	Acid soluble (nmol P_i)	Acid soluble (dpm ^{32}P)	^{32}P (dpm)
Control					
6 hours	0.523	23.1	30.6	1.61×10^6	6,685
8 hours	0.463	21.7	25.5	1.26×10^6	10,115
+ dThd	0.508	22.2	28.0	1.51×10^6	12,670
Oestradiol					
6 hours	0.869	27.9	45.0	2.75×10^6	8,885
8 hours	0.876	28.6	43.6	2.63×10^6	16,780
8 hours + dThd	0.793	29.0	41.1	2.47×10^6	18,056

[a] Experimental groups (column 1) are depicted as control and oestradiol (5×10^{-9} M). Within each group 6 hour and 8 hour subgroups refer to the time of labelling with [^{32}P]P_i. In the 8 hour plus dThd subgroup cells are labelled for 8 hours with [^{32}P]P_i and for the last 2 hours with [^{3}H]dThd. Columns 2 and 3 refer to the protein and DNA content of the sonicate. Columns 4 and 5 refer to the mass and radioactivity of phosphate in the acid soluble fraction and are determined as described previously (Lippman and Aitken, 1980a, 1980b). Column 6 applies to radioactivity detected in DNA (eluted from hydroxylapatite columns). Standard deviations are not presented but were in the range of 10–15% of presented values.

TABLE VIII
Effects of Oestrogen and Thymidine on DNA Synthesis in MCF 7 Cells transformed to Mass Units of Incorporation[a]

Group	Protein (mg/mg DNA)	P_i (nmol/mg)	^{32}P (dpm/pmol P_i)	[^{32}P]P_i (pmol/mg protein)	[^{32}P]P_i (pmol/mg DNA)
Control					
6 hours	22.6	58.5	52.6	127.1	2,822
8 hours	21.4	55.1	49.4	204.8	4,492
8 hours + dThd	222.8	55.1	53.9	235.1	5,361
Oestradiol					
6 hours	31.2	51.8	61.1	145.4	5,536
8 hours	30.6	49.7	60.3	278.2	8,513
8 hours + dThd	27.4	51.8	60.0	300.9	8,245

[a] Column 1 refers to experimental groups as described in the text. Columns 3 and 4 present the mass and specific activity of phosphate in the acid-soluble pool. Column 5 refers to the mass of precursor incorporated into DNA during the labelling period indicated in column 1. Mass units are derived by dividing the observed dpm for each precursor by its known or presumed specific activity ([^{32}P]P_i = value presented in column 4).

TABLE IX
Effect of Oestradiol and Thymidine on Net DNA Synthesis in MCF 7 Cells[a]

Group	P_i/mg protein	P_i/mg DNA
I. Control	77.7	1,670
Control + dThd	108	2,539
Oestradiol	132.8	2,977
Oestradiol + dThd	155.5	2,709
II. dThd/Control	1.39	1.52
Oestradiol/Control	1.71	1.78
Oestradiol + dThd/Control	2.00	1.61

[a] Column 1 refers to experimental groups. Column 2 refers to the differences in the mass of precursor incorporated into DNA between 6 and 8 hours of labelling. In section II data are still further reduced to a set of ratios relative to appropriate controls. The proper control for [^{32}P]P_i is found in row 1 of section I (control).

D. Hormonal Regulation of Net DNA Synthesis

With this experimental design it is finally possible to rigorously investigate the hormonal regulation of DNA synthesis. The effect of varying concentrations of oestradiol on the incorporation of labelled precursor, [^{32}P]P_i, into DNA is shown in Figure 12. Cells were exposed to hormone for 32 hours. Following treatment there was a dose-related increase in the incorporation of phosphate into DNA of MCF 7 cells which was evident between $10^{-7}$and 10^{-11} M and maximal at 10^{-9} M.

The time course of the effect of oestradiol and tamoxifen on net DNA synthesis in the absence of exogenous thymidine is shown in Figure 13. Values are normalized against the values observed after 8 hours of a given treatment (8 hours is the minimum labelling time which can be used in ^{32}P incorporation studies in MCF 7 cells). It can be seen that control cells present a highly variable background with one peak occurring between 24 and 36 hours after transfer to serum free conditions and a second peak occurring at about 48 hours. The limited ability of MCF 7 cells to survive under serum free conditions precluded the extension of time course experiments beyond 60–72 hours, and it was consequently difficult to determine whether this second wave also represented a partial synchronization of MCF 7 cells or was actually a continuous gradient of DNA synthesis. In the absence of exogenous thymidine the effect of tamoxifen is highly inhibitory within 18 hours of antioestrogen administration. Concurrent administration of oestradiol and tamoxifen resulted in a stimulation of phosphate incorporation well above control levels. It is of interest that the peaks of incorporation of oestrogen treated cells occurred synchronously with those in control cells and differed only in magnitude of incorporation. This general pattern was highly reproducible from one experiment to the next. The time of onset of the first peak varied experimentally between 18 and 24 hours after addition of fresh serum free medium and extended for approximately 12 hours. A second peak was evident in three out of four experiments in control cells and was invariably present in oestrogen treated cells.

Striking effects on the pattern of DNA synthesis described above were observed on addition of exogenous dThd (10^{-7} M, 5 μCi [^{3}H]dThd) to cells, as shown in Figure 14. The effect of thymidine alone is clearly limited in this experiment to early time points (18–30 hours). Oestrogen treatment produced a slight peak at approximately 18 hours and had major effects during later stages of the incubation as values for net DNA synthesis rose progressively up

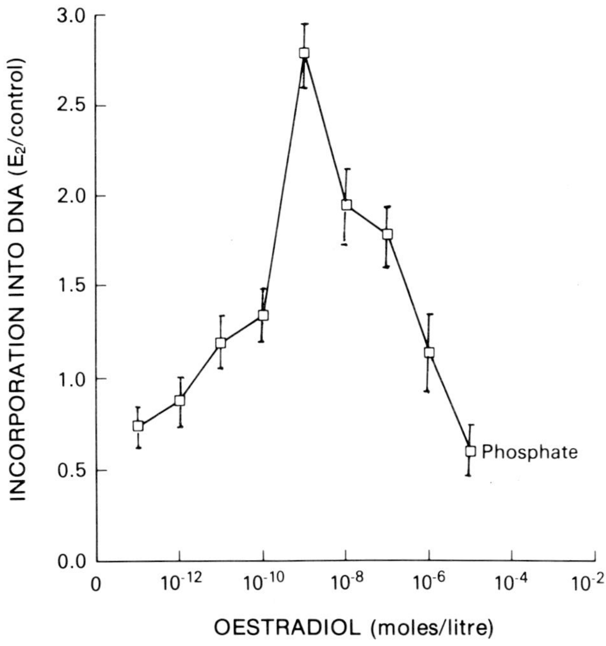

Fig. 12. Effect of varying concentrations of oestradiol on DNA synthesis in MCF 7 cells. Cells were treated as previously described (Fig. 9). Twenty-four or 26 hours after time 0, [^{32}P]P_i (1 μCi/ml) was added to wells. Radioactivity in acid-soluble and DNA fractions was determined as previously described (Lippman and Aitken, 1980a, 1980b). The protein, DNA, and acid-soluble phosphate contents were also determined. Values for incorporation of phosphate (pmol/2 hours) were calculated as previously described and normalized per unit DNA. Results are presented as the ratio to control values.

to five fold over control levels. The coupled effect of oestradiol and thymidine essentially lies in an increase in the magnitude of the early wave of DNA synthesis over either oestrogen treatment or thymidine administration alone. In other experiments (data not shown), the effect of oestrogen plus thymidine on phosphate incorporation varied between a two and four fold increase over controls at the first wave of synthesis. The first wave of synthesis in MCF 7 cells is thus primarily associated with availability of exogenous thymidine and the second with availability of oestrogenic hormones.

Application of similar experimental analysis to tamoxifen administration is shown in Figure 15. It can again be seen that thymidine administration alone (10^{-7} M, 5 μCi/ml) increased net DNA synthesis during early stages of the incubation. Tamoxifen alone profoundly inhibited incorporation of phosphate into DNA. Tamoxifen and this concentration of thymidine (10^{-7}

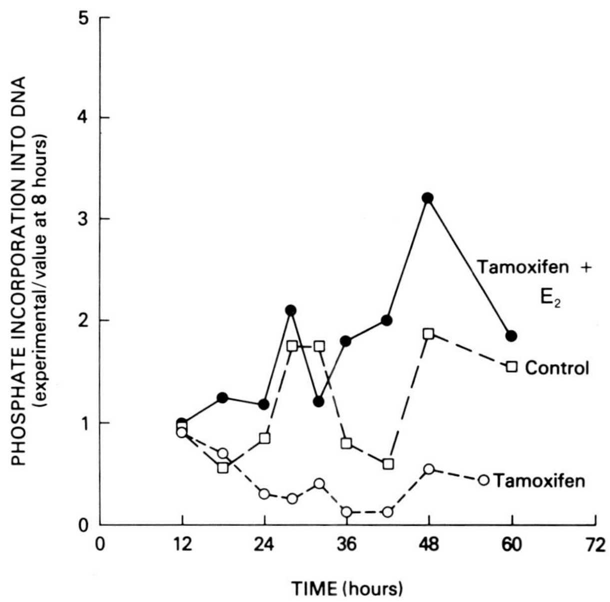

Fig. 13. Effect of hormones on net DNA synthesis in MCF 7 cells in the absence of exogenous thymidine. Eight hours prior to time 0, cells were transferred to 10^{-5} M phosphate medium and at time 0 medium was again replaced ± tamoxifen (2×10^{-6} M) or oestradiol (10^{-8}M) + tamoxifen (2×10^{-6} M). [^{32}P]P_i was added to samples (1 μCi/ml) 8 or 6 hours before the indicated time of harvest. Data reduction to mass units of phosphate (pmol/2 hours) incorporated into DNA was performed as previously described. The presented values were normalized against the value observed within the same experimental group after 8 hours of incubation. Standard deviations were in the range of 10–15% at all represented points.

M) in conjunction consistently permitted recovery of MCF 7 cells from tamoxifen arrest and in the experiment shown here produced an actual increase above control levels during the earlier wave of DNA synthesis. The ability of dThd to reverse tamoxifen inhibition of phosphate incorporation during later stages of the incubation was somewhat variable. In the experiment shown no such ability was evident. In a second experiment, dThd plus tamoxifen treatment elevated incorporation over tamoxifen alone at all stages of the incubation although values were nonetheless lower than those observed in the presence of dThd alone. In this latter experiment, dThd was added at 2×10^{-7} M, 10 μCi/ml, and this higher concentration may have resulted in somewhat greater effects.

In summary, it can be seen that oestrogens and antioestrogens exert powerful regulatory effects on DNA synthesis in MCF 7 cells. The growth fraction is dramatically increased by oestrogen administration. Cells frequently show two major peaks of DNA synthesis, an early wave which is

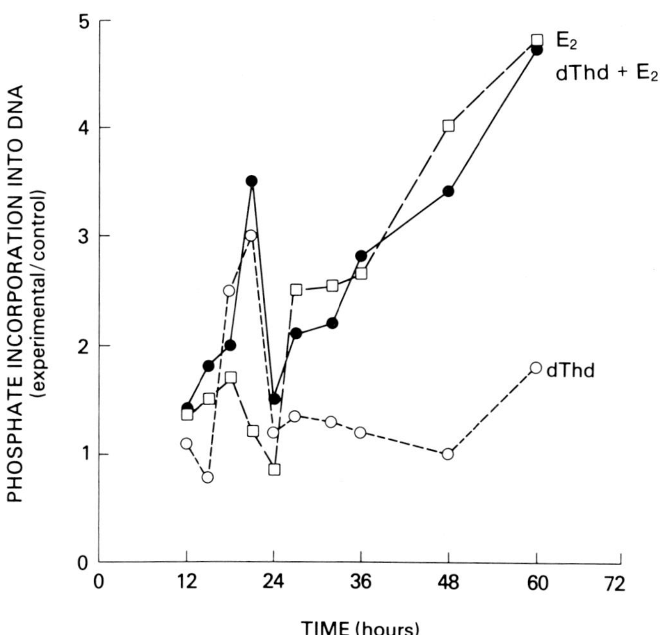

Fig. 14. Effect of exogenous thymidine and oestradiol on net DNA synthesis in MCF 7 cells. Cells were treated with oestradiol (5×10^{-9} M) and/or thymidine (10^{-7} M). Presented values were normalized against the values seen in controls at the same time point. Standard deviations within any experimental group did not exceed 15% of the mean value.

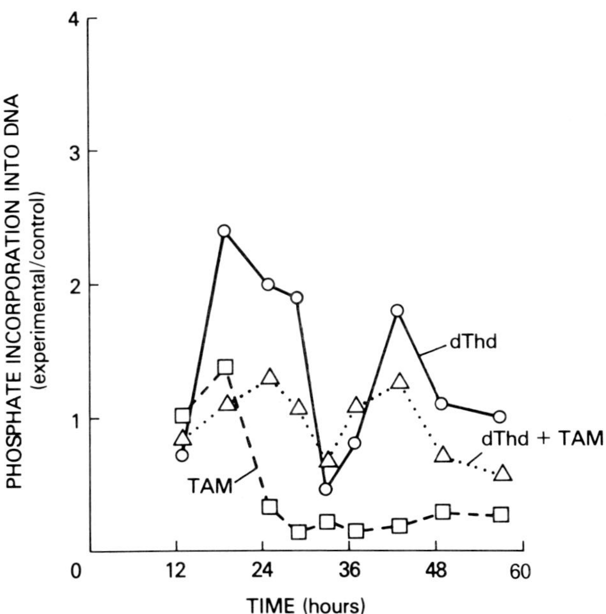

Fig. 15. Effect of exogenous thymidine and tamoxifen on net DNA synthesis in MCF 7 cells. Cells were treated with tamoxifen (2×10^{-6} M) and/or thymidine (10^{-7} M). Data are presented as in Figure 14. Standard deviations are not represented for reasons of clarity but did not exceed 15% of the values presented.

associated with the availability of exogenous thymidine (18–30 hours) and a second wave of synthesis unaffected in magnitude by the administration of thymidine. The effects of oestrogen alone are manifested in an amplification of these waves of DNA synthesis rather than in a change in the time frame within which cells enter DNA synthesis. Oestrogen action relative to controls is especially evident during later phases of the serum free incubation. Tamoxifen administration decreases net DNA synthesis within 18 hours after treatment, and this effect can be reversed by simultaneous exposure to oestradiol. Also, thymidine addition to the medium at concentrations in excess of 10^{-7} M partially reverses the inhibition produced by tamoxifen, and this reversal is most apparent during the early wave of DNA synthesis.

IV. DISCUSSION

It is clear that oestrogen administration results in an increase in the growth fraction of MCF 7 cells. It is not clear, however, whether this is due to

(a) a decrease in cell death, (b) an increased growth rate (decrease in length of the cell cycle), or (c) an increased recruitment of nondividing cells arrested in G_1 (G_0) into the actively dividing population. There is evidence that oestrogen *in vivo* acts as a trophic hormone under physiological conditions by recruitment of cells from G_0 to G_1, as, for example, in the induction of uterine growth (Hamilton, 1968; Epifanova, 1971). However, it has also been reported that oestrogen administration to MCF 7 cells does in fact decrease cell cycle time, and increased growth was attributed in this case to a specific decrease in the length of the G_1 phase of the cell cycle (Weichselbaum *et al.*, 1978). In addition, oestradiol has been observed to increase the mitotic index of MCF 7 cells by 51% (serum free conditions, 2×10^{-9} M oestradiol, 72 hours) and by 72–240% (1% charcoal treated calf serum, 2×10^{-9} M oestradiol, 24–48 hours). The mitotic index was observed to vary between 1.28% and 15.34% depending on the circumstances of growth and incubation time (see Table I).

The fact that MCF 7 cells represent a transformed cell line may be of considerable significance in the interpretation of data relating to cell cycle kinetics. Transformed cells are known to exhibit dormancy, being recruited from the actively dividing population into the nondividing population. However, the depth of their arrest is considered to be slight and they are comparatively easily returned to the cell cycle.

The precise conditions under which oestrogen might act as a required element in the passage of human breast cancer cells through G_1 are unclear. MCF 7 cells represent a transformed line in which we have previously been unable to demonstrate a dependency on oestrogen as a trophic factor. Cells appear to grow equally well in the absence of oestrogen provided other trophic factors (serum, insulin) are present, and it is indeed difficult to demonstrate oestrogenic effects in the presence of optimal amounts of these factors. It is not clear at this time whether the oestrogen produced increase in growth fraction of these cells is due to increased cell multiplication or decreased cell death or a combination of both. There is also some question about the known reduced ability of transformed cells to arrest in G_1(G_0) under adverse conditions, a fact which can result in differential cell death of cancer cells relative to normal cells in response to some forms of chemotherapy. If transformed cells such as the MCF 7 or ZR 75 lines must indeed divide or die, cell growth and cell death are not necessarily independent phenomena and increase in growth ensures a decreased rate of cell loss from the population. Conversely, failure to divide ensures an increased rate of population attrition.

In the experiments described above MCF 7 cells display an apparent partial synchronization of phosphate incorporation into DNA following transfer to serum free medium (Fig. 13). Neither oestradiol nor tamoxifen administration affected the timing of observed waves of DNA synthesis with respect to controls. The causes of this partial synchronization of the cell population are unknown. Nutritionally arrested cells are known to respond to addition of serum or critical nutrients in a synchronous fashion (Doida and Okada, 1972). Observations in MCF 7 cells could reflect a similar phenomenon. However, cells were actively growing and not in growth arrest at the time of medium transfer. It is conversely possible that the replacement of serum supplemented medium with fresh serum free medium resulted in a depletion of cell produced growth factors which must then reaccumulate in order to stimulate mitosis.

Regardless of the mechanisms of this synchronization, the fact that oestrogen treatment did not discernably decrease the delay period required for DNA synthesis suggests that the primary effect of oestrogen may not be a decrease in cycle time but rather an entry of cells not scheduled to divide into the actively growing population. The possibility that oestrogen additionally decreases cell cycle time is not necessarily precluded. However, the two to five fold increases in phosphate incorporation observed during pulse labelling in a synchronized population make the latter possibility remote as the sole mode of oestrogenic action in MCF 7 cells. Since phosphate incorporation into DNA is normalized versus either protein or DNA content, a two fold increase in incorporation infers that the likelihood of a given cell being in S is twice as great in an oestrogen treated population as in controls. Two to five fold reductions in cell cycle time seem improbable.

The pattern of net DNA synthesis in MCF 7 cells and the effects of exogenous thymidine on that pattern yield some interesting suggestions about the possible role of salvage and *de novo* pathways of pyrimidine production in MCF 7 cells and the potential mechanisms by which oestrogen may increase the rate of DNA synthesis in hormonally responsive systems. It is of interest that the early wave of DNA synthesis in MCF 7 cells is modulated by the availability of exogenous dThd. Thymidine administration increases DNA synthesis at early time points in controls; oestrogen treated cells have a greater ability to utilize thymidine as a trigger for net DNA synthesis than do controls. Tamoxifen treated cells which had been profoundly inhibited were rescued by exogenous thymidine during this early stage of the incubation and actually showed a stimulation above control levels in one experiment. The activity of thymidine kinase is known to be increased by oestrogens and decreased by antioestrogens in MCF 7 cells (Lippman *et al.*, 1976d). The increase in net DNA synthesis in oestrogen treated populations relative to controls at early incubation stages could therefore be due to increased thymidine kinase activity. However, the ability of thymidine to reverse tamoxifen inhibition implies that, although thymidine kinase activity is decreased, there is no functional impairment of salvage activity (at least at the high levels of thymidine employed in these experiments, 5×10^{-8} to 2×10^{-6} M). During later stages of the incubation, effects of thymidine on net DNA synthesis were not as apparent, possibly indicating an increased dependency in MCF 7 cells on *de novo* pyrimidine production. Such a dependency may reflect either a depletion of available salvage sources of thymidine in the earlier wave of DNA synthesis or an oestrogen dependent induction of critical *de novo* or intermediary enzymes.

REFERENCES

Allegra, J. C., and Lippman, M. E. (1978). *Cancer Res.* **38**, 3823–3829.

Doida, Y., and Okada, S. (1972). *Cell Tissue Kinetics* **5**, 15–26.

Edwards, D. P., Murthy, S. R., and McGuire, W. L. (1980). *Cancer Res.* **40**, 1722–1726.

Engel, L. W., and Young, N. A. (1978). *Cancer Res.* **38**, 4327–4339.

Engel, L. W., Young, N. A., Tralka, T. S., Lippman, M. E., O'Brien, S. J., and Joyce, M. J. (1978). *Cancer Res.* **38**, 3352–3364.

Epifanova, O. I. (1971). *In* "The Cell Cycle and Cancer" (R. Baserga, ed.), pp. 143–182. Marcel Dekker, New York.

Hamilton, T. H. (1968). *Science* **161**, 654–661.

Hayashi, I., and Sato, G. H. (1976). *Nature* **259**, 132–134.

Hayashi, I., Larner, J., and Sato, G. (1978). *In Vitro* **14**, 23–30.

Lippman, M. E., and Aitken, S. C. (1980a). *In* "Regulation of Initiation of DNA Synthesis and Differentiation in Cultured Animals Cells" (J. DeAsua, L. Montalcini and S. Iacobelli, eds)., pp. 3–19. Raven Press, New York.

Lippman, M. E., and Aitken, S. C. (1980b). *In* "Hormones and Cancer" (S. Iacobelli, R. J. B. King, H. R. Linder, and M. E. Lippman, eds), pp. 1-20. Raven Press, New York.

Lippman, M. E., Bolan, G., and Huff, K. (1976a). *Cancer Res.* **36**, 4595–4601.

Lippman, M. E., Bolan, G., and Huff, K. (1976b). *Cancer Res.* **36**, 4602–4609.

Lippman, M. E., Bolan, G., and Huff, K. (1976c). *Cancer Res.* **36**, 4610–4618.

Lippman, M. E., Bolan, G., Monaco, M. E., Pinkus, L., and Engel. L. (1976d). *J. Steroid Biochem.* **7**, 1045–1051.

Lippman, M. E., Monaco, M. E., and Bolan, G. (1977). *Cancer Res.* **37**, 1901–1907.

Lippman, M. E., Allegra, J. C., and Stobl, J. S. (1979). *Cold Spring Harbor Conferences on Cell Proliferation* **6**, 545–555.

Osborne, C. K., Bolan, G., Monaco, M. E., and Lippman, M. E. (1976). *Proc. Natl Acad. Sci., U.S.A.* **73**, 4536–4540.

Osborne, C. K., Monaco, M. E., Lippman, M. E., and Kahn, C. R. (1978). *Cancer Res.* **38**, 94–102.

Richter, A., Sanford, K. K., and Evans, V. J. (1972). *J. Natl Cancer Inst.* **49**, 1705–1712.

Soule, J. D., Vazquez, J., Long, A., Albert, J., and Brennan, M. (1973). *J. Natl Cancer Inst.* **51**, 1409–1413.

Strobl, J. S., and Lippman, M. E. (1979). *Cancer Res.* **39**, 3319–3327.

Thompson, E. B., Anderson, C. V., and Lippman, M. E., (1975). *J. Cell. Physiol.* **86**, 403–411.

Weichselbaum, R. R., Hellman, S., Piro, A. J., Nove, J. J., and Little, J. B. (1978). *Cancer Res.* **38**, 2339–2342.

23

Effects of Antioestrogens on the Growth and Cell Cycle Kinetics of Cultured Human Mammary Carcinoma Cells

M. D. GREEN, A. M. WHYBOURNE, I. W. TAYLOR AND R. L. SUTHERLAND

I. INTRODUCTION

A number of different endocrine therapeutic regimens, including endocrine ablation (hypophysectomy, adrenalectomy and ovariectomy), high dose steroid administration (androgens, glucocorticoids and oestrogens) and, more recently, administration of the antioestrogen tamoxifen induce regression of many malignant tumours of the human breast (McGuire *et al.*, 1975; Mouridsen *et al.*, 1978). Such regression is almost invariably confined to

NON-STEROIDAL ANTIOESTROGENS
ISBN 0 12 677880 9

those tumours which express the specific oestrogen receptor protein, suggesting that these endocrine effects may be mediated through the oestrogen receptor mechanisms of oestrogen responsive tumour cells (DeSombre *et al.*, 1974; McGuire *et al.*, 1975; Mouridsen *et al.*, 1978). Little is known, however, of the mechanisms by which changes in the endocrine environment influence the rate of mammary tumour cell proliferation or cell death and it is probably naive to assume that such a wide range of endocrine manipulations mediate their effects in identical ways. In this laboratory we have recently established a research programme to investigate, in more detail, the effects of changes in the endocrine environment on cell proliferation and cell death in monolayer cultures of human mammary carcinoma cells. Such research may lead to a better understanding of the biochemical mechanisms by which these endocrine effects, especially those of oestrogens and antioestrogens, are mediated at the target cell level.

The effects of oestrogens on mammary tumour cells have been studied in some detail both *in vivo* and *in vitro*. Ovariectomy is known to induce regression of a number of different experimental mammary tumours of rats and mice (Huggins, 1965; Gullino *et al.*, 1975; Watson *et al.*, 1977, 1979; Sluyser, 1979), and although this may be due to a direct effect of oestrogen deprivation on oestrogen dependent tumour cells, other indirect effects of oestrogen withdrawal have been implicated. For example, in the DMBA-induced rat mammary carcinoma model it is thought that the reduction of oestrogen induced prolactin synthesis is the principal event in tumour regression (Manni *et al.*, 1977), whilst in other tumour types, reduction of oestrogen induced synthesis of undefined growth factors has been implicated (Sirbasku, 1978).

Tumour regression resulting from high dose oestrogen administration has not been investigated in great detail. An early study with DMBA-induced tumours suggested that large doses of oestrogen directly inhibit stimulation of mammary tumour growth by prolactin (Meites *et al.*, 1971). More recently Tsai *et al.* (1979) reported a significant reduction in the concentration of oestrogen receptors in two different rat mammary tumours (DMBA and R3230AC) following high dose oestrogen administration. Such a decrease in oestrogen receptor concentration may be implicated in the antitumour activity of this treatment.

Attempts to demonstrate direct stimulatory effects of oestrogen on the proliferation of mammary tumour cells *in vitro* were initially inconsistent as far as demonstrating significant increases in cell numbers. However, recent data on two cell lines, MCF 7 and ZR 75–1, have demonstrated significant increases in cell numbers following oestrogen administration *in vitro* (Lippman *et al.*, 1976; Weichselbaum *et al.*, 1978; Allegra and Lippman,

1978). A direct inhibitory effect of high dose oestrogen treatment on cell growth has also been demonstrated *in vitro* (Lippman *et al.*, 1976; Riley *et al.*, 1978; Weichselbaum *et al.*, 1978). This oestrogenic effect appears to be mediated independently of the oestrogen receptor since it is unaffected by inhibitors of RNA and protein synthesis (Riley *et al.*, 1978) and can be induced, at similar concentrations, by ligands which have very weak affinity for the oestrogen receptor, e.g. 17α oestradiol (Lippman *et al.*, 1976). Non-specific effects of hydrophobic steroids on cell membrane and cytoskeleton structure have been suggested as possible primary steps in the inhibition of cell growth by high dose oestrogen *in vitro* (Riley *et al.*, 1978).

The inhibitory effects of a number of synthetic non-steroidal anti-oestrogens on the growth of experimental mammary tumours of rodents have been documented (Terenius, 1971; DeSombre and Arbogast, 1974; Nicholson and Golder, 1975; Jordan, 1976; Tsai and Katzenellenbogen, 1977; Tsai *et al.*, 1979; Sluyser, 1979; Rose *et al.*, 1980). It is generally agreed that tumour regression induced by these compounds is confined to oestrogen receptor positive tumours, which is in agreement with the clinical situation, and has led to the popular belief that these compounds exert their effects by interfering with oestrogen receptor mediated oestrogenic action.

In vitro experiments investigating the direct effects of antioestrogens on the growth of cultured human mammary carcinoma cells have invariably demonstrated growth inhibition and inhibition of the rate of incorporation of tritiated thymidine in oestrogen responsive cell lines (Lippman and Bolan, 1975; Lippman *et al.*, 1976; Horwitz *et al.*, 1978a; Allegra and Lippman, 1978). These inhibitory effects can be reversed by simultaneous or subsequent addition of a 10-fold lower concentration of oestradiol, suggesting that the inhibitory effects of antioestrogens on cell proliferation are oestrogen receptor mediated (Lippman *et al.*, 1976; Horwitz *et al.*, 1978a). Recent experiments with the ZR 75-1 cell line growing in serum free, hormone supplemented medium have shown that tamoxifen can inhibit cell growth below that seen in the absence of oestradiol (Allegra and Lippman, 1978). This may be due to residual effects of cellular oestrogens in control cultures (cf. Strobl and Lippman, 1979) or to an additional effect of tamoxifen which is not influenced by oestrogen and which may or may not be oestrogen receptor mediated.

The above data illustrate that there are well-documented effects of oestrogens and antioestrogens on the growth of mammary carcinoma cells *in vivo* and *in vitro*. However, little is known of the biochemical mechanisms which mediate these effects. In an attempt to understand more clearly the molecular basis for the antitumour activity of tamoxifen, we first investigated the effects of this drug on the growth and cell cycle kinetic parameters of cultured human mammary carcinoma cells.

II. CYTOTOXIC EFFECTS OF TAMOXIFEN ON OESTROGEN RECEPTOR POSITIVE MAMMARY CARCINOMA CELLS

With the exception of the previously unpublished data presented in Figure 4 of Chapter 22 there is no direct experimental evidence that the non-steroidal antioestrogens are cytotoxic, i.e. that they induce their growth inhibitory effects by increasing the rate of cell death. We therefore designed a series of experiments to ascertain whether tamoxifen was cytotoxic *in vitro* and, if so, its specificity (i.e. oestrogen receptor positive versus oestrogen receptor negative cells), dose and time dependence. Preliminary experiments indicated that the effects of tamoxifen on cell growth were related to the concentration of foetal calf serum in the culture medium. Although tamoxifen has not been reported to have high affinity, saturable binding sites on plasma proteins, it appears to be bound with relatively high affinity to non-specific sites in serum and plasma (Sutherland, unpublished observations). As a result, most of the drug is protein bound in solutions containing plasma proteins, and thus the concentration of drug in free solution is dependent upon the protein concentration. In order to minimize the non-specific binding of antioestrogens to foetal calf serum it seemed appropriate to work at reduced foetal calf serum concentrations. For this reason a series of experiments was performed to ascertain the minimal concentration of foetal calf serum that could maintain maximal rates of logarithmic growth in the cell lines under study.

Initial experiments were performed with the much studied MCF 7, oestrogen receptor positive, human mammary carcinoma cell line, (Soule *et al.*, 1973). Cells (2×10^5) in logarithmic phase of growth were plated into 25 cm^2 Falcon flasks in 5 ml of medium (see legend to Fig. 1) containing varying concentrations (1–10%) of normal or charcoal stripped foetal calf serum. Every two days thereafter cells were removed from triplicate plates with 0.05% trypsin, 0.02% EDTA in phosphate buffered saline (PBS), dispersed into a single cell suspension by sucking in and out of a pasteur pipette and counted on a haemocytometer. Mean cell numbers per flask for each treatment were recorded and plotted against time.

When cells were cultured in 5–10% normal foetal calf serum they grew with a mean doubling time of about 30 hours, until a maximum cell density of approximately 3×10^6 cells/flask was reached between 6–7 days (Fig. 1). The medium was not changed in these experiments. In experiments where the medium was changed every 2 days the initial rate of growth was not appreciably affected but a significantly higher confluent density of $6–8 \times 10^6$ cells/flask was attained. Reducing the foetal calf serum concentration to 1% had little effect on the logarithmic phase of growth but appeared to cause a significant lag period (Fig. 1). Although the maximal cell density attained at 6 days was not significantly lower than that seen with 10% serum, the low serum concentration was unable to maintain cultures when the medium was not changed, and cell numbers began to fall subsequent to day 6, presumably due to nutrient deprivation (Fig. 1). Removal of oestrogens and other low molecular weight compounds by charcoal adsorption appeared to increase the lag phase and reduce the maximal cell numbers attained in both 1 % and 10 % foetal calf serum (compare 1 % and 10 % normal serum with 1 % and 10 % stripped serum in Fig. 1). However, the growth rate during the logarithmic phase appeared to be little affected by adsorbing the serum with charcoal. Indeed, following this initial lag period, both MCF 7 and BT 20 cells were able to grow at maximal rates for at least two cell cycles in 1 % stripped foetal calf serum. Since the binding of tamoxifen to serum proteins and the effects of endogenous oestrogens were minimized under these conditions, the effects of tamoxifen on asynchronous cells were subsequently studied in 1 % stripped foetal calf serum, with the additional of drug during the exponential growth phase.

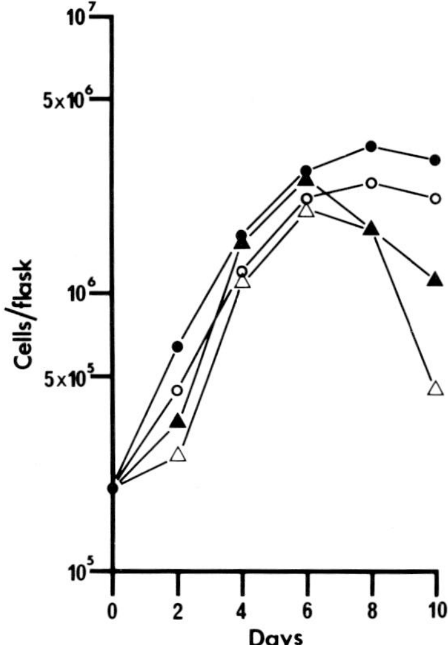

Fig. 1. Effect of concentration of normal and charcoal treated foetal calf serum on the growth of MCF 7 cells. 2×10^5 exponentially growing cells were plated into 25 cm^2 flasks in 5 ml of medium (RPMI 1640 containing 0.34 g/l arginine, 0.63 g/l asparagine and 0.04 g/l folic acid and supplemented with 20 mM Hepes buffer, 14 mM sodium bicarbonate, 6 mM L-glutamine, 20 μg/ml gentomycin and 10 μg/ml insulin) containing varying concentrations of normal or charcoal stripped foetal calf serum. Cell numbers/flask were recorded at 2 day intervals for 10 days. The mean cell numbers from triplicate flasks were recorded for 10 % normal (●), 10 % stripped (○), 1 % normal (▲) and 1 % stripped (△) foetal calf serum.

Addition of tamoxifen to the medium of MCF 7 cells grown under these conditions resulted in a dose dependent inhibition of cell growth. In the experiment illustrated in Figure 2, the lowest dose (2 μM) caused inhibition of cell growth although the cells continued to grow. The similar number of cells recorded for the treated (2 μM) and control groups at 48 and 72 hours was not in agreement with the kinetic data reported in Figures 4 and 5 and can probably be attributed to the difficulties in obtaining accurate cell counts from lines, like MCF 7, which clump and hence do not easily form single cell suspensions. Cultures treated with 6 μM tamoxifen continued to grow but at a significantly reduced rate for the first 24 hours after addition of the drug. Thereafter cell numbers remained static for a further 24 hours, and then began to decline rapidly. At the highest dose (10 μM) cell numbers declined immediately after addition of the drug and all cells were dead by 48 hours.

III. CYTOTOXIC EFFECTS OF TAMOXIFEN ON OESTROGEN RECEPTOR NEGATIVE MAMMARY CARCINOMA CELLS

Since much of the experimental and clinical data suggest that the antitumour effects of tamoxifen are confined to oestrogen receptor positive

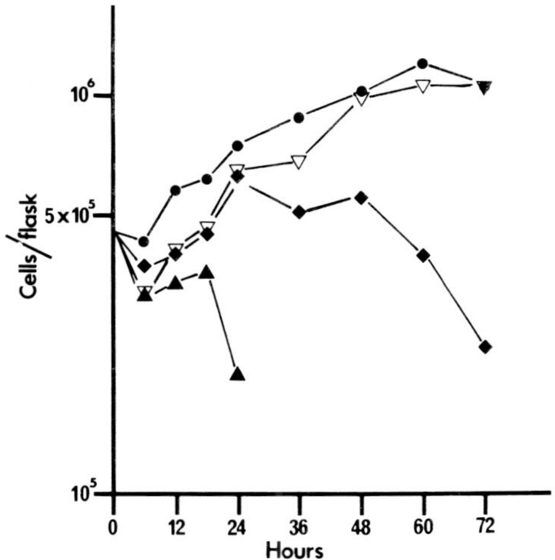

Fig. 2. Effect of tamoxifen on the growth of MCF 7 cells. 2×10^5 exponentially growing cells were plated into 25 cm^2 flasks in 5 ml of medium containing 1 % stripped foetal calf serum. Two days later the medium was changed and tamoxifen added at final concentrations of 0 (●), 2 (▽), 6 (◆) and 10 μM (▲). Cells were harvested with 0.125 % trypsin in PBS at regular intervals during the next 72 hours, cell numbers recorded and samples stained for FCM analysis.

tumours it was of interest to determine whether the cytotoxicity observed with the oestrogen receptor positive cell line MCF 7 was also observed in cells not expressing the oestrogen receptor. For these experiments a well-characterized human mammary carcinoma cell line, BT 20 (Lasfargues and Ozzello, 1958), which has been shown by ourselves and others (Horwitz *et al.*, 1978b) to be oestrogen receptor negative, was used. When BT 20 cells were grown in 1 % stripped foetal calf serum in the presence of varying concentrations of tamoxifen in the range of 1–10 μM, a dose-dependent tamoxifen induced cytotoxicity, similar to that seen with MCF 7 cells, was observed (Fig. 3). These data illustrate that, at micromolar concentrations, tamoxifen can have profound inhibitory effects on the growth of both oestrogen receptor negative and oestrogen receptor positive cells *in vitro*.

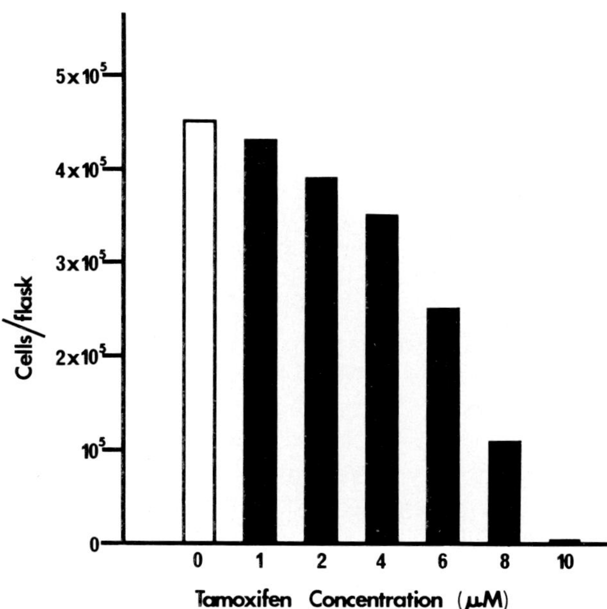

Fig. 3. Effect of tamoxifen on the growth of BT 20 cells. 2 × 10^5 exponentially growing cells were plated into 25 cm^2 flasks in 5 ml of medium containing 1 % charcoal stripped foetal calf serum. Two days later the medium was changed and tamoxifen added at concentrations ranging from 1–10μM. Cells were harvested 48 hours after addition of drug and mean cell numbers from triplicate flasks recorded. No cells remained after 48 hours of treatment with 10 μM tamoxifen.

IV. EFFECTS OF TAMOXIFEN ON CELL CYCLE KINETIC PARAMETERS

Having established that culture conditions could be chosen to demonstrate varying degrees of growth inhibition by tamoxifen, we conducted experiments to test whether this growth inhibition and cytotoxicity were associated with a perturbation in the cell cycle kinetic parameters of antioestrogen treated cells. Experiments were performed with both the oestrogen receptor positive (MCF 7) and oestrogen receptor negative (BT 20) human mammary carcinoma cell lines.

A. Determination of Cell Cycle Kinetic Parameters

Flow cytometry (FCM) is a technique which allows rapid measurement of DNA distribution in large populations of cells (for reviews see Crissman *et al.*, 1975; Mullaney *et al.*, 1976; Horan and Wheeless, 1977). Briefly, this technique uses the stoichiometric binding of specific fluorescent dyes to DNA to measure the DNA content of single cells. By counting a large number of single cells (generally about 50,000) the DNA distribution of the whole population may be determined. Figure 4 shows examples of DNA histograms of MCF 7 cells obtained in this way. The first peak at channel number 50 represents cells with a G_1 DNA content and the second, smaller peak, at twice the fluorescence, i.e. channel 100, represents cells in G_2 + M phase of the cell cycle. Cells in S phase have fluorescence intensities between these two limits. Cell cycle kinetic parameters (i.e. the proportion of cells in G_1, S, and G_2 + M) can be calculated by a number of analytical techniques (for reviews see, Zeitz and Nicolini, 1978; Johnson *et al.*, 1978).

In this study FCM analysis was performed on an ICP22 pulse cytometer (Ortho Instruments, Westwood, MA, USA). Cells to be analysed were first made permeable by detergent treatment and then stained with an ethidium bromide-mithramycin staining solution (Taylor and Milthorpe, 1980). Samples of the stained cells were excited at 360–460 nm and the resulting fluorescence was measured at greater than 550 nm. Estimations of cell cycle parameters were calculated from the resulting DNA histograms using a planimetric method of analysis (Milthorpe, 1980).

B. Effects of Tamoxifen on Asynchronous Cells

The data presented in Figure 2 illustrate the effects of three different doses of tamoxifen (i.e. 2, 6 and 10 μM) on the growth of MCF 7 cells. Cell cycle kinetic parameters were also monitored in this experiment and the data are summarized in Figures 4 and 5. In Figure 4 the DNA histograms for control cells and cells treated with tamoxifen for 36 hours are shown. Treatment with

2 μM tamoxifen resulted in a significant reduction in the percentage of S phase cells from 36% in control cultures to 26% in treated cultures (Fig. 4). This is in agreement with the growth inhibition observed at this dose (Fig. 2). At 6 μM, a dose which completely inhibited an increase in cell number (Fig. 2), the percentage of S phase cells had fallen even further to 15% at 36 hours (Fig. 4). The dose-dependent decrease in the percentage of S phase cells was accompanied by a comparable increase in the proportion of cells in G_1 (Fig. 4). Interestingly, the DNA histogram of the cells treated with the 10 μM dose was not markedly different from that of the control culture despite the dramatic cell loss at this dose. However, there was a small but significant decline in the percentage of G_1 phase cells and increase in the percentage of S phase cells at the 10 μM dose, a trend which was the opposite of that seen at the lower dose.

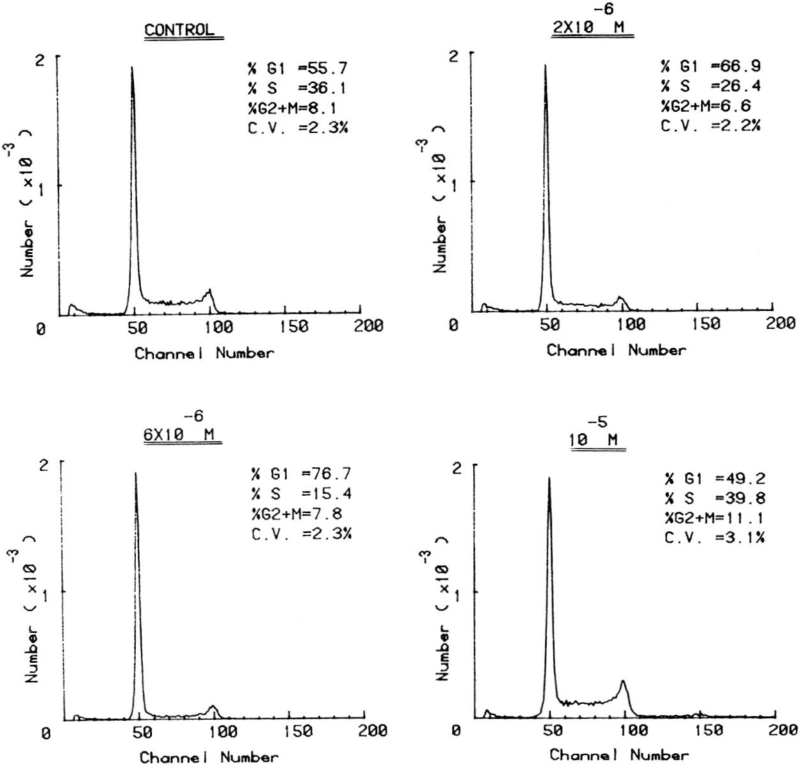

Fig. 4. Effect of tamoxifen treatment for 36 hours on the DNA distribution histograms of MCF 7 cells. The cells were from the experiment described in Figure 2 and the FCM analysis was performed as described in the text.

The time dependence of tamoxifen induced changes in the percentage of cells in the G_1 and S phases of the cell cycle are shown in Figure 5. The percentage of control cells in S phase was constant during the first 36 hours but declined significantly during the next 36 hours as the growth rate declined (see Fig. 2). This was probably due to nutrient deprivation at the low serum concentration. At the two lowest doses of tamoxifen (i.e. 2 and 6 μM) there was little change in the percentage of S phase cells during the first 12 hours, but between 12 and 24 hours of treatment these levels declined rapidly at both

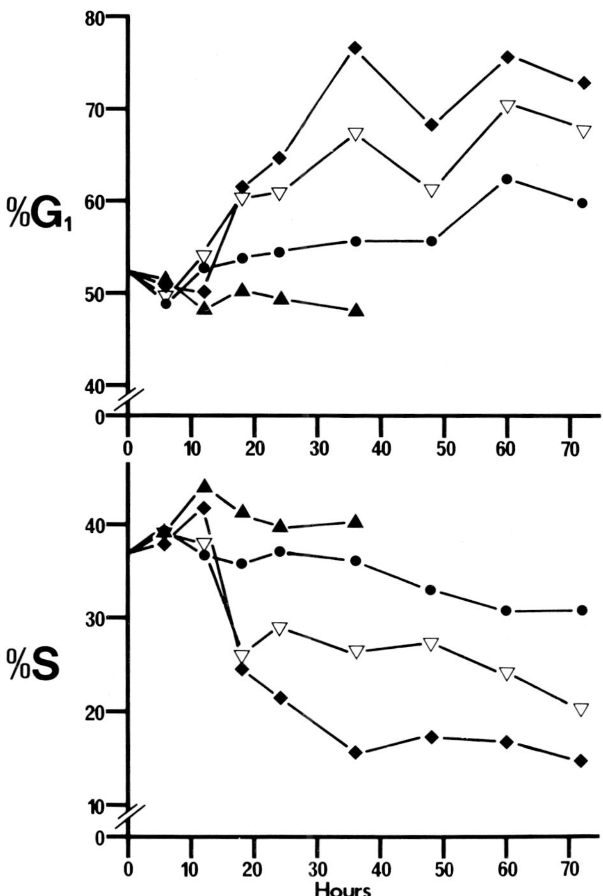

Fig. 5. Effect of tamoxifen on the proportion of MCF 7 cells in the G_1 and S phases of the cell cycle. Cells were grown in 0 (●), 2 (▽), 6 (◆) and 10 μM (▲) tamoxifen and were taken from the experiment described in Figure 2.

doses although the effect was more marked at 6 μM. Thereafter the percentage of S phase cells continued to fall slowly until the end of the experiment at 74 hours (Fig. 5). This decline in the percentage of S phase cells was paralleled by an increase in the proportion of cells in G_1. At the highest dose (10 μM), where cell numbers began to decline by 6 hours after addition of the drug, a small but significant increase in the proportion of S phase cells was apparent by 12 hours and this was maintained during the next 24 hours. After 36 hours of treatment with 10 μM tamoxifen insufficient viable cells remained for FCM analysis. A concurrent significant decrease in the percentage of G_1 cells (cf. control) was observed at this dose (Fig. 5).

Identical experiments with the BT 20 cell line yielded similar results, i.e. the 2 and 6 μM doses were associated with significant time and dose-dependent decreases in the percentage of S phase cells and increases in the percentage of G_1 phase cells, while the cytotoxic 10 μM dose resulted in a small but significant decline in the proportion of G_1 cells and increase in the percentage of S phase cells (data not shown).

C. Effects of Tamoxifen on the Progression of Synchronized G_1 Cells through the Cell Cycle

Since the previous experiments with asynchronous MCF 7 and BT 20 cells had demonstrated that treatment with 2 and 6 μM tamoxifen caused an accumulation of cells in the G_1 phase of the cell cycle, further experiments with synchronized cells were designed to test whether tamoxifen was exerting its effect by inducing a block in G_1 and inhibiting the entry of cells into S phase. Unfortunately the MCF 7 line was not amenable to synchronization due principally to the difficulties of obtaining single cell suspensions of these cells. However, the BT 20 cells could be synchronized by centrifugal elutriation (Meistrich *et al.*, 1977), and since the effects of micromolar doses of tamoxifen were similar in these two cell lines, BT 20 cells were used.

For the experiments described below, exponentially growing BT 20 cells were synchronized by centrifugal elutriation and a population containing about 90 % G_1 cells was obtained. 5×10^5 G_1 cells were then plated into 25 cm^2 flasks in 5 ml of medium containing 2 % foetal calf serum with or without tamoxifen. Flasks were harvested at regular intervals, cells counted and samples prepared for FCM analysis. The increase in foetal calf serum concentration from 1 to 2 % was necessary because of the unacceptably high proportion of control cells which failed to progress through the cycle when subcultured in 1 % serum. To compensate for the increased proportion of the drug bound to serum proteins at the higher serum concentration, the dose of tamoxifen was increased to 10 μM in these experiments. This dose did not result in a decrease in cell numbers during the course of the experiment.

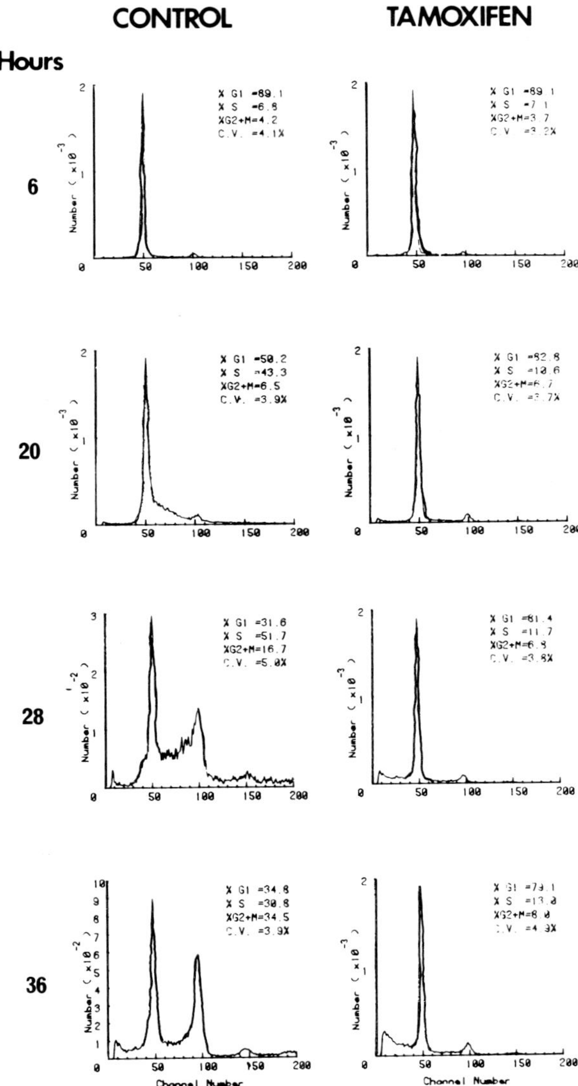

Fig. 6. Effect of tamoxifen on the progression of synchronous G_1 cells through the cell cycle. DNA histograms obtained from FCM analysis of BT 20 cells. A synchronous population of G_1 cells was obtained by centrifugal elutriation of exponentially growing cultures of BT 20 cells. 5×10^5 G_1 cells were then plated into 25 cm^2 flasks in 5 ml of medium containing 2% charcoal stripped foetal calf serum with or without 10 μM tamoxifen. Cells were harvested from duplicate flasks at regular intervals during the next 52 hours and prepared for FCM analysis as described in the text.

When synchronized G_1 cells were plated in 2% foetal calf serum, a large cohort of cells began to leave G_1 after 6 hours, and by 28 hours the proportion of G_1 cells had been reduced from 90% to 30% (Figs 6 and 7). Although the percentage of G_1 cells declined only slightly during the remaining 24 hours of the experiment, the FCM profiles illustrated in Figure 6, show this cohort of cells progessing from early S phase, through S phase to G_2 + M between 20 and 36 hours. The DNA histograms for treated cells were entirely different (Fig. 6). Tamoxifen (10 μM) almost completely inhibited the movement of cells out of G_1 (Fig. 6) with less than 10% of cells leaving G_1 during the 52 hours of the experiment (Fig. 7). A similar concentration of another non-steroidal antioestrogen, CI 628, was less effective than tamoxifen in this regard but was still a potent inhibitor of the progression of synchronized cells out of the G_1 phase of the cell cycle (Fig. 7).

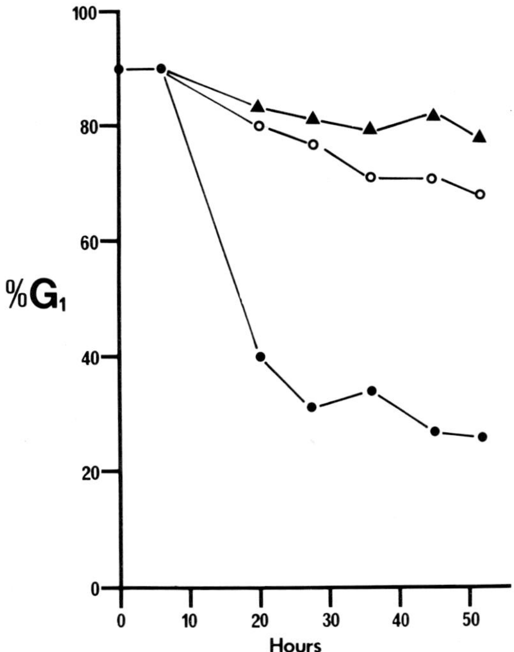

Fig. 7. Effect of tamoxifen and CI 628 on the proportion of BT 20 cells in the G_1 phase of the cell cycle following subculture of synchronous G_1 cells obtained by centrifugal elutriation. Data are from the experiment described in Figure 6. Both drugs were added at a concentration of 10 μM. Control (●), tamoxifen (▲), CI 628 (○).

V. DISCUSSION

These experiments summarize our first attempts to understand the effects of tamoxifen on the growth and cell cycle kinetics of cultured human mammary carcinoma cells using flow cytometry. Since this technique is exceedingly rapid and measures the relative concentration of DNA per cell, it has obvious advantages over time-consuming autoradiographic techniques and methods which rely on interpreting changes in the rates of incorporation of radiolabelled precursors into DNA. Our experience with the well-characterized human mammary carcinoma cell lines, MCF 7 and BT 20, illustrate that both these cell lines are readily amenable to study by flow cytometry. It is hoped that this will lead to an increased understanding of how many physiological and pharmacological agents influence the growth of these cells *in vitro*, and allow us to identify any cell cycle specific effects of such compounds.

In an attempt to understand more clearly the effects of tamoxifen on the growth of MCF 7 cells, three different doses of drug, producing markedly different effects, were studied in detail. The 2 μM dose resulted in a reduction in cell numbers while cells continued to grow. The 6 μM dose caused an arrest of cell growth with cell numbers declining subsequent to 48 hours, while the 10 μM dose resulted in immediate cell death. It was of considerable interest that the same doses of tamoxifen caused similar effects on the oestrogen receptor negative BT 20 cell line since it has previously been demonstrated that tamoxifen inhibition of the incorporation of tritiated thymidine into DNA is confined to oestrogen receptor positive cells (Lippman and Bolan, 1975; Lippman *et al.*, 1976). In other experiments with MCF 7 cells to be published elsewhere, we have demonstrated that while a 10-fold lower concentration of oestradiol can completely reverse the growth inhibitory and cell cycle kinetic effects of 2 μM tamoxifen, oestradiol can only partially reverse the effects associated with 6 μM tamoxifen. This probably indicates that tamoxifen has growth inhibitory effects *in vitro* which are not oestrogen receptor mediated since they are not always reversed by oestradiol in oestrogen receptor positive cells and are also observed in oestrogen receptor negative cells.

The changes in growth induced by 2 and 6 μM tamoxifen were accompanied by significant changes in the cell cycle kinetic parameters resulting in an accumulation of cells in the G_1 phase of the cell cycle and a comparable reduction in the proportion of S phase cells. These effects were dose-dependent since the 6 μM dose, which arrested growth after 24 hours, depleted the proportion of S phase cells to a greater extent that the 2 μM dose where cells continued to grow. Such results are not unexpected in view of the previous demonstration that tamoxifen inhibits the incorporation of tritiated thymidine into DNA in MCF 7 cells (Lippman and Bolan, 1975; Lippman *et al.*, 1976).

There are two likely explanations for this accumulation of cells in G_1. Tamoxifen may either preferentially kill cells in S phase or induce a block in G_1, which does not allow cells to enter S phase. In the experiment with synchronous BT 20 cells, tamoxifen treated cells remained in G_1 during the 52 hours of treatment. Since cell numbers did not change during this period the result cannot be attributed to preferential killing of cells entering S phase and must therefore be due to an arrest of cells in G_1.

In contrast to the situation seen at the lower doses, treatment with 10 μM tamoxifen was not associated with gross perturbation in the DNA distribution histograms obtained by FCM analysis. Since cell numbers declined rapidly at this dose, the drug must kill cells in all phases of the cell cycle under these experimental conditions. The small but significant increase in the proportion of S phase cells and decrease in the percentage of G_1 phase cells observed at this dose could be accounted for if G_1 cells were more susceptible than S phase and G_2 + M cells to the cytotoxic effects of tamoxifen. This seems a likely explanation since unpublished data from clonogenic survival studies on synchronized cells have illustrated that only cells exposed to low doses of tamoxifen during the G_1 phase of the cell cycle will subsequently die.

In summary, the data presented here have illustrated two distinct effects of tamoxifen *in vitro*: a growth inhibitor effect associated with an accumulation of cells in G_1 which may or may not be oestrogen reversible depending on the dose and cell line; and a non-specific cytotoxic effect. The oestrogen reversibility of the phase specific effect requires further detailed investigation before any conclusions relating to its relevance to the antitumour effects of tamoxifen *in vitro* can be made with confidence. Such studies are being actively pursued in this laboratory.

REFERENCES

Allegra, J. C., and Lippman, M. E. (1978). *Cancer Res.* **38**, 3823–3829.

Crissman, H., Mullaney, P. F., and Steinkamp, J. A. (1975). *In* "Methods in Cell Biology" (D. M. Prescott, ed.), Vol. IX, pp. 179–246. Academic Press, New York.

DeSombre, E. R., and Arbogast, L. Y. (1974). *Cancer Res.* **34**, 1971–1976.

DeSombre, E. R., Smith, S., Block, G. E., Ferguson, D. J., and Jensen, E. V. (1974). *Cancer Chemotherapy Reports* **58**, 513–519.

Gullino, P. M., Pettigrew, H. M., and Grantham, F. H. (1975). *J. Natl Cancer Inst.* **54**, 401–414.

Horan, P. K., and Wheeless, L. L. (1977). *Science* **198**, 149–157.

Horwitz, K. B., Koseki, Y., and McGuire, W. L. (1978a). *Endocrinology* **103**, 1742–1751.

Horwitz, K. B., Zava, D. T., Thilagar, A. K., Jensen, E. M., and McGuire, W. L. (1978b). *Cancer Res.* **38**, 2434–2437.

Huggins, C. (1965). *Cancer Res.* **25**, 1163–1167.

Johnston, D. A., White, R. A., and Barlogic, B. (1978). *Comput. Biomed. Res.* **11**, 393–404.

Jordan, V. C. (1976). *Eur. J. Cancer* **12**, 419–424.

Lasfargues, E. Y., and Ozzello, L. (1958). *J. Natl Cancer Inst.* **21**, 1131–1147.
Lippman, M. E., and Bolan, G. (1975). *Nature* **256**, 592–593.
Lippman, M. E., Bolan, G., and Huff, K. (1976). *Cancer Res.* **36**, 4596–4601.
McGuire, W. W., Carbone, P. P., and Vollmer, E. P. (1975). "Estrogen Receptors in Human Breast Cancer". Raven Press, New York.
Manni, A., Trujillo, J. E., and Pearson, O. H. (1977). *Cancer Res.* **37**, 1216–1219.
Meistrich, M. L., Meyn, R. E., and Barlogie, B. (1977). *Exptl. Cell Res.* **105**, 169–177.
Meites, J., Cassell, E., and Clark, J. (1971). *Proc. Soc. Exper. Biol. Med.* **137**, 1225–1227.
Milthorpe, B. K. (1980). *Comput. Biomed. Res.* **13**, 417–429.
Mouridsen, H., Palshof, T., Patterson, J., and Battersby, L. (1978). *Cancer Treat. Reviews* **4**, 131–141.
Mullaney, P. F., Steinkamp, J. A., Crissman, H. A., Cram, S. L., Cromwell, J. M., Salzman, G. C., and Martin, J. C. (1976). *Ann N. Y. Acad. Sci.* **267**, 176–190.
Nicholson, R. I., and Golder, M. P. (1975). *Eur. J. Cancer* **11**, 571–579.
Riley, P. A., Latter, A., and Sutton, P. M. (1978). *Eur. J. Cancer* **14**, 579–586.
Rose, D. P., Pruitt, B., Stauber, P., Erturk, E., and Bryan, G. T. (1980). *Cancer Res.* **40**, 235–239.
Sirbasku, D. A. (1978). *Proc. Natl Acad. Sci. U.S.A.* **75**, 3786–3790.
Sluyser, M. (1979). *Biochim. Biophys. Acta* **560**, 509–529.
Soule, H. D., Vazquez, J., Long, A., Albert, S., and Brennan, M. (1973). *J. Natl Cancer Inst.* **51**, 1409–1416.
Strobl, J. S., and Lippman, M. E. (1979). *Cancer Res.* **39**, 3319–3327.
Taylor, I. W., and Milthorpe, B. K., (1980). *J. Histochem. Cytochem.* **28**, 1224–1232.
Terenius, L. (1971). *Eur. J. Cancer* **7**, 57–64.
Tsai, T. L. S., and Katzenellenbogen, B. S. (1977). *Cancer Res.* **37**, 1537–1543.
Tsai, T. S., Rutledge, S., and Katzenellenbogen, B. S. (1979). *Cancer Res.* **39**, 5043–5050.
Watson, C., Medina, D., and Clark, J. H. (1977). *Cancer Res.* **37**, 3344–3348.
Watson, C. S., Medina, D., and Clark, J. H. (1979). *Cancer Res.* **39**, 4096–4104.
Weichselbaum, R. R., Hellman, S., Piro, A. J., Nove, J. J., and Little, J. B. (1978). *Cancer Res.* **38**, 2339–2342.
Zeitz, S., and Nicolini, C. (1978). *In* "Biomathematics and Cell Kinetics" (A. J. Valleron and P. D. M. Macdonald, eds), pp. 357–395. Elsevier/North-Holland Biomedical Press, Amsterdam.

24

Steroid Receptors and Response to an Antioestrogen in Postmenopausal Endometrial Carcinoma and Metastatic Breast Cancer

P. ROBEL, R. MORTEL, C. LEVY, M. NAMER AND E. E. BAULIEU

NON-STEROIDAL ANTIOESTROGENS
ISBN 0 12 677880 9

I. INTRODUCTION

Target tissues contain specific intracellular receptors for steroid hormones, and receptor concentrations in tumours might be possible indicators of hormone responsiveness (Jensen *et al.*, 1967; McGuire *et al.*, 1977). No effect of hormone can be elicited in cells deprived of receptor. In a few experimental models, the magnitude of hormonal effects has been positively correlated with the concentration of receptor, but in hormone-dependent cancers, in particular breast cancer, the predictive value of receptor measurements has only been established by comparison with the results of hormonal treatment.

Some attempts were made to directly demonstrate the effects of hormones on tumours, using incubations or cultures of tumour explants in the presence of steroid hormones (Tseng *et al.*, 1977; Saez *et al.*, 1978). This *in vitro* approach suffers serious limitations; therefore we have tried to set up an *in vivo* biochemical approach to relate receptors and hormonal response in endometrial and breast cancers.

In recent years, epidemiological, experimental, clinical and therapeutic considerations have suggested that oestrogens are involved in the occurrence and progress of endometrial and breast carcinoma. It is known that a characteristic effect of oestradiol is the increase of progesterone receptor concentration in the uterus (Milgrom *et al.*, 1973). Its measurement may therefore be utilized as a biochemical indicator of the response of tumour cells to oestrogen.

Several compounds of the triphenylethylene series exhibit both oestrogenic and antioestrogenic properties. This is the case for tamoxifen which, in the rodent uterus, has been shown to increase progesterone receptor concentration, while it counteracts oestrogen-induced uterine growth. Since the hormonal control of progesterone receptor in human endometrium seems to follow the same principles as in animal models (Bayard *et al.*, 1975, 1978), we decided to give tamoxifen to postmenopausal patients with endometrial carcinoma. Moreover, tamoxifen has been widely used for the treatment of breast cancer patients with good results, and we consequently found it appropriate to test it in metastatic breast cancers (Namer *et al.*, 1980). In endometrial and breast cancer patients, two tumour samples could be obtained under acceptable ethical conditions, the first one before, and the second one after, administration of tamoxifen. Tamoxifen binds to the oestradiol receptor, and tamoxifen-receptor complexes accumulate in the nucleus. It was anticipated that the exposure of tumour cells to the drug would be indicated by the decrease of available cytoplasmic sites and the increase of nuclear receptor. The tumour response to tamoxifen on the other hand, would be demonstrated by increased progesterone receptor. Finally, this increased progesterone receptor concentration might lead to an improved effectiveness of progestagen therapy.

II. ASSAY PROCEDURES

A. Receptor Measurements

Oestradiol and progesterone receptors were measured in fresh biopsy samples of endometrial cancers collected in ice cold medium and processed less than one hour after removal. The technique utilized allowed measurements of total (filled and unfilled) oestradiol and progesterone receptor sites in the cytosol and nuclei as reported in detail by Bayard *et al.* (1978). The measurement of nuclear receptor sites has been recently improved by the use of a glass-fibre filter exchange technique permitting both exchange and measurement of bound radioactivity without transfer of nuclear suspensions (Levy *et al.*, 1980). Essentially, nuclear preparations containing hormone-receptor complexes were adsorbed onto glass-fibre filters. Receptor sites, both empty and occupied by endogenous hormone(s), were labelled by incubation with [^{3}H]oestradiol or [^{3}H]progesterone in the presence or absence of 100-fold excess of non-radioactive competitor. Buffer containing unbound radioactive hormone was drained, the filters were washed with appropriate buffers, and then transferred into vials. Radioactivity was eluted and counted in a toluene based scintillant after constant shaking for at least 3 hours.

Aliquots of the homogenate and nuclear suspensions were measured for DNA using the technique of Burton (1968). All results were expressed in pmol of hormone binding sites per mg of DNA. Assay sensitivity was such that any value less than 0.09 pmol of nuclear receptors and less than 0.11 pmol of cytosol receptors was considered zero and reported as such in the tables.

In skin metastases of breast cancers, oestradiol and progesterone receptors, readily labelled by radioactive ligands at 0–4°C, were measured only in cytosol fractions, otherwise using a procedure similar to the one of Bayard *et al.* (1978). Results were expressed in fmol/mg cytosol protein. Assay sensitivity was such that any value less than 5 fmol/mg cytosol protein was considered zero and reported as such in the tables. In several cases, measurements were made on biopsies from adjacent nodules, and receptor concentrations were not significantly different.

B. Ornithine Decarboxylase (ODC) Activity

ODC activity was assayed in endometrium samples according to Kaye *et al.* (1971) with minor modifications. The $^{14}CO_2$ produced was trapped in a disposable polypropylene centre well filled with Soluene (Packard). After completion of the reaction, the well was transferred into a counting vial containing 10 ml of scintillation liquid. The conditions of enzyme reaction were verified to yield linear dependence of $^{14}CO_2$ generated when protein concentration varied from 0.5 to 2.0 mg/ml. The results were expressed in pmol of CO_2 produced per hour per mg of DNA.

C. Oestradiol Dehydrogenase (E_2DH) Activity

Enzyme activity was measured in the 105,000 g pellet of endometrial samples according to Pollow *et al.* (1975a). After incubation with [^{3}H]oestradiol, [^{3}H]oestrone was separated by silica gel thin layer chromatography and enzyme activity expressed in pmol of oestrone produced per min per mg of protein.

D. Radioimmunoassay of Serum Hormones

Serum hormone levels were determined by radioimmunoassay. Antibodies were graciously provided by Roussel-Uclaf. Antioestrone antibody N° 3946 cross-reacted slightly with 16α-OH oestrone (~ 4%) and oestradiol (~ 2%). The antioestradiol antibody N° 3341 cross-reacted slightly with oestrone and oestriol (~ 5%). The only significant cross-reactions of antiprogesterone antibody N° 3297 were with 5α-pregnanedione (~ 40%), deoxycorticosterone (~ 4%) 17-OH progesterone (~ 4%), pregnelone and 3α-OH-5α-pregnane-20-one (~ 3%).

Serum samples were extracted with ethyl acetate, defatted and chromatographed on small celite columns (1 g) soaked with formamide: water (1:2 v/w) and equilibrated with hexane. Progesterone, oestrone and oestradiol were recovered in hexane:benzene (85/15), hexane:ethyl acetate (90/10), and hexane:ethyl acetate (80/20), respectively. The appropriate fractions were then processed for radioimmunoassay. All results were expressed in pg/ml of serum.

E. Calculations

Means are presented with a standard error of the mean as the index of dispersion. The non-parametric rank correlation coefficient of Spearman was used to compare data.

III. ENDOMETRIAL CARCINOMA

A. Introduction

Endometrial carcinoma occurs most frequently in post-menopausal women, and epidemiological studies have shown an increased risk in women exposed to prolonged unopposed oestrogenic stimulation (Gusberg, 1976; Richardson and MacLaughlin, 1978; Smith *et al.*, 1975). It is equally well accepted that progestational agents achieve objective remission in 30 to 35% of patients with advanced or metastatic endometrial cancer (Kohorn, 1976; Reifenstein, 1974; Richardson and MacLaughlin, 1978). However, based on clinical criteria, it is not possible to select those patients likely to benefit from hormonal therapy.

Numerous investigators have reported the presence of oestradiol and/or progesterone receptors in human endometrial carcinoma. Quantitative estimates have been published (Crocker *et al.*, 1974; Evans *et al.*, 1974; Gustafsson *et al.*, 1977; MacLaughlin and Richardson, 1976; Pollow *et al.*, 1975c; Tseng and Gurpide, 1972; Young *et al.*, 1976) but due to methodological differences and assay variations results from various studies are barely comparable. In general, these reports deal with determination of oestradiol and progesterone receptors in cytoplasmic preparations. Consequently, no systematic measurements of cytoplasmic and nuclear concentrations of oestradiol and progesterone receptors have been reported in patients with adenocarcinoma of the endometrium.

B. Patients

Forty-three patients with histologically proven adenocarcinoma of the endometrium were seen in consultation and treated at the Institut Gustave Roussy, Villejuif. Their ages ranged from 43 to 75 years with a mean of 62. All patients menopaused spontaneously for at least 3 years; only 3 had a known history of exogenous hormone ingestion after menopause. Every effort was made to obtain enough tissue for receptor studies and histologic confirmation. The degree of tumour differentiation was reported according to the FIGO classification (*Acta Obstet. Scand.*, 1971, **50**, 1). Grade 1: well differentiated, Grade 2: moderately differentiated, and Grade 3: anaplastic tumours.

Two endometrial biopsy samples were obtained from 25 patients, the first at the time of referral, the second during surgery or immediately before radiotherapy. Whenever possible, part of each sample was submitted for histologic confirmation and the remainder for biochemical studies. After the first biopsy, 15 patients took orally 40 mg of tamoxifen daily for 5–7 days (Group 1) and the second biopsy was performed 12–18 hours after the last dose. Ten patients ingested 10 mg 8 and 4 hours prior to the second biopsy (Group 2). The interval between the two biopsies in this last group varied from 1 to 6 days. Receptor concentrations were determined in all biopsy samples and, in addition, the activities of ODC and E_2DH were evaluated before and after tamoxifen treatment.

C. Results

1. *Oestradiol and Progesterone Receptors*

Nearly all tumours contained oestradiol and progesterone receptors, but in variable amounts (Fig. 1). No receptors in either cytosol or nuclei were detected in one tumour examined for oestradiol and in 7 tumours assayed for progesterone.

The total oestradiol receptor concentration (cytosol + nuclear) in the tumours examined was similar to that in the late proliferative phase of normal

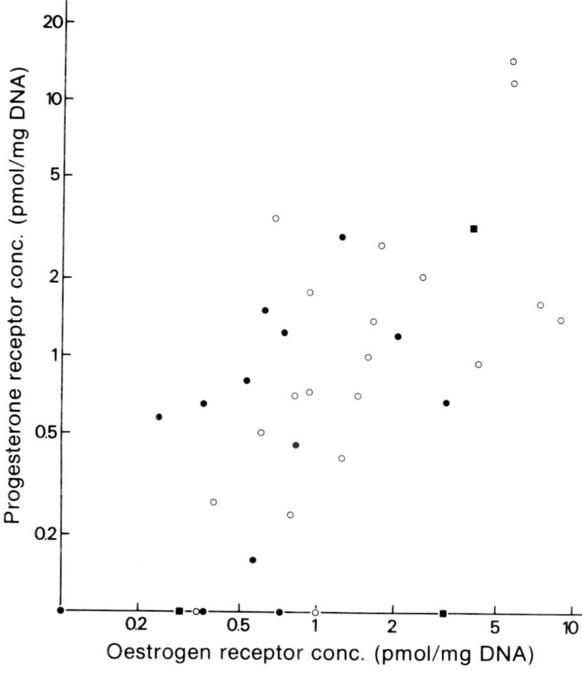

Fig. 1. Correlation of oestradiol and progesterone receptors in endometrial carcinoma. Histologic grading according to FIGO classification. Grade 1 (○), Grade 2 (●), Grade 3 (■).

endometrium (Table I). However, the values for progesterone receptor concentration were relatively low and comparable to those found in the secretory phase of the normal menstrual cycle.

When present, most oestradiol and progesterone receptors were found in the cytosol. However, the receptor concentration was much higher in the nuclear fractions from 6 specimens examined for oestradiol and from 2 tumours tested for progesterone receptor. No attempt was made in this study to determine whether or not nuclear receptors were occupied by endogenous hormone(s).

Although the difference was not statistically significant between the groups, there was a clear tendency for the more differentiated Grade 1 tumours to contain higher levels of oestradiol and progesterone receptors than the Grade 2 carcinomas. The small number of Grade 3 cases allowed no comparison.

2. *Hormonal Correlations of Receptors*

The values for serum oestradiol were comparable to published reports (Benjamin and Deutsch, 1976; Judd *et al.*, 1976; Korenman *et al.*, 1969) and remained lower than those for oestrone (Table II). Serum progesterone levels were low in normal postmenopausal women (De Villa *et al.*, 1972), and the

TABLE I
Oestradiol and Progesterone Receptors in Normal and Malignant Endometrium

Endometrium Status	Receptor concentration (pmol/mg DNA)	
	Oestradiol receptor	Progesterone receptor
Late proliferative	2.2 ± 0.3[a] (21)[b]	3.1 ± 0.3 (21)
Late secretory	0.9 ± 0.2 (56)	1.1 ± 0.1 (56)
Carcinoma G1	2.3 ± 0.5 (21)	2.2 ± 0.8 (21)
Carcinoma G2	0.8 ± 0.2 (13)	0.7 ± 0.2 (13)
Carcinoma G3	2.5 ± 1.1 (3)	0.9 ± 0.7 (4)

[a] Mean ± S.E.M.
[b] Number of cases.

mean progesterone values were identical in the 3 histologic grading groups. Oestradiol values did not change with the degree of tumour differentiation, but a highly significant difference ($p < 0.01$) was observed between the mean oestrone levels of patients with well and those with moderately differentiated cancers.

Linear regression coefficients were calculated between serum levels of the hormones measured and total oestradiol and progesterone receptor concentrations. We found no significant correlation between oestradiol receptor and serum levels of oestrone, oestradiol or progesterone even within the histologically defined groups. Similarly, no correlation was found between progesterone receptor and serum levels of oestrone, oestradiol or progesterone. However, in well differentiated tumours a positive correlation at the limit of statistical significance ($0.05 < p < 0.10$) was observed between serum oestradiol and progesterone receptor concentration.

3. *Effects of Tamoxifen*

a. Receptors. In Group 1, the patients were given 40 mg of tamoxifen daily for 5–7 days. No change occurred in the subcellular distribution of oestradiol receptor. However, in Group 2, where tamoxifen administration immediately preceded biopsy, the ratio of cytoplasmic to nuclear receptor shifted in favour of nuclear receptors, as previously observed in animal model experiments (Sutherland *et al.*, 1977). In Group 1, progesterone receptor sites increased in all but 4 samples (Fig. 2) and the difference was statistically significant at p <

TABLE II
Serum Levels of Oestrone, Oestradiol and Progesterone in Patients with Postmenopausal Endometrial Carcinoma

Endometrial carcinoma	Hormone concentration (pg/ml serum)		
	Oestrone	Oestradiol	Progesterone
Whole series	33.8 ± 2.5[a] (43)[b]	23.6 ± 1.5 (42)	435.6 ± 48.6 (42)
Grade 1	29.3 ± 2.9 (24)	22.0 ± 1.6 (23)	439.9 ± 55.9 (23)
Grade 2	43.0 ± 4.0 (15)[c]	25.6 ± 2.9 (15)	451.0 ± 102.0 (15)
Grade 3	57.2 ± 15.3 (4)	27.2 ± 7.7 (4)	361.0 ± 10.3 (4)

[a] Mean ± S.E.M.
[b] Number of cases.
[c] $p < 0.01$ (nonparametric Wilcoxon rank order test).

0.05. Interestingly, at the same dose, a substantial elevation in progesterone receptor concentration was noted in all tumours where the receptor was not measurable or was present at very low concentration in the samples assayed before tamoxifen treatment. In Group 2 patients no increase of progesterone receptor was generally observed.

b. Ornithine Decarboxylase. ODC activity was measured along with receptor concentrations in 13 tumours, 4 of which came from Group 1 patients, and was determined before and after tamoxifen in 9 other tumours where receptors could not be measured due to limited sample size. The administration of tamoxifen in these additional patients was similar to that of Group 2 patients. No statistical difference was observed in enzyme activity

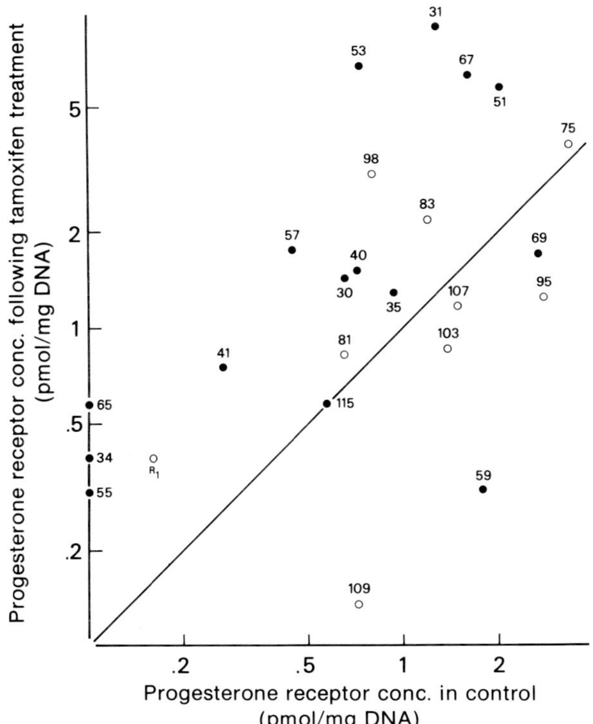

Fig. 2. Total progesterone receptors (PR_T) (pmol/mg DNA) in endometrial carcinoma before and after tamoxifen. Group 1 patients (●) (40 mg of tamoxifen daily × 5-7 days); Group 2 patients (○) (10 mg of tamoxifen at −8 and −4 hours). Patients are designated by their identification number.

before and after tamoxifen treatment (Fig. 3). In 4 tumours of Group 1, ODC values either decreased or were unchanged by the drug. We also found no correlation between tumour grading and ODC activity before or after tamoxifen treatment.

The enzyme was also measured in 6 gestational endometria following voluntary interruption of 1st trimester pregnancy and in 7 endometrial samples obtained from menstruating women undergoing uterine curettage for benign gynaecologic disorders (Table III). Activities were very low in gestational endometrium. No difference was observed between proliferative and secretory endometria. However, the values were much lower than those observed in endometrial carcinoma. Interestingly, the only case of hyperplasia in this group demonstrated an ODC activity lower than cancers but higher than normal endometrium.

c. Oestradiol Dehydrogenase. The activity of E_2DH was measured along with receptor concentrations before and after tamoxifen treatment in 14 tumours of which 9 came from Group 1 patients. In 6 additional patients, (3 receiving the Group 1 treatment) only enzyme activity was determined

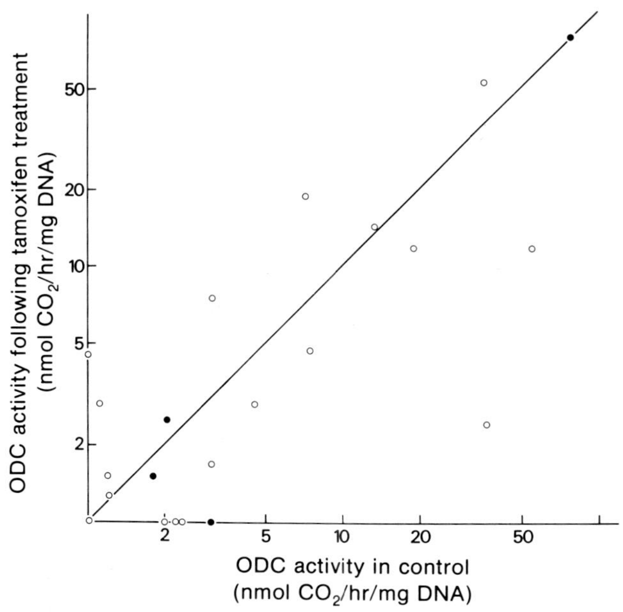

Fig. 3. Effects of tamoxifen on ODC activity. Groups as in Figure 2. Group 1 patients (●); Group 2 patients (○).

TABLE III
Ornithine Decarboxylase (ODC) Activity in Endometrial Samples

Sample	ODC activity (pmol CO_2/hr/mg DNA)
Cancer	8133 ± 2827[a] (22)[b]
Proliferative	1266 ± 292 (4)
Secretory	1106 ± 201 (2)
Hyperplastic	2296 (1)
Gestational	129 ± 72 (6)

[a] Mean ± S.E.M.
[b] Number of cases.

because of limited material. In general, the enzymatic activity was comparable to the values reported for normal proliferative endometrium (Tseng *et al.*, 1977) (Table IV). The activity did not vary significantly between well and moderately differentiated tumours, although it tended to be higher in well differentiated samples. In addition, no significant change was observed in the values obtained before and after the drug in patients who received low doses of tamoxifen. For those given 40 mg daily for 5–7 days, the activity of the enzyme did not follow a clear pattern. When the basal level was low (5 cases), i.e. less than 3 pmol of oestrone/min/mg of protein, activity was slightly increased. Such increases were not considered significant due to the lack of sensitivity and precision of the assay at low activities (less than 10 pmol of oestrone/min/mg protein). When the control activity was greater than 10 pmol of oestrone/min/mg protein, however, large decreases were observed in 5 of 7 cases.

d. Serum Oestrogens and Progesterone. The serum levels of oestrone, oestradiol, and progesterone showed no significant changes in the values at the schedules and doses of tamoxifen used in this study (Table V).

D. Discussion

The mean age (62 years) of our patient population is in keeping with previously reported data (Clark, 1978; MacMahon, 1974; Pfleiderer and Paessler, 1978). However, the few patients with undifferentiated carcinomas averaged 70 years of age. This finding is also in agreement with Wade *et al.* (1967) and Ng and Reagan (1978) who reported that anaplastic tumours occurred primarily in older women.

1. Oestradiol and Progesterone Receptors

Widespread concentrations of oestradiol receptors were measured in 36 of 37 tumours examined. The mean values observed in this study support the findings of Tseng *et al.* (1977) that, in postmenopausal endometrial carcinoma, the level of oestradiol receptors is similar to that in the endometrium of normal women in the proliferative phase of the cycle. Crocker *et al.* (1974) and Pollow *et al.* (1975c) found oestradiol receptors in all endometrial cancer samples, but Grilli *et al.* (1977) and Muechler *et al.* (1975) reported oestrogen receptor in 67–92 % of the specimen assayed. Therefore, it

TABLE IV
Oestradiol Dehydrogenase (E_2DH) Activity in Endometrial Adenocarcinoma Before and After Tamoxifen

Identification number	Grade	E_2DH activity (pmol oestrone/min/mg/protein)		
		Before	Tamoxifen	After
W30	2	0.6		2
W69	1	1		1.5
W57	2	1.2	Group 1	13
W65	1	3	40 mg	5
W34	3	3	daily	4.8
W46	1	19	× 5–7 days	1.8
W35	1	21		1.2
W45	1	48		12
W53	1	67		73
W51	1	74		67
W67	1	99		64
W32	1	273		73
C5	2	1.1		2.3
W95	2	1.2		8
W101	1	4.7	Group 2	12.7
W107	2	4.9	10 mg	6
W81	2	8	at	12
W110	2	8.6	−8 and −4 h	14.4
W89	2	12.8		10.7
W75	1	30		3.6

appears that oestradiol receptors are present in a large majority of endometrial adenocarcinomas.

Of 38 tumours assayed for progesterone receptors, 10 contained undetectable or insignificant amounts of receptors (less than 0.3 pmol/mg DNA). In 6 cases, the concentration was comparable to that of proliferative phase; in the majority of samples, as reported by Pollow *et al.* (1977), the range and mean values were similar to those observed in late secretory endometrium. Consequently, the oestrogen/progesterone receptor ratio in these postmenopausal adenocarcinomas was generally greater than in normal premenopausal endometrium.

Finding the majority of oestradiol and progesterone receptors in the cytosoluble fraction was not surprising considering the low levels of circulating oestrogen and progesterone in these women. However, 5 tumours would have been classified as "oestradiol receptor negative" and 2 as "progesterone receptor negative" on the basis of cytoplasmic receptor measurements alone. Therefore, it appears that simultaneous measurement of both cytoplasmic and nuclear receptor sites is necessary to accurately report the total intracellular receptor concentration and before tumours can be classified as so-called "receptor negative". As an alternative to separate assays

TABLE V
Serum Levels of Oestrone, Oestradiol and Progesterone Before and After Tamoxifen

Hormone	Hormone levels (pg/ml serum)		
	Before	Tamoxifen	After
Oestrone	25.1 ± 3.4[a] (12)[b]	Group 1 40 mg daily – 5–7 days	23.8 ± 3.0 (12)
Oestradiol	20.0 ± 1.6 (12)		18.7 ± 1.9 (11)
Progesterone	521.8 ± 126.3 (12)		317.8 ± 51.2 (12)
Oestrone	38.9 ± 4.3 (8)	Group 2 10 mg at –8 and –4 h	30.6 ± 4.3 (8)
Oestradiol	27.1 ± 3.5 (8)		21.3 ± 2.3 (8)
Progesterone	444.4 ± 101.7 (8)		371.6 ± 52.9 (8)

[a] Mean ± S.E.M.
[b] Number of cases.

for cytoplasmic and nuclear receptors, other investigators (Feil *et al.*, 1979; Tseng *et al.*, 1977) have incubated the whole tissue with radioactive hormone and subsequently measured the hormone tightly bound to nuclei. It should be recognized, however, that this method does not properly measure endogenous nuclear receptors, but determines the total translocated hormone-receptor complexes under *in vitro* conditions.

The relationship between receptor levels and the degree of tumour differentiation has been the subject of conflicting reports (Evans *et al.*, 1974; Feil *et al.*, 1979; Gustafsson *et al.*, 1977; Pollow *et al.*, 1975c; Tseng and Gurpide, 1972; Young *et al.*, 1976). Our study provided no clear-cut answer to this question as no statistical difference was found between the groups. Nevertheless, as reported by other investigators (Gustafsson *et al.*, 1977; Pollow *et al.*, 1975c; Young *et al.*, 1976), this study showed a clear tendency for well differentiated tumours to contain higher levels of both oestrogen and progesterone receptors. Our findings disagree with those of Pollow *et al.* (1977) who reported a progressive increase of oestradiol receptor concentration from well to poorly differentiated tumours.

2. Hormonal Correlations of Receptors

Data accumulated in the evaluation of hormonal correlations of sex steroid receptors in normal endometrium and the lack of corresponding knowledge in endometrial cancer led us to measure serum levels of oestrone, oestradiol, and progesterone in our patients. The observed mean oestrone values were lower than the plasma levels reported by Korenman *et al.* (1969), and Benjamin and Deutsch (1976). However, they correlated well with the serum values published by Judd *et al.* (1976) and Rader *et al.* (1973) and remained higher than serum oestradiol. It is unlikely that the high level of oestrone observed was due to oestradiol metabolism in the tumour since Tseng *et al.* (1977) and Pollow *et al.* (1975b) reported a low 17β-hydroxysteroid dehydrogenase in endometrial carcinoma. Siiteri *et al.* (1974) has suggested the possibility of oestrone playing an important role in the development of postmenopausal endometrial carcinoma. We have no explanation for the unexpected observation that in patients with less differentiated cancers the concentrations of serum oestrone were significantly higher than those observed in patients with well differentiated tumours.

3. Effect of Tamoxifen

The level of receptors at which a tumour will respond to hormone or antihormone treatment is still unknown. Thus a test that directly allows an evaluation of the response to a hormonal challenge is desirable. Gurpide and Tseng (1978), and Pollow *et al.* (1975b) proposed a method based on the measurement of E_2DH before and following medroxyprogesterone acetate administration to patients with endometrial carcinoma. They reported up to a 4-fold increase in enzyme activity and a reduction of oestrogen receptor levels in those tumours responsive to progestins. In addition Pollow *et al.* (1975b) reported the highest values for the enzyme activity in well differentiated tumours. These findings suggest that measurement of E_2DH before and after progestin, along with determination of sex steroid receptor concentrations, may provide a reliable means of selecting those tumours which are likely to respond to progestin therapy. The question remains, however, whether there is a means of converting progesterone receptor negative tumours into tumours with measurable progesterone receptor concentrations.

As described above, we selected tamoxifen for challenging the hormonal responsiveness of endometrium carcinoma. Contrary to the test with medroxyprogesterone acetate which acts via the progesterone receptor, tamoxifen is active via the oestrogen receptor of the tumour. Progesterone receptor is assayed as a biochemical marker of the oestrogenic response. We have confirmed our preliminary results (Robel *et al.*, 1978) and now have evidence that, in human endometrial carcinoma, tamoxifen given at a dose of 40 mg daily for 5–7 days induces or increases progesterone receptor concentration. Such effects were not apparent when the antioestrogen was administered in short term (8 and 4 hours prior to the second biopsy).

ODC is an enzyme whose activity has been associated with a variety of cell proliferative responses (Bulger and Dupfer, 1977; Kaye *et al.*, 1971; Tabor and Tabor, 1976). Following a single dose of oestradiol to immature rats activity starts to rise in the uterus by 2 hours (Kaye *et al.*, 1971), but after prolonged treatment it returns to basal values. We observed no changes in ODC activity in our Group 2 patients and postulated that a rapid or transitory increase may have been missed. We then administered only 10 mg of tamoxifen 8 and 4 hours prior to the second biopsy and again no increase in ODC activity was observed. These results are in keeping with observations that, in the rat uterus and cultured mouse L cells, tamoxifen cannot induce cell division (Jordan and Dix, 1979; Jung-Testas and Baulieu, 1979).

IV. BREAST CANCER

A. Introduction

Sixty to 70% of postmenopausal breast cancers are oestradiol receptor (ER) "positive". Of those about 50% respond to hormonal manipulation whether it be ablative surgery or administration of androgen, oestrogen or progestin and more recently antioestrogen (DeSombre *et al.*, 1979).

Approximately 50% of postmenopausal cancers have measurable concentrations of progesterone receptor (PR) of which more than 90% belong to the ER positive group. There are no experimental data demonstrating the hormonal regulation of progesterone receptor concentration in breast tissue *in vivo*. It was therefore interesting to check whether the increase observed after tamoxifen in endometrial cancer would be also seen in mammary tumours.

B. Patients

Twenty-one postmenopausal women with advanced metastatic breast cancer were investigated at the Centre Lacassagne, Nice. None of them had received any adjuvant therapy. Biopsies were performed on adjacent hypodermic nodules. After the first biopsy, patients received 30 mg of tamoxifen for 7 days, until the second sample was obtained.

C. Results

1. Oestradiol and Progesterone Receptors

Oestradiol receptor was absent or low (less than 20 fmol/mg protein) in 9 cases. All but one ER negative case was also PR negative. Among the 12 remaining ER positive cases, only 2 were PR negative (Table VI). A significant positive correlation was observed between the concentrations of PR and ER in untreated tumours.

2. Effect of Tamoxifen

Whenever present, available ER sites were greatly decreased after tamoxifen (Table VI). This decrease likewise resulted from tamoxifen binding to oestrogen receptors and transfer of the receptor complexes into the nucleus (Robel *et al.*, 1978). No PR receptor change was recorded in cases where ER was less than 20 fmol/mg cytosol protein. Seven of the 12 remaining cases showed an increase of PR of more than 100 fmol/mg cytosol protein.

D. Discussion: Effects of Tamoxifen

The increase of PR after tamoxifen was never observed in tumours with less than 20 fmol of ER per mg of cytosol protein. This is a direct demonstration that a sufficient concentration of ER is required to obtain a biochemical response *in vivo*. Among ER positive cases about one half responded to tamoxifen. This finding is in keeping with the approximately 50% of ER positive tumours which display objective remission after hormonal therapy (DeSombre *et al.*, 1979; Jensen *et al.*, 1967).

V. RESPONSE TO HORMONES AND PROSPECTS OF HORMONE THERAPY

When measurements are made on a small specimen of a malignant tumour, it is assumed that the results are representative of the whole tumour. It is quite likely that several samples of the same tumour may differ in terms of

TABLE VI
Oestradiol and Progesterone Receptors in Breast Cancer Metastases[a]

Identification number	Age (yrs)	Receptor concentration (fmol/mg protein)			
		Before tamoxifen		After tamoxifen	
		ER	PR	ER	PR
1	71	0	0	0	0
2	85	0	0	6	0
3	60	0	0	0	0
4	54	0	30	n[b]	0
5	58	0	0	0	0
6	72	7	0	0	0
7	59	11	0	n	0
8	71	13	0	0	11
9	72	20	7	0	13
10	72	25	20	n	50
11	63	53	92	12	1120
12	70	80	110	17	980
13	80	85	60	7	50
14	69	92	34	11	605
15	77	120	105	0	0
16	57	120	1030	12	1600
17	65	185	190	25	440
18	57	225	0	8	0
19	70	350	65	9	205
20	67	430	n	11	30
21	75	n	0	25	770

[a] Values < 5 fmol/mg cytosol protein were considered as not different from zero.
[b] n = not determined for technical reason.

differentiation, relative amounts of epithelial and stromal elements, proportion of malignant cells, inflammatory or necrotic changes, etc. However, we were reassured by the fact that receptor measurements performed on adjacent skin metastases of breast cancer gave closely similar results. Also, the constancy of ODC activities in endometrial cancer before and after tamoxifen is worth mentioning. A critical point is the possibility that the response of progesterone receptor to tamoxifen might reflect the response of normal cells interspersed in the biopsy samples. However, careful histologic evaluation could be performed on most biopsies and has generally shown that most if not all of the cells were indeed malignant. It should also be recalled that sensitivity of breast cancer cells to hormones has been directly demonstrated in cultures of established cells lines, e.g. MCF 7 (Lippman *et al.*, 1976; Horwitz and McGuire, 1978).

In addition, complex hormonal changes may be elicited at the pituitary, adrenal or ovarian level, following administration of an antioestrogen. However, such changes are unlikely to be prominent in postmenopausal women and no change of plasma sex steroids has been recorded.

In contrast to breast cancers, there is agreement that almost all endometrial cancers contain sizeable and even relatively large concentrations of oestradiol receptor. This observation underlines the importance of a test challenging the hormonal responsiveness using a compound binding to the oestrogen receptor, such as tamoxifen. A significant increase of progesterone receptor was observed in about 60% of cases, with poor correlation with the level of oestradiol receptor in the control biopsy.

In metastatic breast cancer, our results confirm the predictive value of oestradiol receptor. Oestradiol receptor negative cases were also generally progesterone receptor negative, and they did not respond to tamoxifen. The same was true for cases with ER less than 20 fmol/mg cytosol protein, and the tamoxifen test might prove useful in determining objectively the set-point of "receptor negative" cases. About one half of oestradiol receptor positive cases respond to tamoxifen by an increase (or induction) of progesterone receptor. An improved predictive value has been shown for the combined measurement of both oestradiol and progesterone receptors, compared to oestradiol receptor alone (Horwitz *et al.*, 1975; DeSombre *et al.*, 1979). Further improvement might result from the tamoxifen test, although the limited number of cases investigated precludes definitive conclusions. It should be performed systematically when available metastases are present. In the future, the development of microassays, which will be performed on needle biopsies of primary tumours, might lead to an extended use of *in vivo* hormonal challenge.

It is well established that progestins are of definite value in the treatment of patients with advanced or metastatic endometrial cancer (Kohorn, 1976;

Reifenstein, 1974; Richardson and MacLaughlin, 1978). However, one drawback of progesterone therapy is the decrease of progesterone receptor concentration (Jänne *et al.*, 1980). Thus, any product which, like tamoxifen, increases progesterone receptor without enhancing tumour growth would be helpful in increasing the magnitude and/or duration of response in patients with endometrial cancer.

A few investigators have empirically used oestrogen and progestin in patients with endometrial carcinoma. Only one study (Sherman, 1966) reported a 20% increase in response. Failures might have been due to the schedule and/or dosage of the hormones. Recently Vihko *et al.* (1978) recommended addition of oestrogen to progestational agents for long term progestin treated patients. However, because of the mitotic action of oestrogens on the endometrium and their possible role in the aetiology of endometrial hyperplasia and adenocarcinoma, the reluctance of most clinicians may be understood.

Tamoxifen has been widely used for the adjuvant therapy of metastatic breast cancer (Lerner *et al.*, 1976; Morgan *et al.*, 1976; Mouridsen *et al.*, 1978). However, it is certainly too early for an exact evaluation of tamoxifen effectiveness, although the results obtained compare favourably with other forms of endocrine therapy (Edwards *et al.*, 1979). Progestins have been the least used hormonal adjuvant treatments in breast cancer (Segaloff *et al.*, 1967; Stoll, 1967).

Tamoxifen has a promoting effect on progesterone receptor in both breast and endometrium cancers. In addition, it does not appear to stimulate tumour growth. Therefore, the sequential or concomittant administration of tamoxifen and progestational agents may increase the number of responders and improve the duration of response in patients with advanced or metastatic endometrial carcinoma and breast cancer.

ACKNOWLEDGEMENTS

We are indebted to B. Eychenne and M. Synguelakis for their expert technical assistance, and to D. Drouet for statistical evaluation. This work was supported by contract n° 76.5.478.A. INSERM.

REFERENCES

Bayard, F., Damilano, S., Robel, P., and Baulieu, E. E. (1975). *C. R. Acad. Sci.* **281**, 1341–1344.

Bayard, F., Damilano, S., Robel. P., and Baulieu, E. E. (1978). *J. Clin. Endocr. Metab.* **46**, 635–648.

Benjamin, F., and Deutsch, S. (1976). *Amer. J. Obstet. Gynaecol.* **126**, 638–647.
Bulger, W. H., and Dupfer, D. (1977). *Arch. Biochem. Biophys.* **182**, 138–146.
Burton, K. (1968). *In* "Methods of Enzymology" Vol. XII, Part B (L. Grossman, K. Moldave, eds), pp. 163–166. Academic Press, New York.
Clarke, M. (1978). *In* "Endometrial Cancer" (M. G. Brush, R. J. B. King, and R. W. Taylor, eds), pp. 3–9. Bailliere Tindall, London.
Crocker, S. G., Milton, P. J. D., and King, R. J. B. (1974). *J. Endocr.* **62**, 145–152.
DeSombre, E. R., Carbone, P. P., Jensen, E. V., McGuire, W. L., Wells, S. A., Wittliff, J. A., and Lipsett, M. B. (1979). *New Engl. J. Med.* **301**, 1011–1012.
De Villa, G. O., Roberts, K., Wiest, W. G., Mikhail, G., and Flickinger, F. (1972). *J. Clin. Endocr. Metab.* **35**, 458–460.
Edwards, D. P., Chamness, G. C., and McGuire, W. L. (1979). *Biochim. Biophys. Acta* **560**, 457–486.
Evans, L. H., Martin, J. D., and Hähnel, R. (1974). *J. Clin. Endocr. Metab.* **38**, 23–32.
Feil, P. D., Mann, W. J., Mortel, R., and Bardin, C. W. (1979). *J. Clin. Endocr. Metab.* **48**, 327–334.
Grilli, S., Ferrari, A. M., Gola, G., Rochetta, R., Orlandi, C., and Prodi, G. (1977). *Cancer Letters* **2**, 247–258.
Gurpide, E., and Tseng, L. (1978). *In* "Endometrial Cancer" (M. G. Brush, R. J. B. King, and R. W. Taylor, eds), pp. 252–257. Bailliere Tindall, London.
Gusberg, S. B. (1976). *Amer. J. Obstet. Gynaecol.* **126**, 535–542.
Gustafsson, J. A., Einhorn, N., Elfström, G., Nordenskjöld, B., and Wrange, O. (1977). *In* "Progesterone Receptor in Normal and Neoplastic Tissues" (W. L. McGuire, J. P. Raynaud and E. E. Baulieu, eds), pp. 299–312. Raven Press, New York.
Horwitz, K. B., and McGuire, W. L. (1978). *J. Biol. Chem.* **252**, 223–228.
Horwitz, K. B., McGuire, W. L., Pearson, O. H., and Segaloff, A. (1975). *Science* **189**, 726–727.
Jänne, O., Kauppila, A., Kontula, K., Syrjäla, P., Vierikko, P., and Vihko. R. (1980). *In* "Steroid Receptors and Hormone Dependent Neoplasia" (J. L. Wittliff, and O. Dapunt, eds), pp. 37–44. Masson Publishing, New York.
Jensen, E. V., DeSombre, E. R., and Jungblut, P. W. (1967). *In* "Endogenous Factor Influencing Host-Tumour Balance" (R. W. Wissler, T. L. Dao and S. Wood, eds), pp. 15–30. The University Chicago Press, Chicago.
Jordan, V. C., and Dix, C. J. (1979). *J. Steroid Biochem.* **11**, 285–291.
Judd, H. L., Lucas, W. E., and Yen, S. S. C. (1976). *J. Clin. Endocr. Metab.* **43**, 272–278.
Jung-Testas, I., and Baulieu, E. E. (1979). *Expl Cell Res.* **119**, 25–85.
Kaye, A. M., Icekson, I., and Lindner, H. R. (1971). *Biochim. Biophys. Acta* **252**, 150–159.
Kohorn, E. I. (1976). *Gynaecol. Oncol.* **4**, 398–411.
Korenman, S. G., Perrin, L. E., and McCallum, T. P. (1969). *J. Clin. Endocr. Metab.* **29**, 879–883.
Lerner, H., Band, P. R., Israel, L., and Leung, B. S. (1976). *Cancer Treat. Rep.* **60**, 1431–1435.
Levy, C., Eychenne, B., and Robel, P. (1980). *Biochim. Biophys. Acta* **630**, 301–305.
Lippman, M., Bolan, G., and Huff, K. (1976). *Cancer Res.* **35**, 4595–4601.
McGuire, W. L., Raynaud, J. P., and Baulieu, E. E. (1977). "Progesterone Receptors in Normal and Neoplastic Tissues", Raven Press, New York.
MacLaughlin, D. T., and Richardson, G. (1976). *J. Clin. Endocr. Metab.* **42**, 667–678.
MacMahon, B. (1974). *Gynecol. Oncol.* **2**, 122–129.
Manni, A., Trujillo, J., Marshall, J. S., Brodkey, S., and Pearson, O. H. (1979). *Cancer* **43**, 444–450.
Milgrom, E., Luu Thi, M., Atger, M., and Baulieu, E. E. (1973). *J. Biol. Chem.* **248**, 6366–6374.
Morgan, L. R., Schein, P. S., Woolley, P. V., Hoth, D., MacDonald, J., Lippman, M., Posey, L. E., and Beasley, R. W. (1976). *Cancer Treat. Rep.* **60**, 1437–1443.

Mouridsen, H., Palshof, T., Patterson, J., and Battersby, L. (1978). *Cancer Treat. Rep.* **5**, 131–141.

Muechler, E. K., Flickinger, G. L., Mangan, C. E., and Mikhail, G. (1975). *Gynecol. Oncol,* **3**, 244–250.

Namer, M., Lalanne, C., and Baulieu, E. E. (1980). *Cancer Res.* **40**, 1750–1752.

Ng, A., and Reagan, J. (1978). *Obstet. Gynaecol.* **35**, 437–443.

Pfleiderer, A., and Paessler, U. (1978). *In* "Endometrial Cancer" (M. G. Brush, R. J. B. King and R. W. Taylor, eds.), pp. 10–16. Bailliere Tindall, London.

Pollow, K., Lübbert, H., Boquoi, E., Kreuzer, G., Jeske, R., and Pollow, B. (1975a). *Acta Endocr.* **79**, 134–145.

Pollow, K., Boquoi, E., Lübbert, H., and Pollow, B. (1975b). *J. Endocr.* **67**, 131–132.

Pollow, K., Lübbert, H., Boquoi, E., Kreuzer, G., and Pollow, B. (1975c). *Endocrinology* **96**, 319–328.

Pollow, K., Schmidt-Gollwitzer, M., and Nevinny-Stickel, H. (1977). *In* "Progesterone Receptors in Normal and Neoplastic Tissues" (W. L. McGuire, J. P. Raynaud and Baulieu, E. E., eds), pp. 313–338. Raven Press, New York.

Rader, M. D., Flickinger, G. C., De Villa, G. O., Mikuta, J. J., and Mikhail, G. (1973). *Amer. J. Obstet. Gynaecol.* **116**, 1009–1013.

Reifenstein, E. C. (1974). *Gynaecol. Oncol.* **2**, 377–414.

Richardson, F. S., and MacLaughlin, D. T. (1978). *In* "Hormonal Biology of Endometrial Cancer", Vol. 42, pp. 13–14. UICC Technical Report Series, Geneva.

Robel, P., Levy, C., Wolff, J. P., Nicolas, J. C., and Baulieu, E. E. (1978). *C. R. Acad. Sci.* **287**, 1353–1356.

Saez, S., Martin, P. M., and Chouvet, C. D. (1978). *Cancer Res.* **38**, 3468–3473.

Segaloff, A., Duningham, M., Rice, B. F., and Weeth, J. B. (1967). *Cancer* **20**, 1673–1678.

Siiteri, P. K., Schwarz, B., and MacDonald, P. C. (1974). *Gynaecol. Oncol.* **2**, 228–238.

Sherman, A. I. (1966). *Obstet. Gynaecol.* **28**, 309–314.

Smith, D. C., Prentice, R., Thomson, D. J., and Hermann, W. L. (1975). *New Engl. J. Med.* **293**, 1164–1167.

Stoll, B. A. (1967). *Brit. Med. J.* **3**, 338–341.

Sutherland, R., Mester, J., and Baulieu, E. E. (1977). *In* "Hormones and Cell Regulation" (J. Dumont and J. Nunez, eds), Vol I, pp. 31–48. North Holland Publishing, Amsterdam.

Tabor, C. W., and Tabor, H. (1976). *Ann. Rev. Biochem.* **45**, 285–306.

Tseng, L., and Gurpide, E. (1972). *Amer. J. Obstet. Gynaecol.* **114**, 995–1001.

Tseng, L., and Gurpide, E. (1975). *Endocrinology* **97**, 825–833.

Tseng, L., Gusberg, S., and Gurpide, E. (1977). *Ann. NY. Acad. Sci.* **286**, 190–198.

Vihko, R., Jänne, O., Kauppila, A., Kontula, K., and Syrjäla, P. (1978). *J. Steroid Biochem.* **9**, 856.

Wade, M. E., Kohorn, E., and Morris, J. M. C. L. (1967). *Amer. J. Obstet. Gynaecol.* **99**, 869–876.

Young, P. C. M., Ehrlich, C. E., and Cleary, R. E. (1976). *Amer. J. Obstet. Gynaecol.* **125**, 353–360.

25

Changes in Endocrine Status Following Antioestrogen Administration to Premenopausal and Postmenopausal Women

A. MANNI, B. ARAFAH AND O. H. PEARSON

I. INTRODUCTION

A major improvement in the management of breast cancer has occurred with the introduction of non-steroidal antioestrogens. Among them nafoxidine and tamoxifen have been mostly used in clinical trials (European Breast Cancer Group, 1972b; Heuson, 1976). Because of photosensitivity reactions associated with the use of nafoxidine, tamoxifen is now considered

NON-STEROIDAL ANTIOESTROGENS
ISBN 0 12 677880 9

the antioestrogen of choice for clinical use. Since the original report by Cole *et al.* (1972) numerous other investigators have confirmed the efficacy and safety of tamoxifen in the treatment of hormone-responsive metastatic breast cancer (Kiang and Kennedy, 1977; Manni *et al.*, 1979b).

Although extensively studied, mostly in rat uteri and rat mammary cancers, the mechanism of action of antioestrogens is not completely understood. When given as a single injection, tamoxifen has been found to be as potent as oestradiol in producing an increase in rat uterine wet weight (Davies *et al.*, 1979), whereas when repeated injections are given, tamoxifen is unable to produce the full uterotrophic response observed with oestradiol (Jordan *et al.*, 1977). Like oestrogens, non-steroidal antioestrogens have been found to bind to the cytosol oestrogen receptor and promote its migration to the nucleus both in rat uteri (Davies *et al.*, 1979) and DMBA-induced rat mammary tumours (Tsai and Katzenellenbogen, 1977). However, after antioestrogen administration an atypical long-term nuclear retention of the antioestrogen occurs and no replenishment of the cytosol oestrogen receptors takes place, such as that observed after oestrogen administration (Davies *et al.*, 1979).

Inhibition of oestrogen receptor synthesis has indeed been considered one of the main mechanisms by which antioestrogens make target organs insensitive to the trophic action of circulating oestrogens and may cause regression of hormone responsive mammary tumours (Nicholson *et al.*, 1976). This concept, however, has been challenged by the observation that antioestrogens have a long biological half-life in the circulation (Fromson *et al.*, 1973). As a consequence it has been suggested that, although oestrogen receptors may be resynthesized in the cytoplasm, they are rapidly translocated to the nucleus by binding ligands in the blood (Jordan *et al.*, 1978). Recently the effects of oestradiol and tamoxifen on transcription have been compared in rat uteri. It has been observed that, whereas oestradiol produced and maintained significant elevations in RNA polymerase I and II activities, the effects on these enzymes brought about by tamoxifen were less and transitory (Davies *et al.*, 1979), pointing to a basic inefficacy of the antioestrogen-receptor complex. We may conclude that, although antioestrogens are able to promote early tissue responses characteristic of oestrogens, these cannot be sufficiently maintained. In addition antioestrogens, either by inhibiting oestrogen receptor synthesis or by continuously promoting their translocation to the nucleus, make the cytosol oestrogen receptors no longer available for interaction with circulating oestrogens thus inhibiting oestrogen action at the peripheral level.

It is the purpose of this chapter to summarize how, in our opinion, the introduction of antioestrogens has greatly improved our understanding of the endocrinology of human breast cancer. We will primarily review the hormonal changes induced by tamoxifen in postmenopausal and premenopausal patients. The results obtained with tamoxifen after major ablative procedures, as well as the results of endocrine therapy after antioestrogens, will also be reviewed as they give further insight into the endocrine factors affecting tumour growth. Finally, we will report our experience with a new antioestrogen, trioxifene mesylate (Lilly), in which we became interested because of its ability to suppress growth hormone secretion in rats.

II. ANTIOESTROGEN-INDUCED CHANGES IN THE HORMONAL MILIEU

A. Postmenopausal Patients

Early in our trial of antioestrogen therapy of stage IV breast cancer in postmenopausal women we were interested in determining whether tamoxifen administration (20 mg p.o. twice a day) had any effect on pituitary function which could possibly account for its antitumour activity. No effect on prolactin secretion was observed in 8 patients studied. The results in one representative patient are shown in Figure 1. Diurnal variation of serum prolactin with a rise during sleep, suppression after L-dopa administration and stimulation after chlorpromazine injection were similar before and after 9 months on tamoxifen in this patient. Similar results were obtained in 7 other patients. Serum growth hormone levels also measured in the same 8 patients were not found to be affected by chronic antioestrogen administration.

In 16 patients we measured serum oestrogens and gonadotropins before and during tamoxifen therapy. The results are shown in Table I. It can be seen that serum levels of oestrone, oestradiol and oestriol were not affected by antioestrogen treatment, whereas serum FSH and LH were slightly, but significantly, suppressed. In summary, chronic antioestrogen therapy had minimal effects on the hormonal milieu in postmenopausal women, thus suggesting that the antitumour effect of tamoxifen is probably direct at the tumour level through selective inhibition of oestrogen action.

Updated results (Table II) on our series of 113 patients that we have previously reported (Manni *et al.*, 1979b) show that the antitumour activity of tamoxifen in postmenopausal women is about equal to that of surgical hypophysectomy, where in our experience the average duration of remission is 18+ months (Manni *et al.*, 1979a).

Of 55 patients in whom oestrogen receptor (ER) status was known, 49 were ER positive and 6 were ER negative. Response to tamoxifen was significantly higher in ER positive patients compared to patients in whom ER status was unknown (63 % *vs* 44 %) ($p < 0.02$). None of 6 ER negative patients responded to antioestrogen therapy. These results confirm the well-established role of ER measurement in predicting response of metastatic breast cancer to endocrine therapy.

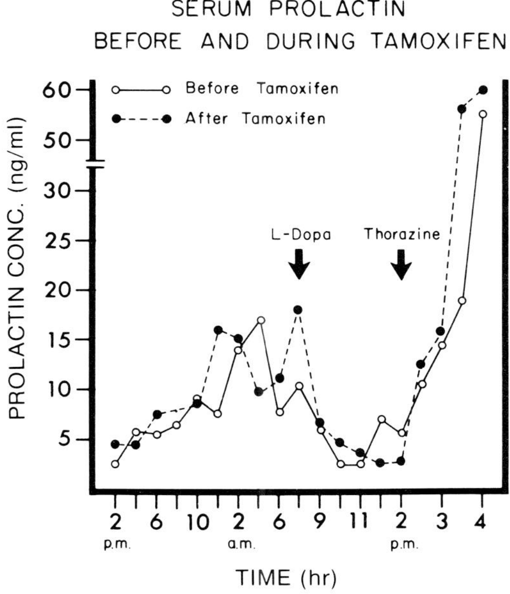

Fig. 1. Serum prolactin levels during the day, at night during sleep, after 500 mg of L-dopa orally, and after 50 mg of chlorpromazine i.m. in a patient with metastatic breast cancer. Studies were done before and 9 months after tamoxifen administration.

TABLE I
Effects of Tamoxifen Treatment on Serum Oestrogens and Gonadotropins in Postmenopausal Women[a]

	Baseline (mean ± S.E.M.)	During treatment (mean ± S.E.M.)
FSH (mIU/ml)	62.3 ± 5.6	48.4 ± 3.9[b]
LH (mIU/ml)	59.6 ± 6.2	47.0 ± 4.0[b]
E_1 (pg/ml)	51.2 ± 8.3	53.3 ± 4.3
E_2 (pg/ml)	31.8 ± 3.9	29.7 ± 3.2
E_3 (pg/ml)	19.5 ± 1.8	24.1 ± 2.3

[a] From Manni *et al.*, (1979b).
[b] $p < 0.05$.

TABLE II
Results of Tamoxifen Therapy in 113 Patients with Stage IV Breast Cancer

	Patients No.	%	Duration (months)	No. still in remission
Remissions	56	50	20+ (4–44+)	7
No progression	8	7	23 (9–45)	0
Failures	49	43	—	—

B. Premenopausal Patients

Preliminary observations by us (Manni *et al.*, 1979b) and other investigators (Heuson, 1976; Pritchard *et al.*, 1978) have indicated that remissions can be obtained with tamoxifen in some premenopausal patients with metastatic breast carcinoma. However, the role of antioestrogen therapy in this category of patients remains to be fully elucidated, in particular its potential ability to replace surgical ovariectomy, which is now the standard endocrine treatment of hormone-dependent breast cancer in menstruating women. We have recently reported our experience with the use of tamoxifen in 11 premenopausal patients with metastatic breast cancer (Manni and Pearson, 1980). An update of our results is shown in Table III. Six of 11 patients obtained significant benefit from antioestrogen therapy with an average duration in excess of 21 months. It is apparent that complete suppression of ovarian function is not necessary to obtain an antitumour effect (Pts 1–4, 6). In an attempt to establish whether larger doses of tamoxifen would induce amenorrhea we have escalated the dose in some patients without noticing any increase in side effects. In 2 patients (Pts 4, 6) (Figs 2 and 3) menses which were irregular while on the lower dose were completely suppressed when the dose was escalated. It should be noted that in some patients (Pts 2, 7–9, 11), due to progression of their disease, the duration of treatment was too short to be able to fully assess the effect of tamoxifen on their menstrual cycles.

A possible explanation of why conventional doses of tamoxifen fail to completely suppress the menstrual cycles in most patients is the observation that antioestrogens markedly stimulate oestrogen production by the ovaries (Manni and Pearson, 1980; Sherman *et al.*, 1979). It is thus possible that the elevated serum oestrogen levels, up to 4 or 5 times the preovulatory peak, might partially counteract the effect of tamoxifen at least at the level of the uterus. The mechanism of this increase in oestrogen production is at present

TABLE III
Results of Tamoxifen Therapy in 11 Premenopausal Patients with Metastatic Breast Cancer

Patient	Age (yrs)	D.F.I.[a] (mths)	Site of metastasis	ER (fmol/mg protein)	Maximum dose/day	Menses	Duration of treatment (mths)[b]	Response	Duration (mths)	Response to ovariectomy
1. EE	46	108	Lung	—	40 mg	Irregular	53 (10)	Remission	10	Remission[c]
2. EM	33	8	Skin, bone	47	60 mg	Regular	9 (4)	Remission	4	Failure[c]
3. AM	53	0	Breast, bone peritoneum	11.5	60 mg	Irregular	15	Remission	15	—
4. MJE	51	54	Pleura	—	80 mg	Irregular→ absent	34+	Remission	34+	—
5. HSW	49	0	Pleura	43	40 mg	Hyster.	22	Remission	22	—
6. BA	45	26	Bone	—	120 mg	Irregular→ absent	40	No change	40	—
7. MM	46	16	Bone	31.4	40 mg	Absent	9 (2)	Failure	—	Failure[c]
8. SML	36	48	Lymph nodes	6.7[d]	40 mg	Regular	2	Failure	—	Failure
9. MLB	48	45	Bone, pleura	Neg[d]	80 mg	Regular	5 (3)	Failure	—	Failure[c]
10. DC	35	0	Bone	Neg/ 7.4[d]	40 mg	Hyster.	2	Failure	—	—
11. MD	32	7	Lung, bone	—	40 mg	Absent	2	Failure	—	—

[a] Disease free interval.
[b] Figures in brackets are months on tamoxifen prior to ovariectomy.
[c] Continued on tamoxifen after ovariectomy.
[d] Done 1–3 weeks after stopping tamoxifen.

not known. It is possible that the hypothalamus and pituitary may sense a lack of oestrogens due to the presence of antioestrogens. This would result in increased gonadotropin output by the pituitary with consequent increase in oestrogen secretion by the ovaries. Serum FSH and LH, however, have been found to be mostly within the normal premenopausal range (Manni and Pearson, 1980; Sherman *et al.*, 1979), although inappropriately high for the level of circulating oestrogens. However in 2 of our patients (Figs 2 and 3), escalation of the dose of tamoxifen caused a rise in serum gonadotropins into the postmenopausal range in the presence of elevated serum oestrogens, definitely indicating an activation of the pituitary gonadal axis.

Whatever the mechanism, the marked rise in serum oestrogens may be a draw-back to the use of tamoxifen in premenopausal women and may have to be counteracted if optimal hormonal control of breast cancer in this category of patients is to be achieved. In support of this possibility are our results with ovariectomy after tamoxifen (Table III). Of 2 patients who had responded to antioestrogens and then relapsed one obtained further remission with

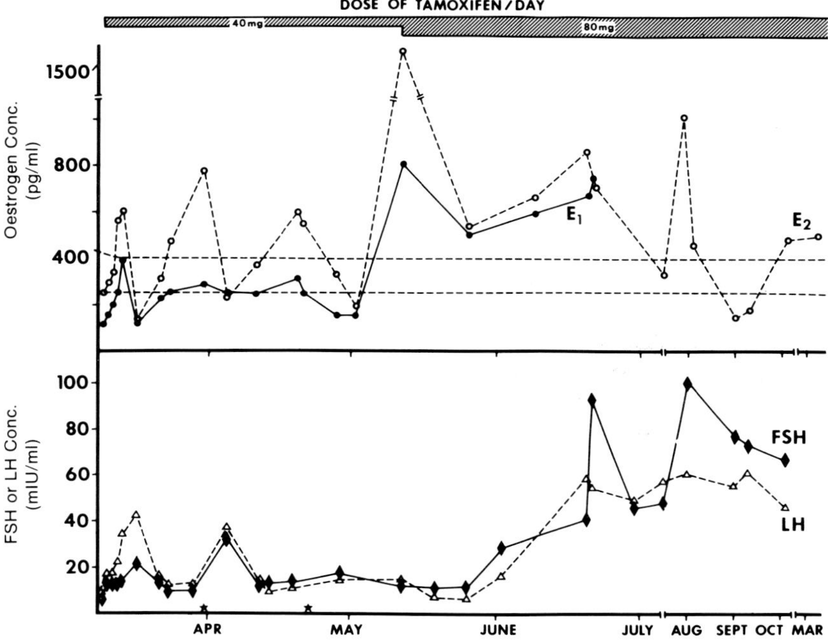

Fig. 2. Serum oestrone (E_1) and oestradiol (E_2) (upper panel) and FSH and LH (lower panel) in a premenopausal patient treated with escalating doses of tamoxifen. Dotted lines indicate the upper limit of normal of E_1 and E_2 for midcycle peak. Menstrual period = (★).

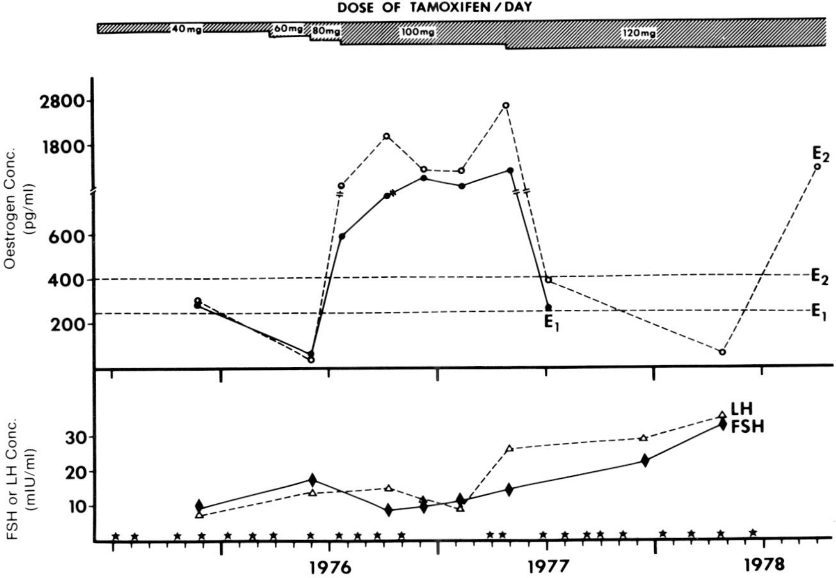

Fig. 3. Serum oestrone (E_1) and oestradiol (E_2) (upper panel) and FSH and LH (lower panel) in a premenopausal patient treated with escalating doses of tamoxifen. Dotted lines indicate the upper limit of normal of E_1 and E_2 for midcycle peak. Menstrual period = (★).

castration (Pt 1). This finding suggests that 40 mg of tamoxifen daily in this patient was insufficient to block all oestrogen action and that ovariectomy, by removing the major endogenous source of oestrogens, permitted more effective antioestrogen action and tumour regression.

It is of interest that of 3 patients who initially failed to respond to tamoxifen none benefited from subsequent ovariectomy. This is in agreement with the report by Pritchard *et al.* (1978) who also found that seven premenopausal patients who failed antioestrogens subsequently failed castration.

If these preliminary observations are confirmed in a larger number of patients, then tamoxifen might be used as the initial treatment of choice in premenopausal patients with hormone responsive tumours. Those who fail to benefit would be treated with chemotherapy without undergoing ovariectomy. Those patients who improve on tamoxifen would subsequently be treated by ovariectomy or radiation castration as a means of compensating for the increased oestrogen secretion by the ovary induced by the antioestrogen. Whether escalation of the dose of tamoxifen might be adequate compensation remains to be determined.

III. ANTIOESTROGEN TREATMENT IN PATIENTS WITH PREVIOUS MAJOR ABLATIVE SURGERY

Table IV illustrates the results of tamoxifen therapy in 29 patients who had undergone hypophysectomy. Completeness of hypophysectomy was documented by undetectable serum growth hormone and prolactin after provocative stimuli (Manni *et al.*, 1979a). Serum oestrone and oestradiol, however, were detectable although in low concentration (5–47 pg/ml). It is apparent that antioestrogen therapy may be quite effective under these circumstances, suggesting that oestrogens, even in small amounts, can directly stimulate tumour growth in the absence of the pituitary gland, and that tamoxifen acts by direct inhibition of oestrogen action at the tumour level. Alternatively, tamoxifen might have an antitumour effect unrelated to its antioestrogenic activity.

Tamoxifen was also able to induce remissions in 2 of 4 patients who had previously undergone ovariectomy and adrenalectomy. Serum oestrone and oestradiol were measurable in these patients, again indicating that ablative procedures are unable to eliminate serum oestrogens completely.

TABLE IV
Results of Tamoxifen Therapy in 29 Patients Post Hypophysectomy[a]

	Patients		Duration	No. still in
	No.	%	(mths)	remission
Remission	8	27	18+ (4–53.5+)	1
No progression	6	21	18+ (11–23)	1
Failures	15	52	—	—

[a] All 29 patients had previously had an objective remission from hypophysectomy.

IV. ENDOCRINE TREATMENT AFTER TAMOXIFEN IN STAGE IV BREAST CANCER

The results presented thus far indicate that tamoxifen is an optimal form of therapy of hormone-responsive metastatic breast cancer at least in postmenopausal women and suggest that oestrogen is indeed the major hormone involved in stimulation of human breast cancer growth, probably acting directly at the tumour level.

We have investigated the possible role of other hormones in supporting tumour growth by sequentially performing hypophysectomy and/or administering androgens to patients who had initially failed or relapsed after antioestrogen.

A. Hypophysectomy

Table V illustrates the results of hypophysectomy after tamoxifen. Sixty per cent of patients who had initially responded to antioestrogens obtained further palliation with removal of the pituitary gland for an average duration of more than one year. It is of interest that 27% of patients who had initially failed tamoxifen responded objectively to hypophysectomy, although with a somewhat shorter duration of response.

These results indicate that, in addition to oestrogens, a pituitary factor may also be involved in the growth of some human breast cancers. Whether it is the suppression of lactogenic hormones, prolactin and growth hormone, that induces tumour regression with hypophysectomy after tamoxifen remains to be determined. The lack of significant palliation in stage IV human breast cancer observed with effective suppression of serum prolactin with the ergot derivative drugs bromocryptine and lergotrile mesylate (European Breast Cancer Group, 1972a; Pearson and Manni, 1978) may be due to the fact that growth hormone in humans is lactogenic, and thus may also need to be suppressed in order to obtain a remission.

B. Androgens

Table VI illustrates the overall results of androgen therapy (Halotestin, 10 mg p.o. twice a day) after tamoxifen. It can be seen that approximately one-third of the patients obtained a remission to androgens after either failing or relapsing on antioestrogen. Of particular interest are the results of androgen

TABLE V
Response to Hypophysectomy after Tamoxifen (Tam)

	No.	Remissions No.	Remissions %	Duration (mths)	No. still in remission	Failures
A. Remissions to Tam	25	15[a]	60	13	0	10
B. Failures to Tam	22	6	27	8.5	0	16
C. Arrest of disease on Tam	10	1	10	20	0	9

[a] In 3 patients only arrest of disease was documented.

therapy in 13 patients who had been previously treated with both tamoxifen and hypophysectomy (Table VII). It is remarkable that 6 of these patients responded to Halotestin, including 2 (Pts 4, 5) who had previously failed to respond to both tamoxifen and hypophysectomy. These results strongly suggest that in this group of patients the mechanism by which androgens induced tumour regression was not an antioestrogenic effect or mediated through the pituitary, but rather a direct effect at the tumour level.

TABLE VI
Response to Androgens after Tamoxifen (Tam)

	No.	Remissions No.	Remissions %	Duration (mths)	No. still in remission	Failures
A. Remissions to Tam	12	5	42	12+	2	7
B. Failures to Tam	12	4	33	8	0	8
C. Arrest of disease on Tam	4	2	50	10+	1	2

V. TRIOXIFENE

Trioxifene mesylate (Lilly) (Fig. 4) has potent antioestrogenic activity in rats. In addition, significant reduction in serum growth hormone (GH) levels were observed at doses of 1–4 mg/kg/day (Fig. 5, unpublished observations, Lilly Research Lab).

Because of the possible role of lactogenic hormones, GH and prolactin (PRL), in sustaining the growth of human breast cancer as discussed earlier, we investigated the effects of trioxifene mesylate on GH secretion as well as other hormones in patients with breast cancer (Arafah *et al.*, 1980). It is possible that effective suppression of GH and PRL secretion might provide a means for medical hypophysectomy when combined with an antioestrogen.

Seven postmenopausal patients (54 to 79 years old) with metastatic breast cancer were treated with trioxifene at a dose of 1–4 mg/kg/day in 2 to 3 divided doses. Treatment was continued for a minimum of 2 months, except in one patient where it was discontinued after 10 days because of the development of hypercalcaemia.

Table VIII is an update of our experience reported earlier (Arafah *et al.*, 1980). Two previously untreated patients obtained objective remissions while one had arrest of her disease during trioxifene mesylate therapy. Two patients (Pts 4, 5) who relapsed on tamoxifen, had further progression of disease during the 2 month trial period with trioxifene. One patient (Pt 1) who

TABLE VII
Response to Androgens after Tamoxifen and Hypophysectomy

Patient	ER (fmol/mg protein)	Response to tamoxifen	Duration (mths)	Response to hypophysectomy	Duration (mths)	Response to androgens	Duration (mths)
1. O.M.	53.9	Remission	9	Remission	29	Remission	18+
2. T.C.[a]	—	Remission	25	Remission	40	Remission	4
3. D.O.	15.5	No change	8	Failure	—	Remission	11
4. C.R.	—	Failure	—	Failure	—	Remission	9
5. E.M.	—	Failure	—	Failure	—	Remission	7
6. D.P.	36	Failure	—	Remission	16	Remission	10
7. A.S.[a]	—	Failure	—	Remission	38	Failure	—
8. V.K.	NEG/14.7	Failure	—	Remission	6	Failure	—
9. L.O.[a]	183	Failure	—	Remission	12	Failure	—
10. C.Mc.[a]	64	No change	21	Remission	21	Failure	—
11. H.Z.	—	Remission	40	Remission	4	Failure	—
12. P.Z.	—	Remission	25	Remission	18	Failure	—
13. G.B.	—	Remission	7	Remission	11	Failure	—

[a] Tamoxifen treatment after hypophysectomy.

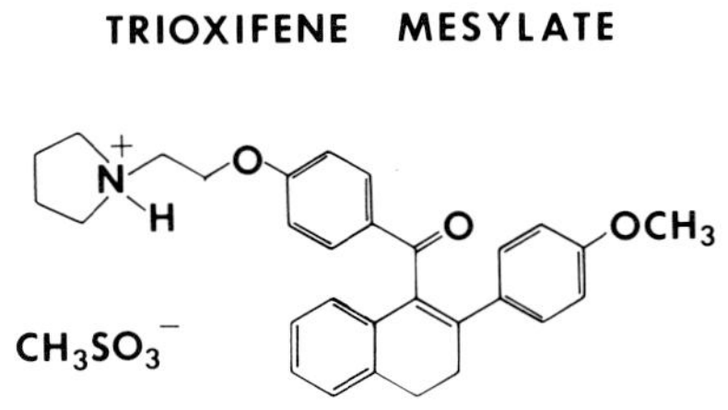

TRIOXIFENE MESYLATE

$CH_3SO_3^-$ OCH_3

Fig. 4. The structural formula of trioxifene mesylate. From Arafah *et al.* (1980).

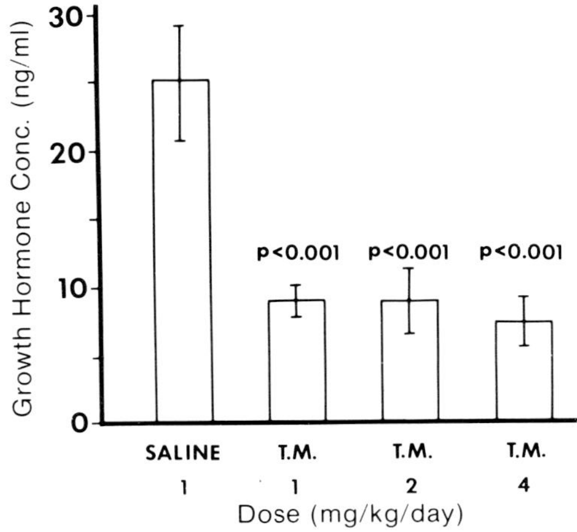

Fig. 5. Growth hormone (GH) levels in rat plasma during treatment with trioxifene mesylate (TM) at a dose of 1, 2 and 4 mg/kg/day for 14 days. From Arafah *et al.* (1980).

TABLE VIII
Results of Trioxifene Mesylate Treatment in 6 Postmenopausal Patients

Patient	Site of Metastasis	Response	Duration of Treatment (mths)	ER (fmol/mg protein)
1	Skin and soft tissue	Remission	8	91
2	Soft tissue and bone	Remission	3+	157
3	Bone	Arrest of disease	12+	ND[a]
4	Bone	Progression	2	ND[a]
5	Lymph nodes	Progression	2	3
6	Bone	Progression	5	90

[a] ND = Not done.

relapsed after 8 months of treatment with trioxifene, showed further progression of disease during a 3 months period on tamoxifen. No side effects were noted in any of these 6 patients during treatment.

There was no effect of trioxifene mesylate treatment on the basal or the sleep related rise in serum GH level in all 6 patients when studied repeatedly at different doses of 1–4 mg/kg/day. However, there was a moderate decrease in the arginine-stimulated GH release in 3 patients noted within one week of treatment with 1.5 mg/kg/day, with no further decrease when the dosage was increased up to 4 mg/kg/day on repeated occasions. The effect in one representative patient is shown in Figure 6. A moderate reduction in the arginine-stimulated glucagon release was also noted in 3 patients within one week of treatment with 1.0 mg/kg/day trioxifene. A minimal further reduction in arginine-induced glucagon release was noted when the dose was increased to 2–4 mg/kg/day. The effect in a representative patient is shown in Figure 7. Basal and arginine-stimulated serum insulin levels were not significantly altered during treatment.

A moderate reduction in serum gonadotropin levels was observed in all 6 patients at all doses studied. Further reductions were noted with prolonged administration of the drug even when the dosage was reduced (Fig. 8). There was no significant effect on serum PRL or thyrotropin levels in all patients.

Further clinical trials are underway to evaluate the effectiveness of trioxifene mesylate as an antitumour agent in women with hormone responsive breast cancer. The effects of trioxifene on GH secretion in humans appear to be minimal under the conditions tested.

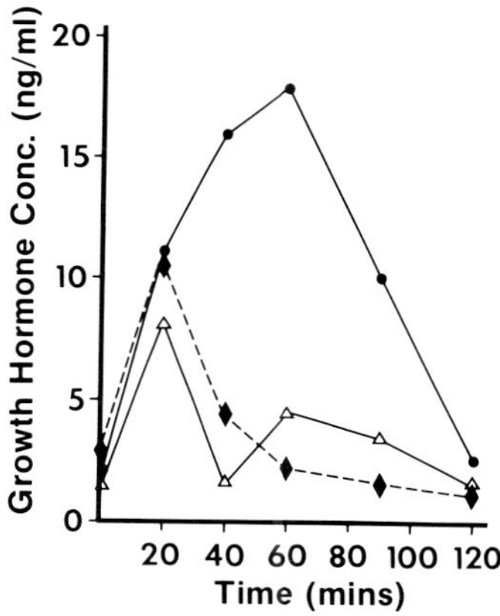

Fig. 6. Serum GH levels during an arginine stimulation test in one patient before (●) and while on trioxifene mesylate, 1.5 mg/kg/day (△) and 4 mg/kg/day (◆). From Arafah *et al.* (1980).

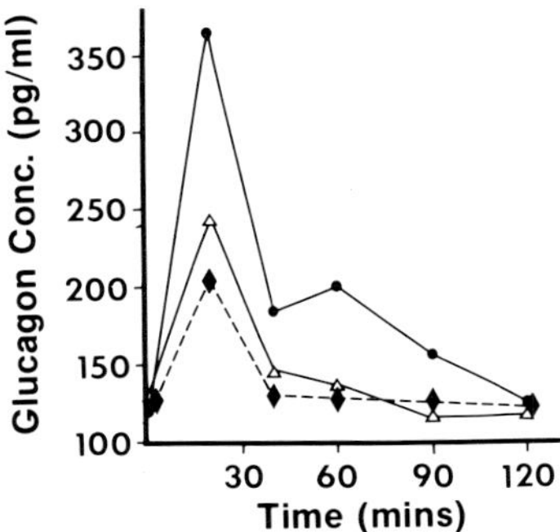

Fig. 7. Serum glucagon level during an arginine stimulation test in one patient before (●) and during trioxifene mesylate therapy at 1 mg/kg/day (△) and 2 mg/kg/day (◆). From Arafah *et al.* (1980).

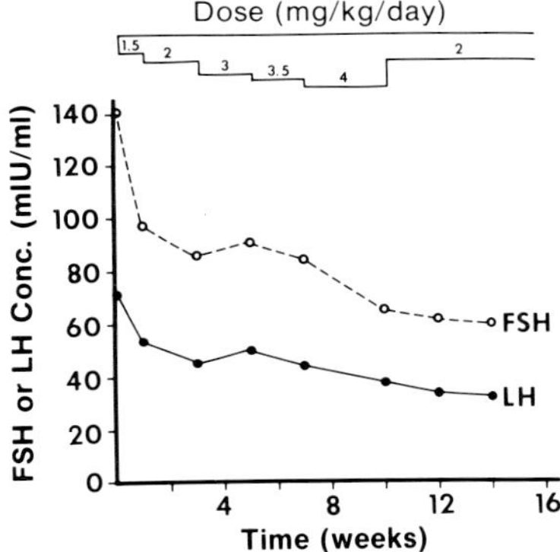

Fig. 8. Serum gonadotropin levels in one patient during treatment with trioxifene mesylate at different doses from 1.5 to 4 mg/kg/day. Each point represents the mean of 6–8 determinations. From Arafah *et al.* (1980).

VI. DISCUSSION

The introduction of non-steroidal antioestrogens has not only proved to be most useful for treatment of breast cancer, but has provided new insights into the endocrinology of human mammary carcinoma. The striking clinical results obtained with tamoxifen indicate that oestrogen is a major hormone involved in sustaining the growth of hormone responsive tumours. In postmenopausal patients, the antitumour effect of tamoxifen does not seem to be indirectly mediated through the pituitary but is more likely to be a direct inhibition of the peripheral action of oestrogens at the tumour level. This concept is particularly supported by the palliation obtained with tamoxifen in completely hypophysectomized patients in whom low levels of circulating oestrogens were detectable. Unless tamoxifen has an antitumour effect unrelated to its antioestrogenic activity, such small amounts of oestrogens must have been able to directly stimulate breast cancer growth in these patients.

Of particular interest are the results of antioestrogen therapy in premenopausal patients. Although data available at present are limited to a small number of patients, it seems that tamoxifen is also a potent antitumour agent in this category of patients. However, a major concern in premenopausal women is the marked stimulation of oestrogen secretion induced by antioestrogen administration either through an activation of the pituitary-ovarian axis and/or increased sensitivity of the ovaries to normal circulating levels of gonadotropins (Sherman *et al.*, 1979). Because of the possibility that the high levels of serum oestrogens might counteract the antitumour action of tamoxifen to some extent, and, in order to obtain optimal hormonal control of tumour growth in premenopausal patients, it may be necessary to combine antioestrogens with suppression of ovarian function. This is usually accomplished at present by either radiation castration or surgical removal of the ovaries. Attractive alternatives in the future for these irreversible modalities include the use of Danazol or LHRH analogues which are now under active investigation and seem to be able to accomplish a reversible medical ovariectomy in experimental animals (DeSombre *et al.*, 1976; Peters *et al.*, 1977). An additional alternative that requires further investigation is escalation of the dose of tamoxifen, which in two of our patients was able to suppress the menstrual cycles, whereas the lower dose was unable to do so.

The antitumour effects of tamoxifen, with its minimal side effects, make this an excellent drug for clinical trials in earlier stages of breast cancer (stage I and II). We have carried out a clinical trial of tamoxifen plus 3-drug chemotherapy (cytoxan, methotrexate and 5-fluorouracil, CMF) versus CMF alone in women with stage II breast cancer (Hubay *et al.*, 1980). Preliminary results indicate that tamoxifen + CMF is more effective in delaying recurrence than CMF alone in women with oestrogen receptor positive tumours. In women with oestrogen receptor negative tumours, there is no significant difference in recurrence noted between the two treatments. Further periods of observation are needed to determine whether earlier use of antioestrogen is more effective than when it is used in later stages of the disease.

The excellent results obtained with tamoxifen raise the question of whether other hormones besides oestrogens play a role in supporting the growth of hormone-responsive human breast cancer. Our results with hypophysectomy and androgens after tamoxifen indicate that other factors besides oestrogens must be involved in regulation of tumour growth. The lactogenic hormones, prolactin and growth hormone, are obviously suspected in view of their well-established role in sustaining the growth of experimental rat mammary cancer (Manni *et al.*, 1977) as well as normal mammary gland. In addition, we have been able to detect prolactin receptors in 51 % of human breast cancer biopsy specimens (Pearson *et al.*, 1978), and we are now in the process of correlating their presence with response to hypophysectomy after tamoxifen. Also a possible direct effect of androgens in tumour growth regulation is suggested by the good palliation observed with administration of pharmacologic doses of androgens to patients who had been previously treated with antioestrogens and hypophysectomy.

In conclusion, tamoxifen has introduced a new concept in breast cancer management, namely antihormone therapy, by which the peripheral action of the hormone is selectively inhibited. This represents a potential advantage over ablative procedures which still leave low levels of circulating oestrogens able to stimulate tumour growth. In addition, antioestrogen therapy, by selectively inhibiting oestrogen action, has enabled us to appreciate the individual and major role that oestrogens play in sustaining the growth of hormone responsive human breast cancer. The development of specific antiandrogens, antigrowth hormone and antiprogestin drugs would be most useful in further elucidating the complex endocrinology of human breast cancer.

ACKNOWLEDGEMENTS

The work was supported by grants from the U.S.P.H.S., CA-05197-20, RR-80, and the American Cancer Society, PDT-48V.

REFERENCES

Arafah, B., Manni, A., and Pearson, O. H. (1980). *In* "Breast Cancer: Experimental and Clinical Aspects". (H. T. Mouridsen and T. Palshof, eds), pp. 281–285. Pergamon Press, Oxford.

Cole, M. P., Jones, C. T. A., and Todd, I. D. H. (1972). *In* "Advances in Antimicrobial and Antineoplastic Chemotherapy, Proceedings of the 7th International Congress of Chemotherapy, Prague, 1971" (M. Hejzlar, M. Semonsky and S. Masak, eds), Vol. II, pp. 529–531. University Park Press, Baltimore, Md.

Davies, P., Syne, J. S., and Nicholson, R. I. (1979). *Endocrinology* **105**, 1336–1342.

DeSombre, E. R., Johnson, E. S., and White, W. F. (1976). *Cancer Res.* **36**, 3830–3833.

European Breast Cancer Group, (1972a). *Eur. J. Cancer* **8**, 155–156.

European Breast Cancer Group (1972b). *Eur. J. Cancer* **8**, 387–389.

Fromson, J. H., Pearson, S., and Bramah, S. (1973). *Xenobiotica* **3**, 693–710.

Heuson, J. C. (1976). *Cancer Treat. Rep.* **60**, 1463–1466.

Hubay, C. A., Pearson, O. H., Marshall, J. S., Rhodes, R. S., Debanne, S. M., Mansour, E. G., Hermann, R. E., Jones, J. C., Flynn, W. J., Eckert, C., McGuire, W. L., and 27 Participating Investigators (1980). *Surgery* **87**, 494–501.

Jordan, V. C., Collins, M. M., Rowsby, L., and Prestwich, G. (1977). *J. Endocr.* **75**, 305–316.

Jordan, V. C., Rowsby, L., Dix, C. J., and Prestwich, G. (1978). *J. Endocr.* **78**, 71–81.

Kiang, D. T., and Kennedy, B. J. (1977). *Ann. Int. Med.* **87**, 687–690.

Manni, A., and Pearson, O. H. (1980). *Cancer Treat. Rep.* **64**, 779–785.

Manni, A., Trujillo, J., and Pearson, O. H. (1977). *Cancer Res.* **37**, 1216–1219.

Manni, A., Pearson, O. H., Brodkey, J., and Marshall, J. S. (1979a). *Cancer* **44**, 2330–2337.

Manni, A., Trujillo, J. E., Marshall, J. S., Brodkey, J., and Pearson, O. H. (1979b). *Cancer* **43**, 444–450.

Nicholson, R. I., Golder, M. P., Davies, P., and Griffiths, K. (1976). *Eur. J. Cancer* **12**, 711–717.

Pearson, O. H., and Manni, A. (1978). *In* "Current Topics in Experimental Endocrinology" (L. Martini and V. H. T. James, eds), Vol. III, pp. 75–92. Academic Press, New York.

Pearson, O. H., Manni, A., Chambers, M., Brodkey, J., and Marshall, J. S. (1978). *Cancer Res.* **38**, 4323–4326.

Peters, G. T., Lewis, J. D., Wilkinson, E. J., and Fuhrman, M. T. (1977). *Cancer* **40**, 2797–2800.

Pritchard, K. I., Meakin, J. W., Myers, R. E., Sutherland, D. J. A., and Mobbs, B. G. (1978). *Ann. Int. Med.* **89**, 721–722.

Sherman, B. M., Chapler, F. K., Crickard, K. C., and Wycoff, D. (1979). *J. Clin. Invest.* **64**, 398–404.

Tsai, T. L. S., and Katzenellenbogen, B. (1977). *Cancer Res.* **37**, 1537–1543.

26

"Nolvadex" (Tamoxifen) as an Anti-Cancer Agent in Humans

J. S. PATTERSON

I. INTRODUCTION

The non-steroidal antioestrogens of the triarylalkene group were the subject of much scientific interest during the 1960s due to their ability to terminate pregnancy by preventing implantation of the blastocyst in rats (Harper and Walpole, 1967). Many of these agents were found to be either ineffective as contraceptive agents in the human or too toxic for this purpose. One agent, Clomid (clomiphene citrate, Merrell) gained widespread usage in the treatment of infertility. Although Clomid and MER-25, a closely related compound, indicated that the antioestrogenic properties predicted by their pharmacological activity in some species (Lunan and Klopper, 1975) were present in man, their toxicity precluded long-term continuous therapy.

Two agents were introduced to clinical usage as potential successors to MER-25 and Clomid. The properties of one of these agents, ICI 46,474, whose

NON-STEROIDAL ANTIOESTROGENS
ISBN 0 12 677880 9

generic name is tamoxifen (USAN tamoxifen citrate) and whose proprietary name is "Nolvadex"* are described in this chapter. It was found to have toxicological advantages over Clomid (Legha and Carter, 1976; Furr *et al.*, 1979). The other, nafoxidine (Upjohn, U 11,100A), will not be discussed further here.

Tamoxifen is the *trans*(Z)-isomer of a triphenylethylene (Z)-2-[4-(1,2-diphenyl-1-butenyl)phenoxy]-NN-dimethylethanamine. The corresponding *cis*(E)-isomer is a compound which is weakly oestrogenic and less than 1 % is present in "Nolvadex". The molecular weight is 563.6 and the molecular formula $C_{26}H_{29}NO.C_6H_8O_7$. The agent is a white, odourless crystalline powder which is only slightly soluble in water. When stored protected from light and moisture it is stable for more than 5 years.

The physical, chemical, biochemical and animal pharmacological properties of tamoxifen have been described in detail by Furr *et al.* (1979). This chapter will summarize the clinical studies, together with the relevant human pharmacology, in relation to its use as an antineoplastic agent.

II. CLINICAL PHARMACOLOGY

The first clinical studies with "Nolvadex" were undertaken by Klopper and Hall (1971) in infertile women. El-Sheikha *et al.* (1972) found that a dosage of 5 mg b.i.d. was only partially effective in causing the disappearance of cystic glandular hyperplasia in patients with menometrorrhagia. In collaboration with Masson, Klopper was able to confirm some of the drug's antioestrogenic properties (Masson and Klopper, 1972). They administered it to amenorrhoeic women and showed that, when administered alone, "Nolvadex" did not induce withdrawal bleeding whilst it was capable of preventing the withdrawal bleeding associated with a short course of ethinyl oestradiol.

This early clinical pharmacology suggested that, in the short term, 20 mg of tamoxifen was the minimal consistently effective dose. Some support for this finding has subsequently emerged from studies by Ricciardi and Ianniruberto (1979) who found that 10 mg "Nolvadex" per day, given to women with cystic breast disease, did not affect the serum gonadotrophins in normal cycling premenopausal women. Boyns and Groom (1972), however, found a significant effect (increase in both FSH and LH) in normal cycling women treated with 20 mg per day. These studies suggest that the threshold for stimulation of pituitary release of gonadotrophins would seem to lie between the daily administration of 10 and 20 mg of "Nolvadex".

*"Nolvadex" is a registered trademark of I.C.I. Ltd.

The situation seems to differ when males are given the drug. Willis *et al.* (1977) found that 10 mg of "Nolvadex" per day was capable of producing a consistent rise in gonadotrophins in normal and oligospermic men. The rise was associated with a secondary elevation of both oestrogen and androgen levels. However, they failed to obtain a significant effect upon the sperm count while Comhaire (1976) obtained a significant elevation of the sperm count using 20 mg (2 × 10 mg daily), and this finding has been confirmed by Bartsch and Scheiber (1979). Both Comhaire (1976) and Willis *et al.* (1977) noted that there was no change in the circulating sex hormone binding globulin in spite of the elevated circulating steroid levels in their male subjects. In contrast, Sakai *et al.* (1978) found that female patients with advanced breast cancer develop increases in both sex hormone binding globulin and the cortisol binding globulin following tamoxifen treatment. Thus, it would appear that "Nolvadex" therapy is capable of producing seemingly opposing activities at different target organs and in the two sexes of one species, namely humans. These early findings of a threshold of consistent activity of "Nolvadex", which lay between 10 mg and 20 mg daily, led to the institution of clinical trials in advanced breast cancer at the higher dosage.

III. CLINICAL STUDIES

A. Single Agent Therapy in Advanced Breast Cancer

Studies in breast cancer were initiated in 1969 at the Christie Hospital, England. The rationale for the use of an antioestrogen was developed from the knowledge that a proportion of breast tumours was oestrogen-dependent. Responses could be achieved by oestrogen withdrawal in both premenopausal and postmenopausal women and by pharmacological doses of oestrogenic agents in postmenopausal women. Tumours which were sensitive to one modality, such as oestrogens, seemed to have sensitivity to other endocrine manoeuvres, such as hypophysectomy or adrenalectomy, performed after remission and relapse. Even the low circulating levels of oestrogens present after the menopause were felt to be sufficient to stimulate hormone-sensitive tumour growth, and antioestrogenic therapy was therefore initiated in postmenopausal women with very advanced disease.

Following the success of the early studies by Cole *et al.* (1971) and Ward (1973), many authors have published papers which cite the use of "Nolvadex" as a single agent in the treatment of advanced (locally inoperable or recurrent or metastatic) breast cancer in the postmenopausal woman. It is difficult to compare the results of many of these studies due to differing criteria for the measurement of response, duration of response and documentation in the studies. Mouridsen *et al.* (1978) have summarized 19 studies from the literature. They noted an overall response rate of 32 % (range 16–52 %) with a further 21 % in the stable disease or "no change" category. The summary by Mouridsen and co-workers was undertaken in an attempt to define the type of patient or tumour which was most sensitive to this antioestrogen therapy. While this type of analysis should, ideally, be undertaken in one large study, there were inadequate numbers in some subgroups, even with over 1000 cases in this survey of the literature. A number of interesting points did emerge which are discussed in this section.

1. The Response in Relation to Other Therapy

Patients previously untreated for advanced disease responded well with a complete and partial response (CR and PR) rate of 118/292 (40 %). Prior chemotherapy alone had no effect upon this propensity to respond with 52/112 (42 %) of such patients also showing remission. A response to previous endocrine therapy, irrespective of modality, improved the chance of a second remission on "Nolvadex" to 31/46 (67 %). In 34 women who failed to respond to previous endocrine therapy, 5 (15 %) achieved a CR or PR on antioestrogen therapy. A small amount of data exists on endocrine responsiveness subsequent to "Nolvadex" therapy and 7/30 (23 %) who failed to respond to this agent subsequently responded to another form of additive endocrine therapy.

Two important points emerge from these data. Firstly, all endocrine therapies cannot be grouped together as "endocrine therapy". Moreover, the assumption that is commonly made, i.e. that failure to respond to one modality will automatically preclude response to another, is untrue. Secondly, response to a first line endocrine therapy is a better predictor of subsequent hormone sensitivity of the tumour than hormone receptor measurement (see Section III, A, 4).

2. The Response in Relation to Age and Menopausal Status

A surprising feature of the studies is that the response to therapy increases with the age of the patient (Table I). It is difficult to explain this finding, as one would expect to produce the greatest effects of an antioestrogen at a time when oestrogen levels are at their highest, i.e. in younger patients. While this might be a feature of selection of the cases, the fact that free cytoplasmic oestrogen receptor (ER) also increases with age may be a related phenomenon (Spaeren *et al.*, 1973). One mechanistic explanation is as follows. It is thought that the antioestrogens act through the free cytoplasmic oestrogen receptor (ER) at the tumour level, and it has been shown, *in vitro*, that tamoxifen exhibits competitive antagonism of oestradiol binding to the ER. As the circulating oestradiol levels fall, with ageing, the tamoxifen (which has an affinity for the ER which is considerably lower than the natural ligand) may thus become a more effective competitor and produce greater antitumour effects.

The foregoing theory, suggesting a relationship of increasing response with the falling circulating oestradiol levels of ageing, becomes untenable when the situation in premenopausal women is examined. Pritchard *et al.* (1979) have published results of an ongoing Phase II study of "Nolvadex" given to premenopausal women. They have shown a response rate of 11/32 (34%) which, at a dose of 20 mg b.i.d. and in the face of normal premenopausal oestradiol levels, might not have been predicted if the drug were only competing poorly with postmenopausal oestrogen levels. This study is backed by sporadic reports in the literature of small numbers of premenopausal women who have been treated with "Nolvadex". There are 139 such cases published or personally communicated to the author. The response rate of 43/139 (31%) lends support to the finding of Pritchard *et al.* (1979). A further argument against the increasing response with ageing in postmenopausal women being due to a falling plasma oestradiol level, leading to a better competitive situation for the antioestrogens, comes with the findings by Manni and Pearson (1979) and Sherman *et al.* (1979) that circulating oestradiol levels are increased, with a doubling of the ovulatory peak, during continuous "Nolvadex" therapy. The levels of oestradiol achieved by these women were 30-fold in excess of the normal postmenopausal plasma concentration. This would have been expected to negate or reduce the effect of the antioestrogen if simple competition were the only factor involved in its activity — unless the antioestrogen were present in a considerable excess. If this excess were present at normal dosages, no increasing response with ageing would be expected in postmenopausal women, as tamoxifen to oestrogen concentrations at the cellular level would be well above the top of the dose response curve.

Neither simple competition between oestradiol and tamoxifen nor a large excess of circulating antioestrogen can be invoked to explain both the premenopausal and postmenopausal findings described here. Other factors, such as nonspecific protein binding of the two ligands or cell membrane effects

TABLE I
Response in Relation to Age of Patient[a]

Age	< 50	51–60	61–70	> 70
CR + PR (%)	40/126 (32)	58/207 (28)	65/189 (34)	60/126 (48)

[a] After Mouridsen *et al.* (1978).

of the antioestrogen or more subtle changes in the endocrine *milieu* of the patient, may be responsible for these findings. The most simple explanation of a change of tumour sensitivity might also be considered.

3. *The Response in Relation to Dosage*

The factors leading to the selection of 20 mg daily as the initial dosage were discussed in Section I. Ward (1973, 1976) has suggested that 40 mg daily is an optimal dosage, and most subsequent studies have adopted therapy within the 20–40 mg daily dose range.

Table II suggests an increase in response rates at dosages above 20 mg but these data are a summation of results from essentially non-comparable studies. No good dose response study has been published although two authors, Westerberg *et al.* (1976) and Elleman (1978, personal communication), have increased the dosage in a number of non-responders with little improvement. The recent pharmacokinetic data on this drug show a long serum elimination half-life, with a consequently wide scatter in steady state serum levels in patients receiving the same dosage. Coupled with the long time taken to achieve a response in some cases (mean of 70 days to achieve PR in responders) meaningful correlations between dosage and response rate require both the long-term observation of the patient and the measurement of steady state serum tamoxifen concentrations. As the proportion of patients responding to the therapy has been surprisingly similar in all studies, considering the many different prognostic variables present, it is clear that large numbers of patients will be required for future dose response studies to be meaningful.

TABLE II
Response to Tamoxifen Related to Dosage[a]

Daily dosage	Response		
	CR + PR	Total	%
20 mg	132	471	28
30 mg	34	75	45
40 mg	170	432	39
30 mg/m^2	19	44	43
80 mg (37)	7	17	41

[a] After Mouridsen *et al.* (1978).

4. *The Response in Relation to the Hormone Receptor Status*

Much has now been published on the correlation of therapeutic response to endocrine therapy and the presence or absence of the cytoplasmic or nuclear oestrogen receptor protein. There has been an increased predictability of a positive response (CR + PR) in receptor positive tumour bearing patients, from around 33% in unselected patients to 50–60% in patients selected for therapy on the basis of a positive oestrogen receptor estimation. These data seem to hold true, irrespective of the additive or ablative endocrine therapeutic regimen.

Whilst there is considerable work in progress attempting to raise the predictability of a positive assay to 100%, very little work is in progress in the receptor negative area in relation to endocrine therapies. Good responses are usually reported to occur in less than 10% of receptor negative tumours. Many of the patients whose tumours are classified as receptor negative will never receive any endocrine therapy. If the patients who achieve disease stabilization are included in the analysis (the "no change" group), the predictability of a response in receptor positive cases rises to over 60%, but the receptor negative group becomes "less resistant" to endocrine therapy with 15% or sometimes more of the patients achieving some effect upon the disease (Cheix *et al.*, 1978). This lack of a complete correlation between receptor status and endocrine response would seem to be particularly true for the antioestrogens (Bishop *et al.*, 1979). While a 10% good response and a further 5% or more disease stabilization would not suggest that these agents are acceptable first line therapies in receptor negative advanced disease, it would seem that they should certainly be considered after the patient has ceased to respond to first line chemotherapeutic agents.

5. *The Response in Relation to Metastatic Site*

The first studies by Ward (1973) and his colleagues suggested that "Nolvadex" was considerably more effective in soft tissue disease than in the treatment of bone lesions. As a consequence, many clinicians selected patients on this basis for their clinical trials. Morgan *et al.* (1976) subsequently reported that more bone disease responded in his series than soft tissue disease. Although he is the only worker to find an increase of bone response over soft tissue response, other workers have confirmed that an antioestrogen may be effective in these lesions. Mouridsen *et al.* (1979) showed that soft tissue lesions responded in 35% of cases while 29% of visceral and 25% of bone lesions also responded. Data from a small study by Westerberg (1980) from the Karolinska Hospital, Stockholm, have recently been presented. This comparative study was aimed at comparing bone responses between fluoxymesterone and "Nolvadex". There was no difference between the androgen and the antioestrogen upon bone disease, confirming the fact that these agents are both to be considered as first line therapy in patients with bone dominant disease.

6. *Side Effects*

The data presented above suggest that approximately one third of untreated patients will respond to therapy with an antioestrogen. Those who respond best are older women with no prior therapy or a known response to endocrine therapy and a hormone receptor positive tumour. Much of the data is similar to that produced by classical endocrine therapy with pharmacological doses of oestrogen. However, Stewart (1979), in her comparative study, has suggested that there is a significant prolongation of survival in the antioestrogen treated group over those who received diethylstilboestrol as first line therapy. An added advantage of the antioestrogen is that premenopausal women also respond to "Nolvadex" therapy.

The major advantage of "Nolvadex" has been its relative lack of severe side effects. At normal dosages, less than 3% of patients are withdrawn from therapy due to intolerance. The commonest cause for withdrawal of the therapy is nausea and vomiting. (Hot flushes are the next most common problem but these do not usually warrant drug withdrawal.) Side effects are very rarely life-threatening and the lack of the common problems associated with oestrogens and androgens has led to the widespread acceptance of "Nolvadex".

Recent attention has focused upon hypercalcaemia during therapy. This did not seem to be a common problem in earlier studies but has recently been reported to occur occasionally in the first few weeks of therapy in patients with bony disease. (Veldhuis, 1978; Patterson *et al.*, 1978; Spooner and Evans, 1979; Villalon *et al.*, 1979). The changing pattern of usage of this drug (as described in Section III, A, 5), with increasing usage in patients with osteolytic disease, may account for the recent number of reports on the subject. It is difficult to assess the incidence of early hypercalcaemia attributable to the drug, in view of the incidence of spontaneous hypercalcaemia in the disease, especially when there is rapid tumour progession. Drug induced hypercalcaemia would not seem to be a common problem in view of the numbers of patients on therapy in over 70 countries and the relatively small numbers of reported problems. Some workers (Arnold *et al.*, 1979) have attributed the hypercalcaemia to a transient disease flare which often predicted a clinical response.

No cases of acute overdosage of "Nolvadex" have been described. One study by Kaiser-Kupfer and Lippman (1978) reported upon four women who received between 120 and 160 mg twice daily for periods in excess of 17 months. Retinal and corneal damage resulted in these cases. Perhaps more remarkable is the fact that the drug was otherwise well tolerated for this length of time by all four patients, one of whom had a serum antioestrogen level (tamoxifen + N-desmethyltamoxifen) in excess of 1500 ng/ml.

B. Combination Therapy in Advanced Breast Cancer

Following the establishment of "Nolvadex" as an effective single agent in advanced breast cancer, a number of investigators have assessed the possibility of the drug being integrated into either a combined endocrine approach or in combination with one or more cytotoxic agents.

1. Combined Endocrine Therapy

The combination of cytotoxic agents which act through different cellular mechanisms has revolutionized the approach to the chemotherapy of breast cancer. Little work has taken place with combination of hormonal agents. Many authors have expressed the view that only a fixed one third of breast tumours are responsive to endocrine therapy — irrespective of the modality employed. The initial experience with combinations employing antioestrogen therapy would seem to lend some support to this hypothesis (Mouridsen *et al.*, 1979; Mouridsen and Palshof, 1980). Ward (1977) demonstrated that the addition of a prolactin lowering agent to the antioestrogen therapy of patients refractory to "Nolvadex" could result in further stabilization of the disease, and 2/45 patients had an objective response. However, Settatree *et al.* (1978) were unable to confirm this finding in women who had not previously received endocrine therapy for advanced disease. The patients in his study received either "Nolvadex" alone or "Nolvadex" plus Parlodel (Bromocriptine). No clear differences between the two arms emerged in this small, but well controlled clinical trial.

One study alone suggests that combination of the androgen fluoxymesterone with antioestrogen therapy may improve the responsiveness of tumours. In this study (Tormey *et al.*, 1976), 18 patients received "Nolvadex" alone and 20 were given a combination of the two therapies. Overall response rates were 5/18 (28%) and 9/20 (45%) respectively ($p > 0.1$). This interim analysis of small numbers of patients suggests a trend in favour of the combined therapy but larger numbers of subjects are required for a conclusive study. As the dosages of the antioestrogen were varied from 2–100 mg/m^2 twice daily against a fixed fluoxymesterone dosage and the study was conducted in an open fashion, a positive result in favour of the combined therapy in the final analysis would require the institution of confirmatory studies.

2. *Combined Antioestrogen and Cytotoxic Chemotherapy*

The combined approach of cytotoxic therapy with an endocrine manoeuvre has the same attractions as the combination of different forms of cytotoxic chemotherapy; that is, it introduces another modality with different dose limiting toxicity and another possible mechanism through which the tumour cell may be attacked. Early uncontrolled studies in advanced breast cancer (Heuson, 1976; Bosch Jose *et al.*, 1977) demonstrated that there is no antagonism between the two classes of agents; in fact, the high response rates suggested that there might even be an additive effect. These results allayed the fears that the cytostatic effects of endocrine therapy might only serve to protect a percentage of the tumour cells from chemotherapy. Furthermore, controlled studies have now been reported confirming the initial impression that cytotoxic chemotherapy could be combined with endocrine therapy (Mouridsen and Palshof, 1980; Tormey *et al.*, 1978; Cocconi *et al.*, 1979). None of the studies is very large, but Mouridsen's (an EORTC study) is ongoing. Tormey's study is interesting in that all patients received dibromodulcitol plus doxorubicin (Adriamycin, Farmitalia) as a second line of chemotherapy, which might account for the relatively low response rate of 36 % achieved with these agents alone, a rate which increased to 64 % in those who received combined "Nolvadex" therapy. The low response rate (32 %) in the CMF (cyclophosphamide, methotrexate, fluorouracil) group of the EORTC study cannot be explained away quite so easily. The increase to 58 %, by the addition of "Nolvadex", would only serve to bring the regimen into the response range claimed by many studies of combination chemotherapy alone. These rates might be explained by the use of stringent response criteria and we must await the publication of the completed study with larger patient numbers before making firm conclusions.

One important question must be answered if the combined approach is to be favoured above the common policy of giving endocrine and cytotoxic chemotherapy in sequence. That question is simply, "Does the patient benefit?". Benefit must be measured in terms of an extension of survival time and the quality of life during that time. It is always assumed that neither therapy is curative. The mean duration of response is in the region of one year for the antioestrogen and rather less for the chemotherapy, and it has been shown (Henningsen and Amberger, 1977) that responders to the "Nolvadex" therapy survive longer than the non-responders. However, long-term responders are very rare and virtually all will die of the disease. A comparison of response rates is inadequate for this exercise as the UICC criteria only require the response to be maintained for 4 weeks. Thus one patient may develop a partial response after 8 weeks of therapy on a regimen and be dead within a few weeks, due to a rapid progression, while another patient may have a stabilization of her condition for two years. Ironically, the former patient will be classified as a responder to the therapy while the latter is regarded as a treatment failure — or at best a disease stabilization.

Many studies have been published combining chemotherapy and endocrine therapy. Only one study has attempted to ascertain if the improved response rate of the combined antioestrogen and chemotherapy is of benefit. Recent results from this study (Cavalli *et al.*, 1978), undertaken by the Swiss cooperative group SAKK, suggest that there is no clear advantage of "Nolvadex" plus combination chemotherapy (3 regimens) over "Nolvadex" alone followed by the same chemotherapies on disease progression. This comparability of both response and survival suggests that the quality of life for the patient might be enhanced by giving the much less toxic endocrine therapy alone, as initial therapy. The reverse of this treatment, chemotherapy followed by endocrine therapy, has yet to be compared with the combined modality approach.

The classical tumour kinetic work of Skipper *et al.* (1965) has led us to endeavour to reduce tumour burden by surgery followed by adjuvant chemotherapy in an attempt to effect a cure. Glick *et al.* (1978) and Morgan *et al.* (1976) have both attempted to evaluate the effects of starting cytotoxic chemotherapy during endocrine response when tumour burden is low. They treated initially with the antioestrogen alone to reduce the tumour load, and then randomly assigned the patients achieving response or stable disease to receive either CMF in addition to the antioestrogen or to continue with the "Nolvadex" alone. Their preliminary results of this so-called stage IV adjuvant therapy were encouraging. Glick *et al.* (1980), have recently updated their results. All patients were selected as ER+ or unknown. They were previously untreated and assessment of response was made arbitrarily at 12 weeks on "Nolvadex" monotherapy. A surprisingly high percentage (71 %) of the 89 evaluable patients showed CR, PR or NC considering that the ER status of 40 was unknown. No differences in survival, response or its duration, emerged between the groups randomized to continue "Nolvadex" plus chemotherapy and "Nolvadex" alone. One interesting feature of this study was that 6/34 (18%) patients assigned to "Nolvadex" alone showed an improvement of their response category after 12 weeks, demonstrating again that responses can appear very late with this drug.

It can be seen from publications cited that there is considerable interest in obtaining the answer to the question "How may a safe, effective antioestrogen be incorporated into the overall treatment policy, to the best advantage of the patient with advanced breast cancer?". Some of the answers have been found or will be forthcoming but many further studies will be required to delineate the place of "Nolvadex" in the overall treatment policy.

C. The Treatment of Male Breast Cancer

The incidence of cancer of the male breast is said to be approximately 1% of all cases of breast cancer. This relatively uncommon tumour would appear to be sensitive to endocrine therapy with responses to orchidectomy occurring in 45–68% of cases (Holleb *et al.*, 1968; Treeves, 1959). Ribeiro (1977) in a retrospective review of 200 cases, reported that 38% of patients had responded to DES with a median remission of 7 years. He saw no remission in those who had bone metastases.

Small numbers of patients have received "Nolvadex" therapy for advanced disease. We have recently reviewed the evidence (Patterson *et al.*, 1980) on data emanating from 16 different centres. 15/31 evaluable cases were classified as responders (CR + PR) and a further 5 had a stabilization of their disease. Responses were seen in visceral, bone and soft tissue dominant disease and the pattern of response was very similar to that seen in the postmenopausal women. Few side effects were seen. Loeber and Mouridsen (personal communication) reported 2 PR and 3 NC in 6 patients they treated with the agent. The data suggest that an antioestrogen is effective in male breast cancer and deserved consideration as a first-line agent in this disease, especially in those men who have ER positive tumours.

D. "Nolvadex" as an Adjuvant to Mastectomy

1. Rationale

The elusive goal of a cure for the patient with advanced breast cancer would seem to be no nearer than it was in 1895 when Beatson performed the first ovariectomy. The early work on animal tumour cell kinetics rapidly established the fact that an experimental cure, with cytotoxic agents, could only be effected when the total tumour load was small. The logical extensions of this work have led to a vast, world-wide programme of investigations. The best approach would be to treat the women before the tumour has become clinically apparent, assuming prevention is not feasible. In the absence of any good markers of subclinical disease, this approach has been limited to screening programmes and health education in order that the tumour may be detected when the total load is still low. The majority of work in "curative" studies has centred around the tumour therapy at the time of presentation and mastectomy. The recognition that many women have disseminated disease with clinically undetectable micrometastatic deposits at the time that the primary tumour is found, has led to the realization that the merits and demerits of various mastectomy techniques are of secondary importance in influencing survival since the disease is already established at a distant site.

Thus, in addition to good local therapy which may include regional radiotherapy and a wide dissection of the lymphatic drainage of the breast, a systemic therapy is required.

There are a number of criteria for this systemic therapy. It is generally believed that it must be an approach which is effective in producing regressions of advanced disease and should, ideally, be non-toxic both in the short and long term if patients with a good prognosis are to be treated. The first adjuvant studies utilized ovarian ablation by radiotherapy or surgery. Although a significant early increase was seen on the disease free interval of the patients following therapy (Cole, 1977) there were no clear effects upon survival and adjuvant ovarian ablation fell into disuse, as even this simple manoeuvre has a morbidity and removes a useful therapeutic approach to the advanced disease. Cytotoxic agents have led the revival of adjuvant therapy in recent years, with encouraging early results from Fisher *et al.* (1975) and Bonadonna *et al* (1976).

Adjuvant endocrine therapy has started to attract considerably more attention again, as it has been postulated that the Milan study of CMF, which seems only to work in premenopausal women, is really producing a chemotherapeutic ovariectomy (Rose and Davies, 1977). Furthermore, it is now known that many women treated in the early studies of ovarian irradiation, received inadequate doses of radiotherapy and continued to produce oestrogens. The demonstration of the peripheral conversion of adrenal steroids to oestrone has also highlighted the incompleteness of the removal by ovariectomy of oestrogenic steroids capable of tumour stimulatory activity. The importance of these adrenal steroids has been emphasized by the recent publication of a Canadian study of combined radiation menopause and prednisone, the latter producing adrenal suppression. In this study, Meakin and co-workers have demonstrated an improved survival for the subgroup of patients receiving prednisone and ovarian radiation (Meakin *et al.*, 1979).

A non-steroidal antioestrogen fulfils many of the criteria for selection as an adjuvant therapy. The efficacy and safety of "Nolvadex" were discussed in Section III, A. It is a systemic therapy which is given orally and is thus easily administered. It has a direct effect at the tumour level. This effect is thought to be mediated, primarily, through the oestrogen receptor and is, therefore, able to antagonize the cellular effects of oestrogens irrespective of their source.

2. *Study Design*

Many practical difficulties are encountered in designing the ideal test of antioestrogen adjuvant therapy. Chemotherapy has been given at doses which are a compromise between minimal efficacy in the advanced disease and the acceptability of side effects. Duration of therapy has ranged from one post-operative course, to two years. The dose and duration of "Nolvadex" as an adjuvant therapy have been decided arbitrarily. Recent work from Jordan (1978) in the DMBA rat tumour has suggested that the drug should be continued for long time periods in relation to the life span of the animal, in order to prevent a regrowth of static but live tumour cells. Most clinical studies have chosen dosing periods of 1–2 years as the best practical approach to the problem. Some recently commenced studies will be utilizing a 5 year therapy regimen. This question of duration of therapy will be resolved when the recurrence and survival curves of these studies are analysed and the data studied for evidence of tumour "rebound" after cessation of therapy.

There are differences of opinion between investigators over the place of the oestrogen receptor measurement in the adjuvant usage of antioestrogen therapy. The studies are split, with the early studies selecting patients irrespective of ER status while some of the more recent have prejudged the issue, based upon the evidence in advanced breast cancer, and are only selecting ER positive or ER unknown patients as candidates for adjuvant endocrine therapy.

Only two group of workers are publishing their early experiences at this time, and neither study has advanced sufficiently to produce evidence of effect upon survival. Palshof *et al.* (1980) has suggested that "Nolvadex" therapy has delayed recurrences in both pre-menopausal and most postmenopausal women, irrespective of ER status. This receptor finding is at variance with the data presented by Hubay *et al.* (1980) at the same meeting. They found that patients receiving CMF had a significantly higher relapse rate at 30 months compared to a group receiving CMF and "Nolvadex". The point of difference is that this improvement was only true for the ER positive tumours (38.5 % vs 10 % recurrences) there being no difference in relapse in the group who were ER negative. These two sets of data give some encouragement to those pursuing other "Nolvadex"-containing adjuvant studies. However, it is clear that large numbers of patients must enter these studies to cater for the various sub-groups such as the ER positive and negative tumours. Furthermore, the dangers of early reporting of transient positive findings must also be avoided. It is likely that the utility of this drug as adjuvant therapy will not be completely clear until the end of the 1980s.

E. Other Tumours

Oestrogen binding activity either with or without clinical evidence of hormonal sensitivity, has been demonstrated in a large number of tissues. Amongst the neoplastic tissues which have been analysed for the presence of a cytoplasmic oestrogen binding protein, positive results have been reported from tumours of the prostate (Wagner, 1975), endometrium (Martin *et al.*, 1979), ovary (Holt *et al.*, 1979), kidney (Concolino *et al.*, 1978), melanoma (Fisher *et al.*, 1976) and the gastrointestinal tract (Alford *et al.*, 1979). Receptor protein has also been found in the rat pancreas (Molteni *et al.*, 1978). The relevance of these findings has not been fully evaluated in any of these tumours and there are no data at all relating to ovarian or pancreatic tumours being treated clinically with "Nolvadex". Some early clinical data in other tumours have now been presented and are discussed in this section.

1. Prostatic Carcinoma

With the exception of breast cancer, there are more data on the effects of "Nolvadex" in prostatic cancer than any other tumour. Nevertheless, data are extremely sparse. There is no published work with "Nolvadex" in prostate tumour models. Previously published work from our laboratories has shown that, at high doses, tamoxifen reduced the weight of accessory sex organs in male rats at doses of 2 mg/kg/day or above, when given orally for 28 days. The effect is more marked upon the seminal vesicle than the ventral prostate (Furr *et al.*, 1979). At 20 mg/kg/day, there was a reduction of testis weight. When this is coupled with a total lack of androgenicity or antiandrogenicity in the rat, this effect may be due to antioestrogenicity or, more likely, to partial oestrogen activity of the compound at this dosage in this species. Furr *et al.* (1979) also commented that tamoxifen has a low affinity for the androgen receptor from the rat prostate *in vitro*.

The rationale for the use of an antioestrogen in prostatic carcinoma has been built up from circumstantial evidence. Both oestrogen and androgen receptors are said to be present in the tumour (Wagner, 1975). The incidence of prostatic hyperplasia and carcinoma increases with ageing as does the oestrogen/testosterone ratio. Oestrogens in pharmacological dosages are effective in this disease. Their effect may be due to a simple suppression of testicular androgen production but there is some evidence, from low dose stilboestrol studies, that the tumour suppression may occur in the presence of testicular androgen secretion. If the effect of stilboestrol is directly upon the tumour cell via the ER, then this is exactly the same situation as in breast cancer, where the antioestrogen is effective but lacks the cardiovascular complications of an oestrogen.

Early studies of "Nolvadex" were performed under strictly controlled conditions on small numbers of patients, as there was the possibility that the effects seen in young males (Comhaire, 1976), with a rise in circulating oestradiol and testosterone secondary to the blockade of hypothalamic feedback mechanisms, would cause a tumour flare as is seen with androgen therapy. The unpublished pilot studies of Robinson and Denis revealed no evidence of this potential problem in a small number of patients with stage III and IV disease. Follow-up studies by Glick *et al.* (1979) and Morgan *et al* (1978) have been published in abstract form. In heavily pretreated males, they reported response rates of 5/22 (23 %) and 4/21 (19 %) respectively. Glick *et al.* found that only two of the five patients showed objective evidence of response, and each investigator reported some subjective decreases in bone pain. Two further case reports exist (Tisman *et al.*, 1976; Osama El-Arini, 1979).

Unpublished observations from three British urological clinics have been made available to us. In small studies (less than 10 cases per centre) increases in bone pain and acid phosphatase soon after the introduction of "Nolvadex" have been seen in patients who were thought to have testicular endocrine function. Studies are in progress to attempt to correlate the endocrine situation to the pain increase. If there is testosterone stimulation, it is possible that further studies of "Nolvadex" in prostatic cancer will have to be limited to orchidectomized males or to patients who receive concomitant anti-androgen therapy.

2. *Endometrial Carcinoma*

Although the rationale for the use of an antioestrogen is probably clearest in the therapy of cancer of the body of the uterus, little clinical work has been undertaken. One of the major stumbling blocks has been the absence of the centralization of therapy for the women with this disease, and the good prognosis for a stage I or II tumour treated by local therapy. Bonte (1979) has shown responses in a small number of women and, more recently, Swenerton *et al.* (1979) has confirmed these findings. The recent findings by Robel *et al.* (1978) of "Nolvadex"-induced induction of progesterone receptor in the endometrium have stimulated further preclinical and clinical interest in this area and a number of prospective studies are in progress.

3. *Other Tumours*

There have been encouraging reports of the effectiveness of endocrine therapy with progestational agents in hypernephroma and an initial report, with responses to "Nolvadex" in 2/3 patients with osseous metastases, was published by Guiliani *et al.* (1978). However, the results of 3 large studies by Mulder and Alexieva-Figuish (1979), Glick *et al.* (1979) and Al-Sarraf (1979) have suggested that there is little or no utility of "Nolvadex" in this disease area.

Macbeth *et al.* (1979) have been unable to demonstrate specific ER binding in 6 cases of malignant melanoma and did not demonstrate any efficacy of "Nolvadex" therapy in these patients. There has been a recent report from Nesbit *et al.* (1979), who have seen objective tumour regressions in 4/26 (21 %) patients treated. Three of the responses were in women (out of 5 women treated) and these responses lasted for more than one year. This study is in accord with anecdotal reports of response to "Nolvadex" therapy from other centres, but is clearly at variance with the Scottish and other, unpublished, impressions.

There are no data from Phase I or II work in ovarian tumours, although a small number of studies have been initiated. Macbeth has been unable to demonstrate any effect of this antioestrogen upon a number of gastrointestinal tumours. There was no evidence of an antitumour effect when "Nolvadex" was given to patients with oat cell carcinoma of the bronchus, although a small number of patients with associated ectopic hormone related gynaecomastia have had a remission of their signs and symptoms (Jefferys, 1979; Fairlamb and Boesen, 1977).

IV. CONCLUSIONS

"Nolvadex" is one of the few novel therapies which have been successfully introduced into cancer therapy in the 1970s. Its presence has added to the therapeutic armamentarium of the clinician in the field of oncology. It has also been shown to be useful in clinical problems unrelated to cancer, such as female infertility. The versatility of this agent has been enhanced by its relative lack of harmful side-effects, which is a facet of a drug which is more and more welcome, in the face of the toxicological problems encountered with the cytotoxic chemotherapeutic agents. The beauty of an antioestrogen is its specificity for the target cell. This is also its limitation, as the number of tumour cells which are truly hormone-dependent is small.

In breast cancer, a clear picture is emerging of the place and time for "Nolvadex" therapy in the course of the disease. In other tumour areas, the fundamental question, "Does this drug have any useful clinical effects?", remains unanswered. The clinic is the arena in which the biochemical and biological questions and theories that are posed by this drug in the laboratory must be solved. The mechanism of action of tamoxifen is by no means clear, although a number of pointers are present. The clinical evidence is much less precise that the laboratory measurements suggest it should be. If new data accrue in the 1980s as rapidly and excitingly as in the past decade, we will have moved a considerable distance towards understanding breast cancer and this must lead to more rational and effective therapies such as "Nolvadex".

REFERENCES

Alford, T. C., Do, H. M., Geelhoed, G. W., Tsangaris, N. T., and Lippman, M. E. (1979). *Cancer* **43**, 980–984.

Al-Sarraf, M. (1979). *ASCO Abstracts* **20**, C–360.

Arnold, D. J., Markham, M. J., and Hacker, S. (1979). *J. Amer. Med. Assoc.* **241**, 2506.

Bartsch, G., and Scheiber, K. (1979). Proceedings of a Symposium "Antihormones, Current Knowledge and Prospective Clinical Relevance in Urology". Innsbruck, December 1979.

Bishop, H. M., Nicholson, R., Blamey, R. W., and Eston, C. W. (1979). *Proc. British Assoc. of Surgical Oncology,* Abstr. 41.

Bonadonna, G., Brusamolina, E., Valagussa, P., Ross, A., Brugnatelli, L., Brambilla, C., De Lena, M., Tancini, G., Bajetta, E., Masumeci, R., and Veronesi, U. (1976). *New Engl. J. Med.* **294**, 405–410.

Bonte, J. (1979). *Reviews on Endocrine-Related Cancer* **3**, 11–17.

Bosch Jose, F. X., Alonso Munoz, M. C., Ojeda Gonzalez, B., and Viladiu Quemada, P. (1977). *Oncologia* **80**, 111–113.

Boynes, A. R., and Groom, G. V., (1972). *In* Proceedings of a Workshop "ICI 46,474 — Work in Progress", pp. 35–41. ICI Ltd., Pharmaceuticals Division, Macclesfield, U.K.

Cavalli, F., Alberto, P., Jungi, F., and Mantz, G. (1978). *Medical Oncology* **5**, Abstr. 17.

Cheix, F., Pemmatau, E., Clavel, M., Mayer, M., and Saez, S. (1978). *Nouvelle Press Med.* **7**, 3633–3635.

Cocconi, F., De Lisi, V., Boni, C., Amadari, D., Poletti, T., and Bertusi, M. (1979). *ASCO Abstracts* **20**, C–45.

Cole, M. P. (1977). *In* "Proceeding of First Tenovus Symposium" (A. P. M. Forrest and P. B. Kinkle, eds), pp. 146–156. E. and S. Livingstone Ltd., London.

Cole, M. P., Jones, C. T. A., and Todd, I. D. H. (1971). *Brit. J. Cancer.* **25**, 270–275.

Comhaire, F. (1976). *Int. J. Fertil.* **21**, 232–238.

Concolino, G., Marocchi, A., Conti, C., Tenaglia, R., Di Silverio, F., and Bracci, U. (1978). *Cancer Res.* **38**, 4340–4344.

El-Sheikha, Z., Klopper, A., and Beck, J. S. (1972). *Clin. Endocr.* **1**, 275–282.

Fairlamb, D., and Boesen, E. (1977). *Postgrad. Med. J.* **53**, 269–271.

Fisher, B., Carbone, P., Economou, S. G., Frelick, R., Glass, A., Lerner, H., Redmond, C., Zelen, M., Band, P., Katrych, D. L., Wolmark, N., and Fisher, E. R. (1975). *New Engl. J. Med.* **292**, 177–122.

Fisher, R. I., Neifeld, J. P., and Lippman, M. E. (1976). *Lancet* **2**, 337–339.

Furr, B. J. A., Patterson, J. S., Richardson, D. N., Slater, S. R., and Wakeling, A. E. (1979). *In* "Pharmacological and Biochemical Properties of Drug Substances" (M. E. Goldberg, ed.), Vol. II, pp. 355–399. American Pharmacological Association, Washington.

Glick, J. H., Creech, R. H., Holroyde, C., Karpf, M., Torri, S., and Varano, M. (1978). *ASCO Abstracts* **19**, C–191.

Glick, J. H., Wein, A., Negendank, W., Harris, D., Brodovsky, H., Padavic, K., and Torris, S. (1979). *ASCO Abstracts* **20**, C–81.

Glick, J. H., Creech, R. H., Torri, S., Holroyde, C., Brodovsky, H., Catalano, R. B., and Varano, M. (1980). *Cancer* **45**, 735–741.

Guiliani, J., Pescatore, D., Gilbert, C., and Martorana, G. (1978). *Eur. J. Urol.* **4**, 342–347.

Harper, M. J. K., and Walpole, A. L. (1967). *J. Reprod. Fert.* **13**, 101–119.

Henningsen, B., and Amberber, H. (1977). *Deut. Med. Wochenschr.* **102**, 713–716.

Heuson, J. C. (1976). *Cancer Treat. Rep.* **60**, 1463–1466.

Holleb, A. I., Freeman, H. P., and Farrow, J. H. (1968). *N. Y. State J. Med.* **68**, 544–553.

Holt, J. A., Caputa, T. A., Kelly, K. M., Greenwald, P., and Chorost, S. (1979). *Obstet. Gynecol.* **53**, 50–58.

Hubay, C. A., Pearson, O. H., Marshall, J. S., Rhodes, R. S., Debanne, S. M., Mansour, E. G., Hermann, R. E., Jones, J. C., Flynn, W. J., Eckert, C., and McGuire, W. L. (1980). *In* "Breast Cancer: Experimental and Clinical Aspects" (H. T. Mouridsen and T. Palshof, eds), pp. 189–195. Pergamon Press, Oxford.

Jefferys, D. B. (1979). *Brit. Med. J.* **1**, 1119.

Jordan, V. C. (1978). *Reviews on Endocrine-Related Cancer* October Suppl., pp. 49–53.

Kaiser-Kupfer, M. I., and Lippman, M. E. (1978). *Cancer Treat. Rep.* **62**, 315–320.

Klopper, A., and Hall, M. (1971). *Brit. Med. J.* **1**, 152–154.

Legha, S. S., and Carter, S. K. (1976). *Cancer Treat. Reviews* **3**, 205–216.

Lunan, C. B., and Klopper, A. (1975). *Clin. Endocr.* **4**, 551–572.

Macbeth, F. R., Calman, K. C., Laing, L., and Leake, R. E. (1979). *Brit. J. Cancer* **40**, 314.

Manni, A. and Pearson, O. H. (1979). *Cancer Treat. Rep.* **63**, 1219.

Martin, P. M., Rooland, P. H., Gammerre, M., Sermont, H., and Toga, M. (1979). *Int. J. Cancer* **23**, 321–329.

Masson, G. M., and Klopper, A. (1972). *In* Proceedings of a Workshop "ICI 46,474 — Work in Progress", pp. 27–34. ICI Ltd., Pharmaceuticals Division, Macclesfield, U. K.

Meakin, J. W., Allt. W. E. C., Beale, F. A., Brown, T. C., Bush, R. S., Clark, R. M., Fitzpatrick, P. J., Hawkins, N. B., Jenkin, R. D. T., Pringle, J. F., Reid, J. G., Rider, W. D., Hayward, J. L., and Bulbrook, R. D. (1979). *Can. Med. Assoc. J.* **120**, 1221–1229.

Molteni, A., Rao, M. S., Reddy, M. K., and Fors, E. M. (1978). *Fedn. Proc.* **37**, 387.

Morgan, L. R., Schein, P. S., Wooley, P. V., Hoth, D., MacDonald, J., Lippman, M., Posey, L. E., and Beazley, R. W. (1976). *Cancer Treat. Rep.* **60**, 1437–1443.

Morgan, L. R., Posey, L. E., and Lanasa, J. (1978). *Proc. 12th Int. Congr. Cancer,* Buenos Aires, **3**, 111.

Mouridsen, H., Palshof, T., Patterson, J., and Battersby, L. (1978). *Cancer Treat. Reviews* **4**, 131–141.

Mouridsen, H., Ellemann, K., Mattsson, W., Palshof, T., Daehnfeldt, J. L., and Rose, C. (1979). *Cancer Treat. Rep.* **63**, 171–175.

Mouridsen, H. T., Palshof, T., Engelman, E., and Sylvester, R. (1980). *In* "Breast Cancer: Experimental and Clinical Aspects" (H. T. Mouridsen and T. Palshof, eds), pp. 119–123. Pergamon Press, Oxford.

Mulder, J. H., and Alexieva-Figusch, I. (1979). *Cancer Treat. Rep.* **63**, 1222.

Nesbit, R. A., Woods, R. L., Tattersall, M. H. N. Fox, R. M., Forbes, J. F., MacKay, I. E., and Goodyear, M. (1979). *New Engl. J. Med.* **301**, 1241–1242.

Osama El-Arini, M. (1979). *Lancet* **2**, 588.

Palshof, T., Mouridsen, H. T., and Daehnfeldt, J. L. (1980). *In* "Breast Cancer: Experimental and Clinical Aspects" (H. T. Mouridsen and T. Palshof, eds), pp. 183–187. Pergamon Press, Oxford.

Patterson, J. S., Furr, B. J. A., and Battersby, L. A. (1978). *Ann. Int. Med.* **89**, 1013.

Patterson, J. S., Battersby, L. A., and Bach, B. K. (1980). *Cancer Treat. Rep.* **64**, 801–804.

Pritchard, K. I., Thomson, D. B., Meakin, J. W., Myers, R. E., Sutherland, D. J. A., and Mobbs, B. G. (1979). *ASCO Abstracts* **20**, C–60.

Ribeiro, G. G. (1977). *Brit. J. Surg.* **64**, 381–383.

Ricciardi, I., and Ianniruberto, A. (1979). *Obstet. Gynaecol.* **54**, 80–84.

Robel, P., Levy, C., Wolff, J. P., Nicolas, J. C., and Baulieu, E. E. (1978). *C. R. Acad. Sci.* **287**, 1353–1356.

Rose, D. P., and Davis, T. E. (1977). *Lancet* **1**, 1174–1176.

Sakai, F., Cheix, F., Clavel, M., Colan, J., Mayer, M., Pommatau, E., and Saez, S. (1978). *J. Endocr.* **76**, 219–226.

Settatree, R. S., Butt, W. R., London, D. R., Holme, G. M., and Morrison, J. M. (1978). *Proc. 12th Int. Congr. Cancer,* Buenos Aires **3**, 79.

Sherman, B. M., Chapler, F. K., Crickard, K., and Wycoff, D. (1979). *J. Clin. Invest.* **64**, 398–404.
Skipper, H. E., Schabel, F. M., and Wilcox, W. S. (1965). *Cancer Chemotherapy Rep.* **45**, 5–7.
Spaeren, U., Olsnes, S., Brernhor, I., Efskind, J., and Pihl, A. (1973). *Eur. J. Cancer* **9**, 353–357.
Spooner, D., and Evans, B. D. (1979). *Lancet* **2**, 413–414.
Stewart, H. J. (1979). *Reviews on Endocrine-Related Cancer,* October Suppl., pp. 51–55.
Swenerton, K. D., Shaw, D., White, G. W., and Boyes, D. A. (1979). *New Engl. J. Med.* **301**, 105.
Tisman, G., Kellon, D. B., Wu, S., and Safine, G. E. (1976). *Clin. Res.* **24**, 381A.
Tormey, D. C., Simon, R. M., Lippman, M. E., Bull, J. M., and Myers, C. E. (1976). *Cancer Treat. Rep.* **60**, 1451–1459.
Tormey, D. C., Falkson, J., Falkson, G., and Davis, T. E. (1978). *AACR Abstracts* **19**, 34 Abstr. 134.
Treeves, N. (1959). *Cancer* **12**, 820–832.
Veldhuis, J. D. (1978). *Ann. Int. Med.* **88**, 574–575.
Villalon, A. H., Tattersall, M. H. N., Fox, R. M., and Woods, R. L. (1979). *Brit. Med. J.* **2**, 1329–1330.
Wagner, R. K. (1975). *Acta Endocr. Suppl.* **193**, 52.
Ward, H. W. C. (1973). *Brit. Med. J.* **1**, 13–14.
Ward, H. W. C. (1976). *In* Proceedings of a Symposium on "Hormonal Control of Breast Cancer", pp. 53–58. ICI Ltd., Pharmaceuticals Division, Macclesfield, U.K.
Ward, H. W. C. (1977). *Clinical Oncology* **3**, 91–95.
Westerberg, H., Nordenskjöld, B., De Schryver, A., and Notter, G. (1976). *Acta Radiol. Ther. Phys. Biol.* **15**, 513–518.
Westerberg, H. (1980).*Cancer Treat. Rep.* **64**, 117–121.
Willis, K. J., London, D. R., Bevis, M. A., Butt, W. R., Lynch, S. S., and Holder, G. (1977). *J. Endocr.* **73**, 171–178.

27

Modes of Action of Antioestrogens *in Vivo* and *in Vitro*: Summary and Future Prospects

R. L. SUTHERLAND AND V. CRAIG JORDAN

I. INTRODUCTION

In this volume an attempt has been made to collate and summarize data relating to the present level of understanding of the mechanisms by which the synthetic non-steroidal antioestrogens antagonize the effects of oestrogens. Naturally, it has been impossible to summarize the entire world literature relating to this group of compounds; therefore, as the editors and many of the authors are primarily interested in antioestrogens as antineoplastic agents, the book has been largely devoted to this area. In addition, several chapters contain data on the molecular pharmacology and molecular mechanisms of action of these drugs, an understanding of which is imperative if the molecular basis of their antitumour activity is to be fully understood.

NON-STEROIDAL ANTIOESTROGENS
ISBN 0 12 677880 9

In a work of this type, which includes contributions from a large number of leading researchers in the field, there must inevitably be some repetition and gaps in the presentation of data. Although we feel that this has been minimal in the present case, it seems appropriate to briefly summarize what has been presented in the foregoing chapters and make some recommendations on what we, the editors, see as priorities for future research.

Two important points need to be stressed from the outset. Firstly, because of the large species differences in the biological properties of different synthetic non-steroidal antioestrogens it is not possible to have a single simple definition of an antioestrogen, nor is it likely that there is a single fundamental molecular mechanism by which they mediate their antagonism of oestrogenic action. Secondly, it is important to realize that hundreds of compounds in this series have been synthesized although only two, clomiphene and tamoxifen, are currently widely used in the clinic. Naturally, the data presented in this book refer only to those few compounds which drug companies have made available to research workers but, as was pointed out by Emmens in Chapter 2, these may not necessarily be the most active nor the best tools for investigative purposes.

II. METABOLISM AND PHARMACOKINETICS

With the exception of the recent studies with tamoxifen (Chapter 4) and trioxifene (Nelson *et al.*, 1979) in man there is virtually no data on the pharmacokinetics of non-steroidal antioestrogens. Preliminary studies (Chapters 4, 7, 11) indicate that tamoxifen and CI 628 have very slow plasma clearance rates compared with oestradiol, and this undoubtedly enhances their competitive efficiency at the target tissue level. The recent development of sensitive techniques for measuring the extracellular fluid and tissue concentrations of these drugs and the recent synthesis of a high affinity, tritiated ligand ([^{3}H]monohydroxytamoxifen) will hopefully yield much needed data on differential tissue uptake, retention and clearance of at least some of these compounds.

The recent interest in antioestrogen metabolism by a number of research groups has already yielded valuable data (Chapters 4, 6, 7). Studies with at least three compounds, tamoxifen, CI 628 and U 23,469, have indicated that it is the polar metabolites and not the parent compounds that are associated with the nuclear oestrogen receptors following a single injection of the tritiated compound. However, one should be warned against extrapolating this to the clinical situation where tamoxifen is administered chronically and where the polar metabolite, 4-hydroxytamoxifen, represents a minor portion (about 1 %) of the total plasma constituents under steady state conditions. It therefore seems extremely important to know the relative concentrations of metabolites present in the tissues and the relative proportions associated with receptors and other saturable binding sites under conditions of chronic administration, before an assessment of the role of polar metabolites in the mechanisms of action of antioestrogens as antitumour agents can be made. The studies reported in Chapter 3, using analogues of tamoxifen which cannot be metabolized, illustrate that metabolism facilitates but is not essential for antioestrogenic action.

Although it is generally believed that the majority of antioestrogen metabolism takes place in the liver (Chapter 4), Rochefort (Chapter 6) has suggested that peripheral metabolism may also occur in some tissues, e. g. chick oviduct and lamb uterus but not in rat uterus. Differential tissue metabolism may influence the selectivity of these drugs and should be investigated further. Interestingly the much studied human mammary carcinoma cell line, MCF 7, appears not to metabolize tamoxifen (Horwitz *et al.*, 1978) indicating that studies with the other two human plasma metabolites, 4-hydroxytamoxifen and N-desmethyltamoxifen, are essential in this *in vitro* system.

Species differences in the metabolism of tamoxifen have been noted, with 4-hydroxytamoxifen and N-desmethyltamoxifen being the major plasma metabolites in rats and humans, respectively. In view of the species and tissue differences in the response to antioestrogens a detailed study of metabolism in different species and tissues seems warranted.

The recent interesting observation that tamoxifen increases the survival of rats treated with cyclophosphamide (Jordan *et al.*, 1980; Ip *et al.*, 1980) may indicate that tamoxifen influences the metabolism and pharmacokinetics of this and perhaps other cytotoxic drugs. Since tamoxifen is becoming increasingly more popular in combination chemotherapeutic regimens, it would be interesting to study both the effects of cytotoxic drugs on tamoxifen metabolism and the effects of tamoxifen on the metabolism and pharmacokinetics of some cytotoxic drugs.

III. NEW RESEARCH TOOLS

Two recent developments should have enormous implications for future research on the mechanisms of action of oestrogens and antioestrogens.

A new antioestrogen, LY 117018 (Fig. 1), has been shown to be antioestrogenic in ovariectomized mice and have a fraction of the partial uterotrophic activity of tamoxifen or trioxifene in the immature rat (Black and Goode, 1980). Interestingly, the compound is dihydroxylated and has a rigid structure so there is no complication with geometric isomerism (see Chapter 3). If, as might be predicted, LY 117018 has a high affinity for the oestrogen receptor, then in a radiolabelled form it would be very useful for the study of antioestrogenic mechanisms.

In this regard, the synthesis of [^{3}H]monohydroxytamoxifen (Fig. 2) with high specific activity (42 Ci/mmole) has permitted the direct study of antioestrogen binding to receptors and target tissues. [^{3}H]monohydroxytamoxifen binds directly to the 8S oestrogen receptor derived from human breast carcinoma (Jordan *et al.*, 1981) and rat uterus. Using rat uterine oestrogen receptors the dissociation constant (K_d) for [^{3}H]monohydroxytamoxifen at 4°C was 2.8×10^{-11} M compared with 3.2×10^{-11} M for [^{3}H]oestradiol. Preliminary studies *in vivo* have demonstrated that [^{3}H]monohydroxytamoxifen binds specifically to rat uterus and vagina and this binding is inhibited by both oestrogens and antioestrogens. Compared with [^{3}H]oestradiol, [^{3}H]monohydroxytamoxifen is slowly accumulated in the uterus and is retained for longer (Jordan, unpublished observations).

The potential of [^{3}H]monohydroxytamoxifen in elucidating antioestrogenic mechanisms is obvious. Most importantly, the physicochemical properties of the antioestrogen-oestrogen receptor complex can now be studied with confidence due to the markedly decreased rate of dissociation of this ligand from the receptor site.

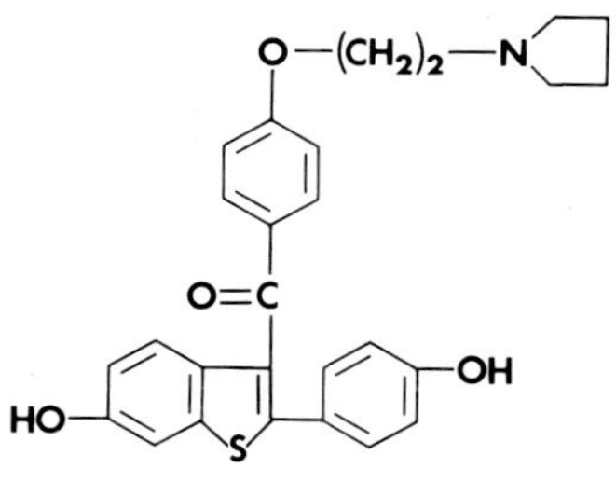

Fig. 1. Structure of the new synthetic antioestrogen LY 117018.

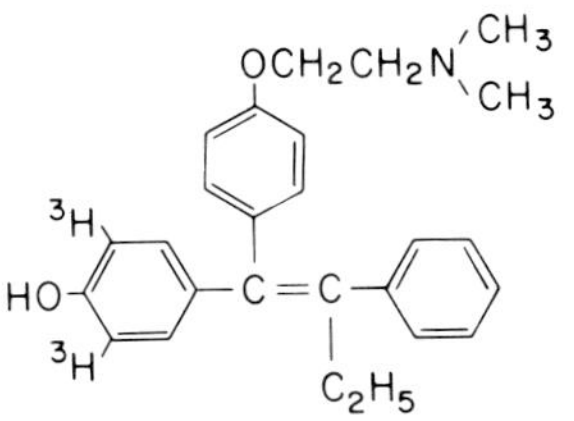

Fig. 2. Structure of tritiated monohydroxytamoxifen showing the positions of the radiolabel.

IV. EXTRACELLULAR AND INTRACELLULAR BINDING

Unlike the situation found with many steroid hormones, high affinity, saturable plasma binding sites have not been reported for the non-steroidal antioestrogens. However, some plasma proteins bind tamoxifen extremely tightly but in a non-saturable manner so that less than 1% of tamoxifen is in free solution at plasma concentrations of 5% (v/v) or greater (Sutherland, unpublished observations). This plasma binding will clearly have profound effects on the plasma concentration and clearance of the drug, and thus a more detailed study of the binding of antioestrogens to proteins in extracellular fluid seems necessary even if such binding is non-specific. Similarly the binding of antioestrogens to foetal calf serum poses problems in interpreting results from tissue culture experiments *in vitro* and extrapolating them to the *in vivo* situation. In future it seems imperative that documentation of the binding to foetal calf serum accompany information on the dose-dependence of antioestrogen effects in tissue culture systems, especially when different foetal calf serum concentrations are being used.

Antioestrogens may also influence the overall endocrine environment by influencing the plasma binding of some steroid hormones. Tamoxifen has been reported to increase the concentration of plasma corticosteroid binding globulin and sex hormone binding globulin (Sakai *et al.*, 1978) and to displace androgens from their binding sites on sex hormone binding globulin (Habib *et al.*, 1979). Clearly, changes in the concentration of specific plasma binding proteins for steroids should be taken into account when attempting to evaluate antioestrogen induced changes in plasma steroid hormone levels.

There is now considerable evidence to suggest that the synthetic non-steroidal antioestrogens mediate much of their antagonistic activity through the specific oestrogen receptor molecules of oestrogen target tissues. A summary of the intracellular interactions of antioestrogens is presented in Figure 3. Antioestrogens and their metabolites appear to enter cells by free diffusion and are retained in oestrogen target tissue cells due presumably to their binding to oestrogen receptors and perhaps the specific antioestrogen binding site (Chapter 19). Interactions with the oestrogen receptor may be weaker, e.g. tamoxifen, or tighter, e.g. monohydroxytamoxifen, than interactions between the receptor and oestradiol itself. The weaker affinity of some ligands, e.g. tamoxifen and CI 628, has been attributed to their faster dissociation rates from the receptor (cf. oestradiol). Studies with the high affinity ligand [^{3}H]monohydroxytamoxifen illustrate that this antioestrogen and oestradiol bind to the same 8S peak on sucrose density gradients (Jordan *et al.*, 1981) and that the antioestrogen-cytoplasmic receptor complex undergoes the same activation phenomenon that has been described for the oestradiol-cytoplasmic receptor complex (Mester *et al.*, 1981). Numerous studies have demonstrated that the antagonist-receptor complex is finally located in the nuclear compartment.

Little is known of the role, if any, of the antioestrogen binding site described in Chapter 19, in mediating the effects of antioestrogens at the target tissue level. The presence of this site in both normal and neoplastic tissues has recently been confirmed (Jordan *et al.*, 1981; Faye *et al.*, 1980). Interestingly, the latter group has presented data which indicate that the concentration of the site may be under hormonal control, an observation in agreement with our own results (Sutherland, unpublished observations). Full investigation of this site from both a physicochemical and functional point of view is keenly awaited.

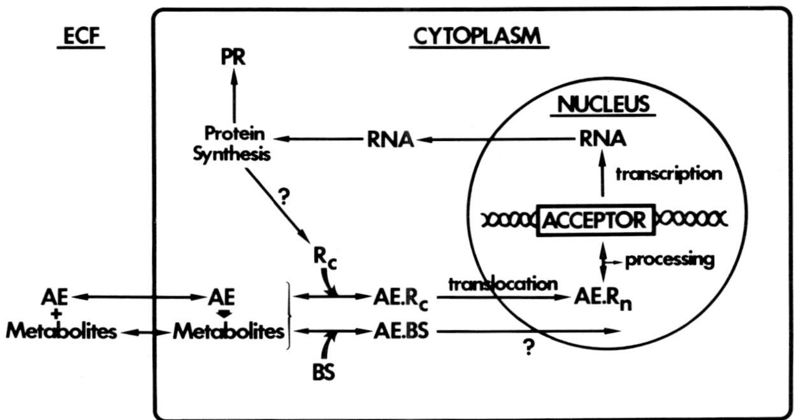

Fig. 3. A model of antioestrogenic action at the target tissue level. Antioestrogens (AE) and their metabolites appear to enter cells by free diffusion and are retained in oestrogen target tissues by forming complexes with the cytoplasmic oestrogen receptor (R_c) or the antioestrogen binding site (BS). The fate of the antioestrogen following interaction with the cytoplasmic antioestrogen binding site is unknown. The antioestrogen-cytoplasmic oestrogen receptor complex (AE.R_c) is translocated to the nucleus to form a nuclear receptor complex (AE.R_n) which interacts with binding sites on chromatin (Acceptor). These chromatin binding sites may or may not be the same as those for oestrogen-nuclear receptor complexes. The subsequent fate of the nuclear oestrogen receptors is unknown but with tamoxifen nuclear "processing" of these receptors occurs.

In some mammalian systems, e.g. rat uterus and MCF 7 cells, the interaction of the antioestrogen-nuclear oestrogen receptor complex with chromatin is associated with increased activity of RNA polymerases, increased RNA synthesis and increased protein synthesis, including the synthesis of the progesterone receptor (PR). These events are qualitatively similar but quantitatively different from those induced by oestrogens. In avian systems no events distal to to the interaction of antioestrogen-receptor complexes with chromatin have been documented.

The effect of antioestrogens on the concentration and subcellular distribution of oestrogen receptors has been investigated in detail in rat uterus, chick oviduct and human mammary carcinoma cells (Chapters 3, 6, 7, 11, 12, 20), but unfortunately the species differences in the biological properties of these compounds have not allowed the development of a unified theory on the role of receptor changes in the mechanisms of oestrogen antagonism. Data with low doses of antagonist in rats (Gardner *et al.*, 1978) and observations in chick oviduct (Sutherland *et al.*, 1977) have shed serious doubt on the previously popular theory that inhibition of cytoplasmic oestrogen receptor synthesis is the primary event in oestrogen antagonism by non-steroidal antioestrogens (Clark *et al.*, 1974). It now seems probable that some impairment of the antioestrogen-nuclear oestrogen receptor complex, either in its interaction with "acceptor sites" on chromatin or in its nuclear "processing", is responsible for the antagonist properties of these molecules. A much greater understanding of these processes is required, and initial progress in this area has been reported in Chapters 14, 15, 20. A detailed study of the interactions between antioestrogen-oestrogen receptor complexes with DNA and synthetic polynucleotides may be a useful approach in view of the interesting data obtained by Dickerman and his colleagues with oestradiol (Thanki *et al.*, 1978). As far as *in vivo* systems are concerned, the avian systems, i.e. chick oviduct (Chapters 11, 12, 15) and chick liver (Chapter 13), appear to be the most attractive from a mechanistic point of view since a great deal is known of the molecular biology of oestrogen action in these systems and because the non-steroidal antioestrogens are pure antagonists.

V. MODELS FOR STUDYING ANTITUMOUR ACTIVITY *IN VIVO*

Study of the mechanisms of action of antioestrogens as antitumour agents has centred mainly on carcinogen-induced animal models. Much effort has gone into studying hormone receptor systems in the dimethylbenzanthracene (DMBA)-induced rat mammary carcinoma model but, as discussed in Chapter 16, these effects may be of secondary importance since tumour growth is dependent upon prolactin. Antioestrogens produce many direct effects on the tumours and on the endocrine system (Fig. 4) which may all contribute to tumour regression. For this reason, the DMBA-induced rat mammary tumour model is perhaps limited in its usefulness for the study of control mechanisms involved in the growth of human tumours and also suffers from the fact that unlike the human disease it does not metastasize.

The report that rat mammary tumours induced by N nitrosomethyl urea (NMU) readily metastasize (Gullino *et al.*, 1975) stimulated interest in this new laboratory model. However, a recent report (Rose *et al.*, 1980) has not confirmed the original observations. NMU-induced tumours are hormone dependent, but the degree of hormone dependence appears to be related to the schedule of carcinogen administration (Rose *et al.*, 1980). The tumours contain oestrogen, progesterone and prolactin receptors and tumour regression occurs in response to ovariectomy or tamoxifen treatment. However, like the DMBA-induced tumour, the predictive value of hormone receptor analysis in NMU-induced tumours in determining their response to subsequent endocrine therapy appears to be tenuous (Ruzicka *et al.*, 1980). Clearly the basic hormone dependence of NMU-induced tumours has to be adequately described before this system can be used with confidence to study antitumour activity at the tissue level. In this way, over-extrapolation of results to the treatment of human breast cancer can be avoided.

An advantage of a transplantable tumour like the LMC_1 rat mammary carcinoma is that it metastasizes (Dixon and Speakman, 1979), however tumour refractoriness to ovariectomy and tamoxifen therapy (Jordan *et al.*, 1979) restrict its usefulness as a model for antioestrogen research. In contrast, the ovarian independent transplantable R3230AC tumour is responsive to antioestrogen therapy (Chapter 18). Should the effects of antioestrogens be found to be the result of a direct insult in the tumour then this model deserves further investigation.

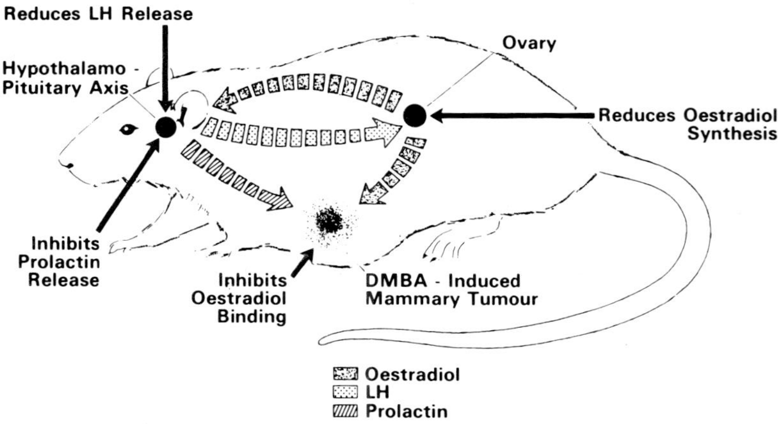

Fig. 4. A summary of the endocrine effects of tamoxifen in the rat.

Recently antioestrogens have been found to be active in controlling the growth of transplantable, hormone-dependent DMBA-induced mammary tumours (Barai *et al.*, 1980) and androgen-dependent R3327 rat prostatic tumours (Ip *et al.*, 1980). Although direct effects of antioestrogens on the oestrogen receptor system can be demonstrated, the indirect effects of reducing circulating prolactin (Jordan *et al.*, 1980) and testosterone (Ip *et al.*, 1980) respectively, are probably the reasons for a reduced rate of tumour growth.

A tumour model system that is directly dependent upon oestrogen is necessary for studying the antitumour effects of antioestrogens *in vivo*. For this reason tumours of the endometrium may, in the future, be studied in more detail. A DMBA-induced rat uterine model has been described *in vivo* (Taki and Iijima, 1963; Sekiya *et al.*, 1972, 1979). The tumour cells respond to progesterone *in vitro* and a combination of antioestrogen and progesterone is synergistic in inhibiting growth (Sekiya and Takamizawa, 1976). This observation is probably related to the ability of antioestrogens to stimulate progesterone receptor synthesis which in turn may sensitize the tissue to progestagens. These data have clear therapeutic implications and warrant further study.

Although encouraging, work on carcinogen-induced endometrial tumours has been slow, principally because there is a long induction period before the appearance of tumours. Another approach which induces endometrial tumours in hamsters by high dose diethylstilboestrol administration (Chapter 10) may not only provide valuable information about hormonal transformation of normal to neoplastic tissue but may also provide a useful model to study the direct control of cell proliferation by antioestrogens *in vivo*.

A number of mouse mammary tumours containing steroid hormone receptor proteins have been described (Sluyser, 1979), but there is little data on the effect of antioestrogens on these tumours. The conventional non-steroidal antioestrogens are predominantly oestrogenic in mice, and thus any antitumour effects may be related to the effects of high dose oestrogen therapy rather than to the direct inhibition of oestrogenic action. This should be further investigated and the new antioestrogen LY 117018, with its much lower intrinsic oestrogenic activity, may be a useful tool for this purpose.

The recent reports of the successful growth of human breast carcinoma biopsies (Giovanella, *et al.*, 1978; Rae-Venter and Reid, 1980) and a number of human breast cancer cell lines in nude mice (Engel and Young, 1978; Ozzello and Sordat, 1980) introduce a potentially useful model system for studying the effects of antioestrogens on human breast cancer cells in an *in vivo* experimental situation. However the oestrogenic effects of antioestrogens in the mouse may be related to some, as yet unknown, peculiarities of metabolism and pharmacokinetics, and these factors should obviously be considered when studying the antitumour activities of these compounds in nude mice. Despite this potential limitation the nude mouse is a model system which needs thorough investigation.

VI. MODELS FOR STUDYING ANTITUMOUR ACTIVITY *IN VITRO*

A recent review of human breast carcinoma cells in continuous culture revealed that in 1978 there were 47 cell lines for which data had been reported and about half of these (22) were shown to be from human, non-HeLa donors and to have epithelial morphology (Engel and Young, 1978). Six lines were shown to be oestrogen receptor positive but only three (MCF 7, ZR 75-1 and ZR 75-27) have been reported to respond to oestrogen with increased macromolecular synthesis and/or cell growth. Only the MCF 7 cell line has been studied in detail in a number of different laboratories. Unfortunately these cells behave differently in different laboratories indicating that different clones of the MCF 7 line probably exist. The lack of a spectrum of oestrogen responsive human breast cancer cell lines has naturally retarded studies on the differential sensitivity of breast cancer cells to antioestrogen treatment. However the recent observation that tamoxifen can inhibit the growth of both oestrogen receptor positive and negative mammary carcinoma cells *in vitro* (Chapter 23) indicates that a study of the differential sensitivity of currently available breast cancer lines to tamoxifen may be fruitful. Similarly, it is important to know whether the cytotoxic phenomenon described in Chapter 23 is confined to human mammary carcinoma cells or is a general nonspecific *in vitro* cytotoxicity.

Despite the relatively wide range of non-steroidal antioestrogens now available there is no data on the differential sensitivity of breast cancer cells to structurally different antioestrogens. Not only may this yield valuable information on structure-function relationships with respect to antitumour activity but studies with metabolites, e.g. 4-hydroxytamoxifen and N-desmethyltamoxifen, may reveal the relative importance of the parent drug and its metabolites in mediating antitumour effects at the target tissue level.

To date, studies on the effects of antioestrogens *in vitro* have been confined to the use of relatively simple cell biology techniques, e.g. changes in cell numbers and rates of incorporation of labelled precursors into protein, RNA and DNA (Chapters 23, 24). The recent application of flow cytometry to studies on the antitumour effects of tamoxifen (Chapter 23) illustrate the potential of this technique in shedding light on the action of antioestrogens. Such a tool should facilitate the elucidation of cell cycle effects in this group of drugs. Many of the questions relating to cell cycle effects are best answered with the use of synchronized cells, but it has been our experience that this is not easily achieved with many human breast cancer cell lines, especially MCF 7 (Sutherland, unpublished observations). Perhaps more detailed studies of the general biology and growth kinetics of breast cancer cells in culture would facilitate the design of better experiments involving antioestrogens.

Experiments which only record the nett changes in cell number following antioestrogen treatment may mask more subtle effects of the drug. For example, a sublethal effect of the drug may allow the cells to survive for an appreciable period but inhibit their ability to divide. Such effects are best tested in clonogenic assays, but there is no published data on the effects of antioestrogens on the clonogenic survival of cultured human breast cancer cells. A number of these human cell lines are known to clone *in vitro* (Engel and Young, 1978) but in general the cloning efficiency is not high. For this reason mouse mammary carcinoma cells, which exhibit high cloning efficiencies, may be more useful, but again work is limited by the number of suitable cell lines currently available.

Clearly work *in vitro*, on the antitumour activity of antioestrogens in mammary carcinoma cells, is severely hampered by the lack of suitable numbers of cell lines that respond to oestrogen with increased rates, and to antioestrogen with decreased rates, of cell proliferation. Other oestrogen receptor positive and oestrogen responsive cell lines derived from rat (Sekiya and Takamizawa, 1976) and human (Ishiwata *et al.*, 1977) endometrial carcinoma have been described, but little data on the effects of antioestrogens is available. Obviously this is a model system which needs more detailed study in the future.

VII. TREATMENT OF HUMAN TUMOURS

The successful introduction of antioestrogens for the treatment of breast cancer has provided us with new therapies with which to observe the biology of the disease. Although there is a wealth of information to indicate that tamoxifen exerts its antitumour effects via the oestrogen receptor, this should not prevent the study of other potential mechanisms. Tamoxifen is primarily used in the postmenopausal patient, but recent results demonstrate efficacy in the premenopausal patient (Chapter 26). With these trials has come information, often conflicting, about the many effects of tamoxifen upon the human endocrine system. These data are summarized in Figure 5. Clearly, some of these associated hormonal effects may modify tamoxifen action at the tumour level.

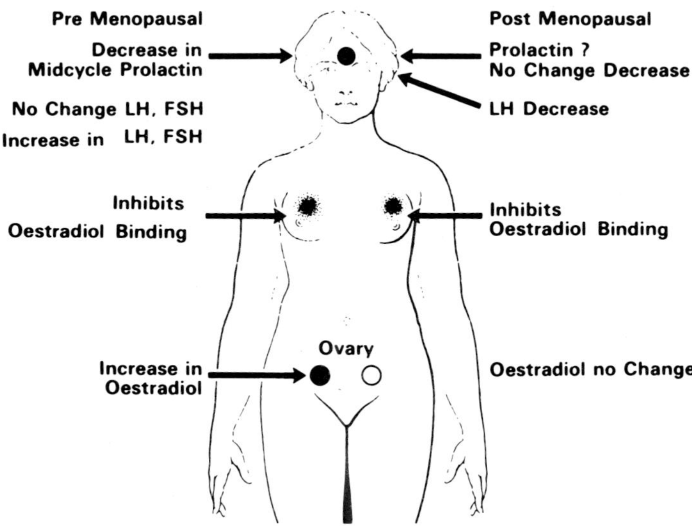

Fig. 5. A summary of the effects of tamoxifen on the endocrine status of premenopausal and postmenopausal women.

In a recent report (Thompson *et al.*, 1980), the response to tamoxifen in premenopausal patients was highly predictive of subsequent response to ovarian ablation. Furthermore the authors claimed that in their group of patients the response to tamoxifen was more strongly predictive than the oestrogen and progesterone receptor status. Of interest was the observation that patients who initially responded to tamoxifen and then failed generally responded to subsequent ovariectomy. It is possible that, in this situation, tamoxifen has increased ovarian oestrogen secretion (Chapter 25) which in turn competitively reverses the action of tamoxifen in the tumour. These observations would have important implications in the future strategy of breast cancer therapy and require confirmation.

Another finding of interest is the success of a second hormone therapy after tamoxifen failure in the postmenopausal patient. A combination of tamoxifen and halotestin (Tormey *et al.*, 1976) or halotestin after tamoxifen (Chapter 25) is more effective than tamoxifen alone. This probably indicates that polyhormonal therapy is not mediated through a single mechanism, i.e. the oestrogen receptor.

The development of antioestrogens with other antihormonal actions may be a useful next step in breast cancer therapy. The new antioestrogen trioxifene inhibits the release of growth hormone in the rat but unfortunately it does not seem to have this action in the human (Chapter 25). Nevertheless, trioxifene is undergoing clinical testing in advanced breast cancer and results should be available in the next few years. The basic biology, pharmacology and antitumour activity of trioxifene have not, as yet, been reported in detail.

The acceptance of low toxicity antioestrogen therapy has come at a time when there is a change in the basic approach to the treatment of breast cancer. Many adjuvant therapy trials, including the Ludwig Breast Cancer Trial, are using a short (1 or 2 year) treatment period with tamoxifen. Preliminary findings have demonstrated that tamoxifen is a useful therapy but recurrence is only controlled as long as treatment is continued. This result may, in principle, reflect the finding that a short treatment period is not as effective as a long treatment period for inhibiting the appearance of carcinogen induced rat mammary tumours (Chapter 16). As a consequence, up to 5 year tamoxifen treatment regimens are being considered as a new approach to adjuvant therapy.

The widespread use of tamoxifen alone or in combination with other chemotherapeutic agents provides a unique opportunity for studying the pharmacokinetics and differential metabolism of these drugs in existing trials. This information coupled with data from laboratory studies of the cell cycle effects of tamoxifen in combination with new and existing chemotherapeutic agents, should be invaluable for planning future clinical trials.

VIII. CONCLUSIONS

The 1970s have witnessed the introduction of a member of an existing series of non-steroidal antioestrogens as an effective non-toxic antitumour agent in the treatment of human breast cancer. In step with the renewed clinical interest in these compounds has come an increased research effort into understanding their mechanisms of action. Although much has been acheived during the past decade a greater effort is required before a full understanding of the mechanisms by which these compounds exert their antioestrogenic effects, and especially their antitumour effects, can be fully understood. With the 1980s should come an increased research effort in this area not only with the existing series of antioestrogens but with new series of compounds having different biological properties, e.g. reduced oestrogenicity, increased anti-oestrogenic activity and perhaps broader antihormonal and/or cytotoxic activity. Hopefully an increased understanding of the molecular mechanisms of action of these compounds will not only lead to their more effective use in the treatment of human disease but will increase our understanding of the central hormonal control mechanisms in reproductive biology and hormone dependent neoplasia.

REFERENCES

Barai, B., Lee, C., and DeWys, W. (1980). *AACR Abstracts* **21**, 1212.

Black, L. J., and Goode, R. L. (1980). *Life Sci.* **26**, 1453–1458.

Clark, J. H., Peck, E. J. Jr, and Anderson, J. N. (1974). *Nature* **251**, 446–448.

Dixon, B., and Speakman, H. (1979). *J. Royal Soc Med.* **72**, 572–577.

Engel, L. W., and Young, N. A. (1978). *Cancer Res.* **38**, 4327–4339.

Faye, J. C., Lasserre, B., and Bayard, F. (1980). *Biochem. Biophys. Res. Commun.* **93**, 1225–1231.

Gardner, R. M., Kirkland, J. L., and Stancel, G. M. (1978). *Endocrinology* **103**, 1583–1589.

Giovanella, B. C., Stehlin, J. S., Williams, L. J., Lee, S. S., and Shephard, R. C. (1978). *Cancer* **42**, 2269–2281.

Guillino, P. M., Pettigrew, H. M., and Grantham, F. H. (1975). *J. Natl Cancer Inst.* **54**, 401–414.

Habib, F. K., Rafati, G., Robinson, M. R. G., and Stitch, S. R. (1979). *J. Endocr.* **83**, 369–378.

Horwitz, K. B., Koseki, Y., and McGuire, W. L. (1978). *Endocrinology* **103**, 1742–1751.

Ip, M. M., Milholland, R. J., and Rosen, F. (1980). *AACR Abstracts* **21**, 60.

Ishiwata, I., Nozawa, S., and Okumura, H. (1977). *Cancer Res.* **37**, 4246–4249.

Jordan, V. C., Dixon, B., Prestwich, G. and Furr, B. J. A. (1979). *Eur. J. Cancer* **15**, 755–762.

Jordan, V. C., Tormey, D. C., Clifton, K., Pandya, K., and Gilchrist, K. (1980a). *AACR Abstracts* **21**, 1275.

Jordan, V. C., Fischer, A. H., and Rose, D. P. (1981). *Eur. J. Cancer* **17**, 121–122.

Mester, J., Sutherland, R. L., Binart, N., Catelli, M. G., Wolfson, A., Seeley, D. H., Yang, C. R., and Baulieu, E. E. (1981). *In* "Hormones and Cell Regulation", Vol. 5 (J. Dumont and J. Nunez, eds.), Elsevier/North Holland, Amsterdam. (In Press).

Nelson, R. L., Dyke, R. W., and Crabtree, R. F. (1979). *AACR Abstracts* **20**, 54.

Ozzello, L., and Sordat, M. (1980). *Eur. J. Cancer* **16**, 553–559.

Rae-Venter, B., and Reid, L. M. (1980). *Cancer Res.* **40**, 95–100.

Rose, D. P., Pruitt, B., Stauber, P., Erturk, E., and Bryan, T. (1980). *Cancer Res.* **40**, 235–239.

Ruzicka, F., Rose, D. P., Pruitt, B., Menting, A., and Fischer, A. H. (1980). *AACR Abstracts* **21**, 152.

Saki, F., Cheix, F., Clavel, M., Colan, J., Mayer, M., Pommatou, E., and Saez, S. (1978). *J. Endocr.* **76**, 219–226.

Sekiya, S., and Takamizawa, H. (1976). *Br. J. Obstet. Gynaecol.* **83**, 183–186.

Sekiya, S., Takamizawa, H., Wang, F., Takare, T., and Kuwata, T. (1972). *Am. J. Obstet. Gynaecol.* **113**, 691–695.

Sekiya, S., Kikuchim Y., Katoh, T., Kobayaski, W., Takeda, B., and Takamizawa, H. (1979). *Gynaecol. Oncol.* **7**, 291–297.

Sluyser, M. (1979). *Biochim. Biophys. Acta.* **560**, 509–529.

Sutherland, R. L., Mester, J., and Baulieu, E. E. (1977). *Nature* **267**, 434–435.

Taki, I., and Iijima, H. (1963). *Am. J. Obstet. Gynaecol.* **87**, 926–934.

Thanki, K. H., Beach, T. A., and Dickerman, H. W. (1978). *J. Biol. Chem.* **253**, 7744–7750.

Thompson, D. B., Pritchard, K. I., Meakin, J. W., Myers, R. E., Sutherland, D. J. A., and Mobbs, B. G. (1980). *ASCO Abstracts* **21**, C–350.

Tormey, D. C., Simon, R. M., Lippman, M. E., Bull, J. M., and Myers, C. E. (1976). *Cancer Treat. Rep.* **60**, 1451–1459.

Index

N

1 2 3 4 5 6 7 8 9 0
A B C D E F G H I J